ATOMIC
MEDICINE

ATOMIC MEDICINE

EDITED BY

CHARLES F. BEHRENS, M.D., F.A.C.R.

Rear Admiral, MC, U. S. Navy, (ret.); Roentgenologist, Yater Clinic, Washington, D. C.; Consultant and Lecturer in Radiology, U. S. Naval Medical Center, Bethesda, Maryland; Formerly: Director, Atomic Defense Division, Bureau of Medicine and Surgery, Navy Department; Commanding Officer, Navy Medical Research Institute, National Naval Medical Center, Bethesda, Maryland.

Third Edition

1959

THE WILLIAMS & WILKINS COMPANY

Baltimore • 1959

First Edition
©, 1949
Thomas Nelson & Sons

Second Edition
©, 1953
The Williams & Wilkins Co.

Third Edition
©, 1959
The Williams & Wilkins Co.

Made in the United States of America

Library of Congress
Catalog Card Number
59–5699

Composed and Printed
by the
WAVERLY PRESS
Baltimore 2, Md., U.S.A.

DEDICATION

To the pioneers in radiology, many of them martyrs to science, who have made possible the
manifold benefits to medical science in this field.

Preface to Third Edition

The events of the last few years include rapid advances in all research and development fields as well as the advent of thermonuclear weapons. The latter have brought still another fantastic increase in the order of magnitude of violence and increased perils from radiation hazards. With regard to these there is much keener and disquieting appreciation of long-range evils to the human race. Thus a new edition of this text became essential.

In meeting the challenge of new developments, all but a few chapters have required extensive revision or called for rewriting; and a few new chapters have been added. The chapter on general bomb effects has been rewritten with greater emphasis on radiation hazards. The chapters on acute whole-body radiation effects are largely new and additional chapters have been added on skin lesions from fallout and the results to the body of radioisotopes which gain internal access. On the score of medical and biological applications of radioisotopes the chapter on tracers has been rewritten with closer orientation to medical fields and the chapter dealing with the problems and methods of administration has been rewritten with emphasis on details of practical techniques. The chapter on particle accelerators has been rewritten; also to a large extent, the chapter on research.

A number of new authors make their appearance in this edition, a few replacing contributors who have left the fields they originally covered and others serving as collaborators. They are all extremely well qualified. It is a temptation to list them here but the general list of contributors will serve better to acquaint the reader with those concerned.

In general, the editor trusts that this edition will continue to serve as usefully as have its predecessors, and in addition, provide a greater measure of practical information of clinical value.

Deeply sincere appreciation is extended the contributors. They have given unselfishly of their time and energy in the midst of very busy lives to make this revision possible.

Appreciation is also extended the publishers and in particular Mr. Dick M. Hoover for kind cooperation and great patience.

A final word now about the title: The term "Nuclear" is now the favored one and of course the basic phenomena pertaining to reactors, bombs and radioactivity are of nuclear origin. Nevertheless, orbital electrons also play important roles in characteristic radiation, photoelectric effects, annihilation reactions and various others. Thus it does not appear entirely amiss to retain the title "Atomic Medicine" especially since that is the original and familiar designation of this text.

Acknowledgments

Great thanks are due Commander I. V. King, MSC, U. S. Navy for help with the manuscript.

With regard to illustrations, special mention is due HMC Haddon, U. S. Navy, who made many of the diagrams and illustrations used in the first chapters. In general the illustrations are from numerous sources and those not specifically accredited are by courtesy of the Navy Medical Department.

Responsibility

The opinions or assertions contained herein are the private ones of the writers and are not to be construed as official or reflecting the views of the National Military Establishment or other governmental agencies.

Preface to First Edition

THE ATOM KNOCKS AT THE DOCTOR'S DOOR

The relentless tide of human events and scientific progress has engulfed the medical profession in a flood of problems, largely unfamiliar, related to the use of atomic energy. Such answers as we have for these problems are widely scattered in textbooks on nuclear physics, physical chemistry, radiation biology and therapy; also in countless individual articles in periodicals and special publications. Hence this book.

An earnest effort has been made to assemble such of this material as is appropriate to the needs of the medical and allied professions, and to present it as clearly as possible, steering a middle course between a presentation suitable only to specialists in the fields of radiation biology and physics and one unduly elementary. A number of authors have contributed chapters and since the subjects are closely related, there is unavoidably some overlapping. This is felt to be an advantage rather than the opposite, since the approach and implications will be different in each presentation.

Deep appreciation is extended by the editor to the contributors who have made this volume possible. They have given generously of time and effort, difficult to spare, from full and busy lives.

Contributors

CHARLES F. BEHRENS, M.D., F.A.C.R.; Rear Admiral, MC, U. S. Navy (ret); Roentgenologist, Yater Clinic, Washington, D. C.; Lecturer and Consultant in Radiology, National Naval Medical Center, Bethesda, Md. (*Chapters 2, 3, 5, 14*; Revision of *Chapters 15 and 16*).

GORDON C. BELL, B.S.; Commander, MSC, US Navy; Head, Radiological Safety Branch, Special Weapons Division, Bureau Medicine and Surgery, Navy Department, Washington, D. C. (*Chapter 21*).

VICTOR P. BOND, M. D., Ph.D.; Division of Medical Physics, Brookhaven National Laboratory, Associated Universities, Inc., Upton, L. I., N. Y. (*Chapters 9, 10, 11, and 13*).

CLARENCE J. BROWN, M. D.; Vice Admiral, MC, U. S. Navy (ret); Medical Consultant, Department of Youth Authority, State of California, Sacramento, Calif. (*Chapter 1*).

FRANCIS W. CHAMBERS, JR., B.S., M.S.; Commander, MSC, U.S. Navy; Head, Radiological Technology Division, Naval Medical Research Institute, Bethesda, Md. (*Chapter 6*).

STANTON, H. COHN, Ph.D.; Division of Medical Physics, Brookhaven National Laboratory, Associated Universities, Inc., Upton, L. I., N. Y. (*Chapter 12*).

ROBERT A. CONARD, M.D.; Scientist, Experimental Pathology Division, Brookhaven National Laboratory, Upton, L. I., N. Y.; Head of Navy Medical Team for Annual Medical Survey of Marshallese Exposed to Fallout in 1954 (*Chapters 9, 10, 11 and 13*).

MURRAY M. COPELAND, M.D., D.Sc.; Professor of Oncology and Director of Department, Georgetown University Medical Center, Washington, D. C.; Consultant to Clinical Center, National Cancer Institute, Bethesda, Md. (*Chapters 19 and 20*).

EUGENE P. CRONKITE, M.D.; Head, Division of Experimental Pathology, Medical Department, Brookhaven National Laboratory, Upton, L. I., N. Y. (*Chapters 9, 10, 11 and 13*).

R. HAROLD DRAEGER, M.D.; Captain, MC, U. S. Navy; Special Assistant for Medical Effects, Special Projects Office, Bureau of Ordnance, Navy Department, Washington, D. C. (*Chapter 24*).

MAYNARD EICHER, A.B.; Physicist, Navy Medical Research Institute, Bethesda, Md. (*Chapter 6*).

FRIEDRICH ELLINGER, M.D.; Chief Radiation Biologist and Head Pharmacology Division, Naval Medical Research Institute, Bethesda, Md.; Member Radioisotope Board and Consultant to Tumor Board, U. S. Naval Hospital, Bethesda, Md. (*Chapter 7*).

JAMES A. ENGLISH, B.S., D.D.S., M.S., Ph.D.; Captain D.C., U. S. Navy; Science Liaison Officer, Office of Naval Research, London, England (*Chapter 23*).

CHARLES F. GESCHICKTER, M.D.; Professor of Pathology, Georgetown University Medical Center, Washington, D. C. (*Chapters 19 and 20*).

HARRY H. HAIGHT, M.D.; Captain MC, U. S. Navy; Commanding Officer, U. S. Naval Medical Field Research Laboratory, Camp Lejeune, N. C. (*Chapter 4*).

R. D. JORDON, A.B.; Lt. MSC, U. S. Navy; U. S. Naval Medical Field Research Laboratory, Camp Lejeune, N. C. (*Chapter 4*).

E. R. KING, M.D.; Captain, MC, U. S. Navy; Director, Department of Nuclear Medicine, U. S. Naval Medical School and Nuclear Medicine Branch, U. S. Naval Hospital, Bethesda, Md. (*Chapter 22*).

LAWRENCE H. LANZL, M.S., Ph.D.; Assistant Professor (Medical Physics), Department of Radiological Physics and Argonne Cancer Research Hospital, U.S.A.E.C., University of Chicago, Chicago, Ill. (*Chapter 17*).

W. S. MAXFIELD, M.D.; Lt., MC, USNR; Head Radioisotope Section, Nuclear Medicine Branch, U. S. Naval Hospital, Bethesda, Md. (*Chapter 21*).

THOMAS G. MITCHELL, B.S., M.S., Lt., MSC, U. S. Navy; Medical Nuclear Physicist, Radioisotope Laboratory, U. S. Naval Hospital, Bethesda, Md. (*Chapter 22*).

JAMES S. ROBERTSON, M.D., Ph.D.; Medical Physics Division, Medical Department, Brookhaven National Laboratory, Upton, L. I., N. Y. (*Chapter 12*).

OSCAR SCHNEIDER, M.D.; Captain, MC, U. S. Navy; Medical Representative to Assistant Secretary Defense for Research and Engineering, Pentagon, Washington, D. C. (*Chapters 15 and 16*).

RICHARD P. SPENCER, A.B., M.D.; Post Doctoral Fellow, National Science Foundation, Department of Biochemistry, Medical Science Division, Harvard University; Formerly Assistant Director, Radioisotope Laboratory, U. S. Naval Hospital, Bethesda, Md. (*Chapter 18*).

JOHN L. TULLIS, M.D.; Pathologist, New England Deaconess Hospital, Boston, Mass. (*Chapter 8*).

SHIELDS WARREN, M.D.; Scientific Director, Cancer Research Institute, New England Deaconess Hospital, Boston, Mass. (*Chapter 24*).

Contents

1▸

Scope and General Background of Atomic Medicine

CLARENCE J. BROWN, M.D.

1.1 General Considerations

This volume represents an effort unique in the annals of medicine. That it treats, in one volume, of a force which scientifically applied, produced the world's greatest man-made catastrophe and history's most exquisite weapon of mass destruction, and of the further application of the same force, in minuscule amounts, for the beneficent purpose of investigating life processes and aiding human ills, is somewhat incongruous, certainly unusual, and quite startling. For never before in history have the interests of the weaponeers and those who practice the healing arts been so closely related.

This explosive, in conception, manufacture and technical perfection, is the result of the genius of the modern international scientific world; of a group of physical scientists who were unavoidably, because of the irresistible seductiveness of a scientific void, caught in a whirlpool of possibilities relating to nuclear fission. They were drawn inextricably into the turbulent vortex of events culminating in the unbelievable power of the atomic bomb.

That there is apparent in the writings and the discourses of atomic scientists, and of others, an undercurrent of mental disquietude, a certain uneasiness as to moral premises, with respect to their part in the development of the weapon, is understandable, even though one may not agree as to its necessity. The bomb, representing the ultimate fruition of a series of basic experiments having to do with the greatest force available to man, was inevitable.

It is fortunate indeed that the men of medicine do not need to carry this particular burden. This triumph of the physical scientists, this masterpiece of weaponeering, of demonstrated efficiency and deadliness is not of medicine's contriving. Hippocrates need not stir uneasily in his shroud, in gentle reproach of his favored crew of earthly disciples.

The cloud which rose above Bikini does not dissipate; it hangs like a pall on the minds and councils of men—it permeates all the sancta of the mighty as well as the ecclesiastic cloisters of the Christian and pagan worlds.

The advent of atomic energy has brought to medicine, more than to any other profession, a bewildering array of new problems, brilliant prospects and inescapable responsibilities.

1.1.1 *Atomic Defense.* The application of this force in war, where it is exhibited in its most horrendous manner, has provided us already with our greatest challenge—the necessity for providing adequate medical care for the victims of mass destruction—the necessity that we must somehow find the means and so organize ourselves that in one or all of our industrial areas we can attend the needs of the thousands of casualties resulting from the fire and blast of atomic bombing. This is the basic problem in civil defense which must be faced and, if possible, resolved. Within this vast organization must be developed the units which will be required to deal with the peculiar hazards associated with atomic explosion and with the other special weapons of war. This is an effort of great magnitude, and in the very heart of it will be the doctors, the nurses, the nurses' aides and all those who possess any knowledge useful to medicine. Physicians, and all who engage in pursuits allied or ancillary to medicine, will be called upon increasingly, as the civil defense organization is developed, for their counsel, their specialized knowledge and their leadership. We cannot be found wanting in this important undertaking.

Indoctrination in the principles of atomic defense should begin now; much may be accomplished in our medical schools, colleges and universities, and even in our secondary schools. Many facets of the subject are highly interesting to young and old alike. Enlightenment will do no harm and will accomplish much to dispel certain fears and apprehensions which may arise. Even now, some quite erudite people fancifully speak of an atomic neurosis, although it seems to be difficult to convince the public of its presence. This type of activity is misdirected effort and the employment of the power of suggestion in this instance is contrary to the public interest. Let us not add still another diagnosis to our elaborate psychiatric nomenclature.

1.1.2 *Radioactive Isotopes.* While the enlightened physician will recognize his obligations in the highly important sphere of national defense, much closer to his professional heart will lie the hopes, the dreams and the boundless horizons associated with the application of the products of atomic energy to the study of biologic processes and the diseases of mankind. Here, indeed, are the opportunities.

To the scientist in his laboratory, to the clinician, to the diagnostician, to the surgeon, even to the armchair philosopher—here is a new and entrancing field for speculation, for investigation and for practical application of a new and formidable tool in the biologic sciences.

The opportunities are unbounded to those who will prepare themselves in the basic knowledge required.

Isotopes may be created at will, in quantities sufficient to satisfy any reasonable demands; the world's supply of radioactive materials, formerly almost priceless and measured in grams in the case of radium, is now available by the ton; throughout the land are men, and mostly they are young men, who, as part of their daily work and with all the insouciance of a garage man repairing a motor, deal with material emanating thousands of curies of radiation and manipulate machines which project nuclear particles at unheard-of velocities.

Across this continent and in a host of foreign laboratories men and women are learning the technics and the methodology of the tracer substances, and are familarizing themselves with the elements and the transmutations created by the atomic pile. From these studies it is hoped that many of the phenomena of life itself may be explored. All the processes, physical and chemical, may be studied, not only for the purpose of advancing our basic knowledge, but—more important—for the exploitation of this basic knowledge in the direction of our survival and the prolongation of our lives and the lives of those yet to come. Man was born not to die, but to live, and it may be, once we know a great deal more about him, that he can be made stronger and far more durable.

The production of radioactive substances in large quantities, and the availability of their use in human application, has provided medicine with new methods of applying radiation in the treatment of certain diseases, methods of far greater selectivity and specificity than are possible with roentgen rays, associated with less discomfort and, if properly used, with less hazard to the patient. Internal radiation by radioactive material, through the medium of the circulating blood and lymph streams, has already been found helpful in a number of baffling conditions.

However, we have made only a beginning. A vast amount of research, including animal experimentation, will be necessary before we learn enough about the substances themselves—before we can realize to the ultimate degree the benefit from their application.

1.1.3 *Radiologic Safety.* A word of caution is necessary concerning the direct application of these substances in the treatment of specific diseases. While scientists everywhere are working with this new tool, the experience of the past four years cautions us against overenthusiasm, for many of the roseate pictures presented to the public in early days have been found premature. As with many discoveries seized upon as possible panaceas for all our ills, we have already determined that medicine has not been and probably will not be revolutionized, at least not at an early date.

The painstaking work with these dangerous elements, the precautionary measures which must be taken, the concentration of knowledge in so few persons preclude the rapid advances for which we hope. We should expect medical science to move slowly and deliberately in this new field, if the interests of our patients are to be conserved.

That this great force should have resulted in so little of practical benefit to mankind since the epochal demonstration in the desert of New Mexico, in 1945, has been disappointing to many. However, we should not be impatient, for the same phenomena characteristic of nuclear fission which make the bomb the deadly instrument it is, lead investigators to proceed with caution and circumspection in delving into the biologic secrets of man. And that is as it should be.

It should be remembered also that during the years of greatest increase in knowledge of the possibilities of nuclear fission, the energies and the intellects of the world's most eminent scientists were devoted, with directed singularity of purpose, to the evolution of the weapon. Six years of development of scientific knowledge applicable to medicine are lost to us.

Whether, in history, the beginning of the atomic age will date from the discovery of the Curies, the researches of Rutherford, the first fission of the atom by Hahn and Strassmann or from the detonation of the first bomb will probably never be determined to the satisfaction of everyone. Similarly, we must also be somewhat indefinite concerning the origin of atomic medicine. It may be said to have had its inception as a new type of medical philosophy sometime between the first click of the counters in the stadium at Chicago, when the first nuclear pile was activated, and the magnificent experiment in the desert of Alamogordo.

Somewhere during this period a new concept of medicine was born, evolutionary in its progress—a concept which has become increasingly intricate and complex.

Everything that has been done with the bomb materials and its product has brought new problems to medicine, some of them quite unforeseen. Many of them are still unsolved, and there will be many more that will require the greatest ingenuity and basic research.

For example, we little thought that from the material mined in Canada, refined at Oak Ridge, transmutated at Hanford, assembled into a bomb at Los Alamos and detonated in the western sea there would descend upon our shoulders a veritable cascade of weird, and for the most part wholly unanticipated, problems having to do with the immediate and remote hazards of plutonium. Indeed, we are told that had it not been for the second bomb tested at Bikini, which was detonated beneath the surface of the lagoon, it is quite possible that we should have gone on for years in the atomic age without any knowledge of the possibilities of underwater explosions in the harbors and streams of industrial areas.

The industrial hazards to workers in our great atomic plants are formidable—the avoidance of radiation has become a way of life. The most meticulous type of incessant watchfulness is essential. The handling and manipulation of radioactive materials by physicians and scientists require a highly intelligent appreciation of the hazards to which they and their patients are exposed, as well as a knowledge of the manifestations and the effects of radiation illness.

Unfortunately, a book on atomic medicine must be concerned with the applications of atomic power in war as well as its applications in the peaceful art of medical practice. This volume treats not of high policy, of ethics, of strategy or of international control; as physicians, these matters are not for us. It attempts to set forth, most undramatically, the authoritative information the physician and all those concerned with civilian defense should have at their disposal at this time. In this broad and constantly expanding field this volume is but the forerunner of many others.

It is the first text on atomic medicine written in the atomic age. Because it is the first it must be authoritative and timely. It is written by persons eminently well qualified to write it, all of them outstanding leaders in this special field, and it should serve as a good foundation upon which to build the emergent structure of atomic medicine.

2▸

The Atom Family and Associated Physics

CHARLES F. BEHRENS, M.D.

2.1 Early Theory

Nowadays most of us take the atom for granted and scarcely ever reflect that the existence of atoms is a matter of theory. We cannot see an atom or pick it up and turn it about to examine it individually; and if some hard-headed skeptic should challenge us with a declaration that there is no such thing as an atom, many of us might have great difficulty in proving its existence.

The concept of atoms as the building blocks of substance is far from new. It tends to be derived from everyday experience in which we build up large aggregations out of small units, and, furthermore, we tend to feel that there is a limit to practically everything, including the divisibility of matter.

Various conjectures on the subject were made by the ancient Greeks, and are worthy of note since their beliefs influenced thought profoundly up to relatively modern times. It appears that an atomic theory of some sort was taught by Kanada about 1000 B.C. Thales at about 600 B.C. conceived of water as the main basic constituent of the universe and pictured the world as a flat disk floating on water. Anaximenes and Leucippus thought in terms of earth and air, to which concept Heraclitus, about 500 B.C., added the notion of fire as an element. Empedocles a little later taught the "earth, air, fire, water" hypothesis, and by 400 B.C. Democritus, who is most often mentioned as the original proponent of the atomic theory, taught that all that existed was comprised by atoms and space, the numbers, sizes and types of aggregations of atoms determining the manifold characteristics of varied sorts of matter. As to general types of atoms, these were of the earth, air, fire, water varieties. Plato added to this the idea of definite geometric patterns—an apt premonition of the science of crystallography.

Aristotle (384–322 B.C.), who was a pupil of Plato, abandoned the notion

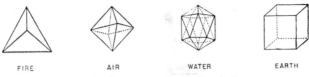

FIG. 1. Ancient concepts of atomic forms

of atoms and simplified the scheme of things to a single basic substance or quintessence, which was called *Hyle* and to which various attributes such as wetness, dryness, coldness and hotness could be added. The Roman naturalistic poet Lucretius (96–45 B.C.) theorized in his classic "De Rerum Naturae" that solid objects were made of hooked atoms and fluids of smooth rounded atoms. However such was the prestige of Aristotle that atomic theories made little headway for many centuries.

2.2 Dalton's Law of Multiple Proportions

The atomic theory was not revived until about the 17th century when men such as Francis Bacon, Robert Boyle and Sir Isaac Newton aroused interest in it again. Lavoisier, in the 18th century, noted conservation of mass and listed some 28 substances as elemental. Dalton early in the 19th century proved the law of multiple proportions, which states that in any given chemical compounds the elements concerned will always be present in precisely the same proportions. It is readily derivable from this that definite units or atoms of the elements concerned must combine with each other in fixed proportions. In fact, on any other basis it would be difficult to explain why definite proportions, rather than variable, exist in chemical compounds.

Beyond these considerations it is also to be noted that certain substances defeat any efforts to break them into simpler components. Thus, by use of heat and chemical action, metallic iron can be derived from various ores, but it is not possible to break iron down into anything else. One may attack any of the innumerable compounds we have at hand to the limit of conventional methods and invariably end with certain substances which cannot be simplified further.

2.3 Scintillations and the Spinthariscope

Finally, we can deduce the existence of atoms from the phenomena associated with familiar radium dials. A view of one through a simple lens will reveal innumerable scintillations rather than a glow effect, and it can be shown that these scintillations are the result of tiny particles of helium of a characteristic atomic mass striking zinc sulfide. A simple apparatus called the spinthariscope and containing a zinc sulfide screen, a

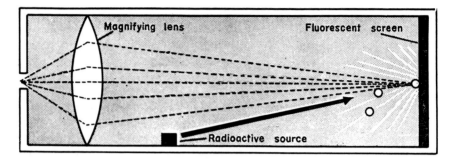

FIG. 2. Spinthariscope: alpha particles produce scintillations on zinc sulfide screen

simple lens and a speck of radium will show the individual splashes of light.

Granted that matter is atomic, let us inquire into the nature of atoms and how they differ from one another to form the 92 elements found in nature and the additional transuranium elements lately prepared.

2.4 The Cathode Ray

For a time there was no reason to suppose that the elemental chemical units or atoms were other than some type of relatively simple building blocks, but toward the end of the last century some peculiar phenomena related to radiations made this facile notion untenable.

Under ordinary atmospheric conditions, air and various gases show considerable resistance to passage of electric currents, and when the resistance is overcome the current usually passes over with a snapping spark; when this occurs on the grandiose scale of nature's operations, there is the flash of lightning and the crash of thunder. When, however, pressure is lowered, as by evacuation of a suitable glass tube to a pressure of about a few millimeters of mercury, then instead of intermittent sparks there are beautiful glow effects in the attenuated gas, such as we see in neon signs. When pressure becomes extremely low the bright glow is eventually replaced by a faint greenish fluorescence which pervades all the glass of the tube except behind the negative electrode cathode where the tube remains dark. It is evident that something is being emitted or radiated from the cathode which causes the glass to fluoresce, and this something is called the cathode ray. Extensive study soon showed that it was particulate or corpuscular in nature and negatively charged so that it could be deflected by electric and magnetic fields.

2.5 X-rays

Roentgen, in 1895, found further that the cathode ray was associated with another ray of totally different type that was exceedingly penetrat-

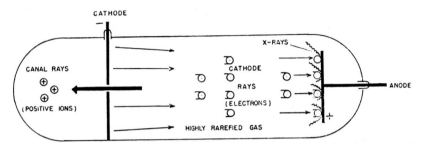

FIG. 3. Important phenomena in an evacuated tube subjected to high potential

ing and not affected by magnetic fields. This ray was, of course, our familiar x-ray and it was soon ascertained that it arose when energetic cathode rays struck a target.

It was calculated very early that each cathode particle has a mass about 1/1800th that of a hydrogen atom and possesses a single negative charge. In fact, these particles were found in connection with so many electrical phenomena that they came to be regarded as particles of negative elec-tricity and so were termed electrons. When thought was given to their origin, it was realized that they must be derived from the gas in the tube, for when a tube is exhausted to a practically complete vacuum no cathode ray can be obtained unless we supply a heated filament. As most of us know, a metal filament heated to incandescence "boils off" electrons and is used as the source of such in modern x-ray tubes by placing it in cup-shaped cathodes.

2.6 Canal Rays

Going a step further, it is evident that when electrons are derived from the atoms of gas, then the atoms so affected should show positive charges; and such is the case. Under electrical stress, electrons are pulled from atoms of the gas remaining in the tube and, in accordance with the familiar law of repulsion of like charges, the electrons near the cathode are hurled off to form the cathode ray. The positively charged atomic residues are attracted to the cathode and if a hole is present in the cathode, some of these, having gained considerable momentum, will pass through to form what are aptly called canal rays. These being positively charged can be deflected by electric and magnetic fields. We can now see that the atom, instead of being a simple homogenous building block, appears to have charged particles entering into its composition.

2.7 Natural Radioactivity

The scientific world, rubbing its eyes with astonishment, was just be-ginning to cope with x-rays and cathode rays when Becquerel presented it with natural radioactivity. He found that there were radiations from uranium ores which affected photographic plates somewhat as do x-rays. Taking the almost unpardonable liberty of telescoping prodigious amounts of earnest work, we can relate that after a few years the radioactive elements radium and polonium were isolated and identified by the Curies. It then became known that by a process of natural decay these elements were emitting what were first termed Becquerel rays; later they were found to be a complex formed by what are now termed alpha (α), beta (β) and gamma (γ) rays.

Relating these facts to our previous findings, we note the significant fact that the beta rays are identical in type with the cathode ray or streams of electrons in evacuated tubes. We have here another indication that the electron should prove an atomic constituent.

2.8 Analyses of Natural Radioactivity

We can gain additional insight by a fairly simple experiment. A small, deep hole is drilled in a block of lead and a speck of radium is placed in the bottom of the block so that the radiations will emerge from a small opening where strong magnetic fields may be applied. The result is that one ray will deviate toward positive polarity rather markedly; another will deviate slightly toward the negative polarity; the third will be unaffected. Analysis shows that the first is the beta ray, already noted as being similar to the cathode ray. The ray with slight deviation toward the negative polarity is the alpha ray and was soon shown to be made of heavy particles with double positive charges and with a mass about four times that of a hydrogen atom; in fact, it was soon identified as being composed of helium atoms which had lost two electrons. The undeviated ray, designated as gamma, was found to be identical in nature with the x-ray.

This was far from all. Intense and exacting studies soon showed that radium in the course of this mysterious activity was disintegrating into other substances in an intricate, long-drawn-out pattern affording sure proof that the atoms themselves are complexities built up of simpler components.

2.9 Radioactive Families

Radium is a member of the uranium series or family. This group undergoes transmutation as follows: Uranium, thorium, protactinium, radium, emanation, polonium, bismuth, thallium and lead. Some changes occur over millions of years, others in a matter of minutes or seconds.

There are also thorium and actinium families which end with lead. Another family tree worked out since the discovery of U^{233} and called the neptunium family, ends with Bi^{209}.

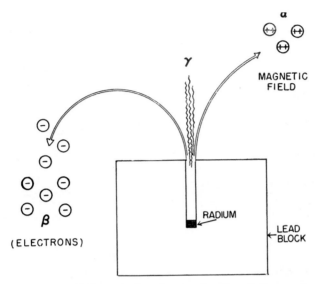

FIG. 4. Differentiation of natural radioactivity

It is interesting to note that when the mass numbers of the thorium series are divided by 4, we have no remainders. With the uranium series the result is always some number plus 2; hence the designation $4n + 2$ for this series. The actinium group yields $4n + 3$. The neptunium family provides $4n + 1$ figures. This last group does not occur naturally probably because the half lives are not long enough.

2.10 The Bohr Atom

At this point we can confidently assert that beta particles or electrons must constitute one of the units of atomic structure. However, it is different with alpha particles. These have an atomic weight about four times that of hydrogen and so would scarcely be building blocks for that gas. Hydrogen suggests itself as a building block, since it is the lightest element known and shows single positive charges when electrons are stripped off. Such hydrogen nuclei are termed protons and heavier elements, on this basis, may be visualized simply as being composed of protons and electrons packed together like so many beans in a bag. Indeed, this was an early concept, and, although plausible, it soon ran into trouble. Early in the century, Lord Rutherford tried the experiment of shooting alpha particles at a very thin gold foil, the expectation on the basis of the "bean bag" atom being that many would get through but would show considerably less velocity and slight dispersion. Instead of this some really amazing things happened. Most particles went through as though practically nothing

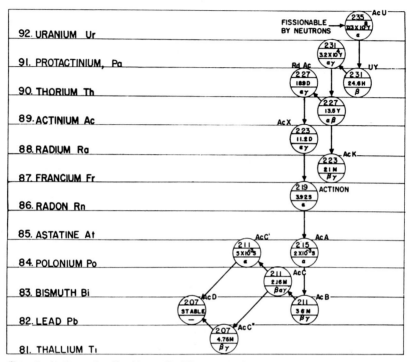

92. URANIUM Ur

91. PROTACTINIUM, Pa

90. THORIUM Th

89. ACTINIUM Ac

88. RADIUM Ra

87. FRANCIUM Fr

86. RADON Rn

85. ASTATINE At

84. POLONIUM Po

83. BISMUTH Bi

82. LEAD Pb

81. THALLIUM Tl

FIG. 5. Actinum family $(4n + 3)$. Element 86 is now termed "Emanation, Em"

were in the way. A few others, however, were greatly deflected, even to the point of being bounced back. The seemingly solid foil of gold acted in the manner of a lattice. Careful study and the application of mathematics indicated that the dispersion pattern could be possible only if atoms were chiefly empty space with practically all the mass concentrated in a tiny dot in the center. On this basis, Bohr developed the modern concept which bears his name and for which he was awarded the Nobel prize in 1912. This concept places a positively charged nucleus containing protons at the center with electrons moving in orbits with diameters approximately 10,000 times that of the nucleus. The diameter of the nucleus is calculated to be approximately $1/10^{12}$ or 10^{-12} cm., and the diameter of the whole atom approximately $1/10^8$ or 10^{-8} cm. (the minus sign indicates that the figure belongs in the denominator). Such figures mean little as thus stated, but when visualized on a scale of more familiar distances the picture becomes startling. Thus, if one imagines a nucleus 1 foot in diameter, then the orbit of an electron reaches out to a diameter of 10,000 feet or almost 2 miles. Again, if we visualize the nucleus as a 1 mm. dot, the orbit becomes 10 meters in diameter. On this basis we can picture an atom as equivalent

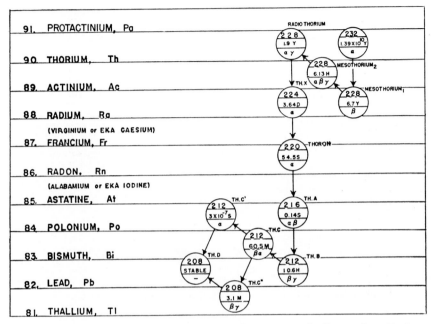

Fig. 6. Thorium family (4n). Element 86 is now termed "Emanation, Em"

to a large spherical room over 30 feet in diameter with a dot in the center, smaller than a BB shot, for the nucleus.

The unit of nuclear diameter is the *"Fermi,"* 10^{-13} cm. and recent work suggests a nuclear radius of $1.18 \times \sqrt[3]{\text{mass number}}$ for elements of A40 or more (See 2.12) and 1.35 × this cube root for lighter elements. It also appears that nuclear borders fade out through a fuzzy skin-like zone 2.4 fermis thick for the heavier group. In this zone charge density drops from 90 to 10 per cent. Protons fade to zero, 1.4 fermis from the center.

2.11 Neutrons

The next heavier gas after hydrogen is helium, with an atomic weight of about 4; when stripped of orbital electrons it has a double positive charge. We have already met helium nuclei as alpha particles. The double positive charge argues for two electrons in the orbit and two protons in the nucleus, but poses the problem of accounting for an atomic weight of 4, when we remember that protons have an atomic weight of about 1 and electrons have relatively negligible mass. The first answer was to postulate a nucleus with four protons, two of which are neutralized by electrons within the nucleus. However, it is not likely that electrons exist as such in a nucleus. Instead they are better thought of as combining with protons to

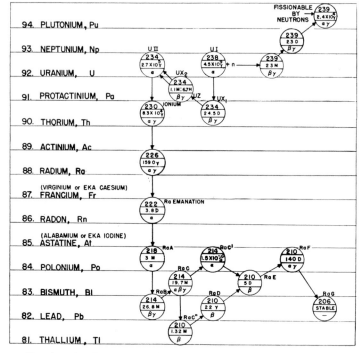

Fig. 7. Uranium family $(4n + 2)$. Element 86 is now termed "Emanation, Em"

form neutral particles termed neutrons. Thus the helium nucleus is visualized as having two protons and two neutrons.

The existence of neutrons was eventually verified. In 1930 Bothe and Becker noted that some extremely penetrating rays were produced when alpha particles struck beryllium, and thought they were dealing with gamma rays. However, in 1932 Joliot and Curie found that these rays behaved differently from gamma rays. They passed through lead too easily but, on the other hand, were readily absorbed in paraffin or hydrogenous material with emission of protons. In the same year, Chadwick showed that they were not affected by magnetic fields, and had a speed of one-tenth that of light so that they could not be gamma rays. He determined further that the rays were particulate, the mass of each particle being virtually the same as that of a proton. This work won him the Nobel prize in 1935.

2.12 Notations

It is appropriate now to describe the notations used to characterize atoms. The number of protons is indicated by a figure placed below and

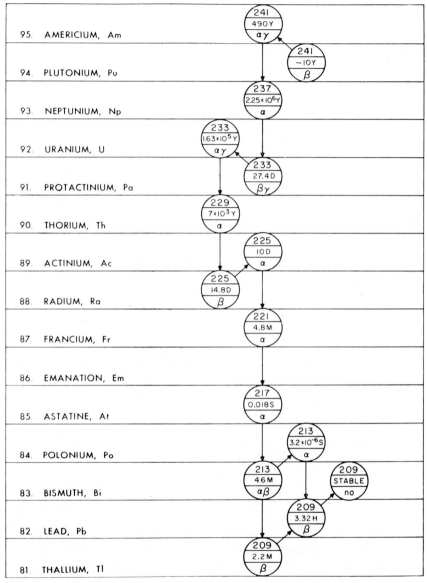

FIG. 8. Neptunium series $(4n + 1)$

to the left of the symbol for the element. The total number of particles, both neutrons and protons, is indicated by a figure placed above and to the right of the symbol. The abbreviations are as follows:

Z = number of protons in the nucleus; this also indicates the usual number of orbital electrons since they are present in the same number to balance the positive charges of the protons.

N = number of neutrons in nucleus.

A = mass number or sum of both neutrons and protons ($A = Z + N$).

n = symbol for neutron.

p = symbol for proton.

e = symbol for electron.

Coming back to the derivation of neutrons from beryllium, the process is as follows: $_4Be^9 + {}_2He^4 \rightarrow {}_6C^{12} + {}_0n^1$.

Here we have a transmutation whereby the light metal beryllium becomes carbon with incidental emission of neutrons; it should be noted that the numbers for both Z and A balance.

The first indications of artificially induced radioactivity noted by Joliot and Curie also involved alpha bombardments as in the following reactions:

$$B^{10} + {}_2He^4 \rightarrow N^{13} + n; \text{ or in briefer form, } B^{10} (\alpha n)N^{13}$$
$$Al^{27} + {}_4He^4 \rightarrow P^{30} + n; \text{ or } Al^{27} (\alpha n)P^{30}$$

In the abbreviated form noted above, the first symbol in the parentheses indicates the bombarding particle and the second the resulting radiation. Both N^{13} and P^{30} are unstable.

At this point we find the atoms possessing nuclei made up of neutrons and protons and provided with orbital electrons corresponding in number to the protons. Atoms, therefore, must differ from each other by reason of variations in the number and arrangement of nuclear particles and orbital electrons.

2.13 Limitation of Nuclear Size

There is a limit, however, to the number of particles that can be crammed into a single nucleus; this will be taken up in more detail later. For the present we will only note that in nature we find the heaviest element to be uranium which usually shows an atomic weight of 238 from 92 protons and 146 neutrons. In addition, by artificial methods we have formed a few so-called transuranic elements which are still heavier, namely, 93 Neptunium (Np), 94 Plutonium (Pu), 95 Americium (Am), 96 Curium (Cm), 97 Berkelium (Bk), 98 Californium (Cf), 99 Einsteinium (E), 100 Fermium (Fm), 101 Mendelevium (Mv), 102 Nobelium (No).

These have been produced by high energy bombardments of heavy nuclei with nuclear particles and also nuclei of lighter elements. Elements 99 and 100 were also found in the fallout and filter debris from the 1952 thermonuclear tests.

All are unstable and it is evident that these nuclei have become overstuffed, which fact is related to atomic fission (which will be considered in the next chapter) and lack of elements heavier than those just mentioned.

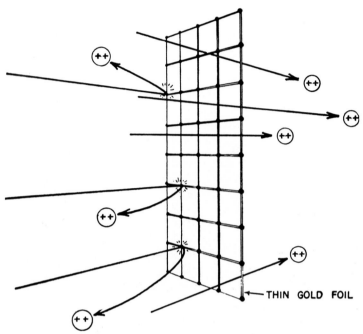

Fig. 9. Rutherford dispersion experiment (schematic diagram). Most particles slip through with little dispersion; a few are greatly deflected.

Since the atomic number reaches 102, electrons up to the same number must find orbits about the nuclei. How they arrange themselves is an extremely complex matter, but a few notes should make the matter sufficiently clear for our purposes.

2.14 Orbital Electron Patterns

We start with a single orbital shell which in the case of hydrogen has a single electron and in the case of helium two. This orbital region will accept no more electrons and thus another zone or shell must be established beyond it for lithium, which has three protons and three electrons. This new shell will hold up to eight electrons and then a third shell becomes necessary. This process goes on until we have seven shells which are usually designated by letters beginning with K for the inner, L for the next and so on. Numbers are also used at times. As each outer shell reaches saturation with eight electrons, we have recurrence of element type in the way of an inert gas. Then as new shells start with a single electron, we find recurrence of alkali metals.

The foregoing agrees well with diagrams of orbital electrons in concentric circles. Spectroscopy however, points to orbital shells containing elliptical

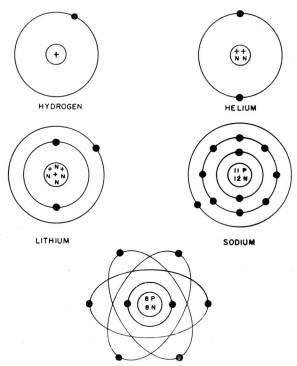

Fig. 10. Schematic atomic diagrams. Electrons in outer orbital shells tend to form orbits with two electrons each, as diagrammed in the case of oxygen.

orbits each containing no more than 2 electrons. *Pauli's Exclusion Principle* applies, which states that no two electrons in an atomic structure can have the same set of *quantum numbers*. These characterize electrons as follows: n, principle number indicating energy state; 1, azimuthal number relating to angular momentum; m, orbital number for spatial orientation; s, spin. In effect this means that orbits can contain no more than 2 electrons and then only if of opposite spins.

Spectroscopy also indicates a series of energy levels characteristic for each element and designated as follows: s, corresponding to sharp lines; p to principle lines; d to diffuse series and f to fundamental. These energy levels and their subdivisions are intimately related to the number of electrons permissible in each shell.

There is a tendency for outer electron shells, except for the first (which will only accept two), to acquire eight electrons. When this cannot be accomplished directly owing to lack of nuclear protons, atoms tend to combine with each other to produce the same result. This causes formation of molecules and various chemical compounds. It accounts in large measure for chemical valence and also has to do with crystallography.

It must be noted too, that although eight is the saturation point for outer shells, yet before the fourth shell fills beyond a few electrons, the third takes on 18 electrons; in similar fashion, the fourth shell acquires up to 32 and the fifth 18. This curious phenomenon is responsible for the large families of metals and of rare earths. Finally it remains to note that two elements exceed the limit of 8 for the outer orbit namely Palladium and Iridium.

One may well ask here why hydrogen atoms do not combine with each other to form He. The answer lies in the repulsion between protons and the need of converting two protons to neutrons. This reaction can take place but not under usual terrestrial conditions. Hydrogen must be subjected to huge pressures and a temperature of millions of degrees, such as is found in the sun and stars, before its atoms will combine to form helium. We have many analogous situations in the case of familiar combustibles. Thus coal will not burn until considerable heat is applied and O_2 furnished.

2.15 Periodic System

The recurrent pattern of 1 to 8 electrons in the outer orbital shell is associated with recurrent changes in chemical behavior as we go up the atomic scale. This results in what is termed the Periodic System (diagrammed in fig. 11, next page).

Relationships between atomic weights and properties were noted by various observors early in the 19th century, culminating in "the law of octaves" propounded by the English chemist, J. A. R. Newlands in 1865; the reports on periodicity by S. Meyer in Germany in 1864–1869; and the systematic tables of the Russian scientist, Mendelejeff (or Mendeleef), published in 1869 and 1871. Many gaps were then present, and no adequate explanation. These gaps have now been filled in and the modus operandi greatly clarified by atomic research and quantum mathematics. It is time now to look into what is our main concern, namely, the associated radiation physics.

2.16 Quanta and Photons

A puzzling discovery of modern physics is that light and other radiations exhibit both wave and particulate behavior. Refraction, diffraction and interference are wave phenomena but photoelectric effects are of particulate type. In these, high frequency radiations eject electrons from certain orbits as though by a billiard ball type of collision; and changes in the intensity of the radiation affects only the number of electrons ejected, not their energy.

| ORBITAL SHELLS | \multicolumn{8}{c}{NUMBER OF ELECTRONS IN OUTER ORBITAL SHELL} | | | | | | | | SPECIAL NOTATIONS |
	1	2	3	4	5	6	7	8	
I	H 1	He 2							
II	Li 2-1	Be 2-2	B 2-3	C 2-4	N 2-5	O 2-6	F 2-7	Ne 2-8	
III	Na 2-8-1	Mg 2-8-2	Al 2-8-3	Si 2-8-4	P 2-8-5	S 2-8-6	Cl 2-8-7	A 2-8-8	
IV	19K:24Cr 29Cu:	20Ca:21Sc 22Ti:23V 25Mn:26Fe 27Co:28Ni 30Zn:	Ga 2-8-18-3	Ge 2-8-18-4	As 2-8-18-5	Se 2-8-18-6	Br 2-8-18-7	Kr 2-8-18-8	

Corresponds to group 8 due to saturation of orbit →

			49	50	51	52	53	54	
V	37Rb:41Nb 42Mo:44Ru 45Rh:47Ag 48Cd:	38Sr:39Y 40Zr:43Tc	In 2-8-18-18-3	Sn 2-8-18-18-4	Sb 2-8-18-18-5	Te 2-8-18-18-6	I 2-8-18-18-7	Xe 2-8-18-18-8	46 Pd falls in this group numerically but has 4 shells and 18 outer electrons. 2-8-18-18
			81	82	83	84	85	86	
VI	55Cs:78Pt 79Au:	56Ba:57-71* 72Hf:73Ta 74W:75Re 76Os:80Hg	Tl 2-8-18-32 18-3	Pb 2-8-18-32 18-4	Bi 2-8-18-32 18-5	Po 2-8-18-32 18-6	At 2-8-18-32 18-7	Rn or Em 2-8-18-32 18-8	77 Ir has 5 shells and 17 outer electrons. 2-8-18-32-17
	87								
VII	Fr 2-8-18-32 18-8-1	88Ra:89Ac 90Th:91Pa 92Ur:93Np 94Pu:95Am 96Cm:							89-96 Forms Actinide Series.

* Lanthanide Series of Rare Earths
57La:58Ce:59Pr:60Nd:61Pm:62Sm:63Eu:64Gd:65Tb:66Dy:67Ho:68Er:69Tm:70Yb:71Lu.

Fig. 11. Periodic table of elements with electron patterns

On the other hand if frequency is sufficiently low there will be no dislodgments no matter how great the intensity. There is no summation of wave effect in photoelectric phenomena such as should free at least a few electrons of low energy, if we were dealing with wave effect. Thus the idea came to acceptance that light, x and gamma rays must come in discrete packets of greater or less energy quanta, to which the term *photons* has been given.

2.17 Planck's Constant

Planck laid the foundation of the quantum theory in work on discrepancies involving radiations at various temperatures, the so-called "Black Body" radiation, which is that from a source theoretically perfect in emission and absorption. He theorized in 1901 that radiation energies could not assume a continuous series of values, but had to be integral multiples of an amount derived from the frequency of the oscillating source and a constant (Planck's constant, h, 6.625×10^{-27} erg/sec.). Thus we have the equation $E = h\nu$ where E represents the energy, h Planck's constant and ν (nu) the frequency. Put in another way the energy of radiations divided by the frequency is always a constant.

2.18 Photoelectric Equation

Einstein worked out the energy relationship still further in his photoelectric equation which is based on the fact that the energy of the incoming photon ($h\nu$) must equal the energy needed to remove the electron plus the kinetic energy given the electron assuming complete absorbtion of the photon's energy. Thus we have $h\nu = \phi + \frac{1}{2} mv^2$ where $h\nu$ is of course Planck's constant times frequency; ϕ is the energy needed to eject the electron and $\frac{1}{2} mv^2$ the familiar formula for kinetic energy, to wit, one half the mass times the square of the velocity.

By reverse application, an incident electron of sufficient energy may produce photons with frequency in accordance with $\frac{1}{2} mv^2 = h\nu$ (ϕ in this instance is relatively so small as to be usually negligible).

2.19 Mass and Waves

It is difficult to visualize light and x and gamma rays as being both particulate and a species of waves but it may help to think of photons in terms of particles possessing pilot waves. It is also notable that in accordance with wave mechanics, every object has associated wave patterns often characterized by the term *"DeBroglie"* in honor of the scientist who pioneered in these wave studies. The wave lengths are held to be in accordance with a definite mathematical relation to energy and mass. Thus, the wave length of any object may be calculated from the equation, lambda $(\lambda) = h/mv$ where lambda $(\lambda) =$ wave length, h Planck's constant, and mv mass times velocity. We can see from this that as mass increases, the wave length diminishes, and becomes relatively insignificant for sizeable objects. Accordingly, for a mass of a gram the order of magnitude becomes 10^{-33} cm. For a high energy proton of 9 mev it becomes 9.5 $\times$ 10^{-13} cm. or roughly the diameter of a nucleus. For a neutron moving at the same speed as gas molecules under ordinary conditions, i.e., a "thermal" neutron, the wave length becomes 1.46×10^{-8}. For a low speed electron at a mass of 10^{-27} and V of 10^5 cm./sec. it becomes 10^{-6} cm. For comparison it might be noted that visible light ranges from 7.6×10^{-5} to 4×10^{-5} cm.; gamma rays usually average about 10^{-10}.

Wave characteristics are of enormous importance in the atomic and nuclear worlds as they clarify phenomena otherwise inexplicable if not incredible. The mathematical background is often spoken of as *"Schroedinger's Wave Mechanics"* since he worked out the fundamental equations involved.

2.20 Relationship of Light and X-ray to Atoms

By classical theory, one would expect revolving electrons to set up electromagnetic fields which would dissipate energy so that the electron would quickly fall into the nucleus. Instead they stabilize in definite orbital zones at fixed energy levels of which there are a number for each atom and between which there are no gradations. Just how they do this is not readily visualized, though it should be pointed out that orbital electrons probably do not correspond to the conventional diagram of little spheres. Instead they might be thought of as vaguely defined regions of electric charge spread about the orbits and showing something akin to standing wave patterns.

Be that as it may, the orbital electrons show what are called stationary states or levels of energy which can be expressed in multiples of a factor based on Planck's constant. Thus, the momentum of an orbital electron must always be an integral multiple of a quantity determined by dividing Planck's constant by the orbital circumference $(h/2\pi r)$.

The lowest energy level is the ground state where the orbit is closest to the nucleus. When energy is supplied as by collision with other atoms, electrons or photons, the orbital electrons are jolted into bigger orbits or even detached. Then, depending on which of these has occurred, almost immediately the electron either drops back to its ground state or is replaced by another electron. In either case, as this occurs, energy is released in the form of a photon or quantum of radiant energy. When an electron is jolted into higher energy levels it may either fall back in several steps giving off a corresponding number of photons of appropriate energy, or in a single jump producing one photon of high energy. Definite spectroscopic lines corresponding to these energies are noted and the concept of energy levels explains the discrete lines and indicates why we do not have a continuous spectrum. It might be noted that hydrogen shows a series of lines in the visible spectrum and others in the ultraviolet, the visible group comprising the Balmer series and the ultraviolet group the Lyman series.

The more complex atoms show a greater variety of orbital energy levels and a correspondingly larger number of spectral lines. In general, the outer electrons are most easily disturbed and certain of their oscillations to and fro between various energy levels produce visible light. When energy is such that the wave length of the resulting photons drops below 100 Ångstrom units we begin to enter the x-ray field where we find greater and greater penetration as the wave length decreases. To obtain these high energy photons, high velocity electrons are directed against a dense target. In this type of action inner orbits, as well as outer, are often disturbed, and when the innermost or K orbit is involved by the catapulting out of an electron, the resultant energy pulse or photon produced when another electron drops into the orbit is in the x-ray zone and characteristic of the element just as visible spectrum lines are.

Other x-ray photons will vary in energy, frequency and wave length with the velocity of the incident electron, and that is, of course, the reason for the use of high voltage apparatus when the more energetic and penetrating x-rays are desired.

2.21 Spin

Electron spin may be in either of two opposite directions and as noted makes possible two electrons in a given orbit. In the case of hydrogen which has only one electron it follows that there are two varieties (ortho and para) depending on spin direction. They differ very slightly. Electron spin also causes an electron moment quantizable in terms of the *Bohr Magneton*, $h\,e/4\,\pi\,m\,c$ where h is Planck's constant, e electron charge and c velocity of light. Value is 0.92732×10^{-20} erg/gauss.

Nucleons also have spin which is related to radioactive behavior (See 2.29).

Orbital rotation, although not a "spin" also causes magnetic moments productive of slight variations in spectroscopic detail—the *Zeeman Effect*.

2.22 Molecular Magnetism

Secondly, there is a matter of molecular magnetism. When two atoms, differing considerably in atomic number, unite, the molecule is asymmetrical and the pole of the resultant positive charge does not coincide with the pole of the resultant negative charge. Molecular spin imparts a rotary motion to such centers of charge distribution, which may be considered analogous to the flow of an electric current in a closed conducting circuit. A miniature bipolar magnet is thus formed.

2.23 Nuclear Surface Tensions

The theory of a nucleus we have been considering brings up a pertinent question as to why the repulsion of like charges does not make close association impossible. How can as many as 100 odd protons be jammed into a tiny nucleus? The fact is there is still much to be learned about it. It is obvious when protons are forced closely enough together, repulsion forces cease to preponderate and other forces, including a surface tension type of effect, take over. Thus we can speak of nuclear fluid and, in fact, nuclei behave as though they are formed of fluid, albeit a fluid of such density (10^{14} gm./cc.) that it has been calculated that one drop would weigh some millions of tons. The surface tension is 10^{19} ergs/sq. cm. as compared to 75 for water. This is still not enough to account for the coalescence and adhesion of nuclear particles and so it has been calculated that another factor must be concerned which has been called "exchange forces."

2.24 Exchange Forces and Mesons

Neutrons and protons are probably not clearly defined as such in nuclei. Instead it is conjectured that there may be some type of intermediary form (nucleon) resulting from charges which are "exchanged" or held in common between the neutrons and protons. On mathematical grounds it has been calculated that such a charge should equal that of an electron but be associated with a mass about 200 times as great. Since particles of such type (known as mesons) have been identified in cosmic rays (see par. 5.15) and produced in cyclotrons, the theory of exchange forces probably has validity. However, the whole meson theory is still subject to perplexities and for practical purposes we still think and speak in terms of neutrons and protons in characterizing nuclei. We bear in mind that they can exchange identities under certain conditions and, as will become apparent later, that such exchanges are closely related to radioactivity.

2.25 Isotopes: Discovery and General Background

One would ordinarily expect atomic weights to be practically even multiples of the weight of a proton but instead, on the basis of O = 16, we find chlorine with a weight of 35.46, neon 20.2, magnesium 24.32, mercury 200.61, etc. After much perplexity and study the factors involved were finally tracked down. See paragraph 5.15.

It will be recalled that in the course of electrical discharges in evacuated tubes, positively charged ions of the rarefied gases were attracted to the cathode with such force that many would shoot through where an

opening was provided. Streams of positive ions can thus be obtained and
are termed canal rays. Magnetic fields naturally deflect these charged particles, the amount of deflection being greater for light particles and small
for heavy, in accordance with familiar laws. Calculation of mass and charge
thus becomes possible by this means.

When this method of study was applied to neon by Thompson and Aston,
a surprise was encountered. Two beams were obtained—one corresponding
to an atomic weight of 20 and the other to one of 22, the type with 20 being
most intense. Studies with chlorine demonstrated two varieties with atomic
weight of 35 and 37; Mercury vapor studies turned up a family with weights
of 198, 199, 200, 201, and 204.

Regardless of variation in atomic weight, chemical behavior remains the
same for each element and the individual variants are spoken of as isotopes.
The differences in weight are due to differences in the number of neutrons,
the number of protons being unaffected. Accordingly, there is no change
in the orbital electron patterns of the isotopes and their combining ten-
dencies. There are, however, slight differences in physical characteristics,
such as specific gravity and melting points. There are also, as we shall see
later, effects on stability involving radioactivity. These stability factors
limit the number of isotopes although they are numerous enough in all
truth and probably too numerous (about 1000) for the harrassed student.
Even hydrogen has two isotopes, namely, deuterium with a neutron added
to its proton and tritium with three particles, two of them neutrons.
Deuterium occurs naturally to the extent of 0.02 per cent. Water made from
it is called "heavy water." It is worthy of note that helium lacks an isotope
with five particles as it will not accept a fifth particle in the nucleus.
The four particles exhibit complete saturation and form a most stable
aggregate, so that a fifth particle would have no place to go or anything
to hang on to in way of exchange forces. This stability for a group of four
probably accounts in part for the tendency of heavy elements to throw
off such aggregates in the form of alpha particles.

2.26 Additional Radioactive Isotopes in Nature

Finally, it might be noted that aside from the radioactive families previously described other naturally occurring radioactive isotopes are now
listed:

K 40, Rb 87, In 115, La 148, Nd 144, Sm 147, Lu 176, W 180, Re 187,
Pt 190 and Bi 209. C 14 might well be included but is in a different category. It is present only by reason of constant replenishment by action of
cosmic rays on nitrogen. Its half life is 5600 years whereas that of the
others is reckoned in many millions and radioactivity very feeble.

K 40 produces almost half a million disintegrations per minute in the human body of average size, C 14 about 2500. This appears a large amount but is actually trifling in comparison with the astronomical number of atoms in the body.

2.27 Avogadro's Number

Avogadro's well-known rule, that equal volumes of gases have equal numbers of molecules, has been applied to all substances in the guise of "Avogadro's number." This concept indicates that when *quantities* of substances are such that their units of weight are numerically equal to their atomic or molecular weights, then they will contain the same number of atoms or molecules as the case may be. When the weight is in grams the number is the unimaginably huge one of 6.025×10^{23}. This is known as Avogadro's number and is the number of atoms to be found in about 1 gm. of hydrogen, 16 gm. of oxygen or 200 gm. of mercury. Again the same number of molecules will characterize 2 gm. of hydrogen, 18 gm. of water, 32 gm. of oxygen, etc. It therefore becomes obvious that half a million beta particles in comparison to the number of atoms in the body shrink to insignificance.

While on the subject, it is appropriate to note here that the term applied to the appropriate number of grams concerned with Avogadro's number is the gram atom or "mole" in the case of atoms, or gram-molecule in the case of molecules, the former being numerically equal to the atomic weight and the latter to the molecular weight. It is also of interest to note by way of comparative figures that 1 cc. of a gas under standard conditions contains 2.688×10^{19} molecules and that 1 mole of any gas measures 22414.6 cc. in volume or approximately $22\frac{1}{2}$ liters.

2.28 Isobars and Isotones

The same and neighboring elements show variations in the distribution of nucleons resulting in three types:

Isotopes, same Z different N
Isobars, same A different Z
Isotones, same N different Z

(Z = proton number; N = neutron number; $A = Z + N$)

The main interest in this chapter relates to effects on stability and radioactivity.

2.29 Neutron Proton Ratios and Stability

Surface tension and exchange forces have already been mentioned (2.23, 2.24) as responsible for holding nuclei together. Instability and radioactivity occur nevertheless and a brief discussion of factors concerned becomes essential (See also Chap. 3).

2.29.1 *Isobaric Effects.* Isobars that differ by one proton usually show radioactive transmutations whereby the nucleus of heavier weight changes to the nucleus of lighter weight and less energy. This occurs in various ways: Neutrons may become protons by electron emission (β decay); protons may become neutrons by capture of orbital electrons or by positron emission. Beta decay is more common and results in a nucleus with one more proton, the atom moving up one number in the atomic scale. Electron capture and positron emission cause the opposite effect since the resultant atom has one less proton. As the result of such changes, isobars differing by one proton are rarely stable. Only three such are listed and of these, two are in dubious status leaving only one pair apparently stable, $_{51}Sb^{115}$ and $_{52}Te^{115}$.

There are several sets of triple isobars in which the middle one is radioactive, e.g., $_{18}A^{40}$, $_{19}K^{40}$ and $_{20}Ca^{40}$. In this instance, $_{19}K^{40}$ becomes $_{20}Ca^{40}$ by beta decay and $_{18}A^{40}$ by electron capture.

There are four sets of stable triple isobars and many stable pairs in which Z differs by two; which brings us to the odd-even factor.

2.29.2 *Odd-Even Abundance.* The instability of isobars differing in Z by 1 as contrasted to stability when Z differs by 2 indicates that stability is favored by the balance produced by pairing. This is reflected in the ratios found in naturally occurring isotopes.

Even Z, Even N	163
Even Z, Odd N	57
Odd Z, Even N	50
Odd Z, Odd N	5

The odd-odd elements are $_1H^2$, $_3Li^6$, $_5B^{10}$, $_7N^{14}$ and $_{23}V^{50}$. Four of these are light elements with equal N and Z. The fifth has a "magic number."

2.29.3 *Magic Numbers.* The inert gases are such by reason of closed outer orbital shells. We can thus derive "magic" stability numbers for orbital electrons from He 2, Ne 10, A 18, Kr 36 and Xe 54, the number being the total numbers of electrons in the various orbits. In the case of nuclei, there is more complexity but it appears that particularly stable nuclei result when either N or Z equals 2, 8, 20, 50, 82 or 126. It seems that nuclear shells exist and that something akin to the Pauli exclusion principle applies.

2.30 Artificial Nuclear Transformations

Aside from natural radioactivity and transformations, a few of artificial variety have been mentioned, e.g., the $_4Be^9$ (αn) $_6C^{12}$ reaction; also the production of transuranic elements. Hundreds of artificially induced transmutations are known, reactions being dependent largely on the type and energy of the bombarding particles, susceptibility or "cross section" of the target nuclei for the reaction and the nature of the resultant nuclei.

Compound nuclei result but usually decay in about 10^{-13} sec. due to the great instability caused by absorption of the kinetic and binding energies of the bombarding particles. These short-lived nuclei are not listed in the reaction descriptions. However, some last for measurable and occasionally considerable periods of time with the result that we find two or more energy states for certain nuclei of the same Z and A, the higher termed the *meta-stable* and the lower the *ground state*. Such nuclei are termed *isomers* and show transition from the higher to the lower energy state by gamma emission. This is called *isomeric transition*. Each of such isomers may have its own decay scheme as in one of the first instances discovered. Thus, metastable Br^{80} shows a 4.4 hr. beta activity as well as isomeric transition to Br^{80} of ground state which shows an 18 min. beta activity. Both beta decays result in Kr^{80}. The explanation for delayed transition to ground states is thought to relate to differences in the angular momenta of the nuclear particles involved, resulting in more or less "forbidden" transitions, some of them highly so. In some cases the ground state is stable.

There are thus three types of *nuclear isomers*: (a) those showing isomeric transition with both states actively radioactive, (b) both radioactive but with little or no detectable isomeric transition, and (c) isomers with stable ground states.

2.30.1 *Reaction Types.* (a) Photon reactions except in a few instances require energies of 6–100 mev and more. Cross sections are low. The (γn) reaction is frequent. (b) *Slow neutrons* frequently undergo capture followed by gamma emission. They cause fissioning of certain heavy nuclei which is, of course, one of the most important of all reactions in nuclear reactors and bombs. (c) *Fast neutrons* often cause the (n, p) reaction and also cause fission of certain nuclei. Neutrons are of special medical importance since neutron fluxes in reactors make possible many of the radioactive isotopes used in medical practice. (c) *Protons* are important in thermonuclear reactions (see 3.4) and produce a variety of reactions. (e) *Deuterons*, the nuclei of heavy hydrogen ($_1H^2$) also produce a variety of reactions and exhibit a peculiarity due to the ease with which their protons and neutrons can be separated. In bombardments by deuterons, the protons are often held back by the *"Coulomb"* repulsion of like charges while the neutrons slip through the potential barrier into the nuclei in what is termed the *"Oppenheimer-Phillips"* reaction. A concentrated beam of high energy deuterons, because of the holding back of protons, may result in a beam of neutrons emerging from the opposite side of the target in what is known as the *"stripping process"*. (f) *Alpha reactions* comprise (α, p) and (α, n) types, the latter being characteristic with light elements. Alpha particles of very high energies also produce mesons (see 5.15) and are used in meson research. (g) *Spallation reactions*, as signified by the term, are those in which a series of light fragments are splintered off by high energy bombardments. An example mentioned (Lapp and Andrews, page 310) is: $_{33}As^{75}$ (d, 9 p, 12 n) $_{25}Mn^{56}$; the deuteron (d) is the bombarding particle.

2.31 Mirror Nuclei

Among the positron emitters we find a number which, following decay, become nuclei with precisely the reverse numbers of protons and neutrons— "mirror images" so to speak, of the originals. Thus $_6C^{11}$ with 6 p and 5 n becomes B^{11} with 5 p and 6 n. Such pairs are termed *mirror nuclei*.

SUMMARY

Atoms are shown to be mostly empty space with tiny dense nuclei forming cores about which electrons of very slight mass form orbital shells; the orbital characteristics determine chemical and crystalline behavior. Over 100 elements with about 1000 isotopes are found in groups with recurring characteristics. Nuclei behave as though formed of exceedingly dense fluid and their particles, protons and neutrons are held together by surface tension and exchange forces.

Stability factors limit the number of isotopes and size of atomic nuclei and are concerned with radioactivity.

Radiations show both wave and particulate characteristics; and light, x-rays and gamma rays act as though they come in discrete packets of energy (quanta or photons).

Further details of the physics will be found in appropriate places in succeeding chapters. More extensive consideration will be found in various textbooks; those given in the following list of references are suggested for additional reading and study.

REFERENCES

CORK, J. M.: *Radioactivity and Nuclear Physics*. Third Edition. New York: D. Van Nostrand Co., 1957.

GAYNOR, F. (editor): *Pocket Encyclopedia of Atomic Energy*. New York: Philosophical Library, Inc., 1950.

GHIORSO AND SEABORG: The Newest Synthetic Elements. *Scient. Am. 195(6):* 67–80, December, 1956.

GLASSTONE, S.: *Sourcebook on Atomic Energy*. New York: D. Van Nostrand Co., 1950.

LAPP, R. E.: *Atoms and People*. New York: Harper, 1956.

LAPP AND ANDREWS: *Nuclear Radiation Physics*. Second Edition. New York: Prentice-Hall, Inc., 1954.

RUTHERFORD, E., as already listed viz: *Radio-active Substances and Their Radiations*. New York: Putnam, 1913. (Historic interest.)

SLATER, J. C.: *Modern Physics*. New York: McGraw-Hill, 1955.

THOMPSON, J. J.: *The Corpuscular Theory of Matter*. London: A. Constable & Co., 1907. (Historic interest.)

NOTE: See also references after Chapter 3 and Chapter 5.

3▸

Nuclear Reactors and Bombs

CHARLES F. BEHRENS, M.D.

3.1 Stability Factors

Fission of atoms into two major fragments is the basic phenomenon (see also par. 2.29) involved in the energy output of nuclear reactors and the fission bomb. This must of necessity be related to nuclear stability and accordingly it is necessary to take up briefly some related nucleonics and energy factors.

Opposing factors affect the stability of atomic nuclei as already indicated. Strong electrical repulsion on the part of the positively charged protons which tends to disrupt nuclei is counteracted by the extreme surface tension effects of dense nuclear fluid and also by what we call exchange forces which tend to cause coalescence.

3.1.1 *Surface Tension Effect.* (See also par. 2.23 and 2.24.) The surface tension factor decreases in relative effectiveness as the atoms increase in size owing to the familiar fact that the volume of a sphere increases more rapidly than the surface area. For instance, a surface area-volume ratio of 3 to 1 will become 3 to 2 when 8 drops are combined into 1. Accordingly, the bursting strain on the nucleus increases with the atomic weight, since the repulsive effect of the similarly charged protons increases with the number of protons in a nucleus, whereas the other factors fail to show a corresponding gain.

3.1.2 *Exchange Forces.* (See also par. 2.24.) Extremely small distances are involved in nuclei as may well be realized from the approximate nuclear diameter 1×10^{-12} cm.; and at such distances it has been calculated that the usual electrical repulsion effects or coulomb forces must be overcome by some species of attraction which is spoken of as resonance or exchange forces. The nature of exchange force is quite obscure but shows the following characteristics:

1. Range of operation is very short, probably 1×10^{-13} cm.
2. It fades out rapidly beyond that short range.

3. It binds nucleons together as though by an electrical charge shared or "exchanged" between them, the charge being that of an electron, associated however, with a mass about 200 times that of an electron.

4. It shows saturation effects so that there is a tendency for nucleons to pair off and for four nucleons to form a sort of closed system as seen in the helium nucleus or alpha particle of two protons and two neutrons.

3.2 Neutron-Proton Ratio and Beta Decay

For each atomic number there are, as noted in the previous chapters, isotopic varieties with different numbers of neutrons. There is, however, in each instance, a limit to the number of neutrons that can accepted without loss of stability. Neutrons are a trifle heavier than protons and are not stable by themselves. When in excess they tend to give up their extra mass in the form of electrons. This loss of mass and negative charge causes the neutron to become a proton, whereupon the nucleus advances one in the atomic scale, owing to the extra proton so acquired.

The electrons emitted in this process form the beta ray and the whole phenomenon is spoken of as beta decay. The number of neutrons relative to protons, although showing in most instances more or less latitude, shows a general increase as we proceed up the atomic scale to the heavier elements.

The common form of hydrogen of course shows no neutrons, as its nucleus is formed by a single proton. In helium we find equal numbers of neutrons and protons. In the middle of the atom family the ratio of protons to neutrons becomes about 1 to 1.3. When we reach the uranium group the ratio becomes 1 to 1.6. We can thus see that if a heavy nucleus breaks in two there will be an excess of neutrons. For example $_{92}U^{235}$ has 143 neutrons, whereas two atoms of $_{46}Pd^{106}$ show 120 neutrons. Uranium does not break precisely in two, as we shall see later, but it is obvious that a little flux of neutrons should be liberated whenever a large nucleus breaks into major fragments; in addition, we can see why these fragments themselves might tend to have too many neutrons for stability.

3.3 Mass and Energy Equivalence

The labors of many years have brought us precise values as to the masses of protons, neutrons and virtually all atoms. However, when we start making comparisons between atomic weights and masses of individual particles we find curious discrepancies. For example, if we add up the weights of the protons and neutrons which go into the formation of helium we obtain the figure of 4.033 mass units. However, the actual measured mass of the helium nucleus is 4.0028 mass units, indicating a loss of 0.03 mass units, equivalent to approximately 28.28 mev. Thus a similar number of grams of matter would vanish in the formation of about 4 gm. or a "mole" of helium from nuclear particles. This is not in accordance with the classic law of the conservation of matter, but instead agrees with the concept of Einstein formulated in 1905, which correlates matter and energy. According to this view, one should think of matter as being a measure of the energy potential or content of a given system. If more energy is bound up in a system, its mass will be greater; if the energy is less, the mass will be less. This does not mean that we can interconvert them entirely at will or that we can "burn" matter to manufacture energy. It really means that whenever energy is dissipated a certain mass of matter disappears; and that whenever energy is captured there is an increase in mass. The equation expressing this is: $E = mc^2$ where m is mass, c the velocity of light and E the energy. If m is 1 gram and c expressed in cm./sec. we obtain a truly astronomical figure for the energy equivalent of 1 gram; viz., 9×10^{20} ergs which in turn is equal to about 25 million kilowatt hours, or more precisely, and in accord with the present-day mode of expression, 25.02×10^6 KWH. If we consider that in the ordinary combustion of carbon, it requires 1 pound or about 454 gm. to produce 4 KWH, we can see that nuclear reactions involve a new order of magnitude well beyond that of other reactions by a factor of millions. Even a single nucleon or mass unit with a weight of 1.66×10^{-24} gm. is equivalent in energy content to 931 million electron volts which would be the energy imparted to an electron by a potential of that degree. In comparison, ordinary combustion of a carbon atom releases energy equivalent to about 1 electron volt.

3.4 Derivation of Solar and Stellar Energy

However we do not ordinarily find matter disappearing as though by a type of crude combustion. Instead we find transmutations in which there are huge releases of energy which we can relate to mass changes. The most important instance of this for us is seen in the case of the sun. We have noted that mass disappears when nucleons combine to form helium. In accordance with this, a huge amount of energy should appear if hydrogen nuclei, or protons, could be converted to helium. It is beyond our power to accomplish this in our laboratories*, but in the sun and stars, where enormous pressures prevail along with temperatures reaching millions of degrees, such conversion of hydrogen to helium is not only possible but actually provides the energy which keeps the universe "going" and makes life possible on the earth. The mass loss of 0.031 gm. per mole of helium formed in this manner equates with an energy release of 2.8×10^{19} ergs or 2.7×10^9 BTU (British thermal units). This is a tremendous amount

* At least on a practical scale; however intensive research is now in progress to accomplish this.

of energy from a small amount of matter but even so, it has been calculated that the energy production of the sun costs it a loss of nearly five million tons per second and that the earth gains 150 tons per day from this radiant energy. It is quite in keeping with this theory of the source of solar energy to note that hydrogen and helium constitute 99 per cent of the matter found in the universe. The figures are: 55 per cent hydrogen, 44 per cent helium and 1 per cent other elements.

Thermonuclear reactions, i.e., those dependant on high temperatures, are involved and a number of possibilities are mentioned.

(1) C—N cycle of Bethe and von Weizsacker (hotter areas): $_6C^{12} + _1H^1 \rightarrow _7N^{13} + \gamma$ (7×10^9y); $_7N^{13} \rightarrow _6C^{13} + e^+$; $_6C^{13} + _1H^1 \rightarrow _7N^{14} + \gamma$ (2×10^5y); $_7N^{14} + _1H^1 \rightarrow _8O^{15} + \gamma$ ($<3 \times 10^7$y); $_8O^{15} \rightarrow _7N^{15} + e^+$ (2m); $_7N^{15} + _1H^1 \rightarrow _6C^{12} + _2He^4$ (10^4y).

(2) p—p cycle: $_1H^1 + _1H^1 \rightarrow _1H^2 + e^+$ (7×10^9y); $_1H^2 + _1H^1 \rightarrow _2He^3 + \gamma$ (10s); $_2He^3 + _2He^3 \rightarrow _2He^4 + 2 _1H^1$ (3×10^5y)

(3) $_3Li^7 + _1H^1 \rightarrow _2He^4 +$ energy (17 mev.) (Red giants).

(4) These various reactions produce huge amounts of energy (often termed "Q") by consumption of hydrogen. When this is sufficiently depleted, such reactions decrease and contraction takes place. Then gravitational increase in temperature should develop whereby direct union of three $_2He^4$ to form $_6C^{12}$ becomes possible with release of 7.3 mev of energy.

(5) With depletion of helium it is thought that further gravitational contraction should occur with probable formation of heavier elements. Of these, Be^7 with a half life of 53d could liberate energy with extreme rapidity (on a stellar scale of energy liberation) and produce flare-ups such as characterize supernovae.

3.5 Mass Defect and Binding Energy

Atomic weights as actually measured are, as we have seen in the case of He, less than those obtained by adding of the weights of their constituent particles. These discrepancies are related both to energy levels and stability. The loss of mass is usually referred to as the mass defect and symbolized by "delta" (Δ). The energy equivalent to this weight loss is usually expressed in terms of millions of electron volts since nuclear energy is so often given up in the forms of radiations whose energies are most conveniently designated in such terms. As noted previously, one mass unit equates with 931 mev. The energy equivalent is also usually spoken of as "binding energy" as it affords a measure of the energy that would have to be applied to pry the nucleons apart again. Another method of dealing mathematically with the mass discrepancy is by means of the so-called "packing fraction." This is nothing but the approximate mass loss or "decrement" per nucleon, multiplied by 10,000 to obtain convenient figures.

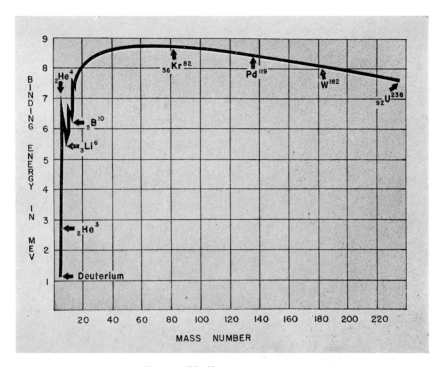

FIG. 1. Binding curve energy

Each nucleon is assigned a value of 1 and the number of nucleons or mass number thus becomes the approximate total weight. Then this is subtracted from the standard atomic weight based on 16 for $_8O^{16}$, to obtain the total mass decrement. This figure is then divided by the mass number and multiplied by 10,000. Thus, for example, in the case of hydrogen we have $\dfrac{1.00778 - 1}{1} \times 10,000 = 77.8$. On this basis, since the elements beyond oxygen and until we pass a mass number of 200 show an atomic weight less than the mass number, the packing fraction is usually negative. This means that in comparison to oxygen these elements have smaller energy potentials. The heaviest elements, however, show positive packing fractions indicating higher energy levels and greater tendency to instability. The packing fraction conception is perhaps useful but it is more satisfactory to dea directly with the binding energies based on actual mass defects. A partial table of these is given on the opposite page.

It will be seen that except for some individual discrepancies there is a general increase in binding energy per nucleon as the atomic weights increase until we reach element 36 of the atomic family, which is $_{36}Kr^{82}$.

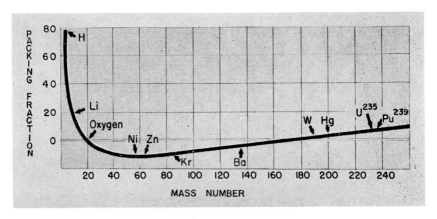

Fɪɢ. 2. Packing fraction curve

After this there is a general decrease in mass defect per nucleon and binding energy per nucleon. This is related to the fact that disruptive electrical effects continue to increase as nuclei become larger. It appears that the opposing forces balance each other most evenly in the middle zone, $_{36}Kr^{82}$ showing the greatest binding energy.

What all this means is that if we tally up our figures we will find that the mass per nucleon of our heavy weight fissionable elements is greater than the mass per nucleon of the fission products. Thus it is apparent that when the heavy uranium or Pu nuclei break in two there is sure to be some dissipation of mass, because the same number of nucleons in the lighter nuclei will weigh less. This in turn means that this loss of weight will be equated with the appearance of energy in accordance with the well-known equation $E = MC^2$, calculations indicating a release of about 200 mev of energy per atom fissioned.

3.6 Activational Factors

One might well conjecture now that all elements should undergo trans-mutation to that element whose nucleus has given up a maximum amount of energy and nucleons attained minimum weight. However, this does not happen any more than diamonds become CO_2 spontaneously, even though energy would be released thereby. Activation energy is required to start the process.

Much energy is required to start most transmutation reactions, just as on the enormously smaller energy scale of chemical combustion heat must often be supplied to initiate the reaction. This factor is usually pictured in mountain crater type of analogy: water or other object in a crater well above ground level will have considerable potential energy that can be made operative and put to work by letting gravitation pull the ob-

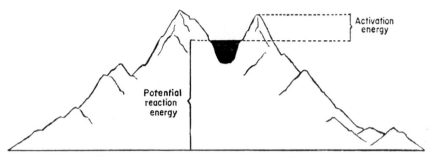

FIG. 3. Crater-type analogy of activation and potential energy

ject downhill. First, however, we must lift the object over the rim of the crater. The energy required to do this is analogous to activational energy. We can think of the unstable elements as having extremely shallow craters and the stable elements as having deep ones. However, there is a discrepancy here, in that unstable elements have such severe internal stresses that the nuclei cannot retain this energy indefinitely and it surges out in one form or another at a definite statistical rate, even without the addition of activation energy. This is somewhat at variance with normal expectations, although it can be considered as roughly analogous to the slow oxidation of rusting and similar chemical phenomena. However, as is often the case with analogies, the similarity is only superficial and in this instance involves only the time factor. A new concept has to be introduced which is related to the wave characteristics of matter.

3.7 Barrier Permeability

Certain elements show spontaneous radioactivity of a type seemingly impossible. Thus, U^{238} emits alpha-particles through a potential barrier much higher than the potential available, which seems about as reasonable as for a man in a deep well to fly out.

The explanation is that because of the wave characteristics of atomic particles, barriers are not completely impermeable. Wave mechanics and related statistical probabilities permit tunnelling or leaking out at rates characteristic for given species of nuclei. Calculations for U^{238} indicate that nucleon aggregations for alpha-emission appear at the nuclear surface at an average of 10^{21} times/s/atom with escapes averaging once in 10^{38} times.

In the case of a single atom the time of such escape is unpredictable but for the huge numbers of atoms involved in our customary procedures, the statistical averages are quite accurate.

3.8 Uncertainty Principle

It is worthy of note here that the uncertainty as to the behavior of an individual atomic nucleus in the matter of radioactive decay, in contrast to an accurate average for large numbers, is a widespread characteristic of physical and chemical phenomena. For instance, one cannot say precisely where a given electron orbit will be; instead there is a zone of probable locations and physicists like to speak of orbital zones and energy levels instead of precise orbits. This takes the edge off the classical rigidity which was formerly thought to apply to all physical phenomena and brings into everything elements of probability or, as it is often put, indeterminism. The scientific generalization of an "uncertainty" or "indeterminancy" principle was formulated by the German physicist Heisenberg in 1927 and involved difficulties with data on electrons in motion. It was noted that precise determination of both position and momentum of a particle at any particular instant is impossible because in the process of determining one, the other alters. Again, when determining the position of an electron or other particle, it must be dealt with as a particle, whereas when momentum is being investigated, wave characteristics are used. Wave and particulate characteristics are complementary and not contradictory and so although the various particles and also photons may act as either waves or particles, they cannot act as both at the same instant. One might well conjecture that the type of behavior depends on particular conditions, and one might even note a very rough analogy in everyday life where we find familiar substances such as water showing three types of behavior depending on whether they are in gaseous, fluid or solid state. Correspondence is most inexact, but it serves to remind us that familiar things also show startling shifts in characteristics.

3.9 Discovery of Fission

Of practical moment is the fact that the radiations from unstable nuclei show the greatest energy when the decay period is shortest and the least when it is longest, in accordance with a definite ratio. Thus a slow alpha particle with a range of 1 cm. in air corresponds to a half life of 2×10^{11} years, whereas an alpha particle of high energy and a range of 6 cm. corresponds to a half life period of 10^{-3} sec. (1/1000). The term "half life," you will remember, refers to the length of time required for a given amount of an unstable element to be reduced by a half.

It should be noted that each alpha-emitting isotope shows a number of characteristic ranges for these particles, thus forming a type of spectrum analogous to that of light, and corresponding to the various energy levels within the nucleus.

For many years we knew of no practical way to influence the rate of decay except on a tiny scale by shooting various particles at the atoms, whereby an occasional one out of thousands of these missiles would score a "bulls-eye" on a nucleus and nick off a fragment or effect some other type of transmutation. Nor were there any widespread hopes of accomplishing more than this. The situation altered, however, when Hahn and Strassman in Germany found that neutron bombardment of uranium caused that element to split into two major fragments. This aroused intense interest not only on its own score but because it brought up the possibility of a chain or continuous reaction. Lighter elements contain a smaller proportion of neutrons than uranium and, as already pointed out, neutrons should be and are liberated when fission occurs. Thus since neutrons occasion fission, it was realized that if enough neutrons were emitted and if enough suitable atoms were available, a spreading type of chain reaction should be possible under proper circumstances. Therefore, despite the fact that nothing like that took place naturally in uranium, it was felt that some method could be found to make it possible and that investigation was clearly in order. Thus the huge gamble of the Manhattan Project was decided on and carried through to success during the past war.

3.10 General Factors Concerned in Fission

The first difficulty in the way of a chain reaction was found in the fact that fission of uranium is practically limited to the U^{235} isotope which is present in natural uranium in only a small percentage. Natural uranium is composed of 99.3 per cent U^{238}, 0.7 per cent U^{235} and a trace of U^{234}. Let us consider now why U^{235} is highly fissionable and the other uranium isotopes refractory in this regard.

Fission does not necessarily take place whenever a neutron strikes a heavy nucleus. Activation energies are concerned. According to wave mechanics, a slow or "thermal" neutron of very slight energy (0.03 electron volts) will be accepted by a U^{235} nucleus: it simply "leaks" in by resonance and in so doing contributes an energy equivalent to 6.4 million electron volts to the nucleus. Therefore, since the critical energy for fission of U^{235} is only 5.2 mev, fission becomes the favored possibility. In the case of U^{238} a slow neutron of about 24 electron volts kinetic energy will be accepted by resonance capture but will only add 5.4 mev energy to the nucleus. Since the critical energy for fission in this case is 5.9 mev, a simple capture is favored which we will describe in detail later. Now if a fast neutron with great kinetic energy crashes into a U^{238}, fission will occur about once in five times, but in general this nucleus finds it easier to disgorge such a neutron again without undergoing fission. Again it may be that, dense as nuclei are, very fast neutrons may be able to pass through. It might be noted also that thorium can be fissioned but is even less obliging than U^{238}. Out of 25 neutrons which gain access only one will cause fission, the others being thrust out again.

3.11 Uranium Piles and Reactors

The all-important characteristic of U^{235} is that it tends to capture thermal or very slow neutrons better than U^{238}. It has what is called a larger cross section for capture. Cross section in this sense does not mean actual diameter but the effective diameter for capture.* This affinity of U^{235} for thermal neutrons is the key factor in making the uranium pile possible.

It is easily seen from the foregoing that the large preponderance of U^{238} in natural uranium prevents any chain reaction in nature and this feature is aggravated by the fact that most impurities are also fond of neutrons. Thus it is apparent that some special arrangement would be essential if a self-propogating or "chain reaction" in uranium was to become possible. The fact that when neutrons liberated by fission are slowed down enough, capture by U^{235} is favored, became the point of attack.

Various substances were considered for the job of slowing neutrons and nearly all were unsuitable because of various difficulties, such as absorption of too many neutrons, unavailability in sufficient quantity and trouble with purification. Eventually it was found that carbon in the form of pure graphite would answer very well. The way in which it is used is as a matrix or "moderator" in which pieces of uranium are embedded in lattice fashion.

The amount and disposition of the graphite are designed to permit numerous collisions, averaging over a hundred, whereby the neutrons reach "thermal speed" or that due only to the molecular jostlings consequent upon the degree of heat present. When the neutron, now at thermal speed, wanders back into a uranium mass, capture by U^{235} becomes the favored possibility. With something over 6 tons of uranium embedded in a carbon matrix, the chain reaction becomes possible to and beyond the critical point, where each uranium atom that fissions will result in the fissioning of another.

The first reactor was constructed at the University of Chicago and was built of layers of graphite bricks; the bricks in alternate layers contain the uranium or uranium oxide. This pile took the form of an oblate spheroid and was brought up to an energy output of about 200 watts. The initial successful operation was 2 Dec. 1942.

This pile was later removed and reassembled at the Argonne Laboratories near Chicago and operates at about 2 kilowatts with occasional boosts to 100. At the level of 2 KW, consumption of U^{235} is about 0.002 gram per day. This is a low power pile without cooling system.

3.11.1 *Control.* Chain reactions once past the critical level build up to destructive levels with extreme rapidity unless controlled because nearly all fission neutrons are of prompt type emitted within a millisecond. For-

* Measured in "Barns" (σ, sigma), 10^{-24} cm^2.

tunately about 0.8 per cent of the neutrons are of delayed type ranging from 0.05 to 55.6 seconds plus a few ranging to 12.5 minutes. This blunts the critical level sufficiently to grant time for operation of control mechanisms. These function by absorbing neutrons and so reducing the fission rate.

The elements usually used are Cd and B, reactions being:

$$_{48}Cd^{113} + _{0}n^1 \rightarrow {}_{48}Cd^{114} \quad \text{and} \quad _{5}B^{10} + _{0}n^1 \rightarrow {}_{3}Li^7 + {}_{2}He^4$$

Cross sections for n capture in "*barns*" are: Cd^{113}, 2500; B^{10}, 4000. The more abundant isotope of Boron, B^{11} has a low value.

Mechanisms are normally of "servo" type and provide regulation by the degree of insertion of control rods containing the above listed elements.

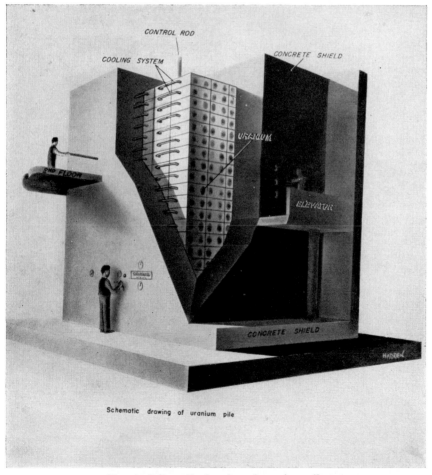

Schematic drawing of uranium pile

FIG. 4. Schematic drawing of uranium pile

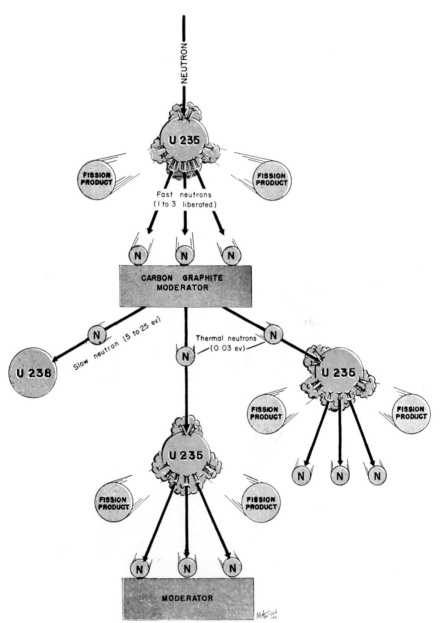

Fig. 5. Chain reaction in pile

3.11.2 *Notes on Present Day Reactors.* Reactors of varied type have been built and are being designed. Some of the factors involved are as follows:

U^{235} is fissionable by fast neutrons as well as thermal.

U^{238}, by neutron capture, becomes the source of another fissionable element, Pu^{239}. (See par. 3.13.)

Th^{232} may possibly prove a source of U^{233} which is also fissionable. The reaction is:

$$_{90}Th^{232} + n \rightarrow {}_{90}Th^{233} \xrightarrow[\text{23.5 min.}]{\beta^-} {}_{91}Pu^{233} \xrightarrow[\text{24.1 days}]{\beta^-} {}_{92}Ur^{233}$$

Heavy water is an excellent moderator. In fact it requires less than one fourth the number of collisions to slow neutrons than is the case with graphite. It is now available in large amounts at reasonable cost and is widely used.

Beryllium is an excellent moderator but is brittle and hard to fabricate. Its dust is highly provocative of granulomatous lesions.

Organic chemicals of the diphenyl and terphenyl groups are being tried as moderators; also polyethylene.

Enrichment of natural uranium with U^{235} or Pu^{239} makes possible faster reactors, the use of ordinary water as a moderator and even dispensing with a moderator.

High temperature operation is possible and is coming into wide use for heat and power.

3.11.2.1 *Some major types of reactors.* The original reactor described above is of *heterogenous type,* the term signifying non-uniform dispersion of uranium in the moderator. The uranium is used in the form of slugs, rods or plates usually jacketed in Al, Zr, or stainless steel (SS); or it may be used in alloy form. Assemblies may be designed for immersion in a fluid moderator. When an enriched fuel assembly is used in a large tank of water we have the *"Swimming Pool"* type.

When uranium is evenly dispersed in the moderator we have the *homogenous* type. Solutions or slurries are generally used. One modern variety designed for educational purposes has the uranium dispersed in polyethylene. Reactors employing a small core containing a homogenous solution of enriched uranium and cooled by water pumped through coils are known as *"Water Boilers."*

Reactors designed to produce more fissionable material than consumed are termed *"Breeders."*

Power Reactors may be compact fast units or large slower types. In England, natural uranium reactors of large size are featured at Calder Hall. In Russia, 5 per cent enriched power reactors are listed. Some degree of Pu production and recovery is usually a feature of power reactors. The value and dependability of power reactors has been well demonstrated in the highly successful submarine *U. S. S. Nautilus*. On the other hand there are engineering problems of new and difficult varieties complicated by radiological safety factors. A great amount of technical data is now available in reports of the 1955 Geneva Conference on "Peaceful Uses of Atomic Energy." Difficulties involve dealing with extremely high temperatures, corrosive and other effects of large neutron fluxes, pile "poisoning" by fission products notably Xenon, dealing with liquefied metals such as Na and K for cooling and many others.

Reactors specifically designed for *MEDICAL AND EDUCATIONAL PURPOSES* are now available and one such has been recently put in operation at the U. S. Naval Hospital, Bethesda, Maryland. It is of low power type and polyethylene moderated. The main purpose is to make practicable the use of short lived radioisotopes thereby providing a wider range of clinical applications and a reduction in general radiation dosage from certain diagnostic procedures. Thus 25 minute I^{128} should prove of value for thyroid studies and 12.8 hour Cu^{64} for positron scintiscanning of the brain for tumor localization. Cu^{64} may also prove of value in liver and blood volume studies. 37.3 minute Cl^{38} should be of great use in electrolyte work.

A new field of research has opened for the discovery and utilization of additional useful products and procedures for biological and medical applications of radioisotopes.

3.12 Bomb Materials

It is evident that as the relative amount of U^{235} is increased we will have a faster operating and less bulky reactor. Such have been constructed. Finally it is obvious that U^{235} in a pure state cannot continue to exist as such except in masses so small that neutrons from fissioning atoms escape in large measure. Since a few neutrons are always available everywhere resulting from cosmic rays, natural radioactivity and occasional spontaneous fissions, there can be no thought of preventing an overcritical mass of U^{235} from a chain fission reaction by neutrons. Once a mass of this substance passes the critical point, fissioning becomes inevitable at a rapidly increasing rate and with such release of energy as to blow the mass apart. In other words, there would be an explosion or flash effect; with this fact in mind, the possibility of an atomic bomb was envisioned. First, however, the problem of separating U^{235} on a large scale had to be solved.

3.12.1 *Separation of U^{235}*. It was a difficult task and it is worth recounting something of it in brief. Chemical methods were inapplicable since they could not apply to isotopes. On the score of physical methods, various types were possible but gaseous diffusion and mass spectrography were those put to most extensive use.

Diffusion depends on the fact that the molecular speeds of gases are inversely proportional to the square root of the molecular weights, the lighter gas showing greater molecular velocity in accordance with the equation:

$$\frac{V^1}{V^2} = \sqrt{\frac{m^2}{m^1}}$$

where V^1 and V^2 represent velocities and m^1 and m^2 the masses of the molecules. Thus if a semipermeable barrier with minute pores is set up, the lighter gas will diffuse through it more rapidly, so that it will be present in higher concentration on the other side. The differential factor is small, the maximum being 1.0043 theoretically and in practice averaging 1.003, employing the hexafluoride of uranium. Some thousands of cycles through barriers were requisite and a correspondingly enormous plant had to be built in order to make possible separation of U^{235} on a sufficiently large scale. There were also great difficulties caused by the characteristics of uranium hexafluoride which is solid at room temperature, shows corrosive properties when traces of moisture are present and is very poisonous.

These problems were successfully met at the Oak Ridge Plant and in addition the use of mass spectrography became practicable. In the latter the basis is the same as that noted in the early separation of isotopes, i.e., upon the application of strong electromagnetic fields to a beam of uranium ions, naturally deflection is different for atoms of different weight and this can serve as a basis for separation. Huge models were used, termed "calutrons."

3.13 Plutonium

As mentioned previously, U^{238} is able to retain neutrons captured at the resonance level of about 25 ev. There is also possibly another resonance level at 5 ev. Now since (1) this neutron capture eventuates in the formation of plutonium, and since (2) Pu behaves much the same as U^{235} in regard to fission possibilities, and since (3) separation of plutonium is possible by chemical means, it was promptly considered a valuable process for further investigation. When uranium 238 captures a neutron the sequence is as follows:

$$_{92}U^{238} + _{0}n^1 \rightarrow _{92}U^{239}$$

This is unstable, showing a half life of about 23 minutes. One of its neutrons changes to a proton by emission of an electron or, as usually stated, the element undergoes beta decay. Since there is now one more proton, the atomic number is increased by 1 so as to reach 93. We thus have a new element, neptunium, one of the transuranic family, $_{93}Np^{239}$. It is too unstable, having a half life of 2.3 days and again showing the phenomenon of beta decay. Accordingly we find $_{93}Np^{239}$ moving up the scale a notch to become plutonium with 94 protons—$_{94}Pu^{239}$. Plutonium thus formed in uranium piles is a long-lived alpha emitter with a half life of 24,000 years, and fissionable.

It is of course a new element, distinguished from U by chemical behavior and, as noted, offers the attractive prospect of separation by chemical means. This proved relatively so advantageous that it has been carried out on a large scale. The technical problems were enormous and the scale of operation unbelievably huge. This may be grasped from the fact that a pile operating at a level of about 500 to 1000 kilowatts produces only about 1 gram of Pu in 24 hours. Thus a high degree of activity had to be carried on to produce enough Pu, and so much heat was generated in accomplishing this that the water required to cool the piles would have been enough to supply the needs of a fair-sized city. An immense chemical separation plant also had to be put in action, and equipped with much automatic machinery designed to prevent undue exposure of personnel to radiations.

3.14 Atomic Bomb Construction

By the means just described, pure U^{235} and Pu^{239} were obtained in sufficient quantities to make bombs. The amount necessary is, of course, related to critical size. It is obvious that if enough of these pure materials are combined in a single mass the chain reaction can proceed at lightning speed, liberating, explosively, staggering amounts of energy. For an efficient reaction, however, this cannot be carried out in any easy casual manner. There are important considerations to be met, involving not only the combination of the proper amounts of material at the right instant but also minimizing the escape of neutrons and preventing dispersion of too much bomb material before it had a chance to be fissioned. Let us look into the details.

It has been noted that huge amounts of energy are involved. Thus fissioning of each U^{235} nucleus releases about 200 mev of energy. This amount of energy produces expansive pressure estimated at about a million times that of TNT. On this basis it is desirable for the reaction to take place in 10^{-9} seconds but we find that in order for the reaction to spread throughout the estimated 2×10^{21} atoms per gram of uranium, 10^{-6} seconds is required, the discrepancy being a thousandfold. To minimize this handicap and also to lessen the escape of neutrons, an exceedingly dense casing, termed a "tamper," is employed, density being the all-important factor. Success in meeting this condition has made a most powerful bomb possible although efficiency is still far from what is desired. It is theoretically possible for about 5 pounds of U^{235} to equal 20,000 tons of TNT but actually more is necessary.

3.14.1 *Fusion or Hydrogen Bomb Possibilities.* When one reflects that conditions within an exploding U or Pu bomb must approximate for a brief instant those within the sun and stars, the thought promptly arises that

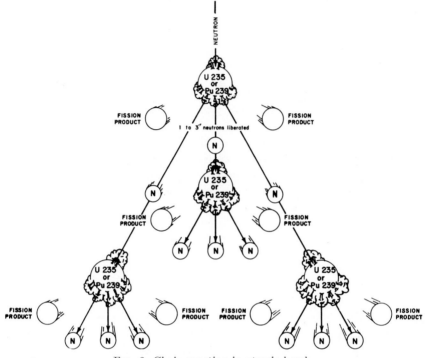

Fig. 6. Chain reaction in atomic bomb

fusion of hydrogen to form helium (see par. 3.4) might well be a practicable means to augment the force of the explosion. This possibility has been realized as is well known. Possible reactions are:

$$_1H^2 + {}_1H^2 \rightarrow {}_2He^3 + n + 3.26 \text{ mev energy or ``Q'}$$
$$_1H^2 + {}_1H^2 \rightarrow {}_2He^4 + \gamma + Q \text{ (low probability reaction)}$$
$$_1H^2 + {}_1H^2 \rightarrow {}_1H^3 + {}_1H^1 + 4.04 \text{ mev}$$
$$_1H^2 + {}_1H^3 \rightarrow {}_2He^4 \rightarrow n \rightarrow 17.6 \text{ mev}$$
$$_1H^2 + {}_1H^3 \rightarrow {}_2He^3 + 2\,n + 10.4 \text{ mev}$$

Reactions between tritons (H^3) and deuterons have a much greater probability factor than those between deuterons.

It is also mentioned (ref. Pocket Encyclopedia) that lithium has theoretical possibilities in accordance with:

$_3\text{Li}^7 + {}_1\text{H}^1 \rightarrow 2{}_2\text{He}^4 +$ energy; or employing the lighter isotope of lithium $_3\text{Li}^6 + {}_1\text{H}^3 \rightarrow 2\,{}_2\text{He}^4 + n +$ energy

3.15 Explosion

In practice the U^{235} or plutonium is kept in such small subcritical masses that the escape of neutrons precludes a spreading chain reaction. Thus in firing the bomb an ordnance problem has to be solved so that the subcritical masses can be fused so firmly and instantaneously as to prevent dispersal of the bomb material in a mere flash. The details of how this is done are necessarily secret, but a suitable type of method can readily be imagined and is usually pictured as a process of shooting the subcritical masses together in a heavy tamper.

Another and very ingenious method now described in the "Effects of Nuclear Weapons" is to make a subcritical mass explosive by reducing its volume. This is accomplished by putting a terrific squeeze on it by *symmetrical implosion* of surrounding charges of high explosive.

In either case a nuclear explosion of tremendous magnitude can be produced. Temperature rises to millions of degrees and a rapidly expanding fireball forms which swiftly ascends into the stratosphere forming as it cools the familiar mushroom figure. An intense flash of light many times brighter than sunlight signals the instant of detonation, and along with the visable light there are intense gamma rays, fast neutrons, and both ultraviolet and infrared radiations. In general radiations account for over a third of the energy of nuclear bombs. Shock waves are violent, prolonged and enormously destructive.

The updraft, in the case of low level bursts, in which the fireball touches the ground sucks up large amounts of debris and again subsurface bursts hurl up large amounts of material. The substances concerned are rendered

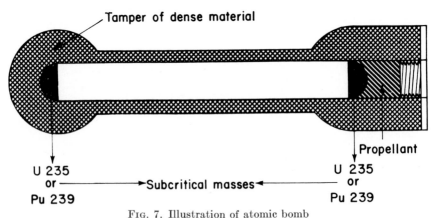

Fig. 7. Illustration of atomic bomb

radioactive by the neutron fluxes and contamination with fission products and, moreover, form large particles with the result that radioactive fallout can constitute a major hazard as has unhappily been well demonstrated (See Chapters 12 and 13). In the case of large weapons it can prove the major hazard to great masses of population.

3.16 Fission Products

Nuclei may be regarded as drops of exceedingly dense fluid and fissioning nuclei as droplets in violent oscillatory agitation. This results in "dumbbell" conformation followed by rupture and suggests that symmetrical division should occur as into isotopes of Pd. Instead we find over 200 nuclides derived from about 60 primary species with mass numbers ranging from 72 to 158. They form a light group centering about 95 and a heavy group clustered about 139. Explanations appear related to nuclear shells, "magic" numbers and mass spectroscopic values.

Fission product nuclei contain too many neutrons for stability (see par. 3.2) and are radioactive showing an average of 3 beta decays often with gamma emission. Some of the more abundant are isotopes of $_{36}Kr$, $_{38}Sr$, $_{39}Y$, $_{40}Zr$, $_{43}Tc$, $_{44}Ru$, $_{52}Te$, $_{53}I$, $_{54}Xe$, $_{56}Ba$, $_{57}La$, $_{58}Ce$, $_{60}Nd$, $_{61}Pm$. Of these, Sr^{90} is receiving great attention and publicity because it is a long lived bone seeker of high yield (19.9 years, 5.3 per cent). Sr^{89}, half life 53 d and yield 4.6 per cent is of importance too, but over a much shorter period.

3.17 Fission Chain Examples

$$_{36}Kr^{89} \xrightarrow[\beta\gamma]{3.2 \text{ min.}} {}_{37}Rb^{89} \xrightarrow[\beta\gamma]{15.0 \text{ min.}} {}_{38}Sr^{89} \xrightarrow[\beta\gamma; \text{ I.T.}]{10 \text{ and } 54 \ d} {}_{39}Y^{89} \text{ (stable)}$$

$$_{36}Kr^{97} \xrightarrow[\beta]{\text{short life}} {}_{37}Rb^{97} \xrightarrow[\beta]{\text{short life}} {}_{38}Sr^{97} \xrightarrow[\beta]{\text{short life}} {}_{39}Y^{97} \xrightarrow[\beta]{\text{short life}}$$

$$_{40}Zr^{97} \xrightarrow[\beta\gamma]{17 \text{ hr.}} {}_{41}Nb^{97} \xrightarrow[\beta\gamma; \text{ I.T.}]{1 \text{ and } 72 \text{ min.}} {}_{42}Mo^{97} \text{ (stable)}$$

$$_{54}Xe^{138} \xrightarrow[\beta\gamma]{17 \text{ hr.}} {}_{55}Cs^{138} \xrightarrow[\beta\gamma]{32 \text{ min.}} {}_{56}Ba^{138} \text{ (stable)}$$

3.18 Bomb Induced Radioactivity

Neutron fluxes and accordingly atomic explosions cause many nuclear transmutations associated with radioactivity. Concern relates largely to the more common substances and fortunately a number of the most vital elements have either a low cross section for neutron capture, or a short half life for the resultant radioactivity. Thus there is little worry on the score of H, N, O, C, S, Al, Mg, Ca and I.

Ordinary salt is important due to formation of 15 hr. Na^{24} and 37.3 min. Cl^{38}, both $\beta\gamma$ emitters. $Si^{28\text{-}30}$ which is common in soil becomes 2.62 hr. Si^{31} a $\beta\gamma$ emitter. P^{31} which is widely distributed becomes 14.5 d P^{32} a β emitter. Sea water and foods can thus be affected more especially by low-level or subsurface bursts. However, duration is not great and food not destroyed by heat and blast would be little affected. Glass due to presence of Na and Si would become radioactive for a time.

Radioactive isotopes of metals that may result include: 12.8 hr. Cu^{64}; B^-, B^+, γ, K and the following $\beta\gamma$ emitters: 45 d Fe^{59}, 2.6 hr./Mn^{56}, 14 hr. and 52 min. Zn^{69}, 12.5 hr. K^{42}, 2.7 d Au^{198}, 48 d Hg^{203}. Hazards from any of these would be restricted to a relatively small area and in general of minor nature. However, 5.2 yr. Co^{60}, a $\beta\gamma$ emitter of high energy could pose a serious threat if cobalt is added to atomic bombs.

REFERENCES

BIEL ET AL.: Compact Low Cost Reactor. *Nucleonics, 9:* 100–103, 1957.

Effects of High Yield Explosions. Statement by Lewis L. Strauss, Chairman and Report by the U.S.A.E.C., 1955. Catalog No. At7: 2N88/6: Government Printing Office, Washington, D. C.

Effects of Nuclear Weapons. Government Printing Office, Washington, D. C., 1957.

KENTON, J. E.: Nuclear Navy Paces U. S. Atomic Industry: *Nucleonics, 15:* 66–71, July 1957.

KING, E. T. ET AL.: The Production of an Medical Application of Short Half-life Radioisotopes. Special Brochure, Department of Nuclear Medicine, U. S. Naval Medical School, Bethesda, Md. 1957.

Peaceful Uses of Atomic Energy. Proceedings of the International Conference, Geneva, 1955. Published in the U. S. by Columbia University Press, New York 27, N. Y. Published in the United Kingdom by H. M. Stationery Office, P. O. Box 569 S.E.I., 16 Vol. See Especially Vol. 2, Physics and Research Reactors; Vol. 9, Reactor Technology and Chemical Processing, and Vols. 10–12, covering Medical and Biological Fields.

Reactor Handbooks. Government Printing Office, Washington, D. C. Physics: No. Y3.At7:8/3645; Engineering: *Ibid.* except 3646; Materials: *Ibid,* except 3647.

RIDENOUR, L. N. The Hydrogen Bomb. *Scient. Am. 182(3):* 11–15, March, 1950.

SMYTH, H. DEW.: Atomic Energy for Military Purposes. Official Report under the auspices of the U. S. Government, 1940–1945. Princeton, N. J.: Princeton University Press, 1945.

NOTE: See also references after Chapter 2.

4▶

General Effects of Nuclear Weapons

CAPTAIN HARRY H. HAIGHT, MC, U. S. Navy (Sections **4.1** to **4.5**) LT. R. D. JORDAN, MSC, U. S. Navy (Sections **4.6** to **4.13**)

4.1 "Nominal" Type Bomb

In previous editions of *Atomic Medicine*, this chapter has been almost entirely a consideration of the so called "nominal bomb" of about 20,000 tons (20 kt) TNT equivalence. Hundreds of articles and publications have considered this type bomb to the point that the subject is about exhausted. The reasons for this overly great devotion to one type of bomb are obvious. The first experimental bomb, known as the Trinity or Almagordo bomb, was of approximately this intensity as were the Hiroshima and Nagasaki bombs. Since these three detonations, especially the latter two, furnished the background for basic studies and calculations, they necessarily retain pre-eminence as bases for practically all further conjecture.

Many bombs have been detonated since those important dates in 1945. England, Russia and the United States have all exploded nuclear "devices" at one place or another around the globe. These latter explosions have been experiments and have been conducted in areas largely devoid of vegetation, obstacles or complex groups of structures. The effort has been to obtain perfect and unobstructed physical measurements and this has somewhat lessened the realistic value for estimates of casualties in numbers or types.

Every effort has been made to prevent danger to human life at all times. In studies *from the medical standpoint*, we must still revert, therefore, to the Japanese bombings which are the only ones which have been well covered from the major standpoints of material damage and casualties.

4.1.1. *Japanese Bombings Studies* (See also **4.6.5**). The Japanese Bombings were studied in minute detail by two groups. First was the "Strategic Bombing Survey" which carefully estimated physical measurements related to material damage at various distances from the epicenter. These figures (Atomic Bombing Casualty Commission) are of fundamental im-

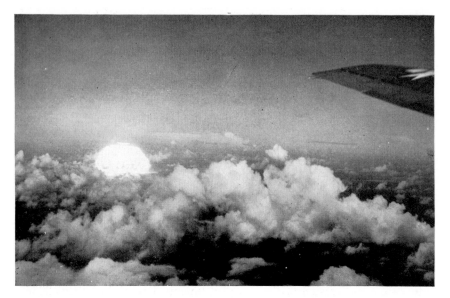

Fig. 1. The "ball-of-fire" at about maximum diameter (Able Day)

portance since they point the finger to the zones of damage caused by blast, heat, etc. They are of limited interest to the medical family (except for planning purposes) because the doctor is primarily interested in treating the casualties rather than in where or how they occurred. This group was accompanied by a medical commission which followed the survey of physical measurements by one of personnel damage. Emphasis was placed on types and numbers of casualties, and the medical care they received both immediately and eventually. Small wonder then, that the nominal bomb is still being used for standard reference.

4.1.2 *High Level Bursts.* Calculations and estimates in the past have mostly been based on the assumption that the most efficient use of the atomic weapon would call for relatively high altitude bursts whereby maximum blast and thermal effects could be obtained and the curse of the little known and fearsome radiation greatly reduced. It was clearly recognized in the first calculations and considerations that blast effects would be at a maximum in the case of a high-level detonation, radiation at a minimum and the thermal effects about equal to blast in casualty production.

It is interesting to note, parenthetically, that the thermal effects of the atomic bomb are primary; that the ignition of combustible material and the subsequent "fire storm" are actually the result of the bomb and not necessarily the result of overturned stoves, broken electrical wiring, etc. It was

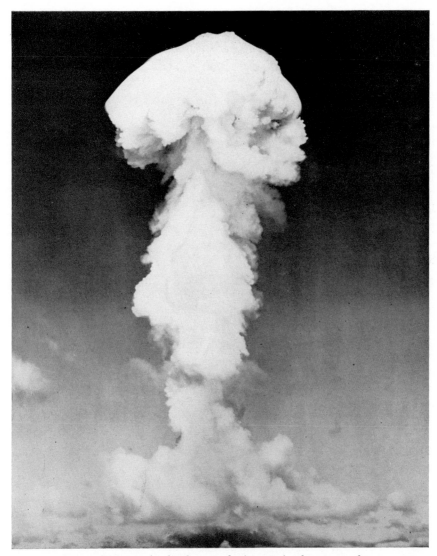

Fig. 2. The atomic cloud; note the ice cap in the stratosphere

particularly interesting to the author to note that in the tornadoes which occurred in Michigan in 1954, a wide swath of destruction was produced by what could well be termed "blast damage" during a tornado. Although the blast damage was so great that it was beyond accurate estimate, there were no fires. It would seem quite evident that the fires produced in the

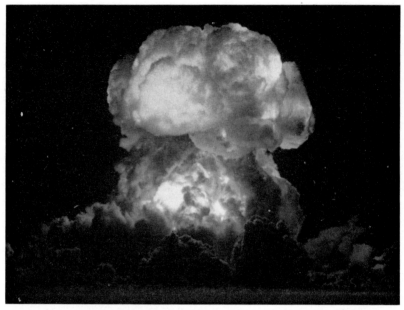

FIG. 2A. Thermonuclear bomb at about 30 miles

only two detonations made in anger, and where careful and detailed assessment of the fire damage have been obtained, indicate that thermal damage
is a very important inherent item of atom bomb destruction.

4.2. Other Types of Bombs

Since the end of the war the United States has done considerable experimenting with various atomic combinations officially called "devices." It
is no secret that these have varied in their size, shape and contour, nor that
some of them can be carried by carrier planes as well as huge bombers; also
that rockets with nuclear war-heads are to be reckoned with in the not too
distant future. Accordingly the "nominal bomb" is only of limited value as
a yardstick for our thinking: We learn from newspaper releases and "The
Effects of Nuclear Weapons" that devices of much smaller and many times
greater strength in terms of tons of TNT equivalence are available for use.
We have learned too, that the U. S. S. R. has detonated a series of bombs
somewhat similar to ours and at least, in a few instances, many times greater
than the nominal bomb; We know that the U. S., Russia and England have
conquered the problems of the so-called hydrogen bomb, the equivalence
of which is expressed in millions of tons (megatons) rather than in thousands.

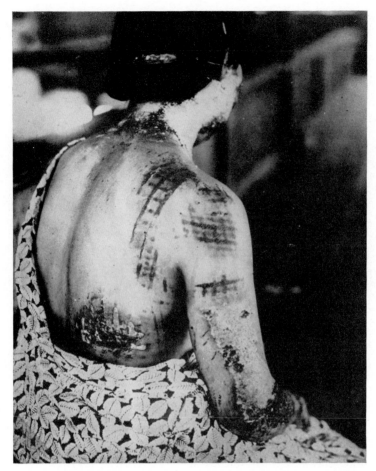

Fig. 3. Pattern burns show the protection offered by light-colored clothing

4.2.1 *Megaton Bombs.* Newspaper releases by the A. E. C., when reporting that an enormous bomb was detonated at the Atomic Proving Grounds in the Marshall Islands, reported that the detonation was probably at ground level. The Director of Civil Defense, then Mr. Val Peterson, reported in an interview in the 8 April, 1955 *"Newsweek"* that a 10 megaton bomb could cause total destruction over a radius of 4 miles with a crater 175–200 feet deep and a mile or more across. (See par. **4.3** and **4.6.1** for more precise data.) Beyond that, severe destruction would extend 4 miles further, moderate damage still another 4 miles, and finally, there would be another 4 miles of light damage: Total radius of damage about 16 miles.

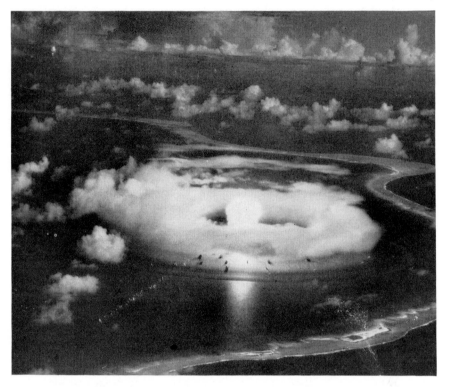

Fig. 4. The "ball-of-fire" (Able Day)

This pictures a smashing blow of staggering magnitude, though in extent of disruption of function and potential threat to multitudes of people, it is likely to be far exceeded by the results of radioactive fallout.

4.3 Comparative Data, 1 kt-20 Mgt. Bombs*

(Derived from data in the "Effects of Nuclear Weapons," 1957)

This book replaces the old "Effects of Atomic Weapons" and contains a wealth of information both general and technical. Space forbids extensive quotation and there is of course a great amount of material beyond the scope of this text. However, in order to provide approximate comparisons in convenient form for the wide range of available nuclear weapons, a chart has been prepared which lists certain effects of medical interest for various distances.

4.3.1 *Blast Damage.* This is presented in terms of the effects on multi-

* 4.3 contributed by the Editor.

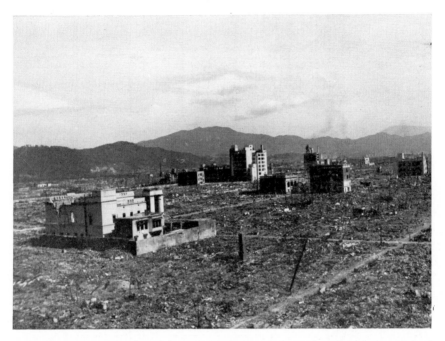

FIG. 5. Note complete destruction of inflammable buildings by "fire storm" (Hiroshima).

story brick apartment buildings. (Fig. 6.41a.)* Such buildings along with various brick dwellings of about similar resistance house a goodly proportion of our people. Aside from the table, comparison with other types is of interest and we find that special windowless blast-proof heavy construction sustains only moderately severe damage from air bursts. Multistory buildings of reinforced concrete and with small windows sustain very severe damage, verging on collapse, up to about 6 miles, from a 10 megaton explosion. The apartments mentioned above would be totally ruined by such a blast up to about 6½ miles and severely damaged up to about 8 miles.

4.3.2 *Flashburns.* These are given in terms of first to third degree as derived from Figure 7.49. The calories/cm² productive of burns vary with bombs of different caliber. The thermal radiation of smaller bombs is concentrated in shorter time intervals than is the case with larger ones and so we find for instance that a 1 kiloton (kt.) bomb causes third degree burns with 6 cal/cm², a 100 kt. bomb requires 8, and a 10 megaton (mgt.) burst 11.

4.3.3 *Fabric Ignition.* Wide variations are shown in Table 7.61 and Figure

* Refers to the "Effects of Nuclear Weapons" as do other similar references in 4.3.

RANGES OF CERTAIN BOMB EFFECTS OF MEDICAL INTEREST IN MILES
(Air Burst) (See Preceding Text)

BOMB SIZE AND TYPE OF DAMAGE	1/4	1/2	1	1½	2	3	4	5	10	20	40	NOTES
1 Kt. BLAST (Apt. Damage)	TOTAL	LIGHT	LIGHT	LIGHT								
1 Kt. FLASH BURNS (Degree)	3	2										
1 Kt. FABRIC IGNITION	MOST (~12 cal/cm²)	FEW (~3.5cal)										
1 Kt. INITIAL RADIATION	LETHAL >3000 REM.	SERIOUS ~300 REM.										
10 Kt. BLAST	TOTAL	TOTAL	LIGHT	LIGHT	LIGHT	LIGHT						
10 Kt. FLASH BURNS	3+	3+	3	2								
10 Kt. FABRIC IGNITION	ALL	MOST (>12cal)	FEW (~7cal)	FEW (~3cal)								
10 Kt. INITIAL RADIATION	LETHAL >3000 REM.	LETHAL ~2000 REM.	SLIGHT ~50 REM.									
20 Kt. BLAST	TOTAL	TOTAL	MODERATE	LIGHT	LIGHT	LIGHT	LIGHT					
20 Kt. FLASH BURNS	3+	3+	3	2-3	1-2							
20 Kt. FABRIC IGNITION	ALL	ALL	MOST (>12cal)	FEW (~7cal)	FEW (~3cal)							
20 Kt. INITIAL RADIATION	LETHAL ~3000REM.	LETHAL ~2000REM.	SLIGHT ~100REM.	SLIGHT ~30REM.								
100 Kt. BLAST	TOTAL	TOTAL	TOTAL	SEVERE	MODERATE	LIGHT	LIGHT	LIGHT				LIGHT DAMAGE TO ~7 MILE
100 Kt. FLASH BURNS	3+	3+	3+	3+	3	2-3	1-2					
100 Kt. FABRIC IGNITION	ALL	ALL	ALL	ALL	MOST >12cal	FEW ~6cal	FEW ~4cal					
100Kt. INITIAL RADIATION	LETHAL >3000REM.	LETHAL >3000REM.	CRITICAL ~700REM.	SLIGHT ~100REM.								
1 MEGATON BLAST	TOTAL	TOTAL	TOTAL	TOTAL	TOTAL	SEVERE	MODERATE	LIGHT	LIGHT			
1 Mgt. FLASH BURNS	3+	3+	3+	3+	3+	3+	3+	3+	1-2			
1 Mgt. FABRIC IGNITION	ALL	ALL	ALL	ALL	ALL	ALL	ALL	MOST >12cal	FEW ~5cal			
1 Mgt. INITIAL RADIATION	LETHAL	LETHAL	CRITICAL ~700REM.	CRITICAL ~600REM.	SLIGHT ~60REM.							
10 Mgt. BLAST	TOTAL	TOTAL	TOTAL	TOTAL	TOTAL	TOTAL	TOTAL	TOTAL	LIGHT	LIGHT		SEVERE DAMAGE TO 8 MILE
10 Mgt. FLASH BURNS	3+	3+	3+	3+	3+	3+	3+	3+	3	3		1st DEGREE BURNS TO 30 MILE
10 Mgt. FABRIC IGNITION	ALL	ALL	ALL	ALL	ALL	ALL	ALL	ALL	ALL	MOST >12cal		
10 Mgt. INITIAL RADIATION	LETHAL	LETHAL	LETHAL	LETHAL >3000REM.	LETHAL ~800REM.	SLIGHT <30REM.						
20 Mgt. BLAST	TOTAL	TOTAL	TOTAL	TOTAL	TOTAL	TOTAL	TOTAL	TOTAL	MODERATE	LIGHT	LIGHT	LIGHT DAMAGE TO 50 MILE
20 Mgt. FLASH BURNS	3+	3+	3+	3+	3+	3+	3+	3+	3+	3	3	2nd DEGREE BURNS TO OVER 30 MILE
20 Mgt. FABRIC IGNITION	ALL	ALL	ALL	ALL	ALL	ALL	ALL	ALL	ALL	MOST >12cal	FEW ~4cal	
20 Mgt. INITIAL RADIATION	LETHAL	LETHAL	LETHAL	LETHAL ~3000REM.	LETHAL ~80REM.							

CHART 1

7.67; and as noted elsewhere in this chapter, color is very important. Certain dark rayons ignite at 1–3 cal/cm², tan cotton shirts ignite at 7 cal for a 10 kt. bomb and 13 for a 10 mgt. burst; rayon gabardine of gold color at 9 and 20 cal/cm² under similar circumstances; tan nylon hosiery at 5 and 10 cal; wool at 16 and 35 without, however, continuing to burn.

4.3.4 *Initial Radiation.* This occurs in the first minute (see par. 4.9.1) and comprises virtually all the dosage of clinical importance from the blast and fireball since in that time the fireball passes out of effective range. It does not include residual or fallout radiation. It is made up of gamma rays (γ) and neutrons (n). These account for about 3 per cent of the explosion energy as contrasted to about 33 per cent for thermal energy.

The contribution of neutrons is of considerable importance with bombs of kiloton type but of minor consequence in megaton bursts, the range of neutrons being notably shorter than those of gamma rays in the latter case, as noted in the following:

BOMB SIZE	NEUTRON RANGES IN MILES		GAMMA RANGES	
	1000 Rem	30 Rem	1000 r	30 r
20 Kt.	0.7 miles	0.9 miles	0.65 miles	1.2
100 Kt.	0.8	1.2	0.8	1.4
10 Mgt.	1.2	1.75	2.1	2.8
20 Mgt.	1.4	1.8	2.3	3.1

Thus the supralethal dose of 1000 r for gamma rays extends about 1 mile further than the equivalent dose of neutrons in the case of 10 to 20 mgt. bombs.

In general, however, the ranges for thermal and indirect blast injuries far outstrip those for serious effects from the initial ionizing radiation. Nevertheless many people in substantial structures or otherwise protected from the former are bound to incur serious radiation exposure. The initial radiation is highly penetrating and about six inches of concrete or one and one-half inches of steel are required to reduce it by a half. Neutrons show more complex behavior but concrete will attenuate them more readily than in the case of gamma rays, producing a 10× reduction by ten inches. Residual and fallout radiations are not so penetrating and two and one-half inches of concrete will reduce gamma rays from those sources by about a half. (Data sources: γ ranges, Figure 8.39; n, Figure 8.72; total radiation 8.82.)

4.4. Fallout

The A. E. C. report (Adm. Strauss), pictures a cigar shaped area some 140 by 20 miles where fallout might be lethal, with a lesser but dangerous contamination extending over something like 240 by 40 miles. A dosage of 2300 r in 36 hours was calculated for a distance of 100 miles, and 1000 r for 125 miles. A city at the 100 mile point would still show 45 r/day a month later. Such figures however, are not realistic in the sense of reflecting necessary exposure. People can and will find shelter. The figures are theoretical possibilities when there is no protection; they are also subject to gross variation depending on the type, power and point of detonation of the bomb as well as vagaries of the weather. They point up nevertheless the likelihood of huge areas of serious radiation hazard.

Cogency is given this consideration by the actual events in the Pacific tests of 1954; and the fact that natives from Rongelap and Rongeric were evacuated from their habitations indicates a strong probability that our previous almost complete preoccupation with blast and thermal effects as the most important factors in an atomic detonation may very well be in error. Various brochures published under the auspices of the A. E. C., indicate that a very large and significant group of natives received a dose of radiation due to fallout (before they were evacuated from their home island), which closely approached the 200 r level. This, by most radiologists, is considered a "Median Sickness Dose" (MSD). It is a published fact that

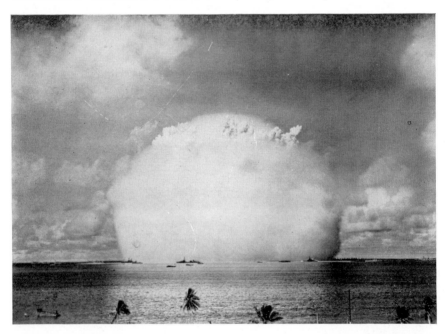

Fig. 6. Underwater blast (Baker Day). Note the fog "doughnut" due to secondary pressure decrease.

none of these natives suffered from radiation illness as such (that is, systemic illness) but that nearly 100 per cent of them did receive localized radiation burns, depilation and obvious recognizable and sometimes painful local lesions. (See Chapter 13.)

Even a casual examination of the map of the Pacific Ocean area serves to indicate that this potentially dangerous fallout pattern covered an area of approximately 5000 sq. miles. (This fact was pointed out in syndicated columns by the Alsop brothers after the calculations of the Physicist, Ralph Lapp.) A recent copyrighted article in the Washington Post and Times Herald, under the International Newspaper Service, quoted a statement from the "Bulletin of the Atomic Scientists" that "there was little chance that 'clean bombs' would ever be used in an all-out atomic war when the greatest devastation can be caused by spraying radioactive debris to the four winds."

4.4.1 *Medical Implications of Fallout.* (See also Chapters 12 and 13.) Assuming that these publicized statements are true, and there is no reason to doubt that they are, the entire perspective of atomic medical defense as we have heretofore considered it, must be changed. We have previously

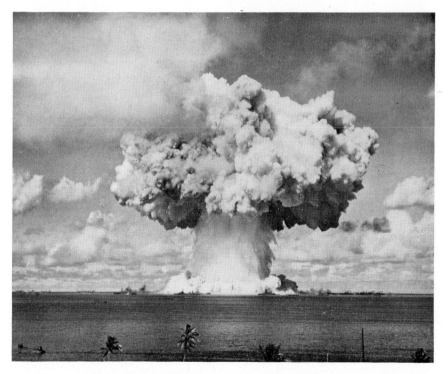

Fig. 7. Underwater blast (Baker Day)

assumed from the figures set forth by the Strategic Bombings Survey that there would be 100,000 casualties per bomb, 50 per cent of which would be fatal and 50 per cent of which would require medical care. Of these, 60 per cent would be traumatic injuries, 60 per cent burns and 15 per cent radiation damage. With the change in concept of strategic or retaliative use of the atomic weapons, it should be evident that these figures are no longer valid. In the case of a surface burst with the newer weapons and with a strong possibility of a dangerous and potentially lethal or disability producing fallout over an area of approximately 5000 square miles or more, the picture has been altered considerably. It was previously hoped and expected that in the case of the high air burst, rescue personnel could be immediately admitted to the area of destruction to carry on fire fighting and rescue activities. This would of course include evacuation to planned medical centers. The problem of properly supplying these areas with equipment and supplies was deemed the momentous one although no one has so far (to our knowledge) perfected a plan or a system by which adequate medical personnel, including nursing service, could be "stockpiled." Dr. Herman Pearse and his colleagues at the University of Rochester calculated the amount of supplies in tonnage and cubage which would be re-

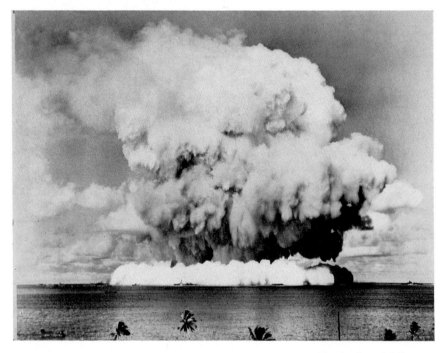

Fig. 8. Underwater blast (Baker Day). Note base surge and beginning of fall-out

quired to treat, properly, 60 per cent of 50,000 casualties who were burned, and came up with astonishing figures. It was calculated that the supplies required would total 8000 tons—more than could be loaded on a World War II liberty ship. This is, for planning purposes, the amount of medical supplies that would be required in the event of a single ordinary bomb drop in a metropolitan area.

Under the new concept the picture becomes extremely complicated. If one should visualize the surface detonation of one of the modern bombs on the city of Washington, D. C. and if one of the "four winds" happened to be from a south southwesterly direction, a dangerous and potentially lethal fallout could occur to the northeast. This fallout would include all of the major eastern cities as far north as New York City. Under such circumstances, all of the fire and rescue plans would be nearly impossible of execution except under extremely well supervised conditions, because of the danger to the rescuers. With proper monitoring it could be possible for the rescue teams to invade the contaminated areas for limited lengths of time without receiving disabling doses of radiation. This would entail, however, careful monitoring and adequate knowledge of the radiation dangers faced by the monitors, unless the rescue teams assume the "go to hell" attitude and completely ignore the dangers. We cannot detect ionizing radiation by any of our five senses.

4.5 Problems and "Ifs"

We come now to the further problem of the "ifs." If we had an adequate alarm system; if there were adequate underground facilities to house a population, and if proper radiation detection instruments were supplied and if capable monitors were available to measure the hazard on the surface of the ground, it might be possible for the populace so protected to reach their underground shelters in time and to remain there without rescue or early resupply for a safe period of time. The stay would depend upon the initial surface readings and the rate of subsequent decay of the radioactive fallout. Conceivably it might extend to one or two weeks for unrestricted egress. Considering the difficulties of progress, the sporadic nature of public interest and the usual apathy, there is little likelihood that any of the "ifs" will be solved adequately in the case of the civilian populations.

In the event of an all-out war at this late date and with the new concept of the use of the bomb, it is essential that all medical personnel, and all other personnel for that matter, become acquainted with the problems of radiation sickness and its treatment. It is true that radiation sickness seldom causes an emergency in the same way as do traumatic injuries and burns, because the serious symptoms of radiation damage usually do not appear for a matter of days or sometimes weeks following exposure. It is also true however that the treatment of radiation sickness is extremely important and far from hopeless. Thus the smug attitude of many a doctor and nurse who assume that it is sufficient if they can cope with the routine types of bomb injury, is no longer valid. The usual types of obvious injury will, of course, be trauma and burns and produce a tremendous and probably insurmountable problem number-wise; but in a little while the care of radiation casualties may constitute the paramount problem over and above the common disaster type which, be it remembered, may be complicated by radiation effects.

It is essential that constant research be pursued in an effort to discover methods of specific treatment for systemic radiation injury of total body type. Considerable time, effort and money have already been expended and some progress made. Details will be found in Chapter 11. It suffices to say here that preparations of spleen and bone marrow have very beneficial results; also platelet transfusions in the hemorrhagic state. They are not as yet, unfortunately, practicable for large scale use. On the score of prophylaxis which under some circumstances may prove an important consideration, it is of value to note that partial shielding is of immense benefit. Also, a whole host of substances exert some beneficial influence, but again they are nearly all impracticable outside the laboratory. One compound, S_2, β-amino-ethylisothiouronium, $Br \cdot HBr$ (AET) is promising and can be taken by mouth. (See Chapter 10.)

It would seem then that the overwhelming emphasis formerly placed on burn and blast casualties and reflected in this chapter in the first two editions of *Atomic Medicine* has become obsolete. In general our thinking and action, medically, must be decidedly reoriented toward increased emphasis on radiation effects. The most hopeful possibility that can be envisioned for the future is that substances will be discovered to counteract radiation damage and sickness which will be both effective and practicable for mass use. Secondly, it is hoped that every effort will be made to insure effective cooperation between all the agencies involved in these problems, notably the F. C. D. A., Department of Defense, Industry and the individual states and municipalities. Therein lies the best possibility that the "ifs" mentioned above will cease to be "ifs"; and that the hazards which presently menace large populations with extermination and still larger populations with serious injuries and genetic damage, will be notably diminished.

4.6 Nuclear Weapon Types

The main effects of various bomb types have already been tabulated and it is now pertinent to supply amplifying data and notes. Since this book is primarily designed for medical groups, the "big picture" and general principles will be presented rather than a wealth of physical data. Most doctors do not care if a 40 per cent burn case received 1 or 100 cal/cm.^{2} at 1 or 10 miles from ground zero. They do wish to know how many of what type case to expect; what the chances are of treating them effectively; what facilities and supplies are requisite and how well they can do under a given set of conditions. However, these in turn call for some knowledge of physical data and so the subject merits at least the brief consideration given here.

4.6.1 *Bomb Size in Relation to Effects.* (See chart.) The technology of modern nuclear weapons has developed to a point where almost any conceivable effect may be expected. The U. S. and her potential enemies have available devices which range in yield from about 1 Kt. (1000 tons TNT equivalent) to 20 mgt. or more. Weapons can be produced varying in yield by a factor well over 1000. Assuming that the cube root holds for intensity (blast and thermal) at any distance for a given yield, it can be seen that the damage radius of a large thermonuclear device may be well over 10 times that of a small nuclear bomb. Since the area is proportional to the square of the radius, variation in area effects a hundredfold or more can be expected.

Total destruction, regardless of shelter, pertains to crater formation. The *Effects of Nuclear Weapons*, Fig. 5.46, indicates that the crater diameter follows roughly the cube root, and the depth the fourth root. A 20 kt. bomb may be expected to produce a crater of 340 ft. diameter, and 53 ft. depth in dry soil; a 20 mgt. bomb, a crater of 3400 ft. diameter by 300 ft. depth.

Effects will also vary enormously depending on point of detonation which may be under water, underground, surface level, low air or high air.

An enemy may also use "clean" or "dirty" weapons, a dirty bomb being one designed or employed to produce a large amount of radioactive fallout as by surface detonation or constructural modifications, or inclusion of substances such as Cobalt in the tamper (Co^{60} which results from neutron fluxes is a potent gamma emitter of about 5 year half life).

For orientation purposes, as already indicated, the nominal 20 kt. bomb forms a convenient point from which to extrapolate. Thus some details of the Japanese bombings will be quoted subsequently from official sources.

A small atomic artillery-type weapon may produce serious blast and thermal effects over an area of less than 1 sq. mile and possibly with little appreciable radiation hazard. The largest thermonuclear weapons are capable of destroying over 700 sq. miles with blast and thermal effects, and in the event of a surface burst, contaminating approximately 7000 sq. miles to a potentially lethal level for unprotected people who do not have or seek shelter.

4.6.2 *Choice of Weapons.* In view of the variety and magnitude of possible effects from nuclear attacks, the types and modes of employment of nuclear weapons become of practical interest as we attempt to visualize medical responsibilities. Some of the main features which appear to affect choice are, in the author's opinion, as follows:

1. Fears of retaliation. These involve, of course, destructive and crippling effects on the enemy's own country. Assuming that an enemy accepts such a gamble, he will have to consider:

2. Essential target areas.

3. Effect desired on target areas; i.e., (a) ruinous blast damage to industrial areas and/or radioactive fallout over large areas to cause enormous casualties, cripple industry, contaminate farm land and handicap transportation, and recovery; (b) limited results in smaller areas.

4. Ability to strike these targets effectively.

5. Risks and costs in personnel and material.

Reasons that can be envisioned for use of small weapons include:

(a) Tactical employment in limited warfare.

(b) Destruction of small target areas such as important industrial plants, transportation centers and troop concentrations.

(c) Greater safety in employment near one's own territory and troops: less general contamination which might interfere with the enemy's own operations.

(d) Greater ease of delivery.

(e) Less expense and less bomb material.

Larger weapons might well involve considerations such as:

(a) Initial knock-out blow to all large cities, industrial areas and major military installations.

(b) Strategic demands related to unrestricted warfare.

(c) Use against a single area of transcendant importance. Such a target might, for instance, be provided by operations similar to those at the allied beachhead in Normandy in World War II. However, in the light of present-day circumstances, operations conducted in that manner would appear most unlikely if the defenders have recourse to nuclear weapons.

(d) An act of final desperation.

4.7 Blast Effects

Casualties may be caused both by direct and indirect effects. However, the direct effects are relatively unimportant in casualty production since humans can be subjected to shock wave pressures of up to 50 psi (pounds per square inch) or more and still survive. Indirect effects, however, provide one of the most serious factors in causing casualties. The range of blast damage varies from a few hundred yards to well over 10 miles radius for fairly serious effects. Air bursts augment these effects, which are, in turn, greatly decreased if weapons are exploded under ground or water. The effects in the latter case are very difficult to predict since they will vary greatly depending on depth.

Blast damage is also greatly affected by terrain and the nature and orientation of structures. Large land masses and well constructed buildings also reflect shock waves. Pressures of 3 to 4 times the value in free air may be produced when a shock wave is propagated into a space of decreasing volume. Reflected shock waves from the earth's surface also add their force to the primary shock wave in what is termed the "*Mach Effect*," producing a substantial increment.

Frame buildings may be expected to withstand a pressure of approximately 3 psi, brick structures 5 psi, and heavy reinforced concrete ones 10 psi, if they have no large areas of unsupported wall near perpendicular to the shock wave front. Windows and insecurely fastened or weak components of buildings generally fail at 1–2 psi and can cause very serious injury to the occupants even though the building is otherwise undamaged. Heavy underground shelters can withstand up to 100 psi.

Most casualties resulting from blast are due to collapsing buildings and flying debris. Many injuries may also be expected from shock waves heaving people against solid objects.

4.8 Thermal Effects

These are predominantly caused by infrared and visible components of the electromagnetic radiations from the nuclear explosion. They constitute the most far-reaching effects of an air burst and can cause temporary blindness up to distances of scores of miles. Retinal damage is possible at ranges where no other injuries result.

The largest thermonuclear devices can produce serious skin burns up to 20 miles or more from ground zero. Fires can be produced at levels which only slightly burn the skin and then, in turn, may cause conventional burns. A sufficient number of fires in a large area may cause a fire storm which can burn an entire city to the ground in the same manner that a large forest fire burns wooded areas. This holocaust phenomenon was observed in the German city of Frankfurt from incendiary bombing during World War II and produced a huge death and injury rate in addition to the devastation of the city. Hiroshima also suffered a fire storm.

Thermal effects are considerably affected by atmospheric conditions. Low clouds and fog can reduce intensity to a few percent of that on a clear day. They are also greatly reduced in the case of underwater and underground shots.

The chances of an individual caught in the open to escape serious flash burns from a nuclear burst is related in great measure to the amount of body covered by clothing and the clothing's color. White or light-colored clothes have a high thermal reflectance and people so clothed may receive little or no injury to the covered arms. (See fig. 3)

The author viewed a perfect example of color protection after a Bikini test "shot." At a distance of several miles from ground zero, large numbers of both black and white terns (tropical birds) were observed flying about. As ground zero was approached, however, the number of black terns decreased until they were no longer to be seen while white birds were still present in abundance.

4.9 Nuclear Radiation Effects

Ionizing radiation effects from nuclear weapons are conveniently divisible into two categories based on time sequence viz: (1) initial and (2) residual phases.

4.9.1 *Initial Phase.* This occupies the first minute after detonation and accounts for approximately one third of the ionizing radiations produced by the fission type bomb. (5 per cent total energy) It includes both the first flash of "*prompt* or *immediate* radiation" from the fission or fusion reactions themselves and subsequent radiation from the fireball. This rises out of range rapidly so that after a minute the initial phase is over.

Initial radiation is composed of gamma rays and neutrons as noted already. Most neutrons are absorbed by substances near the weapon and produce additional gamma rays by $(n \rightarrow \gamma)$ reaction.

Effects in this phase are of importance chiefly to individuals who are protected sufficiently from blast and thermal injuries to survive. People within ranges to be killed by initial radiation are also in the zones where they may well be killed twice before by blast and heat.

4.9.2 *Residual and Fallout Radiation.* This comprises radiation from fission products and from isotopes rendered radioactive by the neutron fluxes as noted in par. **3.18**. Induced radioactivity affects mostly areas in the zone of complete destruction and so is of little concern there. However, in a surface burst much surface material is sucked up by the thermal updraft of the fireball and in addition to being subjected to neutron fluxes is also contaminated with fission products.

The importance of this phenomenon is related to particle size. Fission products themselves are exceedingly finely divided as the result of being vaporized at the moment of explosion. Thus they are readily carried in the stratosphere and fall out very slowly and therefore with greatly diminished activity. Particles sucked up from the earth are much larger and produce prompt and dangerous fallout.

Dr. Libby of the AEC mentions three types.

1. Local fallout of larger particles occurring in the first few hours or days.
2. Diffuse fallout of small particles which remain in the lower layers of

the atmosphere subject to slow settling or being washed out by rain in the course of several weeks and in the same general latitude.

3. Long-term fallout (half or more of total) finely divided from the stratosphere, slowly leaks to earth at a rate of perhaps 10 per cent per year.

4.9.3 *Fallout Hazards.* As noted above the principle immediate hazard relates to the larger particles which reach the earth promptly beginning in a few hours. Considerable variation is possible and of course in the event of subsurface bursts, a deluge of radioactive spray and water or a heavy downpour of contaminated debris will take place almost at once. The most likely hazard however will be that from a surface burst and then the atmospheric conditions, prevailing winds as well as thermal drafts produced by the bomb become exceedingly important especially as regards precautions downwind, evacuation and rescue operations.

The delay is very important not only from the standpoint of such factors but as permitting people in general to seek shelter.

As regards radiation perils these derive from both external and internal dosage. Of these the external are by far the most important. The threat to life relates to gamma rays averaging about 0.7 mev, but beta burns of the skin may be a prominent feature (See Chap. 13).

Radioactive isotopes which gain access to the body pose remote possibilities related largely to Sr^{90} a 28 year beta emitting bone-seeker with potentialities for increasing the incidence of leukemia and bone tumors. This element readily finds its way into plants, livestock, and eventually humans (See Chap. 12).

4.10 Review of Japanese Experience (Hiroshima and Nagasaki)

To provide a point of reference, and remembering the present enormous variation in bomb power, it is useful to present data from the strategic bombing survey of these cities (General Report of the Atomic Bomb Casualty Commission). The bombs used were of approximately 20 kt. in TNT equivalence.

4.10.1 Material Damage

All wooden houses within a radius of 1 km. from the ground center were pulverized in an instant; wooden houses in the area between radii of 1–2 km. were devastated totally; those in 2–3 km. were destroyed severely; those in 3–4 km. were damaged moderately. A severe destruction of the houses means a damaged condition in which nobody can live further. The floor mats were even blown up. Moderate damage means the houses were scarcely available to live in, for all doors and windows are blown off. The roof tiles slip down and the roof leaks heavily. The damage to doors and windows is seen up to 6 km. Slipping down of roof tiles up to 8 km. Breaking of the window glasses extends to around 16 km.

All concrete buildings are more resistant, even in the central area, for only upper roofs are damaged. All furnishings were stirred up completely. Outside a radius of 1 km. from the ground center, there is almost no damage in a concrete building. All window glass was blown out to a distance of 2 km., and window frames toward the explosion center were also destroyed.

The fires caught all wood and concrete buildings in the area within a radius of 1 km. from the ground center. The wooden houses were burned for the most part, in the area between radii of 1–2 km., partly burned in the area of 2–3 km. Some of the well constructed concrete buildings partially escaped from the fires, even in the area within a radius of 1 km. from the ground center.

The official survey of the Hiroshima Prefecture revealed the total number of houses in the city of Hiroshima before the bombing to be 75,000; out of them 55,000 were totally burned (including totally destroyed and burned, and partially destroyed and totally burned), 12,600 partially burned, 6,820 totally destroyed, 3,750 partially destroyed. All damaged houses were counted and found to total 68,170, that is, over 90 per cent of all houses.

In the Nagasaki district, the destructive power seemed to be far greater. There are mountain chains running in a south-north direction, at both the east and west sides of the bomb center. On the bombed side of the mountains the damage was more severe, behind them it was slighter.

At Nagasaki, in the central area, all iron-framed, slate- or zinc-covered factory plants were destroyed; roofs and walls were broken off, iron frames were also deformed and some of them twisted like jelly. This may be due to an influence of the fires, too.

The Nagasaki Prefecture reported; "11,494 houses were totally burned, 2,652 houses totally destroyed (escaped from the fires), 5,441 houses partially destroyed."

A few additional excerpts from the U.S. Strategic Bombing Survey, *The Effects of Atomic Bombs on Hiroshima and Nagasaki*, will add to an understanding of the effectiveness of the atomic bomb in action and of a few of the problems which result from its use:

The electric power transmission and distribution system was wrecked; all utilities and transportation services were disrupted over varying lengths of time. The water reservoir, which was of reinforced concrete and earth-covered, was undamaged; it was nearly 2 miles from the blast center. However, 70,000 breaks of pipe connections in buildings and dwellings were caused by blast and fire effects. No subsurface pipes were crushed and no leaks resulted from blast as a direct cause, though several leaks in underground mains resulted from falling debris. Pressure in the city center dropped to zero because of the connection breaks and the damage to a 16 and a 14 inch water main where they crossed damaged bridges. Six sewer pumping stations were rendered inoperable by fire and blast within a radius of 1 mile. The remaining eight stations were only slightly damaged, but no effort was made to repair or operate them. Fire fighting and rescue units were equally stripped of men and equipment. Father Siemes reports that 30 hours elapsed before any organized rescue parties were observed. In

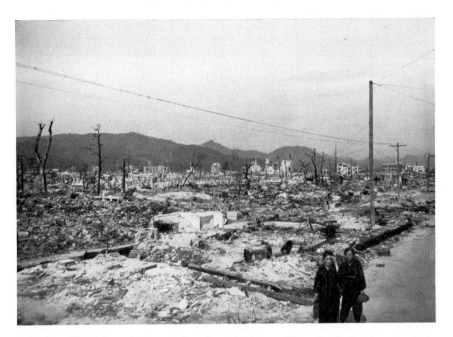

FIG. 9. Hiroshima three months after the blast. Note the lack of progress in clearing the ruins.

Hiroshima only 16 pieces of firefighting equipment were available for fighting the conflagration, three of them borrowed. Effective medical help had to be sent in from the outside, and arrived only after a considerable delay. Of more than 200 doctors in Hiroshima before the attack, over 90 per cent were casualties and only about 30 physicians were able to perform their normal duties a month after the raid. Out of 1,780 nurses, 1,654 were killed or injured. Though some stocks of supplies had been dispersed, many were destroyed. Only three out of 45 civilian hospitals could be used, and two large Army hospitals were rendered unusable. Those within 3,000 feet of ground zero were totally destroyed, and the mortality rate of the occupants was practically 100 per cent. Two large hospitals of reinforced concrete construction were located 4,900 feet from ground zero. The basic structures remained erect but there was such severe interior damage that neither was able to resume operation as a hospital for some time and the casualty rate was approximately 90 per cent, due primarily to falling plaster, flying glass, and fire. Hospitals and clinics beyond 7,000 feet, though they often remained standing, were badly damaged and contained many casualties from flying glass or other missiles.

4.10.2 *Casualties.* (See also Chapter 16.) One 20 kt weapon fired at a 2000 ft. altitude over a city of 100,000 or more would produce approximately 50,000 killed and 50,000 surviving casualties: 60 per cent mechanical; 60 per cent burns; and 15 per cent radiation.

This is an impressive number of casualties especially since some will

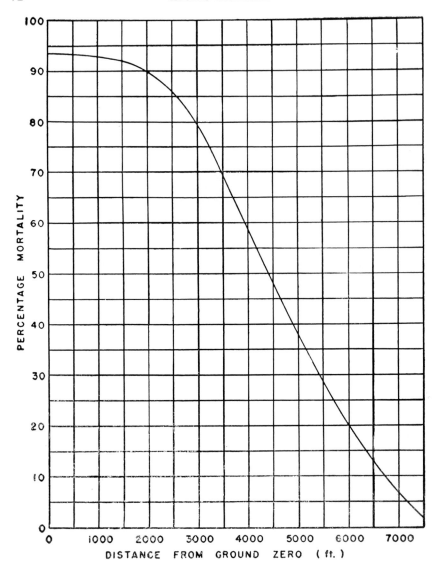

FIG. 10. Percentage mortality as function of distance from ground zero. (From: *Effects of Atomic Weapons.*)

surely be doctors and nurses, and a number of medical facilities will be destroyed.

The congressional report "Civil Defense for National Survival" (No. 2946, 84th Congress, 1956) quotes an estimate from "Operation Alert" of 1955 based on an all-out attack on 60 cities in the U. S. and its possessions with 61 bombs ranging from 5 to 20 mgt. power as follows:* 8¼ million dead, first day; 8 million dead within six weeks of which 3.9 million would be due to fallout; and 12 million injured survivors after the first day with about one-third recoveries.

The use of thermonuclear weapons in an all-out attack would cause millions of dead and injured; and fallout would add radiation victims far beyond the 15 per cent estimated on the basis of Japanese victims.

Reverting to our figures for a 20 kt. bomb, the medical personnel, supplies and facilities needed to treat 50,000 casualties provide huge statistics, as follows (estimate of Dr. Herman Pearse, Professor of Surgery, University of Rochester): 170,000 professional personnel; $10,000,000; and 8000 tons of medical supplies.

Obviously professional personnel in adequate numbers could not be procured in such an emergency for a period of days or weeks under conditions likely to exist, even assuming that other areas had not been hit.

The money factor would certainly be ignored until later, but the supplies would involve handicaps due to destruction of rail and motor transport and general confusion. Many places for emergency treatment in or near the victimized city would also be destroyed. It is encouraging to note that good headway has been made in stockpiling essential emergency supplies in locations readily available.

4.11 Panic

Almost as important as the initial casualty rate would be the panic situation. Many survivors would probably attempt to evacuate the city and a number would become liable to hunger, disease, exposure to the elements, and, still more important, to fallout radiation. This would also reduce the number of people available for first aid, rescue, and damage control.

Therefore from a medical standpoint we have an almost impossible situation. All casualties could not be treated, and treatment in general would be often rudimentary. The call is for much education, indoctrination, and provision for strict controls in all aspects. It must be remembered that, as already indicated, the new devices will surely magnify the figures given probably a hundredfold.

4.12 Solutions†

The three primary principles which must be learned and used are:
1. Survive.

* Contributed by Editor.
† No perfect solutions are possible and huge losses of personnel and vast destruction of property inevitable. Nevertheless much can be done and a hopeless attitude is not justified; but as already indicated resolute action is needed to replace the all too many "ifs" mentioned by Captain Haight, by actual accomplishments.

2. Help others.

3. Dig out and clean up.

These are, of course, simplifications which involve a host of difficult complexities. A wealth of pamphlets and brochures dealing with the many problems are available from the F. C. D. A. and Government Printing Office. Some basic consideration will be found in Chapter 16 and special problems relating to fallout are considered in Chapters 12 and 13.

In connection with the third stage, that of digging out and cleaning up, certain phases can be carried out even during high fallout intensities if proper radiological safety measures are used and teams relayed from sheltered areas. Monitors trained to know the significance of radiac instrument readings will have to be available and the instruments well maintained, properly calibrated and accessible. Such instruments will include those of counter type, i.e., scintillometers, geiger counters and ionization chamber types. Tables for interpreting readings are widely available including nomograms. The *Effects of Nuclear Weapons*, 1957 contain such.

In addition there is need for wide use of personnel dosimeters such as the pencil-type ion chamber, phosphate-glass variety and film badges.

Highly contaminated areas may be entered for limited periods if a few common sense principles are used. In general the less radiation one receives the better, and protective garments and partial shielding appear in order. Emergency doses of up to 100 r may be taken; and if necessity is compelling and some degree of ensuing radiation sickness justified, dosage may be extended even to 200 r.

Planning to reduce the degree of exposure is mandatory and accurate monitoring essential in order to keep such exposure to the least possible; also proper equipment.

4.13 Community Efforts

These are considered in Chapter 16 but a few general principles seem worthy of emphasis here as well.

1. Dispersal.

2. Indoctrination of the public in serious measure.

3. Adequate warning.

4. Underground shelters. The Swedish subway system provides a good example and in addition various expedients are mentioned by civilian defense authorities.

5. Early information regarding fallout zones.

6. Adequately stocked emergency supplies and medical facilities.

7. Adequate provision for administrative control in metropolitan areas especially those which embrace several municipalities and states.

8. Arrangements for mutual support and the housing of vast numbers of evacuees.

9. Evacuation plans.

REFERENCES

HERSEY, J. R. *Hiroshima.* New York: F-R. Publishing Corp., 1946.

Operation Crossroads. Joint Task Force. New York: William H. Wies and Co., 1947.

The Effects of Nuclear Weapons, U. S. Government Printing Office, Washington, D. C. 1957.

U. S. Strategic Bombing Survey, Med. Div. The Effects of Atomic Bombs on Health and Medical Services in Hiroshima and Nagasaki. Washington 25, D. C. U. S. Government Printing Office, 1947.

NOTE: See also references after Chapter 16.

5▸

The Ionizing Radiations

Charles F. Behrens, M.D.

5.1 Ionization Effects

From a medical standpoint the most unique feature of the atomic bomb and of radioactive isotopes is the emission of ionizing radiations. The term "ionizing" is applied because the profound effects produced on living tissue by these radiations are related largely to ionization. All the radiations concerned produce ionization directly or indirectly and practically all of the biologic changes they produce are related to this ionization. The differences in effects are related to degree of penetration, ionization power, dosage factors, tissues involved and secondary factors.

The ionization we are confronted with here is somewhat different from the ionization we are familiar with in solutions where chemical compounds are dissociated into atoms or radicals of opposite charge by electrolytic dissociation. Instead, this ionization affects the individual atoms themselves whereby we have ion pairs formed by dislodgment of electrons. Then instead of neutral atoms we have free electrons with negative charges and atoms with positive charges owing to loss of these electrons.

The energy required to jolt electrons from their orbits varies with elements and the orbital shells affected. Much more energy is required to eject electrons from the inner shells than from the outer, and generally the ion pairs formed in tissue result from ejection of outer electrons at an energy cost estimated to average 32.5 electron volts per ion pair. In terms of energy in its more familiar forms, ionization involves rather slight amounts so that an enormous quantity of radiation would be required to raise the temperature of tissue a fraction of a degree. Accordingly the serious biologic effects we have to deal with are certainly not related to crude energy transformation into heat but to physicochemical changes. These changes are of intense interest and form the object of much research. However, at this point, it is only appropriate to note a few salient facts. Chemical changes are apt to occur in molecules whenever one or more of their atoms is ionized. Such changes affect not only substances dissolved or in colloidal suspension in tissue fluid, that is, water, but in addition the water itself will show chemical changes. Hydrogen and oxygen molecules are often reduced to their atomic form and traces of hydrogen peroxide appear, as well as OH groups and possibly organic peroxides. A great variety of changes may take place due to ejection of electrons concerned in molecular binding. The result is the formation of scattered points of chemical interference with metabolic processes and control mechanisms. Abnormal compounds may also diffuse beyond the site of origin and spread harmful effects. At all events, careful studies reveal such things as depression of cell respiration, some degree of inactivation of enzymes and denaturization of proteins, and slowing down or interruption of mitosis with abnormalities in the chromatin patterns. It might be noted that quantitatively a "roentgen" or "r" unit of ionizing radiation produces 1.6×10^{12} ion pairs per gram of tissue. This seems a tremendous number, but the hosts of atoms and molecules are far more tremendous (see Avogadro's number, par. 2.27). Thus, it is calculated that only about 1 molecule in ten million is affected by a dose of 1000 r. However, damage to large important protein molecules concerned in vital functioning may obviously be fatal to cells, and in mammalian species secondary effects from lowered blood counts, hemorrhage, infection, and GI disturbances are such that fatal dosages mostly range below 800 r.

5.2 Derivation of Ionizing Radiations

The radiations we are most concerned with result largely from nuclear instability, and are emitted as the nuclei revert to more stable forms. We know that most of the elements we are familiar with are stable. However, the isotopes formed as the result of fission or by bombardment in cyclotrons are apt to contain too many neutrons or protons for stability. Thus, as noted before, since the ratio of neutrons to protons is normally lower in the lighter elements, fission products are apt to show an excess of neutrons. Again the bombardment of elements in the cyclotron by various particles, such as protons, deutrons and alpha particles, tends to produce nuclei out of balance. Finally, the sum total of nucleons may be too large as in the case of the heaviest elements; or the nucleus may be too highly energized, with the result that changes take place in the direction of greater stability and with the release of energy involving radioactivity. The type of change depends on the type of in-balance and the excess energy available.

5.2.1 *Alpha Emission and Beta Decay.* In the case of very heavy nuclei there is a pronounced tendency to throw off alpha particles made up of two neutrons and two protons. The nucleus left after one or more alpha emissions is apt to have too many neutrons (since lighter nuclei require relatively

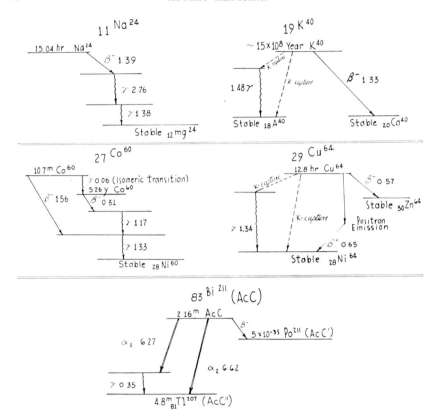

Fig. 1. Examples of radioactive decay. (Adapted from: Diagrams in Nuclear Data, NBS Circular 499.)

fewer) and accordingly the emission of alpha particles is apt to be followed by the conversion of a nuclear neutron to a proton. This takes place by emission of an electron to form the beta ray and so this process is known as beta decay. In the case of lighter nuclei, alpha emission is not favored and is seldom possible. The most frequent process is beta decay.

5.2.2 *Positron Emission.* Occasionally, however, protons are in excess and different mechanisms of stabilization result, bringing us the acquaintance of a new particle, the positron. It is the same order of mass as the electron but has a positive charge and is formed in the course of converting a proton to a neutron. However, another consideration, namely, that of supplying energy, is involved in the change, corresponding to the slightly greater mass of a neutron (1.00759 mass units for a proton versus 1.00898 for a neutron). 1.02 Mev of energy is required and thus the nucleus must be at a correspondingly high energy level or stage of excitation in order to emit a positron. $_7N^{13}$ affords an example: It emits positrons with a maximum kinetic energy of 1.2 mev to form $_6C^{13}$. This is associated with a mass loss equivalent to an energy release of 2.22 mev according to Einstein's equation $E = MC^2$. If we add the 1.20 mev of kinetic energy to the 1 mev needed to form a positron, we obtain 2.20 mev which is a very close approximation to the theoretical 2.22 value and verifies the correctness of the famous equation of energy mass equivalence. However, not every isotope with excess protons has sufficient energy to emit a positron and thus we find still another process at work which is less costly in energy, namely, electron capture.

5.2.3 *Electron Capture.* What happens here is that an electron is pulled into the nucleus from the K or occasionally the L orbit, whereupon the electron unites with a proton to form a neutron. An example is furnished by $_{23}V^{47}$ which by this process becomes $_{22}Ti^{47}$ The electron thus lost is immediately replaced by one from another shell and of course, as we will recollect, this must result in the release of a quantum of radiant energy or photon, in the form of K x-ray, characteristic of Ti^{47}.

The tale is still not told, for it turns out that after K capture some nuclei are still in an excited stage as for instance when Be^7 becomes Li^7 by K capture. The excess energy in this case is given off in the form of gamma rays.

5.2.4 *Gamma Emission.* As just noted γ rays provide a means of disposing of excess energy following emission of particulate rays. In addition the transition of certain nuclei to isomers is accomplished by gamma ray emission. This process is called *isomeric transition*.

5.2.5 *X-ray Emission and Internal Conversion.* It has just been noted that orbital electron capture results in x-ray formation. X-rays are also formed in another manner. In a number of instances nuclear gamma rays dislodge orbital electrons. This process is termed *internal conversion* and of course results in x-ray formation. The dislodged electrons are non-nuclear in origin and are usually designated "e" instead of β^-. (See par. 5.8.)

5.3 Annihilation Reaction and Summary of Reactions

One might well surmise that when a positron is thrust out into a universe where there are numerous electrons available and where there is, according to the physicist Dirac, a sort of state or sea of negative energy, there are apt to be fireworks, and such indeed is the case. In a tiny fraction of a second, the positron and an electron rush together, fuse and disappear in a radiation flash by what is called the annihilation reaction. The "flash" consists of two gamma photons of 0.5 mev energy each, and is of course really invisible to the human eye.

To recapitulate, unstable nuclei revert to stable forms by emission of alpha particles (helium nuclei), beta particles (electrons), positrons (positive electrons), gamma rays and capture of electrons. Sometimes several methods are seen in succession. Thus $_{27}Co^{55}$ changes to $_{26}Fe^{55}$ by positron emission, after which $_{26}Fe^{55}$ becomes $_{25}Mn^{55}$ by K capture.

5.4 Alpha Particle (symbol α, mass 4.0028, charge $+ 2$)

This is the nucleus of the helium atom and consists of two protons and two neutrons. It lacks orbital electrons. It was identified originally in connection with radium but is emitted by a number of elements, virtually all of them of heavy weight. The heavy nuclei, as pointed out already, have relatively less surface area in relation to disruptive electrical effects and are, in general, more apt to permit such a large aggregation to escape. The alpha particles thus produced have speeds varying from about one-twentieth to one-tenth of that of light, depending on energy levels. These levels and speeds are characteristic of the elements concerned, although certain of these elements show more than one level of alpha particle energy. It is to be noted also that the energy and range of alpha particles are related to the half life, the logarithm of the half life being proportional to the logarithm of energy of the emitted particles. Finally, owing to relatively heavy mass and double positive charge, alpha particles have tremendous ionizing power, but, because of their size, little penetration. In air, about 30,000 ion pairs are formed per centimeter, producing a dense columnar streak of ions with infrequent deflections. However, alpha particles can be stopped by a sheet of paper and in tissue their range is measured in microns. Thus they are not able to penetrate the horny layers of the skin and are of little consequence as an external radiation peril. However, when alpha-emitting substances are fixed in the body so as to permit internal action, even these short range effects can prove exceedingly harmful and often lethal.

5.5 Beta Particles (symbol β, or $_0e^{-1}$, mass 0.000549, charge -1)

These are actually electrons, identical with those from other sources such as evacuated tubes and heated filaments. They differ only as regards velocity, direction and focusing. Energies vary from practically zero to 3 mev or occasionally much higher. An important and perplexing difference from the alpha particles comes to light here. Instead of certain discrete and fixed levels of energy and hence velocity, we have a wide, continuous distribution of energy levels between zero and maximum so as to form a sort of continuous spectrum. This is out of keeping with other types of radioactive behavior and also involves discrepancies with the law of conservation of energy. Each beta decay in a given isotope state is associated with the same energy release but obviously, since there is a continuous energy spectrum extending downward from the maximum level (E max), the beta particles do not carry off all of it. Pauli provided a theoretical solution of the problem by postulating the existence of neutral particles, neutrinos, which carry away the unaccounted for energy.

Electrons show greater range and penetration but much less ionizing power (75 per 1 cm. air) than alpha particles. They are also readily deflected. Thus a 3 mev alpha particle shows a range of only 1.7 cm. in air, whereas beta particles of similar energy travel about 13 meters in air. An alpha particle is stopped by about 0.06 cm. of aluminum but an energetic beta particle may transverse 1 cm. Beta particles can thus penetrate and damage skin. Nevertheless, they are of most importance when they are given off within the body following the absorption of a beta-emitting substance.

5.6 Neutrino (Symbol, ν (nu), mass not over $\frac{1}{20}$ that of electrons, charge 0)

Neutrinos are emitted with both β^- and β^+ decay, the total energy being distributed between the beta particles and neutrinos on a statistical probability basis. The neutrino is exceedingly elusive due to slight mass and lack of charge. However, it has recently been detected by an elaborate scintillation technique. Dr. Reines and his associates at Los Alamos succeeded in detecting a neutrino induced reaction involving protons which resulted in formation of a neutron and positron.

5.7 Bragg Ionization Effect

The ionization figure of 75 per 1 cm. of air is an average since electrons, and other charged particles as well, show a curious variation in ionizing power, dependent upon velocity. Thus electrons at a velocity of 0.4 that of light, which corresponds to an energy level of 46,000 electron volts, produce 288 ion pairs per 1 cm. of air. As velocity and energy increase, the amount of ionization decreases so that at the velocity of 0.5 that of light (0.5 c) and energy of 79,000 ev, the ionization rate becomes 185 per centimeter. A velocity of 0.8 c and corresponding energy of 0.34 mev yield 72 ion pairs per centimeter and at a velocity of 0.95 c and energy of 1.125 mev we find the rate 51 per centimeter.

The reason for this effect is thought to lie in the assumption that high speed electrons pass atoms too quickly to exert as pronounced an effect as slower electrons. However, with extreme speeds and energies there is again a slight increase in ionization, apparently dependent upon alteration of the electron's electric field with extension of it at right angles to its path, the result being that there is a slightly wider sweep.

This variation in the amount of ionization is spoken of as the "Bragg Ionization Effect" and the degree as "specific ionization" or "K." Mathematically we find that "$Kt = 46/(v/c)$" where v = velocity of the electron and c the speed of light.

5.8 Non-Nuclear β Rays and Internal Conversion

The electrons which constitute beta rays are largely emitted by the nuclei but not exclusively. Those which produce the continuous spectrum and suggest the existence of the neutrino are definitely of nuclear origin, but there are other beta particles which show discrete energy levels and are associated with rays identical with K and L x-rays. Thus gamma rays from 83 Bi^{214}-(RaC) are similar to the K and L x-rays of bismuth. What happens is that nuclear gamma rays sometimes eject electrons from the K and L orbital shells, thus producing at once K and L x-rays and electrons of orbital origin at definite energy levels. The gamma ray may be completely absorbed in accomplishing this, the phenomenon being known as internal conversion.

5.8.1. *Auger Electrons.* Electrons ejected from inner orbits may in turn bounce electrons from outer orbits. These are known as *"Auger Electrons."*

5.9 Positron (symbol $_0e^+$, mass 0.000549 (same as electron), charge + 1)

These are seen in the case of certain unstable isotopes, cosmic rays and pair production (see par. 5.11.3). They naturally have some ionizing power from their own properties of mass and charge but, as we have already seen (par. 5.3), disappear almost immediately in annihilation reactions with resultant creation of gamma photons.

5.10 Ionizing Electromagnetic Radiations or Gamma and X-ray: General Note

Electromagnetic radiations comprise a huge field extending from beyond the longest radio waves of some hundreds of meters, length to hard gamma rays with a wave length of 10^{-12} cm. The term electromagnetic came to be applied when it was discovered that electric and magnetic fields are not only invariably associated with each other but that changes in them produce wave disturbances. The waves are of complex transverse type and show electric and magnetic components oscillating at right angles to the direction of propagation. This type of wave appears characteristic of the whole group, including, of course, visible light, infra-red, ultraviolet, x-rays and gamma rays. Differences in behavior are related to the frequencies, wave length and energy differences as well as to mass considerations. We are familiar with the fact that radiowaves arise from large oscillating electromagnetic fields and so it should not surprise us that similar oscillating fields should arise on a minute scale from the vibrations or oscillations in the orbital zones of atoms, or affecting nuclear particles, since in these instances, too, electromagnetic fields are involved. Both gamma and x-rays, as already noted, belong to this family of radiations. Most x-rays in general clinical use are of longer wave length and lower frequency than gamma rays but the ranges overlap so that there are soft gamma rays of x-ray type and hard x-rays in the gamma zone. There are no essential differences in fundamental behavior or effects and it is necessary in each instance to know various quantitative and qualitative data in order to deal effectively and safely with this type of radiation, whether "x" or gamma.

5.11 Gamma Rays (symbol γ; mass 0.00107 at 1 mev; charge 0)

It will be noted that mass is ascribed to gamma rays in the subject heading. This is a natural consequence of the particulate behavior these radiations show in certain phenomena. It is also a natural consequence of the energy-mass relationship inasmuch as we have seen that there must be some mass corresponding to the presence of energy levels. Thus not only is it to be expected that radiant energy should show mass effects, but that the greater the energy, the greater the mass. This has been verified experimentally, but it must be pointed out that there are certain differences between the particulate behavior of electromagnetic quanta of energy or photons and that of "true" particles such as electrons, protons and the like.

5.11.1 *Mass-Velocity Equation.* The energy of electrons increases with velocity in a manner we are quite familiar with from everyday experience with macroscopic objects and conventional physics. The new conceptions of physics, however, cause us to look for increased mass with increased energy and such we find to be the case, although this is undetectable within the velocity ranges pertaining to familiar visible objects. Mathematically the relationship is expressed by the equation:

$$M = M_0/\sqrt{1 - (v/c)^2}$$

where M = the mass of the object in motion, M_0 the resting mass of the object, v the velocity of the object, and c the speed of light.

The relationship to the mass of electrons to velocity is shown in the following table:

Electron Mass Changes with Velocity

Velocity Relative to that of light v/c	Electrons Mass relative to mass in resting state M/M_0
0.0	1.000
0.1	1.00005
0.5	1.159
0.9	2.3
0.999	22.3

It is notable here that increase in mass is extremely slight even at a velocity one-tenth that of light, or nearly 20,000 miles per second, and does not become especially marked until velocity approaches that of light. We can, therefore, readily see why verification of the mass increase with velocity is possible only with particles which can be given fantastic speeds.

5.11.2 *Frequency-Mass Equation.* In the case of infra-red, visible light, x- and gamma rays, velocity is the same for all in so-called empty space, even though the energy levels are vastly different. In this case the increase of energy involves increased frequency and shorter wave length, associated with which there are more waves per centimeter and more energy in each wave packet (or quantum or photon). Mathematically a different equation becomes necessary to express the mass energy relationship and so we find the following:

$$M = h\nu/c^2$$

where M is the mass of the photon, h Planck's constant, ν (nu) the frequency and c the speed of light.

The following table affords some interesting figures for comparisons:

WAVE LENGTH	ENERGY	MASS REL TO THAT OF AN ELECTRON
10,000 A (infra-red)	1.2 ev	2.4×10^{-6}
0.1 A (x-ray)	0.12 mev	0.24
0.01 A (gamma ray)	1.2 mev	2.4

We can readily see from these figures why infra-red rays can exert no photoelectric or ionizing effects since it requires more than 1.2 ev to eject even the loosly attached electrons of the elements used in photoelectric cells and, as we have seen, about 32.5 ev to form ion pairs on tissue. It might be noted here that what infra-red, visible light and ultraviolet accomplish in tissue is related to some species of excitation of electronic orbits to higher energy levels rather than to ionization. We can see also why x- and gamma rays are so potent in dislodging electrons and producing ionization.

It was once thought that gamma rays were invariably associated with beta rays, but we know now that such is not the case. However, they are chiefly of nuclear origin and their emission frequently does take care of odd bits of energy left over after the emission of electrons or positrons. Gamma rays, as we have seen, may also produce K and L x-rays and beta particles. They also vary considerably and their wave lengths are characteristic of the elements emitting them. Some of the longest gamma waves are emitted by radioactinium, 3.9 angström units. Some of the shortest are derived from $_{83}Bi^{212}$ (ThC) and $_{83}Bi^{214}$ (RaC), the wave lengths being about 0.0466 angström units (an angström unit [Å] is 10^{-8} cm.).

The penetrating ability of gamma rays is extremely great and, other factors being equal, is inversely proportional to the density of the substance concerned. Range is also great and so it is small wonder that these rays are of greatest importance as an external hazard even though the ionizing power is extremely feeble, averaging only 1.5 ion pairs per centimeter in air. Their penetrating power, range and abundance make them extremely effective biologically and, as we have seen, they were the cause of many deaths in the Japanese bombings. It is certain too that many Japanese victims who died early from burns and various traumatic effects would have succumbed to radiation illness due to gamma rays had they survived their other injuries.

Since gamma rays have no charge, ionization in tissues is largely secondary. Some atoms of course have electrons knocked out by gamma rays acting as particles, and are thus ionized directly. However, the dislodged electrons usually have considerable energy and produce by far the most of the ion pairs resulting from this radiation.

5.11.3 *Absorption of Gamma Rays.* The absorption of gamma and x-ray is related to density and thickness of material involved and is characteristic for each material or substance. The proportionality constant is spoken of as the linear coefficient of absorption and gives the relative loss of intensity per cm. of path. Its relation to the half value layer (or the thickness of a given material required to reduce the intensity of incident radiation by half) can be expressed by:

$$\mu = \frac{0.693}{X_{\frac{1}{2}}}$$

where $X_{\frac{1}{2}}$ represents the half value layer and μ the coefficient. Absorption takes place in three ways depending upon the energy levels of the radiation. Low energy gamma and x-ray photons are absorbed largely by the *photoelectric effect.* The photon gives up all its energy to the electron, only a small part, usually 30 to 50 electron volts, being spent in dislodging the electron, the rest going into kinetic energy. The photon disappears. The energy relations are stated in Einstein's photoelectron equation and involves Planck's constant. It simply states in mathematical terms, for purposes of calculation, the sensible proposition that the energy of the incident photo must equal the energy needed to dislodge an electron, plus the kinetic energy imparted to it. Thus remembering (1) that the energy of the photon is denoted by $h\nu$ where h is Planck's constant and ν the frequency, (2) that kinetic energy equals one-half the mass (m) times velocity (v^2), and (3) representing the energy required for dislodgment of the electron ϕ, we arrive at the equation $h\nu = \phi + \frac{1}{2} mv^2$. Reverse application of the photoelectric effect is also possible so that bombarding electrons can give us photons of frequency and hence wave length, in accordance with this equation.

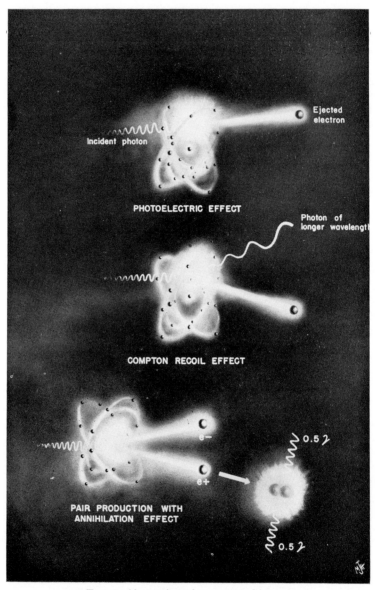

FIG. 2. Absorption of gamma and x-rays

The second mode of absorption is by what is called, in honor of the discoverer of this phenomenon, the *"Compton recoil"* effect, and concerns higher energy rays. In this case, the photon again acts like a miniature billiard ball but fails to give up all its energy and glances off at reduced energy, which means longer wave length and lower frequency. The electron struck by it is dislodged and propelled from the parent atom just as is the photoelectron.

The third method of absorption is by *"pair production"* and involves photons in the high energy ranges beyond 1.02 mev.* This process is of unusual interest as it involves readily apparent transmutations of energy to matter. Certain of the photons which pass very close to the nucleus disappear and in their place electron pairs of opposite charge, i.e, an electron and positron appear. The positron promptly disappears in an annihilation reaction with creation of two gamma quanta of 0.5 mev each, as previously noted (fig. 26; see also par. 14.10).

5.12 X-rays

In the matter of radioactivity, x-rays are overshadowed in importance by gamma rays, but nevertheless they play some part. It has already been noted that they are similar to gamma rays except that, in general, they usually have lower frequencies and longer wave lengths than gamma rays. We have also seen that K and L x-rays are often produced secondarily by gamma rays. There is still another source of x-rays and that is in connection with the atomic bomb. It was discovered some time ago that the frequency of light and accordingly the wave length and color are related to the temperature of the emitting body; indeed, we know this from practical experience. A poker heated in a furnace is noted to have a dull red glow at relatively low temperatures and becomes "white hot" at high temperatures, the dull red glow being of longer wave length than the bright white glow. The relationship is expressed mathematically in what is known as *Wien's displacement law*; the equation for which is $\lambda_m T = K$ where λ_m = maximum wave length, T the absolute temperature and K a constant (0.20 cm. degrees).

When we apply this law to radiation from the sun, we find that, corresponding to the maximum intensity of its visible light being in the green zone, we have a surface temperature of about 6000°C.

In an atomic bomb, the fire ball shows an initial temperature estimated at several million degrees. Applying the equation to this, we find that the resultant radiation should be in the x-ray zone. Thus before the surface T of the fire ball diminishes there are probably a few instants during which

---

* A small amount of high energy X or Y radiation may also be absorbed by nuclei. See 2.30.1

x-rays are emitted purely because of the temperature effect. However the law may not hold true at such temperatures and all initial radiation is attributed to the gamma rays and neutrons.

In the case of x-ray apparatus it is worth noting in passing that in addition to K and L x-rays produced by the incident electrons knocking K and L orbital electrons out of their orbits, x-rays of other frequency may be produced in x-ray apparatus in accordance with the photoelectric equation. This equation, you will remember, is as follows: $h\nu = \phi + \frac{1}{2} mv^2$, where h is Planck's constant, ν the frequency of the radiation, ϕ the energy needed to dislodge the electron and $\frac{1}{2} mv^2$ the kinetic energy of the dislodged electron. In our first mention of this it was indicated that the kinetic energy of an expelled electron is related to the energy of the incoming radiation, and that the equation also applied in reverse. In accordance with this we have: $\nu = (\phi + \frac{1}{2} mv^2)/h$. Thus we can see that the greater the velocity of a bombarding electron, the higher will be the frequency, energy and penetrating power of the resultant x-ray, and hence the shorter the wave length. In practice the figure for $\frac{1}{2} mv^2$ of the electron is so great that ϕ can be disregarded and dropped from the equation. It is apparent from all this why x-ray apparatus has advanced along the line of increasing voltage so as to provide electrons of greater and greater speed. The result is that x-rays can now be produced for therapeutic, industrial and scientific use at frequencies equal to and even surpassing most gamma rays.

5.12.1 *Absorption of X-rays.* Very soft x-rays, such as 10–15 kv x-rays are almost completely absorbed by the photoelectric effect. At the 100 kv level, absorption by the Compton effect accounts for about one-fourth of the energy, and at 200 kv greatly predominates. After 1 mev is passed, pair production begins and increases with the energy of the radiation and also in proportion to the square of the atomic number of the absorbing elements. At about 50 mev it becomes the principal mode of absorption in tissue. See also 5.11.3

5.13 Neutrons (symbol $_0n^1$, mass 1.00898, charge zero)

Since neutrons have no charge, one might at first thought suspect them to be relatively innocuous. However, the sad fact is that, owing to several factors, they are relatively extremely dangerous biologically. Because of their mass, which is about that of a proton or hydrogen nucleus, they have great kinetic energy and, owing to lack of charge, penetrate readily and so reach the nuclei, where they cause ejection of protons from hydrogenous material, and result in the formation of various unstable isotopes. Hydrogen, which is very abundant in living matter, tends to have its nuclei shot out by fast neutrons to form protons; moreover it captures slow neutrons to form deuterium, in which process gamma rays are emitted. Again, in the case of sodium, there is often the reaction: $_{11}Na^{23} + _0n^1 = _{11}Na^{24}$. This form of sodium is radioactive, emitting beta particles. Nitrogen 14 may become C^{14} with emission of a fast proton when struck by neutrons. In similar manner, radioactive isotopes of phosphorus, sulfur, calcium and other elements may be formed. The result of this sort of thing is that the effect of neutrons in tissue is greater than comparative ionization figures, as measured in instruments, would indicate. Thus biologic effectiveness is rated at from two to ten times as great as that of gamma rays, or even more, depending on the tissue concerned. The average increase is usually placed as about a five times factor at the present time and this figure appears likely to be revised upward.

Neutrons are thrown off in large numbers at the time of an atomic explosion, but this will have little bearing on casualty production because their limited range does not extend beyond the zone of lethal effects from other causes. However, neutrons are of great concern in certain cyclotron operations, about uranium piles and in the course of various laboratory studies.

Finally, it is to be noted that free neutrons are unstable and if they escape capture will undergo beta decay. Experiments have indicated a half life of between 9 and 30 minutes with a probable half life of 20 minutes.

5.14 Protons (symbol p_1 or H^1, mass 1.00759, charge $+ 1$)

These are identical with hydrogen nuclei and, although not of biologic importance in atomic bomb explosions, natural radioactive decay or pile operation, they are encountered in the course of scientific work and are produced secondarily in tissue by neutrons. They are potent ionizers by reason of mass and charge and will penetrate well if of high energy. In fact, it is hoped that they may someday have therapeutic applications since there is a marked gain in ionizing power as the speed of the particle lessens, in accordance with the Bragg effect described in the case of electrons. Some figures are interesting here: Penetration to a depth of 10 cm. is possible with an energy of 115 mev. During the last centimeter of travel, ionization is six times that at the surface, and in the last half centimeter, 16 times that value.

It will be noted that the proton has a trifle less mass than the neutron. This correlates with the fact that 1 mev energy must be supplied to make possible the change of a proton to a neutron by emission of a positron and that neutrons by themselves are unstable.

5.14.1 *Antiproton or Negative Proton.* Recent studies reported by the AEC announce discovery of particles of proton mass but negative charge.

They were identified in stacked photographic plates subjected to bevatron radiation by "stars" indicating energy releases of such magnitude as to bespeak annihilation reactions from combination of antiprotons with protons or neutrons.

5.15 Meson or Mesotron (several different masses, charge plus, minus or neutral)

These particles were first postulated by Yukawa in 1935 as being necessary to account for the "exchange forces" involved in holding nucleons together, and later actually identified in connection with cosmic rays. They have also been produced in high energy accelerators. Energies up to Bev levels are used with various particles and target materials. The mesons that result are mostly "*pi*" (π) *mesons or pions*. These are the ones thought to be concerned with the exchange forces that aid in holding nuclei together. Thus they are occasionally spoken of as cosmic glue or cement. Doubtless they serve as such but actually they afford no such static picture. Apparently they oscillate in and out of the nucleons with extremely high frequencies producing a sort of cloud effect and giving nuclei fuzzy borders.

Free pions may show $+$, $-$ or 0 charge; mass 273.5 m_e (mass of electron) (264 for π°); half life 2.5×10^{-8} seconds ($1^{\circ-14}$ seconds for π°). Neutral pions vanish in production of gamma rays. Charged pions decay to *mu* (μ) *mesons* and neutrinos. Mu mesons may be $+$ or $-$; mass 207 m_e; half life 2.15×10^{-6} seconds. Decay is into electrons and neutrinos.

Positive pions are mostly repelled by nuclei and decay. Negative pions and mu mesons readily drop into atomic orbits replacing electrons briefly. Negative pions are captured by nuclei almost at once with shattering effects. They confer about 195 mev of energy and the nuclei explode forming "*stars*" in photo emulsions. Negative mu mesons are not captured by nuclei so quickly and are not as disruptive although they add 107 mev "energy." They usually produce neutron emission instead of "star" formation. It is of interest to note that the orbits of mesons replacing electrons must be very small due to mass effect; and in the case of heavy elements such as Pb, the K orbit actually falls within the nuclear borders.

Negative mu mesons by reason of their relatively long half life and lessened rate of nuclear capture are very penetrating. In fact they constitute the "hard" component of cosmic rays at sea level.

Tau and kappa mesons with masses of about 975 and 1000 m_e respectively have been identified; also particles of about 2200 m_e termed " V " *particles* because of the inverted " V " tracks they cause in cloud chambers.

These heavy particles are far from being well understood. Half lives are very brief and decay about as follows: τ, 3π; K, $\mu+$ $2\gamma(?)$; V particles, nucleons and +pions.

5.15.1 *Notes on Cosmic Rays.* The cosmic rays are a complex of radiations derived largely from the incidence of extremely high energy protons along with some heavier particles with atomic numbers up to 40. As these particles strike the atmospheric atoms, various reactions with production of mesons occur, and the mesons themselves decay with production of electrons, positrons, gamma rays, secondary pair production, and so-called showers or avalanches of lower energy electrons. The origin of the primary particles is not established, although it is speculated that pulsing magnetic fields associated with sun spots might energize the particles. The energies involved appear to average about 6 billion electron volts and probably extend as high as 10^{-17} ev. As might be expected, cosmic radiation becomes more intense at higher altitudes, but biological effects would not be important except beyond 70,000 ft. where most of the radiation would be of the primary type and contain more heavy nuclei.

The hard components of cosmic rays are mainly highly energetic μ mesons of enormous penetrating power. The soft components (absorbable by 10 cm. Pb) are largely electrons and positrons.

5.15.2 *Fusion and Mesons.* Low temperature fusion reactions have been produced by the bombardment of liquefied hydrogen by negative mu mesons. Mesonic deuterium atoms result which unite with ordinary hydrogen atoms to form He^3. The meson is promptly ejected with 5.4 mev energy. (U. of Cal. Rad. Lab. as reported in the "Scientific American," Vol. 196: 2; 59–60, Feb. 1957).

5.16 Secondary Radiations

A few secondary radiations mentioned in the literature are listed below for reference.

1. Delta Rays: A number of secondary electrons produced by ionization have sufficient energy imparted to them to produce ionization themselves. Thus an electron ionization track will often show little offshoots where such has taken place. The subsidiary ionizing electrons which form these tracks constitute the delta rays.

2. Bremsstrahlung Radiation: The absorption of electrons involves a deceleration or "braking" effect. This becomes rapid toward the end of the course and the energy is converted into γ rays. These γ rays are often spoken of as Bremsstrahlung—German for "braking radiation." It might be noted that the usual production of x-rays other than from K or L capture, is also a bremsstrahlung effect.

Finally, in recapitulation the principal radiations may be tabulated as follows:

TABLE OF IONIZING RADIATIONS AND PARTICLES

NAME	SYMBOL	MASS	CHARGE	HALF LIFE	REMARKS
Alpha	α	4.0028	2 Pos.	Stable	Helium nuclei
Electrons Beta*	β, β^- or e, e^-	0.000549	1 Neg.	Stable	Form beta and cathode rays
Positron	β^+ or e^+	0.000549	1 Pos.	Annihilation	Positive electron
Gamma and x-ray	γ or x	No rest mass	0	Stable	High frequency photons
Proton	p or $_1H^1$	1.00759	1 Pos.	Stable	Hydrogen nucleus
Antiproton	p^-	1.00759	1 Neg.	Annihilation	Negative proton
Neutron	n or $_0n^1$	1.00898	0	10 min.	Decay to p by β^- emission
Deuteron	d or $_1H^2$	2.01419	1 Pos.	Stable	Heavy hydrogen nucleus
Neutrino	ν (nu)	½0 mass of electrons	0	Stable	Associated with β and meson decay
Mesons†	π (pi)	264 and 273.5	+, − or 0	2.5×10^{-8} and 10^{-14} sec.	Exchange force mesons
	μ (mu)	207	+ or −	2.5×10^{-6} sec.	Hard component, cosmic rays (μ^-)
	τ (tau)	975	+ or −	10^{-9} sec.	—
	κ (kappa)	1000	+	10^{-10} sec.	—
"V" Particles	V	2200	+, − or 0	3×10^{-10} sec.	—

* See Electron and Positron.
† Star forming mesons sometimes designated "sigma (σ)"; certain other mesons occasionally designated "rho (ρ)."

REFERENCES

NOTE: See references after Chapters 2 and 3.

6 ▶

Detection and Measurement of Radiation

F. W. Chambers, Jr. B.S., M.S. and Maynard Eicher, A.B.

(Revised by F. W. Chambers)

6.1 Introduction

The effects of radiation are more difficult of precise evaluation in the case of living organisms than in other material. There is a variation in response to radiation between species, individuals of the species and components of the individual, as well as delay in observable response. This has made it necessary to measure the radiation by physical means, standardize the measurements and then evaluate the biologic effects on the basis of these standard values. The technics and units for the standardization of ionizing radiations have been established over a period of years. However, many complexities are involved and special training is requisite to deal adequately with them. The purpose of this discussion, therefore, is to acquaint the doctor with the fundamental principles of detection and measurement of ionizing radiation, and the main types of instruments, rather than to give a complete and detailed presentation; this latter would require a volume in itself.

6.2 Methods of Detection and Measurement

Radiation may be detected and measured in numerous ways. Among them are the activation of photographic emulsions, scintillations produced in various materials, coloring of crystals, depositions of colloids, biological effects, ionization in gases and vapors including cloud chamber effects and production of heat (calorimetry). At the present time the ionization and scintillation effects are most extensively used. When radiation in the form of charged particles (alpha particles, beta particles, protons) or photons (x-rays or gamma rays) interact with matter, ionization (ion pairs) is produced in which positively and negatively charged particles or ions are formed. The specific ionization or ionization per unit length of path of the radiation is a function of the energy of the particle or photon, the mass or charge of the particle and the matter with which the radiation interacts. The specific ionization is greatest near the end of the path of the various radiations. The ionization or production of ion pairs under the proper conditions may manifest itself either as an electric current or electrostatic charge. The measurement of this current or charge with proper technics permits the quantitative or qualitative measurement of the radiation. Numerous and complicated factors are involved in making the measurements, and these are dependent in each individual case on the materials and methods of measurement. A discussion of these factors (except in specific cases) is beyond the scope of this chapter. The basic instruments, at present, for the measurement and detection of radiation in medical applications, are the ionization chamber, the Geiger-Muller counter and the scintillation detector. The first two have certain basic similarities but their operation and use are so different that after a brief discussion of general principles applicable to both instruments, they will be taken up individually.

6.3 Geiger-Müller Counter and Ionization Instruments: Basic Principles

Both have a chamber (Figs. 1A and 1B) which contains a gas (air, argon, etc.) and electrodes for collecting the ion pairs produced. The ion pairs which are produced when radiation passes through the gas in the chamber would recombine and form neutral atoms again if some method were not used to collect them promptly. The application of a potential voltage supply (such as a battery) along with a detection device across the electrodes of the chamber answers this purpose as it will permit the collection of the positively and negatively charged ions or particles. Positively charged ions or particles will be attracted to the negative electrode, and the negatively charged ions or particles will be attracted to the positive electrode. If increasing values of voltage are applied to the electrodes while the intensity of the radiation and other factors, such as geometry, are kept constant, the ionization current will increase. This is due to the fact that more and more ion pairs are being collected before they are able to recombine. There is a

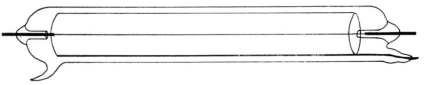

Fig. 1A Geiger-Müller tube

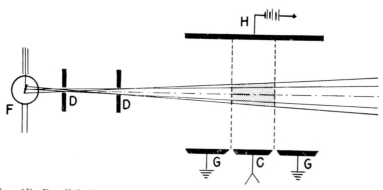

Fig. 1B. Parallel plate type ionization chamber. F, x-ray tube; D-D, limiting diaphragms; H, high voltage supply to electrode; G, ground potential; C, collecting electrode to electroscope.

voltage above which (within limits) there is no significant increase of current with increase in voltage. This provides what is called the saturation current, which is reached when practically all of the ion pairs that are formed by the ionizing radiation are being collected. This voltage is also the minimum that may be used with ionization chamber instruments. It is, however, better to work at a voltage slightly above this minimum, since in this way a fluctuating voltage supply will not affect the saturation current which, of course, forms the basis for measurement either by means of amplification or by proportional discharge of an electroscopic system.

When an increase in voltage beyond the saturation current level is carried to a sufficient degree, a point will be reached at which the charged particles (ion pairs) will begin to be accelerated to such an extent that they in turn will act as ionizing agents and form still more ions in addition to those from the primary radiation and its secondary effects. This effect is called ionization by collision. The net result is that when proper adjustments are made a single ionizing particle or photon entering the chamber can produce an avalanche of ions.* This is the basis of Geiger-Müller tube operation. The voltage is usually 1000 to 2000 volts, the cathode forming a cylinder within which the anode, in the form of a wire, is mounted.

Finally, if the voltage is increased enough, a continuous gaseous discharge can take place. The geometry of the ionizing volume and the gas used in it are important factors in the response discussed above. It might be noted in this respect, that to keep the "avalanche" effect limited to a sufficiently brief time, Geiger tubes usually have a small amount of organic hydrocarbon vapor added to the gas to produce a quenching effect. A frequent mixture is 10 per cent alcohol vapor and 90 per cent argon at

* Sometimes termed "Townsend Effect or Avalanche".

10 cm. Hg pressure. The alcohol tends to cling to the cathode cylinder, thus cutting off what would otherwise be a heavy flow of electrons from this source.

The point at which the acceleration of the particles first begins to produce cascading fluxes of ions is the point at which we start to consider Geiger-Müller type operation in the proportional zone. When the gas pressure is reduced and the voltage is increased, a tube of the Geiger-Müller type construction will act as a proportional counter in which, for each ionization due to the radiation, there will be produced a certain proportional amount of additional ions by collision. By using this proportional counter region one is able to detect and measure smaller amounts of ionizing radiation with less sensitive measuring instruments.

The number of additional ions produced by collision in the proportional region also increases with applied voltage and at this point it becomes necessary to shift our attention from the formation of ion pairs by the initial radiation to pulses of ionized particles due to the added ionization by collision. In the proportional counting region, the size of the pulse is proportional to the voltage applied "and to the number of initial ionizing events; and thus to the amount of energy expended by an ionizing particle within the sensitive volume of the counter." However, as the voltage is increased still higher, the size of the pulse becomes substantially constant though it is still a function of the voltage on the counter, the gas in the counter, and the geometry of the counter. This region is called the plateau of the Geiger-Müller tube. Here the amount of ionization due to the initial radiation no longer controls the pulse, since a single particle can set off the complete momentary discharge of the tube. This amplification occurs in the customary operating zone of Geiger-Müller apparatus and permits the measurement of extremely small amounts of radiation owing to the fact that it is possible to detect individual ionizing particles. The drawback is that there is no discrimination between energy levels of the incident particles or photons. Finally, if the voltage is increased above this point, there will be a continuous discharge in the tube, which is valueless and may damage the equipment.

We can now see why the Geiger tube gives us counts per minute rather than the original and proportional ionization effect. Figure 13 shows the effect of voltage on the output of the Geiger-Müller tube. The Geiger-Müller tube should be operated toward the low side of the plateau region. The ionization chamber or the Geiger-Müller counter can be designed to detect or measure any type of ionizing radiation, but each has its proper place. For example, the ionization chamber is generally used to measure x- or gamma rays, while the Geiger-Müller counter is used to measure particle radiation from radioactive isotopes. In some cases their fields of use overlap. This occurs in the case of the beta-gamma-emitting isotopes, such as iodine[131]. The ionization chamber can be used to advantage in determining the activity of the iodine to be administered, while the Geiger-Müller counter can be used to advantage in detecting and measuring the very small quantities of radiation in biopsies or excreta. One important point should be brought up here. Both instruments should be calibrated against a standard before they are used.

6.4 Photographic Detection*

Photographic emulsions are used considerably in the medical application of isotopes. They are used in protection measurements and in making radioautographs. Radioactive isotopes produce the same effect on photographic emulsions as do x-rays. A film similar to a dental film is worn by personnel working with radioactive material. This film is partially covered with a material like lead or cadmium, so that it is possible to evaluate, to a certain extent, the relative quantity of beta and gamma radiation the individual received. After a period of time (usually a week) the film is developed, and the darkening effect is measured with a photodensitometer. Readings of the meter are converted by means of beta and gamma calibration curves into REP's in the case of the beta rays and "r" in the case of gamma or x-rays. There is considerable room for improvement in photodosimetry; nevertheless it is a most valuable means of integrating the dose received by individuals working with radiation.

Radioautographs are used to determine the distribution of radioactive materials in a section of bone or tissue, etc. For example, a section of tissue containing radioactive material is placed on a film or slide that has a photographic emulsion on it. The slide is exposed for a certain length of time, depending on the amount of radioactivity in the tissue, and then it is developed. The slide is then stained and it is possible to see the distribution of the radioactive material in the tissue. The visualization of the distribution of the radioactive isotope within a single cell is not yet possible because of the poor resolution due to the graininess of the emulsion and to the diffusion of the radiation. Improvement of technics and materials may eventually make this possible.

6.5 Scintillation Counters

Rutherford and his co-workers developed a technic in the early stages of nuclear research that made use of the scintillations produced by the excitation of fluorescent and phosphorescent screens when they were bombarded by alpha particles. This technic has been recently revived with the advent

* See also par. **15.9.4.**

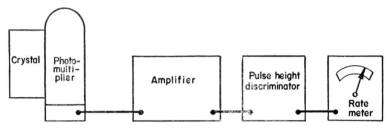

F$_{IG}$. 2. Scintillation counter

of the photomultiplier tube and large transparent crystals which convert the energy of photons or particles into light (Fig. 2).

The photomultiplier tubes generally used at the present time employ 10 or 11 stages with over-all multiplications of greater than 10^6. They are normally operated at total acceleration voltages between 800 and 1200 volts. The most generally used scintillator is thallium activated sodium iodide. This type of detector is much more efficient for gamma counting than the Geiger-Müller tube and can be used with scaling equipment.

Constantly improving photomultiplier designs together with a broader application of scintillator types and physical forms have greatly expanded their field of usefulness. Crystals have been fashioned which wrap around the radioactive samples and thus improve collection efficiency. Such crystals are termed "well counters."

6.6 Wilson Cloud Chamber

Although the cloud chamber (Fig. 3) would be used in very few laboratories devoted to the medical applications of radiation, the instrument has played such an important role in the understanding of nuclear processes that it would be well to describe it briefly.

The cloud chamber permits the visualization of the ionization along the path of a photon or particle as it traverses the chamber. The principle upon which it works is the condensation of water or other vapor on each ion within its sensitive volume by means of the expansion of the vapor saturated gas. The droplets formed scatter light and, therefore, may be observed or photographed.

A simple diagram of this structure of the chamber is shown in Fig. 3. The operational procedure is to compress the gas, then open a valve that permits rapid expansion of the gas, which forms the droplets. A sufficiently bright light to observe or photograph the droplets is turned on at the proper time. If a photograph is made, a synchronizing mechanism turns on the light and exposes the film. Magnetic fields are used to deflect charged par-

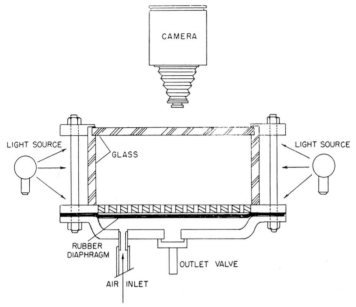

F<small>IG</small>. 3. Wilson cloud chamber

ticles, thereby permitting the determination of their charge, energy and mass relationships.

6.7 Calorimeters

The use of calorimetric technics for measuring ionizing radiations has been limited by the relatively small magnitude of the energy produced and the resultant necessity for extremely sensitive apparatus. They permit the desired direct measurement of energy derived from the absorption of radiation and so are of great scientific interest. They are, however, not yet adaptable to practical clinical work and are beyond the scope of this chapter.

6.8 Units of Ionizing Radiation

Two units have had widespread use in the measurement of radiation· They are the roentgen and the curie. They were established primarily for measuring x-rays and radium. However, they have been unofficially extended to include any radioactive isotope. As was mentioned before, the introduction of artificial radioactive materials has complicated the situation and several new units have been suggested. The "rad" is now coming into use as the unit of absorbed dosage.

6.8.1 *r Unit.* The roentgen was not established to measure the effects of x- or gamma radiation in tissue but rather the ionizing effects of the radiation in an arbitrary medium, air. The roentgen is defined as that quantity of x- or gamma radiation such that the associated corpuscular emission per 0.001293 gm. of air (1 cc. of air under standard conditions) produces, in air, ions carrying one electrostatic unit of charge. The term "associated corpuscular emission" refers to the secondary effects of the x- or gamma radiation in which there are produced photoelectrons, Compton scattering and pair formation. The relative contribution of these various secondary effects varies with the energy of the radiation. One electrostatic unit of charge is produced when 2.083×10^9 ion pairs have been formed. It can be shown that 1 "r" unit also represents the absorption of approximately 87 ergs of energy in 1 gm. of air. The roentgen is not dependent on the time required for the ionization to take place; therefore, the dosage rate of x- or gamma radiation is expressed in terms of roentgens per unit time. A patient receiving 10 r per minute for 10 minutes would accumulate a dose of 100 r.

When the roentgen was extended to include the gamma rays of radium, a correlation was established between the roentgen and a gram of radium or a curie of radon. One gram of radium or 1 curie of radon filtered by 0.5 mm. of platinum produces 0.84 r per hour at one meter.

6.8.2 *Curie.* The curie was established as the unit for measuring the activity of radioactive isotopes formed as a result of the spontaneous disintegration of radium. The International Radium Standards Commission adopted an arbitrary figure of 3.7×10^{10} disintegrating atoms per second per curie for the equilibrium quantity of any radioactive decay product of radium. The term equilibrium quantity was introduced so that it was assured that, at the time the disintegrations were being determined, as many atoms of the element were being formed from the parent element as were disintegrating. In extending the use of the curie to any radioactive isotope, 1 curie of a radioactive isotope decays at the rate of 3.7×10^{10} disintegrations per second. A more frequently used term is the millicurie which is that amount of a radioactive isotope that decays at the rate of 37 million disintegrations per second. If a known number of millicuries of a certain radioactive isotope is to be administered to a patient, it is possible to calculate approximately the amount of radiation he will receive as a result of the dose.

6.8.3 *Rutherford Unit.* A unit has been suggested to replace the curie and has been given the name of the rutherford. The rutherford is defined as that quantity of any radioactive isotope that disintegrates at the rate of one million disintegrations per second. One millicurie of radon would be equal to 37 rutherfords.

6.8.4 *REP Unit.* Since the roentgen by definition is limited to the measurement of photons of x- or gamma radiation, a similar unit was established to measure the ionization of radiation other than x- or gamma rays. This unit is the roentgen equivalent physical. As was mentioned before, it can be shown that 1 r represents the energy loss of approximately 87 ergs by ionization in 1 gm. of air. The roentgen equivalent physical is defined as that quantity of corpuscular radiation which produces in tissue per gram of tissue, ionization equivalent to the quantity of ionization of 1 r of gamma radiation in air. This amounts to an average energy loss of approximately 93 ergs by ionization in 1 gm. of tissue. The term corpuscular radiation is applicable to beta rays, protons, neutrons, alpha particles, and so on. The roentgen equivalent physical cannot be considered equal to the roentgen since the energy loss per roentgen of x- or gamma rays is usually greater in tissue than it is in air. The loss is approximately 95 ergs per gram of muscle, with .825 mev photons.

6.8.5 *Rad Unit.* This is a unit of absorbed dose and equals 100 ergs per gram of the irradiated material. Absorbed dose is the amount of energy imparted to matter by ionizing radiation or particles per unit of the irradiated material at the site of interest. The rad is nearly the same as the average value of the rep in tissue for practical purposes and is not subject to changes as are the values of the rep.

6.8.6 *Rem Unit.* The International Commission on Radiological Protection has suggested that this unit be used when it is necessary to add doeses of different radiations, especially those of differing effectiveness. The letters of the unit bespeak "Roentgen Equivalent Man (or Mammal)" and relate to the amount of radiation equivalent biologically in man to 1 r of gamma or x-rays. It thus is related to the biological effectiveness (RBE); and for practical purposes the dose in Rem is equal to the dose in Rads × the RBE.

6.8.7 *RHM Unit.* The RHM unit, which has been used considerably in the protection measurement and can be used in calibrating radioactive sources, is the roentgen per hour at 1 meter. The roentgen per hour at 1 meter is the quantity of any radioactive substance which emits x- or gamma rays, such that the ionization produced in air by the radiation at a distance of 1 meter from the source is equivalent to 1 r per hour.

6.8.8 *The "n" Unit.* This has been used occasionally in neutron dosimetry as the amount of neutron radiation which produces the same discharge of the 100 r Victoreen chamber as does 1 r of x-ray. This chamber was not designed for neutron dosimetry and chambers of the same sensitivity for x-rays may differ in neutron response. One must therefore be wary of "n" figures. It is now more customary to use the Rem or Rad in neutron dosimetry. Due to high RBE values, 1 n is considerably higher in biologi-

cal effects than 1 r. A value of 2 r has been mentioned as an approximation but the RBE varies depending on whether the neutrons are slow or
fast and also with the tissues irradiated. The RBE of 10 currently listed
for fast neutrons is related to slight cataract formation whereas for lethal
effects the RBE is put at about 1.7 in the *Effects of Nuclear Weapons*, 1957.

6.9 Practical Application of Units and Meters

It is possible to make fairly accurate intralaboratory comparisons of all
gamma ray emitting isotopes using the roentgen per hour at one meter, if
the disintegration scheme of the isotope is known to permit the calculation
of the rhm or if the value of rhm for the particular isotope can be obtained
from a table. These values give a correlation of roentgens and curies of any
gamma ray emitting isotope, the same as the value 0.84 r per hour at 1
meter, gave between the roentgen and the curie of radon.

A suitable portable ionization type instrument such as the Victoreen
Model 247A (Fig. 4) may be used to measure the milli-roentgens per hour
at 1 meter. The procedure would be to calibrate the meter with radium
sources filtered with 0.5 mm. platinum to check the linearity of the scale
and the accuracy of its calibration. If 2 mg. of radium are placed at 1 meter
from the center of the ionization chamber (this can be found by removing
the cover from the meter), the meter should read approximately 1.68
milli-roentgens per hour. If there is a small variation, and it is known that
the meter is working properly, a factor can be used to correct the readings
to the proper values. The radium is then replaced by the radioactive material. Precaution should be taken to assure the absorption of all beta rays
before they have reached the ionizing volume with minimum absorption of
the gamma rays. The problem of absorption, scatter and geometry makes
it necessary for a person trained in the measurement of isotopes to carry
out these calibrations, to be assured of reproducible results. The reading of
the meter is then divided by the value of milli-roentgens per hour at 1 meter
that can be calculated from the table (0.231 milli-roentgens per hour at 1
meter per millicurie in the case of iodine 131) and this value is divided by
the number of cubic centimeters (or milliliters) of the solution to give the
activity in millicurie per cubic centimeter (or milliliter). The correction for
the decay of the iodine 131 from the time it is assayed to the time at which
it will be used, must be taken into consideration. It might be well here to
review the terms *decay scheme* and *decay rate*.

The decay scheme of a radioactive isotope is a diagram or table of the
manner in which it is transformed into another element.* An example is the
decay scheme of Iodine[131]. Approximately 87 per cent of the atoms disinte-

* See Fig. 1 Chapter 5.

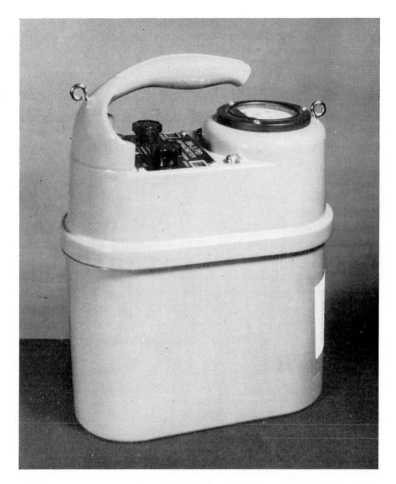

FIG. 4. Portable ionization chamber type instrument

grate by emission of an 0.608 mev beta and either one 0.364 mev gamma or two of 0.080 and 0.284 mev. About 9 per cent decay by emitting one 0.135 mev beta and one 0.637 gamma; 3 per cent by an 0.250 mev beta and 0.722 gamma; 1 per cent via 0.815 mev beta and 0.163 gamma.

The decay constant is defined as the fraction of the sample decomposing per unit time. A more familiar term involving decay of the isotope is the half life, which is the time it takes for one-half the radioactive atoms present at any time to disintegrate. The half life for iodine[131] is eight days. Therefore, if any assay is run on iodine[131] eight days after the previous assay, there will be only one-half the activity. For example, in the case of the calibration discussed above, suppose the value was 1 millicurie per cubic centimeter at 10 A.M. on the eighth of the month. If the material were assayed by the technic described at 10 A.M. on the sixteenth of the month, the value would be one-half millicurie per cubic centimeter. Cobalt 60 can be used as a gamma ray standard giving 1.32 milliroentgen per hour at 1 meter. Cobalt[60] has a half life of 5.3 years, however, and a correction for decay must be made.

The Geiger counter is not efficient as a gamma ray detector, but it is used to measure beta-gamma-emitters, as well as pure beta-emitting isotopes. After the technic has once been established and standards have been prepared or obtained, the procedure for measuring the activity of a radioactive isotope is simple and routine. The background count is taken first. This count is then deducted from any future reading. These counts recorded in the absence of the radioactive sample may be caused by cosmic rays, contamination, etc. Every effort should be made to keep this count as low as possible. After the background is taken, the standard sample is introduced to check and calibrate the counter. The sample to be calibrated is then placed in the counter, and the number of counts taken is compared with the standard to determine the activity of the sample. The procurement of standards, especially of short-lived isotopes, has been a problem. The use of long-lived simulated standards will help this situation.

In measuring alpha particles it is necessary to use a wire mesh window or to introduce the alpha-emitter into the chamber, since alpha particles have extremely short ranges and are easily absorbed by very thin sheets of material. A sheet of paper will absorb most alpha particles. Alpha particle ionization chambers and a special counter called a methane proportional counter are used to measure alpha particles. Portable survey instruments that are sensitive down to 200 disintegrations per minute are used in contamination or protection measurements.

6.9.1 *Ionization Chambers*. The commercial ionization chamber type of instrument is, as a general rule, ruggedly designed, portable, dependable, and little maintenance is required if it receives reasonable care. These instruments are not nearly as sensitive as the Geiger-Müller tube. There are numerous types of ionization chambers and many radiation laboratories build their own special instruments for each application. A superficial discussion of the operation of ionization chambers will be given. More detailed discussions may be found in the literature.

6.9.2 *Lauritsen Electroscope*. The Lauritsen electroscope is an inexpensive type of ionization chamber (Fig. 5). This type of instrument does not need a continuous source of external voltage. It consists of a supported, free to move, conducting coated quartz fiber, scale, a microscope that can be focused to detect the movement of the fiber across the scale and a chamber to enclose the quartz fiber system. The quartz fiber system is insulated from the chamber and a charge is placed on the fiber by applying a potential from the fiber system to the case. The voltage must be high enough so that, at the end of the run, the voltage left on the instrument still will be above minimum saturation voltage. When a charge is placed on the fiber, it moves away from its supports since they both have the same type of charge. There will be a certain drift in the instrument, which is due to background. This is quite reproducible and should not be confused with leakage that might take place because of contamination, humidity or dirt on an insulator.

The instrument is simple to operate; however, caution should be taken in interpreting the results as the deflection is not linear. A calibration curve is necessary or readings should always be taken over the same portion of the scale. The larger the volume of the chamber, the smaller the amount of radiation it will detect. The electroscope in Fig. 6 is for measuring radioactive samples, while the one in Fig. 7 is a protection meter called a pocket dosimeter for measuring the amount of radiation a person receives while working around radiation.

6.9.3 *Victoreen "r" Meter.* Another type of ionization chamber is the Victoreen Condenser r Meter. In this meter the chamber and electrometer are separate (Fig. 8). The chamber is placed in the electrometer and charged; it is then removed and exposed to the radiation which partially discharges it; it is then replaced in the electrometer which indicates the loss of charge due to ionization, which in turn shows the amount of radiation to which it was exposed. The 100 "r" chamber of this instrument has been used to measure neutrons, as well as x- and gamma rays. When measuring anything except x-rays from 90,000 volts (90 kv) to 200,000 volts (200 kv), precautions must be taken. In evaluating the results one must read the literature concerning the use of the instrument for the particular radiation under investigation.

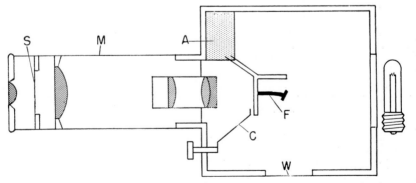

Fig. 5. Lauritsen electroscope: S, scale; M, microscope; A, insulator; C, charging contactor; F, fiber; W, window.

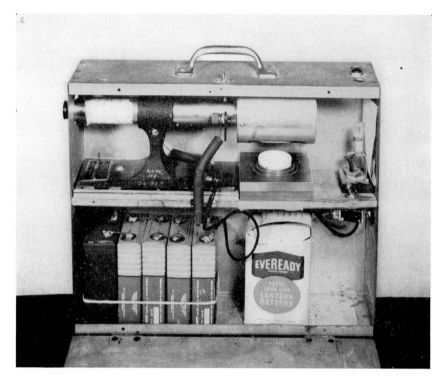

FIG. 6. Electroscope for measuring radioactive samples

A protection meter called the "minometer" has a separate pencil type chamber and electrometer and is used in a manner similar to the Victoreen Condenser "r" Meter. The ionization chamber instruments mentioned above are all of the integrating type in that they record the amount of exposure of the chamber to radiation. Another type of ionization chamber instrument built by Victoreen is a rate meter which indicates the amount of radiation per unit time. This meter can be used to calibrate gamma-ray-emitting isotopes.

6.9.4 *Laboratory Ionization Chambers.* The laboratory type of ionization chamber is designed in many different ways, depending upon the problem involved. Two valuable chambers for laboratory instruments are modifications of the parallel plate type chamber. One design, which is a modification of the Failla type extrapolation chamber, is shown in Fig. 9. One electrode (the high voltage electrode) consists of a thin nylon window which has been coated to make it conductive. It is insulated from, and mounted on, a brass ring with screw threads. The ring screws on to a brass plate which

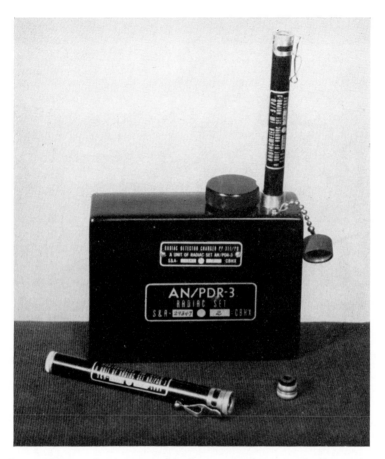

Fɪɢ. 7. Pocket electroscope with charger; used as a protection meter

supports the collecting electrode and guard ring. The guard ring may serve
one or both of two purposes. One is to separate the high voltage electrode
from the collecting electrode, and the other is to produce as uniform a field
as possible between the two electrodes. The screw arrangement permits a
varying volume of air between the electrodes so that the volume can be
extrapolated to zero.

Another modification of the parallel plate type of ionization chamber is
the standard air chamber which was designed and is used at the National
Bureau of Standards. This chamber is a primary standard x-ray ionization
chamber (Fig. 10). A diaphragm limits the beam of radiation which passes
between a parallel plate guard ring assembly. In order to avoid absorption
of the softer components of the x-ray beam, the guard ring is made small

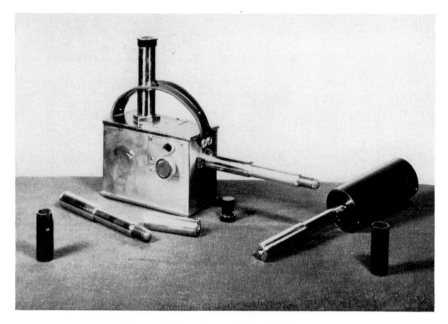

FIG. 8. Victoreen condenser "r" meter

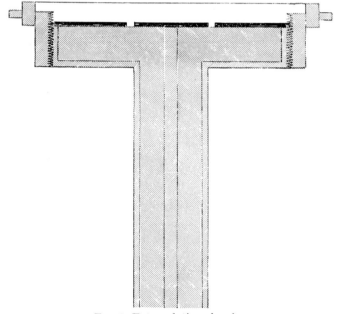

FIG. 9. Extrapolation chamber

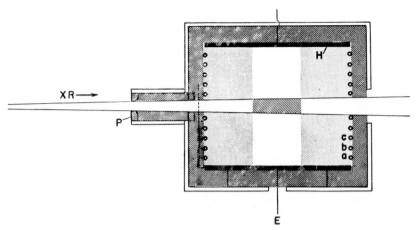

FIG. 10. Standard x-ray ionization chamber: XR, x-ray beam; P, limiting diaphragm; H, high voltage electrode; E, collecting electrode connection to measuring device; abc, guard wires.

and a guard wire system is used to improve the uniformity of the field. The ionization that takes place in the volume formed by the diaphragming of the beam and the collecting electrodes can be detected and measured by means of an electroscope or electrometer.

6.9.5 *Geiger-Müller Counters.* One of the most powerful observing and measuring tools available to the medical scientist is the Geiger-Müller counter. This device approaches an ideal of exact measurement. A direct and finite counting process is used to measure radiation quantity and intensity. For investigative work the Geiger-Müller counter has greatly extended the ability of the physiologist to trace the distribution of elements entering the human body.

The sensitive element of Geiger-Müller counter instruments is essentially a diode, or two-electrode tube, filled with gas at a low pressure. The gas content and voltage applied across the electrodes are so adjusted that entry or release of a single charged atomic particle, proton or electron within a certain volume between the electrodes produces collision ionization in the gas and rapid discharge of a relatively large quantity of electricity across the interelectrode space. The first such counter instrument was developed in 1908 by Rutherford and Geiger at the University of Manchester, in England. With this instrument it was possible to increase the electrical effect of a single alpha particle so that it could be observed directly on an ordinary electrometer. The type of counter tube most commonly used for radiation measurements was produced in 1928 by Geiger and Müller. This is the tube generally referred to as the Geiger-Müller tube. A typical method of construction is shown in Fig. 11. The anode wire is tungsten of

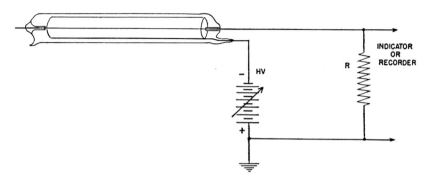

FIG. 11. Geiger-Müller tube with connections to recorder

about .005 in. diameter and is stretched along the axis of a glass cylinder. The cathode is a copper cylinder within the glass with the electrical connection brought out through a seal. Extensive investigations have been made on different kinds and mixtures of filling gases, but ones frequently used are argon and hydrogen, at low pressure.

The operation characteristics of a tube of this general type can be demonstrated if it is connected, as shown in Fig. 11, to a variable source of high voltage DC in series with a resistor R. The output, connected across R, goes to some suitable amplifying or pulse-recording system. If the tube is placed in the presence of some constant intensity ionizing radiation, the counting-rate response can be plotted against the voltage applied between anode and cathode.

The idealized curve of such a plot is shown in Fig. 13. As the voltage is increased from zero to the point A, the tube behaves as an ionization chamber. Ions formed by the incident radiation are swept across the interelectrode space to their appropriate electrodes without producing any multiplicative collision ionization in the gas. This small ion current will not be detected with the amplifier. As the voltage increases from A to B, some pulses will begin to appear, indicating the beginning of the ionization-multiplying process. This region includes that of proportional counter action. Pulses in this region are found to be proportional in size to the initial ionization produced by the characteristic particle. A relatively high sensitivity recording apparatus is required to observe these pulses, so generally the count rate will not noticeably rise until the voltage exceeds the point B. As the voltage goes beyond B, the counting rate rises sharply with voltage and the pulse size may still show some dependence on the characteristic of the initiating particle. At the voltage C the counting rate levels off and the pulses are of uniform size, characteristic of the tube itself. This is known as the Geiger-Müller threshold voltage. At voltages from C

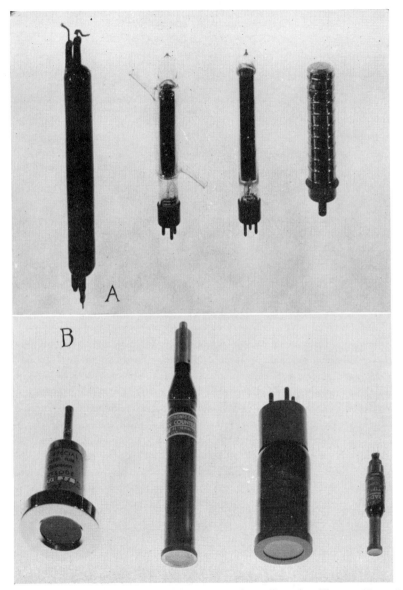

FIG. 12 (A & B). Various types of counter tubes. (See also Figures 11 to 17.) (Bureau of Medicine and Surgery, U. S. Navy.)

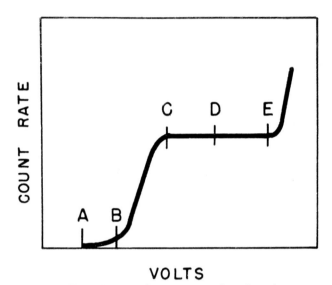

VOLTS

FIG. 13. Geiger-Müller tube counting response plotted against voltage applied between cathode and anode. A, B, proportional counter region; C, D, E, plateau or Geiger-Müller counting region.

to E, the counting rate remains practically constant, with perhaps some upward slope. This region of operating voltage is referred to as the plateau. A wide plateau is decidedly desirable because it minimizes the importance of constancy in the high voltage power supply. A point D in the center of the plateau is generally selected for operation, thus permitting some voltage fluctuations without affecting the counting rate. The plateau for a good counter may be 200 to 300 volts or even longer.

If the electrode voltage is increased beyond E, spurious pulses appear, not due to the incident radiation but arising within the tube itself. At still higher voltages, these pulses increase to a condition of continuous discharge through the tube. The over-all merit of a certain tube is determined by the slope and width of its plateau. Several factors influence these characteristics, including gas pressure, tube geometry and the external measuring circuit.

The exact nature of the mechanism of the discharge within a Geiger-Müller tube is quite complicated and is not completely known. A general qualitative description of counter action can, however, be given. If a high speed ionizing particle enters a counter tube operating on its voltage plateau, collisions will occur with atoms of the filling gas in the cathode cylinder. The ion pairs formed by splitting the neutral gas molecules are positive ions and free electrons of high mobility. These released electrons move toward the anode wire under the influence of the strong electric field applied between the electrodes. As they pick up speed, they produce new ion pairs by collision, leaving many more free electrons in their wake. These newly released electrons in turn produce more collision ionization and ultraviolet photons are released near the anode wire which liberate photo-electrons from the cathode wall. These photoelectrons fall in toward the wire, increasing the intensity of collision ionization. The avalanche of accumulative ionization continues until the potential difference between the electrodes drops to a point where ionization by collision can no longer occur. At this point a full-glow discharge momentarily exists in the counter tube. This entire succession of events lasts about .005 to .1 second. The electrode potential recovers itself according to the time constant of the associated circuit. After the multiple ionization has started until the potential recovers, the tube is insensitive to any newly incident rays. The passage of such rays at this time would be unrecorded by the counter. This period of insensitivity during the discharge cycle results in a counting loss which reduces the efficiency of the counter.

The counting loss becomes a serious factor when radiations of high intensity are measured because many ionizing particles are passing through the tube at one time. The development of self-quenching or fast counter tubes has greatly reduced the counting loss error. Such a tube is made by the addition of a small amount of organic vapor in the gas filling. This increases the instability of the discharge, causing it to terminate much more quickly, thus greatly reducing the time for a single discharge cycle. With proper choice of circuit components, the pulse length can be as short as one micro-second. The mechanism of the discharge in a fast counter is somewhat different from that of the slow counter. After an initial ionizing event has occurred in the fast counter tube, the released electrons start the collision-ionization process in the immediate vicinity of the wire. The discharge spreads along the wire with the high potential field providing the energy necessary for collision ionization toward the wire itself. Apparently no photoelectron emission from the cathode wall acts in the process.

Ionization resulting in a pulse in a Geiger-Müller counter tube can be initiated as indicated by high speed particles such as alpha rays or beta rays. The tube's usefulness is, however, much broader. The other kinds of radiation it will detect include cosmic-ray particles, gamma and x-rays, and, with certain refinements, protons, deuterons, neutrons and the relatively low energy photons of ultraviolet and visible light. The ionization mechanism of alpha particles and high speed electrons has been explained. To permit these particles to enter the counter tube, a sufficiently thin wall must be provided in the glass envelope to offer minimum absorption. The thickness of particle-admitting windows and walls is generally indicated by milligrams per square centimeter of window area. In common use are thin glass side walls of 30 mg/cm² thickness, admitting beta particles having energies above 160 kev. Mica windows down to 0.5 mg/cm² are available, although in normal laboratory work the thin windows run between 1.4 and 4 mg/cm². Mica of 4 mg/cm² is approximately 15 microns thick, and will pass beta particles of energy in excess of 47 kev. For alpha radiation, a mica window thickness of 1.4 mg/cm² has the equivalent stopping power of one centimeter of air. This thickness will also pass all beta radiation in excess of 25 kev when the source is in close proximity to the window. Thin metal wall Geiger counter tubes are widely used in applications not requiring the extremely thin windows. Recent technical developments in mica-to-metal and glass-to-metal sealing have made controlled mass production possible and many manufacturers have entered the field.

For x-ray and gamma ray measurements it is desirable to use metal cathodes of proper absorption coefficient and wall thickness. Part of the energy of incident photon radiation is converted by absorption in the cylinder wall into the energy of photoelectrons or recoil electrons. These electrons, released from the wall into the interelectrode gas, start the trigger-discharge process just as the ionizing particles start it by direct collision. For cosmic rays, x-rays and gamma rays, therefore, the total energy intercepted and available for conversion is approximately proportional to the cross sectional area presented by the cathode to the incident flux.

Detection in the ultraviolet and visible spectral regions is accomplished by the use of quartz windows and by special treatment of the cathode to make it photosensitive. Slow neutrons can be detected by observing the secondary radioactivity induced in the cathode, or in the case of boron-trifluoride-filled counters, the alpha particles released in the gas by the fast neutron induced disintegration of boron. Recoil protons from hydro-

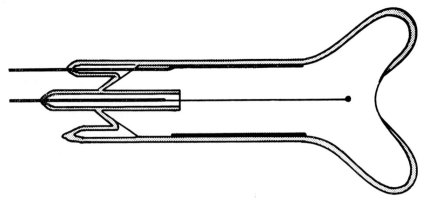

Fig. 14. Thin window Geiger-Müller tube with conductive layer (cathode)

gen containing wall material offer a similar method for detecting slow neutrons.

The wide range of operating conditions of Geiger-Müller counters permits great latitude in constructional dimensions which makes this instrument available for a variety of uses. Tubes as small as a needle up to many inches in cross section have been operated successfully. For measurement of radiation from solutions, immersion-type counters have been developed. Where extremely high sensitivity is desired for detecting minute activity in a gas, the gas can be incorporated in the filling mixture. Flowing liquids such as venous blood can be passed through a special chamber constructed around the counter cathode of the tube, shown in Fig. 16. Probably the most commonly used counter tube for laboratory work is the end-window type. A very thin sheet of mica cemented or fused to a bell-shaped glass envelope can provide a large area, pressure-tight, low-absorption window. Such a design (Fig. 17) is particularly advantageous for measuring radiation from samples placed in flat dishes directly below the window. These are only a few of the many special purpose counters which have been developed.

The operating voltage of most commercial Geiger counter tubes ranges from 600 to 1500 volts. The plateau length is usually 100 to 350 volts. Self-quenching tubes are generally used and when filled with an organic quenching vapor, the life expectancy is of the order of 10^9 counts. Considerable work has been done toward the development of improved Geiger tube fillings. Halogen gas mixtures are among the most promising. Stainless

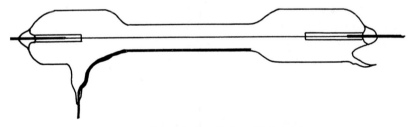

FIG. 15. Thin window Geiger-Müller tube

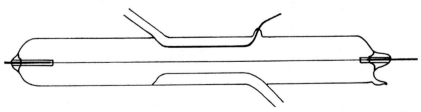

FIG. 16. Geiger-Müller tube designed to measure radiation from flowing solutions

steel cathode tubes have been constructed with the Geiger threshold in the neighborhood of 700 volts, having a virtually flat plateau of several hundred volts. These tubes appear to have an operating temperature range from $-55°C$ to $+75°C$, and a life expectancy of over 5×10^{10} counts.

As has been indicated, a factor to consider in judging the merit of a tube is its counting loss or "dead time." The shorter this is, the greater will be the resolving time of the counter. This is the ability of the tube to distinguish between two ionizing events occurring within a very short interval. High efficiency is particularly important when measuring high intensity levels of radiation. Resolving times of self-quenching counters are of the order of 100 microseconds.

6.9.6 *Scalers and Rate Meters.* Practically all instruments used with Geiger-Müller counter tubes can be classed as either pulse scalers or rate meters. The simplest device to detect or count pulses from a counter is merely a pair of high impedance phones connected through a condenser to the high resistance "R" in Fig. 11. Each pulse will produce an audible click in the phones and high pulse rates a buzz. Measurements in the laboratory

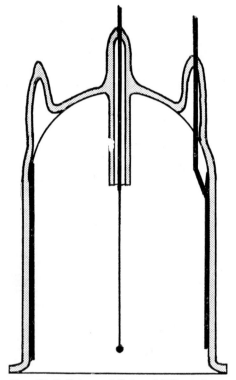

FIG. 17. Bell type of Geiger-Müller tube

require accurate counting of the number of pulses per unit of time. Mechanical counters or registers cannot be driven reliably at rates in excess of 100 times per second, so other means are required to record the high rates of Geiger tube counting, as high as 5000 counts per second, or more. This can be done electronically by a scaling circuit. The pulses are first amplified and shaped to a standard size before entering the first scaling stage. The basic scale-of-two unit is, briefly, an electronic means of storing a pulse until a second one is received. At that time a single pulse is released to the circuit following. Thus it is seen that each scaling stage releases one-half the pulses it receives and by cascading numerous stages the number of pulses finally released to a mechanical register is much less than the counter tube initiated but in a known geometric ratio. For example, six scale-of-two stages emit one count for every 2^6 or 64 counts received at the input. Such a circuit would be called a scale of 64. A decade scaler is a refinement which produces a pulse for every 10, 100, 1000, etc., pulses received. Further additions which are sometimes incorporated in laboratory instruments for the convenience of the operator are: A loudspeaker, electric timer, cut-off

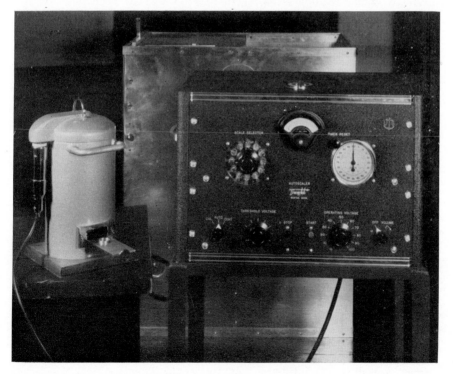

FIG. 18. Laboratory type counting unit

after predetermined number of counts, scale selector, indicator for inter-polation of pulses left within scale units at termination of count, and automatic reset to clear residual pulses before a new count is made. A regulated high voltage power supply is essential to maintain the counter tube voltage in the center of the plateau. In many instruments this voltage may be varied for proportional or Geiger counter action. Scalers are built with special parallel plate chambers for alpha counting, and with propor-tional counters having a continuous flow methane atmosphere for counting alpha particles in the presence of high beta and gamma activity.

The rate meter type of circuit is widely used for portable or survey in-struments. If the pulses from a Geiger counter tube are integrated or rectified, a DC voltage can be developed, the magnitude of which is pro-portional to the rate of pulsing. When amplified by one or more vacuum tube stages, this voltage can be read directly on a meter or recorded on a paper tape. This meter simply reads the rate of arrival of pulses and with rates above ten times normal background the rate is rapid enough so that a steady meter reading is obtained. Much work has been done on the development of portable rate meters for military purposes and ore prospect-ing. These instruments are battery-operated, have a range selection, and the pulses can be monitored with phones or a flashing neon light. A thin wall counter tube can be mounted as a probe at the end of a length of cable, and, for beta-gamma survey instruments, a sliding window provided in the metal housing to admit the beta rays to the tube. Integrating rate meters have applications in the laboratory for measuring and monitoring high intensity radiation or where accuracy does not require the recording of each individual count.

A pre-amplifier vacuum tube quenching circuit is necessary with non-self-quenching tubes and is frequently used with all counters. This circuit reduces the resolving time and permits lower impedance pulses to be fed into the high gain amplifiers minimizing spurious counts and capacity effects in the lead wires. The quenching circuit is usually located as close to the counter tube as possible.

6.10 Laboratory Installation

A laboratory installation for isotope or tracer work is shown in Fig. 18. Accessories to the basic Geiger-Müller counter tube and scaler include a lead-shielded tube chamber to reduce background counts, special cups and holders for the samples, an automatic sample changer, and an automatic timer. A well-type scintillation counter would have a similar superficial appearance.

Laboratory design is treated in Chapter 21 and various types of clinical apparatus and their practical use in Chapter 22.

6.11 Personnel Dosimetry

This is closely associated with radiation protection and widely employed. It is discussed in Chapter 15 where notes will be found on pocket dosimeters, film badges and phosphate glass dosimeters.

6.12 Descriptive Terminology*

In order to facilitate ready comprehension of radiological discussions, it appears appropriate to include a few brief notes on this subject.

6.12.1 *Quality of Radiation.* Gamma and x-rays are described in various terms and so we note that *"soft" radiation* is characterized by low energy, low penetration, low frequency and absorption in superficial tissues, and *"hard" radiation* by the opposite. Most gamma rays are harder than conventional x-rays. The average gamma energy of fission products is about 0.7 mev (millions of electron volts) and that of the gamma rays from the nuclear blast several mev. Cobalt^{60} emits 1.1 and 1.3 mev gamma. Modern apparatus can produce x-rays of 70 mev or more but most diagnostic x-ray equipment operates near 100 kv, and therapeutic units at 250 kv. There are however therapy units of 1 and 2 mv capacity in fairly frequent use and a few betatrons of from 20 to 70 mev capacity. At the other end of the scale some very soft x-rays are used for superficial therapy with energies near 10 kv, the so called *"Grenz Rays."* In radiological parlance, Handbook 59 of the N.B.S. gives the following designations:

Low voltage x-ray: up to 140 kv.

High voltage x-ray: 140 to 250 kv (this is also frequently designated the "deep therapy" range because for some years such x-rays provided the deepest effect possible.

Supervoltage x-ray: 250 kv to 3 mv.

Multimillion volt x-ray: over 3 mev.

A distinction is made between the voltage at which x-rays are produced and the energy of the photons. They are not always the same since in multimillion volt apparatus, x-rays and various ionizing particles are given energies of mev ranges by means of acceleration processes although the actual voltages employed are vastly less (See Chapter 17). The terms kv or mv refer to voltages actually employed in production and the terms kev and mev to photon energies. (K or k is for the prefix kilo—a thousand; M or m for a million.)

The quality of radiation refers to penetration power and as a measure of this, the term *"Half Value Layer"* (H.V.L.) is often used. This is the thickness of a specified material (usually Al, Cu or Pb) which will reduce the dosage rate to a half. The harder, more energetic and penetrating radiations naturally have higher H.V.L.s.

6.12.2 *Specific Ionization.* The biological effectiveness in terms of Rems and RBE is related to the ionization produced in tissue which is spoken of

* Contributed by Ed.

as *"Specific Ionization."* Occasionally when excitation is also important, the total transfer of energy is considered and one finds that the term "Linear Transfer per unit of length" is used (let.). However "Specific Ionization" is the factor of main interest and is usually given in terms of the number of ion pairs produced per micron of water.

6.12.3 *Quantitative Considerations.* These include terms such as MLD, the median lethal dose—the amount likely to produce a 50 per cent mortality (400 to 450 for man). It should be noted however that such terms must be considered in relation to penetrating ability or "quality" of radiation. Usually MLD dosage figures imply that whole-body, high energy, radiation has been employed. One also sees notations such as LD 20 etc., the number referring to mortality percentage.

6.12.4 *Standards.* These involve "Maximum Permissible Dosages" (MPE) and now are related to genetic and other long range effects. They have been stringently revised so that workers subjected to radiation hazards are not to average more than 5 r per year. (See Chapter 14.)

War and other emergency conditions which may call for relation of exposure to acute effects of larger doses involve what are often termed "Calculated Risk Exposures." These are considered in the chapter cited above. Acute exposures up to 25 r are considered relatively negligible at least as far as one such exposure is concerned in limited groups. Again dosages up to 100 r are not likely to prove incapacitating. Beyond that amount an increasing incidence of radiation sickness can be expected to cause casualties and beyond several hundred r fatalities will occur with recovery becoming unlikely at the 600 r level assuming that the whole body is subjected to high energy gamma, x-ray or neutron exposure.

REFERENCES

Cork, J. M.: *Radioactivity and Nuclear Physics.* Second edition. New York: D. Van Nostrand Co., 1950. Third Edition, 1957.

Evans, Robley D.: *Radioactivity Units and Standards.* New York: McGraw-Hill, 1947.

Glasser, O.: *Medical Physics,* Vol. II., Chicago: Yr. Bk. Pub., 1950.

Glasser, O., et al: *Physical Foundations of Radiology.* New York: Hoeber, 1944.

Hine and Brownell: *Radiation Dosimetry.* New York: Acad. Press, 1956.

Hoag and Korff: *Electron and Nuclear Physics,* New York: D. Van Nostrand Co., 1948.

Korff, S. A.: *Electron and Nuclear Counters.* New York: D. Van Nostrand Co., 1946.

Lapp and Andrews: *Nuclear Radiation Physics.* New York: Prentice-Hall, 2nd Ed., 1954.

Radiological Defense, Vol. IV. Armed Forces Special Weapons Project, 1950.

Rossi: *Ionization Chambers and Counters.* New York: McGraw-Hill, 1949.

Strong, John: *Procedures in Experimental Physics.* New York: Prentice-Hall, Inc., 1942.

Yagoda: *Radioactive Measurements with Nuclear Emulsions.* New York: Wiley, 1949.

Note: See also references after Chapters 15 and 22.

7 ▶

Fundamental Biology of Ionizing Radiations

Friedrich Ellinger, M.D.

7.1 Common Features

A survey of the accumulated data on the effects of ionizing radiations on living matter reveals the interesting fact that there exist certain common features in the response of cells and tissues to irradiation, regardless of the nature of the rays, whether they are of the electromagnetic type, like x-ray or gamma rays, or whether they are corpuscular radiations like alpha, beta, neutron or proton rays. It also appears that these effects of irradiation are qualitatively the same, whether the source of rays is outside the body or within.

On first sight this may appear surprising. However, these common features in the response of cells and tissues are easily understood if we view the various natural phenomena called "radiations" under the single concept of "energy."

Radiations, however, may be viewed under a single concept not only from the point of view of the physicist, but also from the standpoint of the biologist. Here it is possible to consider radiations under the single concept of "stimulus." We define as a stimulus "any external change, capable of influencing living matter in such a way that the latter is modified in the course of its vital functions."

7.2 General Manifestations

Having thus obtained a means of understanding for the common feature in the response of cells and tissues to the exposure to radiations, we shall now summarize *the general manifestations of radiations on living matter*:

    1. *Ways of action:* The effect may be a local or direct effect, or a systemic or indirect one.

2. *Time and effect:* The effect may manifest itself immediately after exposure, and is, therefore, called an immediate effect. Frequently, however, a certain amount of time elapses before the effect of irradiation becomes manifest. This period is called the "latent period." The subsequent manifestations of irradiation are called the "late effect."

3. *Quality of effects:* Radiations produce morphologic as well as functional changes in cells and tissues. It is important to realize that radiations like pharmacologic agents "do not create new functions in a cell or tissue; they only modify existing functions, or at most make evident functions which have previously been latent" (Sollmann).

4. *Quantity of effects:* Radiations produce reversible as well as irreversible effects. The latter are also called radiation injuries. Reversibility or irreversibility of radiation effects depend on the radiation dose.

The site of action of all radiations is the cell.—This brings up the question as to the *mode of action of radiation in a cell.*

Absorption of energy by a cell represents the first step in the chain of events which leads to the morphologic and functional changes of a cell.

The cell representing the biologic unit of life is, however, physically considered, a multiplicity, being made up of 10^9–10^{10} of molecules in active motion. Chemically, too, the cell is a multiplicity consisting, in addition to water, of a variety of substances such as proteins, carbohydrates, fats, minerals, etc. The physicist Dessauer considers that 1/100th to one-tenth of the molecules of a cell must be affected before a change in a cell becomes visible.

7.3 Primary Effects

The next question to be answered is, which of the molecules forming a cell are primarily affected by irradiation? that is, we have to discuss *the problem of the primary effect of ionizing radiations.* It is generally believed that the primary process occurs in the large protein molecules and the water of the cell. It is believed that following irradiation a denaturation of the proteins occurs similar to that seen in protein solutions irradiated *in vitro.* Protein solutions show coagulation after exposure to irradiation. To the eye this looks exactly the same as the well known heat coagulation. However, there is a definite difference in that the heat coagulum can easily be re-dissolved by means of certain physicochemical processes, whereas the radiation coagulum is an irreversible precipitate.

The assumption of denaturation of proteins for the explanation of the primary effect of radiations on cells finds support in numerous biologic observations of the irradiated cell. It is interesting to note that physical studies of the irradiated cell also seem to support this contention. Following irradiation, a striking difference in the ultraviolet absorption of cells related to changes in nucleoproteins is observed before a histological change in a cell becomes visible.

The effect of ionizing radiations on proteins offers not only a basis for the understanding of their direct effects on the cell but also for their indirect actions.

It has been demonstrated that irradiation of proteins leads to the formation of toxic substances which in their pharmacologic effects are similar to histamine. They are usually called histamine-like substances (H-substances, for short). We have been able to demonstrate by irradiation with cathode rays the formation of histamine from histidine, an amino acid which forms part of most proteins of the mammalian body. To be sure, histamine is not the only toxic decomposition product of the irradiated proteins. The possibility of its radiochemical formation deserves, however, particular interest because histamine even in minute quantities exercises effects not only on the circulatory but also on the gastro-intestinal and autonomic nerve system. The histamine hypothesis appears, therefore, suitable for the explanation of the indirect or systemic radiation effects.

The action of ionizing radiations on water results in the formation of hydrogen peroxide and other oxidizing agents which may contribute secondarily to the formation of toxic compounds and enzyme inactivation.

7.4 Morphologic Effects

We turn now to a description of *the morphologic changes of the irradiated cell:*

The part of the cell most sensitive to radiation is the cell nucleus, but cytoplasm is also sensitive to radiation.

The morphologic changes consist in:

1. *Pyknosis of the cell nucleus:* This is generally understood as a coagulation of the chromatin. It is sometimes observed only a few minutes after exposure.

2. *Karyorrhexis:* This means disintegration of the cell nucleus. Fragments of nuclear substance are distributed in the cytoplasm.

3. *Liquefaction of the cell mass* with vacuolation; all that ultimately remains are chromatin fragments. It is interesting that sometimes changes in the mitochondria represent the first appreciable alteration of the cell which may be detectable with appropriate staining methods prior to those in the cell nucleus.

It is of great importance to realize that *all these changes depend* on the radiation dose and *are characteristic of but not specific for radiations.*

7.5 Functional Effects

We are turning now to the *changes in vital function*, following irradiation:

1. *Motility* may be restricted, suppressed or remain unchanged. While suppression of cell motility is evidence of cellular death, its survival by no means implies absence of injury by radiation, e.g., irradiated spermatozoa retain their motility, are still capable of fertilization, yet monstrosities may result.

2. *Reproductive power* may be restricted or suppressed. Sometimes irradiation stops mitosis in the equatorial plate stage. In other instances irradiation results in abnormal mitosis (e.g., giant cell formation). If already commenced, mitosis generally proceeds to completion. Then comes a mitosis-free period, following which mitosis may start anew.

3. *Growth* may be restricted or suppressed. The effect on growth usually becomes manifest after a latent period, which is considered to be due to progressive formation of harmful metabolic products. It should be emphasized that the latent period depends upon the intensity of irradiation and not on the speed of proliferation of the irradiated tissue.

4. *Metabolism:* fatty, mucoid or amyloid degeneration may follow exposure to irradiation. Of considerable interest is the effect of radiations on the cell respiration; it is maintained by some that respiration and glycolysis remain unaffected by radiation, and by others that both are depressed. These contradictory results can be explained by the wide variations in the doses applied as well as by the heterogeneous experimental materials used (plant, cells, tissue cultures, organ sections of animals). Attention should be called to those investigations which have shown the possibility of reducing oxygen consumption of normal tissue cells, while causing simultaneous intensification of aerobic and anaerobic glycolysis. In this manner the metabolism of the normal irradiated cell approaches that of a tumor cell, except that glycolysis in the former is not independent of oxygen consumption. These data are of interest in connection with the production of cancers by irradiation.

5. *Permeability:* irradiated cells show a fluctuation of increased and decreased permeability.

6. *Specific cell functions*, e.g., gland secretion may be restricted or suppressed.

7.6 Manner of Action

If an attempt is made to visualize *the manner in which vital functions are affected by irradiation*, a picture somewhat on the following lines may be drawn:

Depending on the dose, the vital energies of cells and tissues are exhausted in a shorter or longer period of time. Irradiation evidently impairs the ability of the cell to maintain metabolic equilibrium, and processes within the cell, therefore, proceed in part at an increased tempo. To some extent the cell becomes prematurely aged.

Observations of an increased tempo of vital processes following irradiation have repeatedly been considered as *stimulation by irradiation*. This is, however, an "erroneous conclusion." What appears as cell stimulation is only a precipitated course of life function ending in cell death.

The problem of cell stimulation by irradiation plays a considerable role in the considerations for the clinical use of radiations. It appears, therefore, worth while to discuss this question in more detail:

The relationship between dose and effect in pharmacology is governed in a number of instances by the so-called *Arndt-Schulze law* which states that small doses exercise a stimulating, medium doses a depressive, and large doses a destructive effect.

Numerous investigators have attempted to prove the general validity of this law also in the field of radiations. There is indeed experimental evidence that small doses of radiations may stimulate certain vital functions of cells as for instance the mitotic cell count. When, however, observations were extended over sufficiently long periods of time, it was noticed that the initial stimulation of the mitotic count was followed by a decline in mitosis, so that the integral value of mitosis over a longer period of observation failed to show any difference between irradiated cells and unirradiated controls.

In conclusion, it may therefore be stated that *experimental radiation therapy has not proved the existence of a true stimulation of cell function*. The accumulated evidence rather indicates that *radiation therapy depends upon the depressant or destructive action of rays*.

7.7 Recovery Phenomena

Recognition of those facts leads us to the *problem of recovery from the effects of irradiation*.

How can we explain recovery from irradiation? The photochemical theory of radiation effects makes the understanding of this phenomenon easy. As mentioned above, radiations produce new substances in the irradiated cells, which have been held to be toxic compounds. According to the photochemical theory, recovery may thus be achieved in two ways:

1. The substances formed photochemically are recombined into their original compounds by reversible chemical reactions. Photochemistry offers a variety of such reactions (methylene blue $\leftrightarrows$ methylene white).

2. The photochemically formed products are removed from the tissues by mechanical means, e.g., by diffusion, or by circulation which has been called the "washing away effect." We have been able to support this theory by experiments using collodium membranes as a cell model.

The phenomenon of recovery divides itself into two distinct biologic groups:

1. The restoration of morphology and function of the individual cell injured by irradiation. This represents *true recovery*.

2. The restoration of morphology and function of tissues and organs by replacement of damaged cells by growth going out from cells which escaped radiation injury. This phenomenon is designated as *pseudo-recovery*.

Cells which on microscopic examination show evidence of radiation injury usually do not recover, though they may complete the process of mitosis.

The problem of recovery of single cells is complicated by the fact that cells may be injured though they appear undamaged. This was demonstrated as early as 1912 by the Hertwigs, using eggs and sperm of the frog and the sea urchin. They found that irradiated eggs were capable of dividing in due time and that irradiated sperm was still capable of fertilizing eggs. In spite of what appeared to be normal functioning, however, the insidious cell injury eventually became manifest, for usually only two to three additional cell divisions took place.

Henshaw has described multipolar cleavage in *Arbacia punctulata* as the consequence of irradiation of either gamete (egg or sperm). This phenomenon too leads finally to cell death.

In experiments with tadpoles, it has been shown that cells which have escaped destruction at the earlier stages of the mitotic processes may succumb, nevertheless, at later stages of division. Reduction of radiation injuries, which may also be considered as recovery from the effect of irradiation, results from lowering of the temperature of exposed cells and tissues. Packard believes that the common factor in these cases of apparent recovery is "the low productive and metabolic rate of the cells following cooling."

7.7.1 *Genetic Factors.* The term "true recovery," as already noted, includes complete restoration of cell morphology and function. Of the utmost importance for the determination of "true recovery" is the discovery, made by H. J. Muller in 1927, that x-rays are capable of producing hereditary effects, the so-called "x-ray mutations."

Muller's observations were made on the fruit fly, Drosophila. They have since been confirmed by numerous investigators in various forms of animals and plants. As the result of these studies it can be stated:

1. Radiation mutations may not manifest themselves before the third generation;

2. The frequency of these mutations, the so-called mutation rate, is directly proportional to the radiation dose;

3. There is no threshold dose for the occurrence of mutations. The total

amount of ionizing radiations received by the germ cells (egg cells and spermatozoa) during the lifetime of an individual are accumulated.

It is true that these results cannot be directly applied to higher forms of life, but it is known from genetics that results obtained in lower forms of life apply at least in principle to man as well. Their importance for medicine and public health cannot, therefore, be overemphasized at a time when larger and larger segments of our population are exposed to ionizing radiations during diagnostic or therapeutic procedures or in the laboratory during research or production work. The strictest observation of recognized safety standards is, therefore, an absolute necessity.

This review of various aspects of the recovery of individual irradiated cells shows that the problem is a knotty one. No doubt "true recovery" of irradiated cells has been demonstrated, but so far only under special experimental conditions which can hardly be reproduced in the mammalian body.

7.7.2 *Recovery in Tissue Cultures.* The recovery of tissues has been successfully studied in tissue cultures. By this method the indirect influence of circulation and nerves is eliminated. Experiments along this line with a variety of materials (embryonal fibroblasts, embryonal choroidea, osteoblasts, etc.) have shown that after a latent period, the irradiated tissue cultures show inhibition of growth for a varying period of time (seven to 20 days) after which the rate of growth in the irradiated and control cultures is the same.

Investigations in which a certain dose of radiation was given with low intensity (long exposure) showed that the effect was less pronounced than when the same dose was given with high intensity (short exposure). This suggests an active repair process in the cells of the tissue cultures during irradiation. Some light has been thrown on the mechanism of this recovery by experiments in which it was demonstrated that subcultures from tissues irradiated with a dose sufficient to check growth, will grow if the explantation is done shortly after irradiation, or if the piece of tissue used for the explantation is first washed with Ringer's solution. These experiments seem to support the hypothesis that the effect of irradiation is due to the formation of toxic substances from cell decomposition. The recovery observed in these experiments would then represent a typical "washing away effect."

7.7.3 *Conclusions on Recovery.* From the foregoing facts, the following conclusions may be drawn. True tissue recovery is conceivable, but the recovery which occurs *in vivo* and *in vitro* and without experimental interference by such procedures as washing, etc., is to be designated as "pseudorecovery," i.e., restoration due to growth occurring in undamaged cells.

Such recovery depends on the reproductive (regenerative) power of the irradiated tissue, the dose of irradiation, the time in which this dose is given and the blood supply of the tissue. In accordance with this view is the fact that tissues most capable of recovery are those with a high power of regeneration, for example, skin and testis.

7.8 Radiosensitivity

Having outlined so far the various morphologic and functional changes produced by irradiation in a cell, the question arises whether or not all cells respond equally to the same dose of radiation. This means that we have to discuss *the problem of radiosensitivity.*

Before starting a detailed discussion of radiosensitivity it will be well to consider what is actually meant by this term.

Radiosensitivity may be defined as the relative response of two cell types, tissues, or organs to a given dose of radiation.

We shall now discuss the *factors influencing the radiosensitivity of cells and tissues:*

1. *The mitotic activity:* In multicellular organisms, cells that actively divide are generally more radiosensitive than cells that do not divide.

2. *The stage of mitosis:* The rise of sensitivity commences in prophase, increases during segmentation and migration of the segmented nucleus and attains a first maximum before division. Radiosensitivity then falls again and reaches a second maximum in the gastrula stage. The increased radiosensitivity during mitosis could be explained by the fact that chromatin exposes a larger surface to the action of rays during mitosis.

3. *The degree of differentiation:* Embryologic and immature cells are in general more radiosensitive than adult cells to which they give rise.

4. *Metabolism:* Increased cellular metabolism is accompanied by an increase in radiosensitivity. A direct parallelism between glycolytic power and radiosensitivity was demonstrated by Chevremont in the thymus and in mouse adeno-carcinomata for nucleic acid metabolism by Goldfeder.

Clinical and experimental evidence has not only brought to light the variation of radiosensitivity of cells of the same type but also considerable differences in the response of cells of different types in their reaction to irradiation. In the order of diminishing sensitivity they may be grouped as follows:

1. Lymphocytes
2. Erythroblasts, granulocytes
3. Myeloblasts
4. Epithelial cells
   (a) Basal cells of testis
   (b) Basal cells of intestinal crypts

(c) Basal cells of the ovary
(d) Basal cells of the skin
(e) Basal cells of secretory glands
(f) Alveolar cells of the lungs and bile ducts
5. Endothelial cells
6. Connective tissue cells
7. Tubular cells of the kidneys
8. Bone cells
9. Nerve cells
10. Brain cells
11. Muscle cells

The factors influencing the radiosensitivity of cells and tissues were recognized as early as 1906 by two French scientists in whose honor the summary of these facts is called the *law of Bergonié and Tribondeau*; it states: The radiosensitivity of a tissue is proportional to its reproductive capacity and inversely proportional to its degree of differentiation.

7.9 Response of Tumors to Radiation

After discussion of the response of normal cells and tissues to irradiation we shall now enter into a brief consideration of *the response of abnormal cancer tissue to irradiation.*

The particular radiosensitivity of malignant tumor cells accounts for the success of radiation therapy in this field. The law of Bergonié and Tribondeau offers the means of understanding the important role of radiations in the irradiation of malignant tumor cells.

It thus appears that the same general principles govern the radiosensitivity of normal and malignant tumor cells. But a *brief outline of the details which account for the special radiosensitivity of tumor cells seems to be necessary*:

1. *The tissue of origin:* A tumor arising from a radiosensitive tissue, e.g., a lymphatic tissue, usually is radiosensitive. These tumors are called constitutionally radiosensitive tumors. A tumor arising from a radioresistant tissue, e.g., bone tissue, is usually radioresistant and is called a constitutionally radioresistant tumor.

2. *Cataplasia:* By this is understood the sum of morphologic and biologic atypia of the tumor tissue; less differentiated tumors (that means increased metabolism!) are usually more radiosensitive.

3. *The size of a tumor:* Small tumors are usually more radiosensitive because of a better blood supply, which in turn means a more active metabolism.

4. *The site of the tumor:* e.g., squamous cell carcinoma of the larynx may behave differently from that of the uterus.

5. *The age of the patient:* Histologically similar tumors are usually less radiosensitive in older people.

6. *The general health of the patient:* Radioresistance increases in cachectic individuals.

7. *Circulation:* Anemia diminishes radiosensitivity.

8. *Hormones:* Exercise the same influences as on normal tissues.

9. *Coexistent infections,* as tuberculosis or lues, diminish radiosensitivity.

10. *Previous treatment:* Exposure to radiations not killing the tumor tissue may render even a constitutionally radiosensitive tumor radioresistant.

11. *Genetic make-up of the tumor host:* Histologically identical tumors arising at the same site of two different animal strains may differ in their radiosensitivity as much as 100 per cent (Goldfeder).

From the data presented it appears that the radiosensitivity of tumor cells and tissues is an exceedingly complex phenomenon. This makes classification of tumors in terms of absolute radiosensitivity for all practical purposes impossible.

For clinical purposes a classification according to their relative sensitivity to normal tissues is customary. From the standpoint of the clinician, a tumor is considered radiosensitive if it can be made to disappear without connective tissue necrosis, and all tumors for which the dose required for their disappearance exceeds the limit of tolerance of the connective tissue are regarded as radioresistant.

Finally, it should be emphasized that the radiosensitivity of a tumor and its malignancy do not go hand in hand, nor do radiosensitivity and radiocurability of tumors run parallel. Here, specific clinical considerations enter the picture, but their discussion is beyond the confines of this review.

The data presented in this chapter form the basis for an analysis of the more complicated actions of radiations on organ systems and the body as a whole. The detailed discussion of the organ effects will follow in the chapter on The Pathologic Anatomy of Total Body Irradiation.

REFERENCES

Note: For pertinent literature the reader is referred to F. Ellinger, *Medical Radiation Biology.* Charles C Thomas Publisher, Springfield, Illinois, 1957.

8 ▸

The Pathologic Anatomy of Total Body Irradiation

JOHN L. TULLIS, M.D.

8.1 Dosage Factors

The effects of ionizing radiations on normal and pathologic anatomy have received considerable attention in the literature. In the past most of the interest has been concerned with the results of sectional irradiation, but the use of the atomic bomb has centered attention on total body irradiation. It is important to grasp the significance of total body irradiation in contrast to localized irradiation since an amount of radiation that is well tolerated when given to a portion of the body might be sufficient to kill if administered simultaneously to the total body. For instance, 10,000 r of penetrating x-rays may be given in divided doses to a small tumor with no general reaction whatsoever and individual doses of up to 400 r may be given to an area as large as 20 x 20 cm. with no more than transient radiation sickness; but it is estimated that 200 to 600 r of total body irradiation in a single acute dose is the range of lethal dosage for man.

The lesions discussed in this chapter were produced by single exposures of the total body of human beings to large amounts (the 50 per cent lethal dose (LD_{50}) or more) of gamma radiation from an atomic bomb source and various experimental animals to large amounts (LD_{50} or more) of gamma and supervoltage X-radiations. The duration of exposure was such that there was not appreciable recovery of the tissue during the elapsed time of irradiation. The gamma and X-radiations used were of hard or penetrating type and produced similar lesions in a given species.

The biologic effects of ionizing radiations are indistinguishable qualitatively, irrespective of their mode of application, i.e., whether an external radiation or radiation from internally deposited radioactive material; and again whether of high or low voltage, provided that ionization within the tissue (absorption of energy) is achieved. Quantitative differences are due to differences in specific ionization patterns (density of ionization).

8.2 Anatomic Lesions

The anatomic lesions resulting from exposure of the total body to large doses of ionizing radiation fall into three main categories: tissue necrosis, multiple hemorrhages and secondary infections.

8.2.1 *Tissue Necrosis.* The immediate and primary effect of irradiation is the production of cellular injury, probably by means of ionization of some components of the cell. Recovery is possible if the injury is slight, but if the injury is extensive cell death occurs. While no tissue is entirely immune there are marked differences in sensitivity among the various tissues. For purposes of this discussion radiosensitive tissues are considered to be those which reveal the earliest occurring and most extensive necrosis in response to irradiation. Thus the hematopoietic and lymphoid tissues, the immature germ cells and the epithelial lining of the gastro-intestinal tract are examples of more radiosensitive tissues, while the highly differentiated tissues such as bone, nerve and muscle are more radioresistant.

8.2.2 *Hemorrhage.* There may be no external evidence of hemorrhage after low doses of radiation, but after high doses this manifestation of injury is common, particularly late in the course of the disease. The appearance of purpura in the skin and bleeding from the nose, mouth, urethra and anus are grave prognostic signs which usually first appear one or two days prior to death. Hemorrhages into the internal organs occur at about the same time and are conspicuous necropsy findings. Thrombocytopenia, increased capillary permeability, and, in the terminal stage of the disease, bacteremia, are associated with and are probably jointly responsible for the bleeding tendency or the so-called hemorrhagic phase of the disease. Only where there is erosion or ulceration of tissue, usually the result of necrosis and trauma, can actual disruption of blood vessels be seen. Such areas in the alimentary and urinary tracts are the source of external hematic loss.

8.2.3 *Infections.* Anemia, destruction of hematopoietic elements with resultant leukopenia, toxemia resulting from the accumulation of tissue breakdown products or absorption of substances or agents from the intestinal tract, and possibly interference with the antibody mechanisms act jointly to lower the resistance of the body to disease. Secondary infections are natural sequelae in this chain of events and terminal bacteremias are found consistently in untreated animals which are allowed to die spontaneously. Hemorrhagic, agranulocytic, necrotizing pneumonias were commonly seen in the Japanese and in experimental animals beginning about two weeks after irradiation. The Japanese also often developed multiple skin abscesses.

8.2.4 *Relative Radiosensitivity of Cells.* It is interesting that there is a marked difference in the ability of the various cells to withstand a given amount of ionizing radiation. It is generally conceded that lymphocytes and erythroblasts are the most sensitive cells in the body. On the other hand, the cells which are even lower in the developmental scale, the stem cells, particularly the reticular cells of bone marrow and lymph nodes, the "indifferent" cells of the swine testis, the primordial ova of the ovary, and the "resting" ameloblasts of developing teeth are among the most radioresistant cells in the body. Thus we have a situation in which the most primitive cells and the most fully developed or adult cells are the most resistant cells in the body, while the developing blast cells, those undergoing rapid change and growth, are the most sensitive to injury by ionizing radiation. It would seem that the law of Bergonié and Tribondeau, which states in general that the more highly differentiated the cell, the more radioresistant it is, should be specifically modified to include among the radioresistant cells the most undifferentiated of all cells, i.e., the primitive stem cells. The reasons for the differences in radiosensitivity are not understood.

8.3 Specific Lesions

With the foregoing comments to serve as orientation in and introduction to the subject, the specific pathologic anatomy of lesions produced by total body irradiation will be reviewed by individual organs or organ systems. Unless otherwise stated, the following remarks are applicable alike to human beings exposed to atomic bomb bursts and to certain experimental animals exposed to ionizing radiations either from atomic bombs or from high voltage X-ray sources.

8.3.1 *Bone Marrow.* Heavy doses of total body irradiation produce an effect on the bone marrow which is detectable microscopically within a few hours after exposure. Dilatation of sinusoids and cell necrosis, including pyknosis, karyorrhexis and karyolysis of nuclei, are among the early changes. All types of hematopoietic cells are involved but the blast cells are the most radiosensitive. Megakaryocytes are more sensitive than erythrocytes and granulocytes, but are probably less sensitive than myelocytes. The reticular cells are radioresistant.

The damage becomes progressively more extensive (Fig. 1). Within two weeks the marrow is depleted of most all hematopoietic cells except the reticular cells. At this time, the marrow appears red, as if it were hyperplastic, but on microscopic examination hyperemia in an aplastic

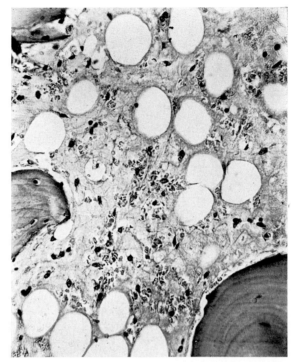

FIG. 1. Bone marrow from a Bikini swine which died 11 days following total body exposure to the ionizing radiations of the atomic bombing (Test Baker). Note the marked cellular depletion and the absence of hematopoiesis. Reticular cells, fat cells, erythrocytes and bone spicules are apparently unharmed. (× 300.)

marrow is found to be the cause of the redness seen grossly. If death does not supervene, recovery of the marrow begins before the fourth week after exposure and by the sixth week a hyperplastic marrow may be found (Fig. 2). Hyperplasia may be confined to primitive blood cells which fail to progress in the development cycle to maturity. If there is adequate marrow regeneration, survival of the host is possible, provided that secondary infections can be kept under control. However, if the bone marrow remains aplastic for as long as six weeks death almost invariably takes place.

8.3.2 *Lymph Nodes.* At first the lymph nodes may shrink below normal size, but by the end of one week they are edematous and gross hemorrhages are present in the pulp, particularly around the periphery (Fig. 3). Lymphocytes are the most radiosensitive cells in the body. Necrosis and fragmentation of these cells begin shortly after exposure to irradiation and rapidly progress for eight to ten hours after which there is only minimal further destruction. The debris is phagocytosed by macrophages which successfully

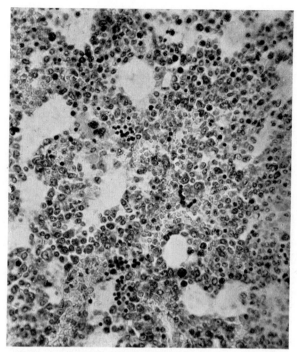

FIG. 2. Necropsy specimen showing regeneration of bone marrow in a Japanese male about nine weeks after bombing. (× 300.) (Tissue section by courtesy of Dr. S. Warren.)

clean up the nodes within twenty-four to thirty-six hours. Following the period of destruction and phagocytosis, there is an attempt at repopulation of the lymph nodes with lymphocytes, which are apparently, in part at least, newly formed cells. The recovery effort is feeble after high doses of radiation, but is appreciable after low doses. Lymph nodes in all regions of the body are involved to some extent in the destructive process, but the cervical, mediastinal, aortic and mesenteric nodes show most extensive changes.

After about one week when hemorrhages occur and the sinuses are dilated and contain numerous macrophages, phagocytosis of erythrocytes by the tissue (fixed) and circulating (free) macrophages is found in most of the nodes (Fig. 4). This process continues and is excessive for at least four weeks. It is not uncommon to find macrophages containing normal-appearing erythrocytes and clumps of blood pigment granules lying side by side. Blood pigment granules are also found lying free in areas of old hemorrhage.

The prominence of the reticular cells in the lymphocyte-depleted nodules

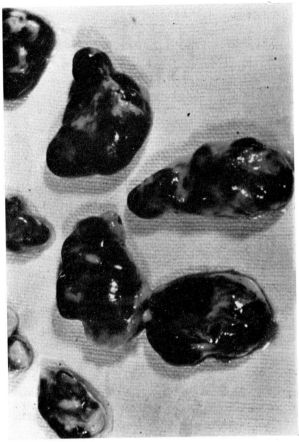

Fig. 3. Enlarged, edematous, hemorrhagic lymph nodes from a swine which died eight days after total body exposure to ionizing radiations from the atomic bombing at Bikini (Test Able).

is probably due to the destruction of the lymphocytes that ordinarily, because of their abundance, tend to obscure these cells.

After the first few days the pathologic picture may be confused as a result of lesions in other parts of the body affecting the lymph nodes. This is particularly true of regional nodes in cases of pneumonia, abscesses and oral and gastro-intestinal ulcerations. Such modifying factors must be taken into consideration when evaluating the changes. In most cases, however, the hemorrhage, edema and at least partial lymphocyte depletion persist for several weeks (Fig. 5), and even in cases which recover the lymph nodes may retain grossly visible blood pigment deposits for at least three months.

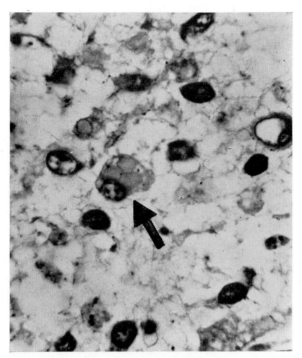

Fig. 4. Lymph node from the animal shown in Fig. 1. The arrow points to a macrophage which contains three visible erythrocytes. (× 900.)

8.3.3 *Spleen.* Grossly the spleen appears about normal in size and shape. There may be a few scattered irregular hemorrhages in the pulp. The cut surface is usually dark red and dry. After the first week malpighian corpuscles are often too small to see grossly. Microscopically the sinuses may be slightly dilated and engorged. There is a more than normal abundance of blood pigment granules deposited in the pulp. Accumulation of cellular debris rapidly followed by phagocytosis and depletion of lymphocytes in malpighian corpuscles and cords of Billroth occur in about the same manner as in the lymph nodes but to a slightly lesser degree and after a greater time lag (Fig. 6). Excessive or abnormal erythrophagocytosis is not uncommon for at least the first month after irradiation.

8.3.4 *Other Lymphoid Tissue.* The thymus, tonsils and lymphoid aggregations in the bowel (Peyer's patches) also show a marked and rapid response to irradiation because of their high lymphocyte content. The cellular depletion is similar to that seen in lymph nodes but, as in the spleen, the reaction is not quite as marked or as rapid and regeneration apparently does not begin as soon after injury, nor is it so complete. Hemorrhages

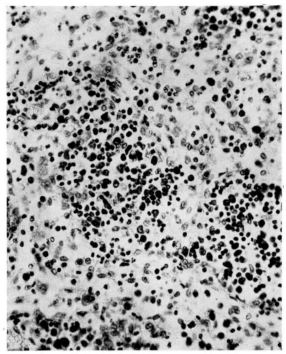

Fig. 5. A lymph node, edematous and markedly depleted of lymphocytes, from the case shown in Fig. 2. (× 300.) (Tissue section by courtesy of Dr. S. Warren.)

in the form of petechiae or small ecchymoses are frequently observed in these organs beginning usually one or two days prior to death.

8.3.5 *Mouth, Oropharynx and Nasopharynx.* In swine, as early as the fifth day after supra-lethal doses of radiation, and in human beings, in the period from three to six weeks after heavy but not overwhelming doses of radiation, agranulocytic ulcerations frequently develop in the mucous membranes. The gingival margins, buccal mucosa, and the pharyngeal tonsils are favorite sites for the shallow, ragged ulcers (Fig. 7). Microscopically the necrotic bases of the lesions contain considerable cellular detritus, perhaps some fibrin stands, but few if any inflammatory cells except when the lesions develop late. If the individual lives for four to six weeks after irradiation and the hematopoietic tissue has regenerated, there may be a low-grade cellular response to the necrosis. The ulcers are not well walled off, yet they do not ordinarily penetrate deeper than the submucosal layer.

8.3.6 *Gastrointestinal Tract.* The mucous membrane from esophagus to anus shows gross evidence of irradiation within one or two days after exposure. Vascular alterations ranging from multiple petechiae to diffuse

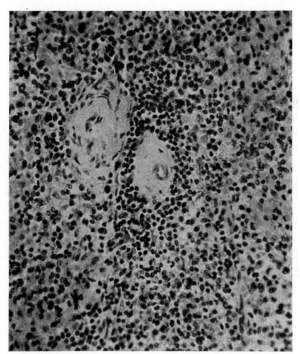

FIG. 6. Spleen from case seen in Figs. 2 and 5, showing depletion of lymphoid elements in the lymphoid nodules and marked thickening and hyalinization of the walls of the two small arteries. (× 300.) (Tissue section by courtesy of Dr. S. Warren.)

congestion appear in the lamina propria and submucosa at this time, particularly after very high doses of radiation. The walls of the stomach and the intestine become edematous, especially in the submucosal and sub-peritoneal layers. Hemorrhages and edema of the wall may occur in any part of the gastrointestinal tract (Fig. 8). Ulcerations in the epithelium may also occur anywhere, but are more likely to be in the large bowel or stomach. They sometimes appear before the fifth day in swine, but may be delayed until the sixth week after irradiation in human beings. In contrast to the gastrointestinal ulcerations that sometimes appear after intensive abdominal radiotherapy, the ulcerations resulting from total body irradiation usually extend no deeper than the muscularis mucosae or submucosa and do not perforate. The margins of the ulcers are ragged and irregular. The hemorrhagic necrotic base may be covered with a 2–3 mm. thick adherent fibrinous membrane. The intestinal ulcers tend to be elongated in the longitudinal axis of the bowel, while the stomach ulcers tend to have elevated, clearly demarcated, roughly circular margins.

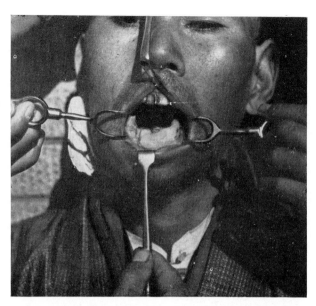

FIG. 7. Necrosis of gum and underlying mandible in a 38-year-old Japanese 12 weeks after the bombing. (Photograph reprinted from the United States Strategic Bombing Survey, "The Effects of Atomic Bombs on Health and Medical Services in Hiroshima and Nagasaki," March 1947, Fig. 49, Courtesy of the National Archives.)

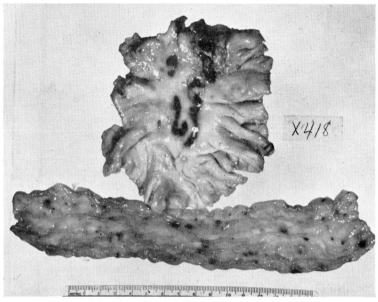

FIG. 8. Edematous large bowel, spotted with hemorrhages and edematous mesentery containing hemorrhagic lymph nodes. From a swine which died 15 days after 400 r in air, total body, 1000 kv x-irradiation, delivered bilaterally.

140

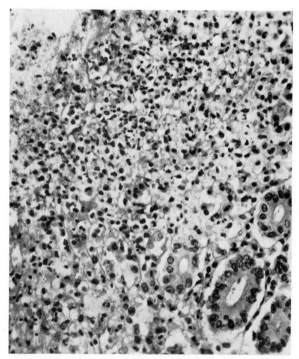

FIG. 9. Margin of an ulcer in the large intestine showing necrosis of glands and a poor cellular response to the lesion. Note also the edematous fibrin network over the ulcer bed. From a Japanese male who died about 11 weeks after the bombing. (× 300.) (Tissue section by courtesy of Dr. S. Warren.)

Microscopically the bases of the early ulcers contain practically no cellular infiltration, but after four to six weeks a few granulocytes are present (Fig. 9). The vessels of the submucosa and lamina propria in the vicinity of the ulcerations are dilated, and usually contain agglutinative or fibrin thrombi. However, there is no known relationship or sequence pattern between the ulcerations and the thrombi; in fact, no reason for the specific location of the ulcerations is apparent. Microscopic examination also discloses degenerative changes in the epithelium of the intestinal glands. This reaction begins within four hours after exposure, reaches a peak at about eight hours, and subsides before twenty-four to thirty-six hours. By this time the cellular debris has been removed and the next generation of glandular epithelium has been laid down. Vacuolation of cytoplasm or nucleus, distortion of shape and variation in size are characteristic of the epithelium in the recovery period following the acute degenerative process. These abnormalities may persist for at least four weeks in swine andt a least three months in human beings. The variation between cells in the same or neighboring glands is quite striking and these changes may take place in the absence of hemorrhage or ulceration. The large vacuolated nuclei with peripheral distribution of chromatin and prominent central nucleoli are sometimes called "owl's eye" nuclei and are characteristic of irradiated cells.

The ability of the intestinal epithelium to partially or completely recover, even after an amount of radiation that is fatal for the individual, is an interesting feature of the injury. Where severe damage to the epithelium including superficial ulceration occurs, regeneration and repair are likely to be accomplished within two weeks. If ulceration of the full thickness of epithelium, extensive hemorrhage, or overwhelming infection occur, local regeneration is, of course, not possible.

A characteristic delayed change takes place in the connective tissue cells in the submucosa (Fig. 10). About the fourth week and thereafter the fibrocytes assume bizarre, often triangular, shapes. They are larger than normal and contain two or three nuclei which are usually hyper-

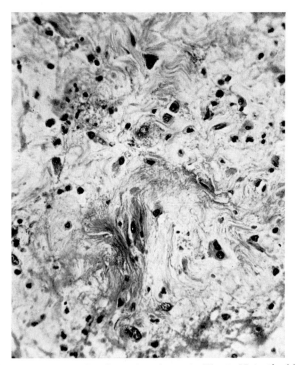

Fig. 10. Submucosa near the ulceration shown in Fig. 9. Note the bizarre, giant, multinucleated fibrocytes, edema and beginning hyalinization of the connective tissue fibers. (× 300.) (Tissue section by courtesy of Dr. S. Warren.)

chromic. Another delayed tissue reaction which may occur simultaneously with the formation of bizarre fibrocytes is hyalinization of the fibrous tissue of the submucosa. The cohesiveness of connective tissue fibers and their collection into amorphous refractile bundles is well established by the sixth to eighth week.

Early in the course of the disease before the onset of hemorrhagic manifestations the lamina propria shows a depletion of lymphocyte population and may perhaps be slightly edematous, but otherwise it is normal. Plasma cells which are relatively radioresistant become the predominent cells in the lamina propria. Later hemorrhage and ulceration entirely distort the pattern of the lamina propria.

The muscle fibers are uninvolved or contain only a few small scattered hemorrhages.

8.3.7 *Gonads.* Both the testis and the ovary are among the more radiosensitive organs in the body. The acute gross lesions in the testis are multiple petechial hemorrhages which are scattered through the interstitial tissue. Later the hemorrhages may be more extensive and impart a diffuse red color to the entire testis. Edema during this period may cause slight swelling. In the chronic stage the testis atrophies and becomes small, firm and fibrotic. Microscopically destruction of spermatogonia is evident soon after irradiation, but spermatocytes, mature sperm and Sertoli cells are more radioresistant. It should be pointed out that, in swine at least, in the immature testis the indifferent (stem) cells undergo no morphologic changes. Two or three months after irradiation thickening of the basement membrane of the tubules with hyaline changes in the connective tissue occur. At this stage the sperm that survived the original injury have been expelled and, owing to the absence of spermatogenesis, are not replaced. The tubules in the chronic stage, therefore, consist of thickened hyalinized membranes and a few Sertoli cells but no germ cells (Fig. 11). The interstitial cells of Leydig do not appear altered. When the testis shrinks as a result of atrophy the interstitial cells are prominent owing to their close proximity. They do not appear increased in absolute number.

The ovary is less radiosensitive than the testicle. Grossly there may be no changes, but occasionally there are a few scattered hemorrhages. The histologic changes consist chiefly of atresia or pyknosis of the nuclei of the developing ova. Morphologically the primordial ova are altered slightly if at all. The stroma may be slightly edematous, but the cells appear normal.

It should be emphasized that ordinary histologic methods do not disclose alterations in the chromosomes. A germ cell, for instance, may appear normal after irradiation until numerous mitoses have taken place, after which the original injury becomes apparent. The normal histologic appearance of a cell does not, therefore, guarantee absence of injury.

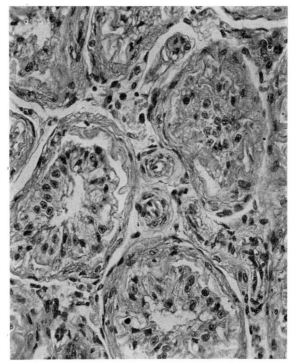

Fɪɢ. 11. Testes from the case seen in Figs. 2, 5 and 6. Note the thickened basement membrane with hyaline changes in the seminiferous tubules and the absence of germ cells. Sertoli cells and the interstitial cells of Leydig survive. (× 300.) (Tissue section by courtesy of Dr. S. Warren.)

8.3.8 *Skin.* Epilation of the scalp in the Japanese began about the second week after irradiation (Fig. 12). Epilation of the axillae, beard, pubes and eyebrows followed in that order but occurred much less commonly. Atrophy of the hair follicles occurs and is accompanied by loss of definition and merging of the several epithelial layers around the shaft and thickening and hyalinization of the basement membrane and surrounding collagen fibers. Regeneration of some of the follicles begins about the third month after irradiation, but the process is extremely slow and may extend over months or years.

Other changes observed in the skin after total body irradiation include vacuolization of nuclei and cytoplasm of the germinal layer of epidermis and, after three to six months, the appearance of bizarre, triangular, multi-nucleated giant fibrocytes in the corium. Also blood vessels in the dermis, after an initial temporary period of dilatation, contract, after which they may become permanently dilated. However, the development of permanent

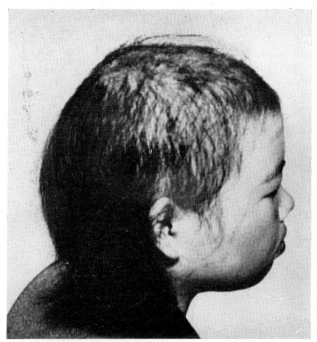

Fig. 12. Generalized epilation in a 19-year-old Japanese who had suffered generalized radiation sickness. (Photograph reprinted from the U. S. Strategic Bombing Survey, "The Effects of Atomic Bombs on Health and Medical Services of Hiroshima and Nagasaki," March 1947, Fig. 48, courtesy of the National Archives.)

dilatation of the blood vessels is more likely to be the long-term result of chronic, repeated, small-dose exposures to radiation. The skin lesions, such as atrophy of the epidermis with flattening of the rete pegs, atrophy of the sweat and sebaceous glands and permanent dilatation of the blood vessels, are the result of repeated exposure to radiation. A single dose of total body radiation sufficient to cause those changes would almost certainly kill the patient before sufficient time had elapsed to allow the changes to become manifest.

8.3.9 *Lungs.* The lungs almost always show evidence of pulmonary edema or bronchopneumonia at autopsy following death from total body irradiation. Grossly the lungs are firm, heavy, wet and contain numerous hemorrhages. Bloody fluid drips from the cut surface and the bronchi and trachea contain abundant pink froth. The chief characteristics of the lesions studied microscopically are their variability in different parts of the lung and the absence of inflammatory cellular response. The alveolar septa are usually congested and somewhat thickened (Fig. 13). The alveoli may be air-filled,

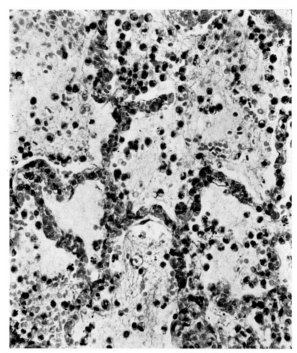

Fig. 13. Pneumonia from the case seen in Figs. 9 and 10. Note the congestion in the alveolar walls and fibrino-serous exudate in the alveoli. Macrophages are the predominant cells in the exudate, but there are also some erythrocytes and a few segmented cells. ($\times$ 300.) (Tissue section by courtesy of Dr. S. Warren.)

but most often contain serous or coagulated fluid, numerous erythrocytes and perhaps a few macrophages. Polymorphonuclear leukocytes do not appear in numbers until after the fourth to sixth week when the hematopoietic tissue, if it is going to at all, has begun to recover. The lesions are distributed in a random fashion and certain areas may contain several different types. Necrosis of the alveolar septa occurs soon after massive doses of irradiation and may occur within two weeks after the LD_{50} dose.

The bronchioles contain cell debris and exudate similar to that in the alveoli. The bronchiolar and bronchial epithelia are fairly radioresistant although some cells are desquamated. The cilia remain intact on the adherent epithelium. The peribronchial tissue may be edematous. The trachea responds in a fashion similar to the bronchi.

The pleural cavities sometimes contain clear or blood-tinged fluid but usually not in great amounts. Fibrin is present in some cases. The pleura itself is either unaltered or contains an acellular fibrinous exudate with easily separated adhesions between opposing surfaces.

In cases receiving massive amounts of radiation, the intercostal muscles are frequently the site of fairly extensive hemorrhages which are readily seen through the parietal pleura. This type of hemorrhage does not usually provoke a reaction in the parietal pleura, probably because death occurs too soon after the injury to permit much reaction to it.

8.3.10 *Heart.* Late in the course of the disease the cardiac muscle usually is spotted with hemorrhages of various sizes and of recent origin (Fig. 14). Both atria and both ventricles are involved, with no consistent preference for one area over another. Grossly the heart muscle tends to become soft and flabby, but microscopically the muscle fibers show little change.

The pericardial sac may contain a slight excess of free fluid.

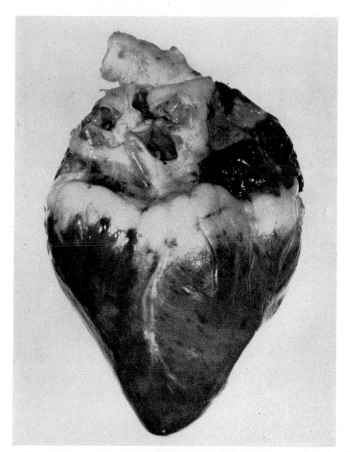

Fig. 14. Heart from a swine which died 16 days after exposure to 600 r in air, total body, 1000 kv x-irradiation, delivered bilaterally. Fresh hemorrhages are present in the myocardium of the atria and ventricles.

8.3.11 *Adrenal Gland*. Beck and Meissner, and Warren and DeCoursey have noted the loss of adrenal lipoid in the Japanese. Histologically the cells are granular and non-vacuolated. They seldom exhibit necrosis. There may be scattered hemorrhages in the cortex or medulla, but these are usually very small.

8.3.12 *Kidneys, Ureters and Bladder*. The glomerular and tubular epithelia appear to be radioresistant. Hemorrhages from the interlobular vessels may secondarily involve the adjacent tubules, but such lesions are rarely extensive. The epithelium lining calyces, pelves, ureters and bladder is less radioresistant and often appears vacuolated or desquamated. Hemorrhage into the loose lamina propria of the urinary tract is often extensive, and leads to death of superficial epithelium with subsequent erosion. This accounts for the hematuria in the last few days of life, and the blood clots found at necropsy in the kidney pelves or urinary bladder (Fig. 15).

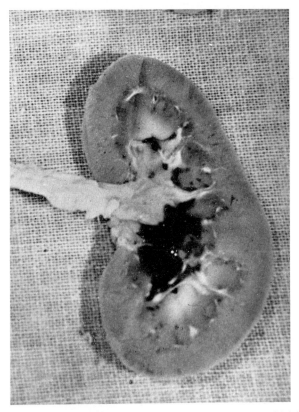

Fig. 15. Kidney from the same swine as in Fig. 3. Note the petechial hemorrhages in the cortex and medulla and the large blood clot in the pelvis.

8.3.13 *Liver and Gall Bladder.* The terminal picture in the liver following total body irradiation is usually not remarkable but infarcts and small focal necroses are sometimes seen. Reversible accumulations of sudanophil fat in the liver have been noted in many animal species. This and other observations lead Ellinger to conclude that the liver is a relatively sensitive organ.

Hemorrhages are sometimes found along the interface between the liver and the gall bladder and in the wall of the gall bladder. The epithelium of the gall bladder may show partial desquamation, but it cannot be considered as specific following irradiation. Edema of the gall bladder wall is often very extensive.

8.3.14 *Brain and Meninges.* The brain itself usually appears normal at necropsy. The dura and pia, however, may contains numerous petechial hemorrhages (Fig. 16) and occasionally there is considerable extravasation

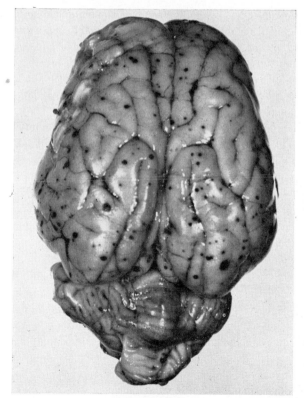

Fig. 16. Multiple petechial hemorrhages are seen in the pia-arachnoid in this brain. From a swine which died 28 days following exposure to 600 r in air, total body, 1000 kv x-irradiation delivered bilaterally.

of blood into the subarachnoid space. Microscopically there may be a few small perivascular hemorrhages and, rarely, necrosis of a nerve cell. Where the subarachnoid hemorrhage has been extensive, the underlying cortex undergoes secondary pressure necrosis.

8.3.15 *Thyroid, Salivary Glands, Pancreas, Epididymis, Fallopian Tubes, Uterus, Smooth and Striated Muscle, Bone, Cartilage and Nerve Fibers.* These organs or tissues rarely show any anatomic effects other than an occasional small hemorrhage. Since the hemorrhages are a function of capillary permeability and thrombocyte deficiencies, their presence should not in itself influence evaluation of the radiosensitivity of the organ under consideration.

8.4 Relation of Symptoms to Lesions

8.4.1 *Toxemia.* The symptoms of nausea, vomiting, headache, weakness, anorexia, edema and multiple petechial hemorrhages common to most cases of total body irradiation disease suggest toxemia. It may be assumed that the toxic substance or substances are produced by tissue necrosis which, in turn, may produce the release of histamine substances, alterations of enzyme and antibody systems and accumulation of breakdown products. There is no conclusive proof for any of these hypotheses.

8.4.2 *Anoxia and Anemia.* The pattern of shock as described by Moon, which includes in sequence capillary atony, increased capillary permeability, hemorrhage into the tissue spaces, hemoconcentration, and tissue anoxia, is probably one of the mechanisms underlying the development of the late manifestations of total body radiation disease. Anemia, resulting from a combination of cessation of erythropoiesis in the bone marrow, hematic loss into the tissues and externally through the alimentary and urinary tracts, and erythrophagocytosis add to the circulatory and cell-respiration distress. Injury to the conduction system in the myocardium is probably the terminating event in some cases.

8.4.3 *Agranulocytosis.* Indisputably evident is the cause and effect relationship of granulocytopenia to lowered resistance to disease, development of secondary infections and agranulocytic ulcerations. Less clear is the relationship of lymphocytopenia to the altered body defense mechanism. Injury to the lymphocytes may alter either antibody storage or antibody formation and thus disturb the humoral resistance to disease.

8.4.4 *Gastrointestinal Damage and Symptoms.* Injury to the gastrointestinal mucosa may play a direct part in the production of nausea, vomiting and anorexia, and it is highly probable that injury to the intestinal epithelium disturbs absorption and excretion phenomena in the alimentary tract.

8.4.5 *Sterility.* The direct relationship of the injury to the gonads and various degrees of diminution of fertility is obvious.

8.5 Diagnosis in Relation to Pathology: Summary

The lesions produced by 50 per cent or more of the lethal dose of total body irradiation are not individually pathognomonic, but when several characteristic lesions occur simultaneously, particularly when there is a known exposure to ionizing radiation, the diagnosis can be made with a fair degree of certainty. The gross necropsy findings where death occurs within a 30-day period as a result of total body irradiation include (1) one or more ulcerations in the mucous membrane of one or more parts of the alimentary tract, (2) hemorrhages ranging from petechiae to fairly extensive ecchymoses in the thoracic and abdominal viscera, (3) clotted blood in the lumen of the gastrointestinal tract and urinary tract, and (4) pulmonary edema or hemorrhagic bronchopneumonia. Histologic study reveals severe injury to the hematopoietic elements except the reticular cells, and to the intestinal and germinal epithelia. Bacterial colonies of terminal origin are found scattered through many of the tissue sections. The bone marrow appears aplastic until about the fourth week when it may begin to regenerate. Ulcerations show necrosis without inflammatory cellular response until after the bone marrow begins to regenerate when there is a poor cellular response. When pneumonia occurs the inflammatory alveolar exudate contains serum, fibrin, red blood cells and perhaps scattered macrophages, but lymphocytes and polymorphonuclear leukocytes are difficult to find. The similarity of these lesions with the lesions in cases of agranulocytosis is obvious.

8.5.1 *Pathologic and Lethal Effects.* Deaths late in the acute phase are usually the result of intercurrent infection. If survival is prolonged, there is evidence of healing in the acute lesions and alterations of a chronic nature take place. These include the lesions usually associated with repeated small doses of x-rays, namely, thickening and hyaline changes in connective tissue, the formation of bizarre giant, multinucleated fibrocytes, permanent dilatation of capillovenules and atrophy of skin and testis.

After large doses of total body irradiation, however, the chronic manifestations are at a minimum simply because life is not prolonged sufficiently for their development. The great majority of the Bikini animals died within 30 days or recovered. There were no deaths even remotely attributable to the irradiation after 90 days. The same is true of animals exposed to single, large doses of penetrating X-radiations delivered to the total body. In the Japanese radiation deaths reached a peak in three to four weeks and occurred only infrequently after eight weeks.

In general the extent and severity of the lesions produced by irradiating the total body are functions of the size of the dose administered, the energy of the source of radiations, which in turn affects the absorption and distribution of the radiation through the body, and the tolerance or resistance of the individual irradiated. Within limits the greater the dose and the energy of the source and the lower the tolerance of the individual irradiated, the shorter the latent period before signs and symptoms appear, the stormier the course, the more extensive the lesions and the more likely death will terminate the illness. Under more favorable conditions there is a better chance for repair of the injury and survival of the individual.

The great significance of severe injury to the bone marrow is indicated by the fact that the leukopenia, bacteremia, multiple hemorrhages and anemia which play such a prominent role late in the course of the disease are primarily the sequelae of hematopoietic injury. It would seem obvious that efforts to reduce mortality resulting from acute total body ionizing radiation injury should be directed toward protection and early restoration of the hematopoietic tissues.

8.6 Lesions Resulting from Radioactive Fallout

(See also Chapter 13.)

An incident has recently occurred in which a number of persons were exposed to sublethal amounts of beta and gamma radiation from a thermonuclear source. A high yield nuclear explosion in the Pacific Proving Grounds in March of 1954 resulted in a fallout of radioactive material on some of the distant downwind Marshall Islands. The inhabitants of four of the islands received a significant amount of total body radiation. As indicated in the reports of the emergency medical team which responded to the accident, a group of 64 Marshallese living on the Rongelap Atoll received a calculated air dose of gamma radiation of 175 r. Three other groups received gamma doses calculated to be 78, 69 and 14 r. The 175 r group experienced symptoms of radiation sickness and hematologic changes (see Chapter 9) similar to those noted in the low-dose casualties among the Japanese who were exposed to atomic bomb gamma radiation in 1945. Because the fallout material tended to cling to skin and hair there were manifestations of localized beta radiation injury in some of the more heavily exposed persons who did not take proper steps to decontaminate themselves. Skin lesions and epilation occurred in about 90 per cent of the 175 r group. The reactions varied depending on degree of contamination of the exposed body surface. Some were superficial epithelial lesions which became depigmented and desquamated, but tended to heal rapidly with repigmentation. Others were deeper lesions (about 20 per cent of the total) which progressed to ulceration, secondary infection and delayed healing.

Histologic study of the deep lesions biopsied in the third or fourth week after injury showed the necrosis, edema, pleomorphism, early atrophic and vascular changes characteristic of recent severe radiation damage. Pigment aberrations and some atrophic changes were present at the site of the deeper lesions one year after the injuries were sustained. Subsequent periodic medical evaluation of the exposed persons has led to the conclusion that they are in "generally good health." It is believed that no long term hazard exists. However, the Atomic Energy Commission plans to continue to evaluate the medical and genetic status of the group at intervals in an effort to establish the facts.

8.7 Delayed Effects of Exposure to Radiation

(See also Chapter 14.)

The discussion thus far has dealt chiefly with the acute pathologic effects of single, large doses of total body radiation delivered in a short period of time. Emphasis has been placed on the study of the sequence of pathologic events which culminate in the death of the exposed subject. However, not all subjects exposed to single doses in the lethal range die. The more resistant individuals tend to gradually recover from their initial illness. Other individuals survive the accumulation of large doses of radiation received in small increments by means of repeated exposures. Although exposed-recovered cases may enjoy a fair state of health for some years, the possibility of delayed radiation effects developing after single sublethal, or repeated or chronic small doses of radiation is a very real one.

8.7.1 *Shortening of Life Span.* The commonest of the late effects are those associated with an accelerated aging process and the development of diseases which are more usually found in the aging organism. Vascular and connective tissue changes in target organs result in such lesions as fibrosis of the skin, chronic pneumonitis, nephrosclerosis and focal fibrosis of myocardium, lymphoid organs and endocrine glands. Atrophy and hypoplasia are particularly prominent in skin, lymphoid organs, bone marrow and gonads. Alterations in pigment deposition are found in epidermis, hair, and internal organs such as liver and heart. Shortening of life span following single and repeated doses of radiation has been clearly shown in experimental animals. It is the result partially of the accelerated aging processes of the general nature outlined above but is also related to the induction of other diseases. Some of these such as the formation of lenticular cataracts varying from a tiny vacuole of little consequence and even reversible, to total opacity resulting in blindness, do not necessarily shorten the life span of the involved patient. Of greater consequence is the development of nephrosclerosis which may lead to hypertension with its many complications which then directly affect the life span. Also radiation injuries produced in the embryo, in germ plasm and those which lead to the induction of neoplasms have a pronounced effect on the life span of either the individual or his offspring.

8.7.2 *Genetic and Embryologic Effects.* The embryologic and genetic effects of irradiation form the subject of special study and are here mentioned only in passing. The brief treatment of the subject does not reflect the importance of this aspect of the radiation problem. The individual may sustain only a state of reduced fertility or may be rendered permanently sterile by the action of radiation on the gonads. The gametes and their precursors may be destroyed outright or may be so injured that they are incapable of fertilization or of producing a viable fetus. When the injury is such that the chromosome structure is altered but fertilization and development of the fetus are possible then genetic mutations in the offspring become possible. It is the slight but genetically transmissible injury to chromosomes which is of greatest concern to future generations and the survival of the race. The extent and magnitude of the problem are not fully understood, particularly with regard to human beings.

We are on somewhat firmer ground when considering the effects of radiation on the embryo. It has been known for some years that pregnant mothers whose gravid uteri were irradiated might deliver abnormal or malformed infants. Of 4400 pregnant women exposed to irradiation from the atomic bomb, 33 were delivered of children with microcephaly. This type of deformity which is associated with mental retardation in many cases may also occur following relatively small amounts of x-radiation directed to the pregnant uterus. If the original injury is too extensive, death of the embryo with abortion or miscarriage results. Hicks has worked out a "developmental timetable" by means of irradiating experimental animals at precise stages of their embryonic development. The type and degree of malformations in offspring depend upon the stage of development at the time of exposure to irradiation and the dose of radiation received.

8.7.3 *Induction of Tumors.* Numerous laboratory investigations have proved beyond doubt the cause-and-effect relationship of ionizing radiations and a wide spectrum of neoplasms. Furth and his colleagues have written several reviews which summarize the literature in this field. Only a few pertinent points will be mentioned here.

Pioneers in the medical uses of x-rays and early research workers using radio-active materials sometimes exposed themselves, particularly their hands, with abandon to what were at first considered to be harmless radiations. It was soon discovered, however, that after repeated exposures and a variable time lapse the skin develops a painful, refractory dermatitis. The involved skin is apt to break down and ulcerate. The ulcers are slow to heal and if healing is accomplished there is marked fibrosis and atrophy of dermis and epidermis. There is a tendency for persisting x-ray ulcerations to become malignant. The first radiation-induced epidermoid carcinomas of the skin in a radiologist were described in 1902 just seven years after the discovery of x-rays. Many others among the pioneer workers with the then new diagnostic and therapeutic agent died from the cancers that developed as delayed effects of the ionizing radiations. That many years may lapse between the time of radiation exposure and the development of malignant neoplasms is an evident but unexplained fact. After latent periods of 15 years or more following the first exposure, bone tumors developed in some of the radium dial painters who repeatedly ingested very small amounts of bone-seeking radium and thorium by repeated "tipping" of their brushes between their lips. Cancer of the lung ranks high among the causes of death in the pitchblende miners of Joachimsthal and Schneeberg. The average latent period before development of the tumors is 17 years. Iatrogenic tumors have been related to the use of radium waters in the treatment of arthritis and the use of thorotrast for diagnostic purposes. To date, no carcinomas that can be directly related to exposure to atomic bomb radiation have been discovered among the Japanese.

8.7.4 *Induction of Leukemia.* This subject is fully discussed together with other hematologic sequelae in Chapter 9. For the sake of completeness mention is made here of the fact that the Atomic Bomb Casualty Commission survey in Japan has disclosed a significant increase in the number of leukemias in the bombed as compared with the control population. Two other studies emphasize the leukemogenic properties of ionizing radiations in man. Warren's recent survey of the incidence of leukemia among radiologists strongly suggests that it is for them an occupational hazard of significant proportions. Further, a recent report from England indicates that patients treated for ankylosing spondylitis with intensive wide-field x-radiation of the spine have a significantly higher incidence of leukemia than the general population.

8.8 Summary of Delayed Effects

It is obvious that tissue responses to radiation may become evident after variable latent periods following exposure. Like the acute effects, the delayed effects depend upon the interaction of many factors including the dose, dose rate, physical type, energy and site of action of the radiations and the resistance of the host. The onset may be insidious with the clinical effect becoming apparent only after a multitude of minor alterations have accumulated in sufficient number over a period of time to effectively tax the physiologic reserve of the host. The accelerated aging process is a mechanism of this type. Some late lesions are readily observable from the onset as in the skin. Because they interfere with the host's comfort or body economy early in their development, as is the case in the formation of cataracts, the latent period can be established with some degree of certainty. The facts remain, however, that the dose-latent period-effect relationships are not well understood. We do not know what a safe dose of radiation is, if indeed, any dose however small is truly innocuous. Nor do we know how long it may take for certain radiation effects to make themselves known. This is particularly true when we consider the germ plasm and injuries to it of a degree that is genetically transmissible and not outright lethal.

Ionizing radiations are potent agents capable of producing a wide range of tissue reactions. Many of these reactions are not understood, some are unknown, others will not become apparent until several generations after the injury. The great boon to the health and welfare of mankind that became available when x-rays and atomic energy became available will remain a boon, in the physicians' usage, only so long as the agents are employed with skill, knowledge, care and when fully justified by the medical needs of the particular case at hand.

REFERENCES

General:

BERGONIE, J. AND TRIBONDEAU, L.: *Compt. rend. Acad. sc., 143:* 983–985, 1906.

CRONKITE, E. P. AND BOND, V. P.: Effects of radiation on mammals, *Ann. Rev. Physiol., 18:* 483–526, 1956.

DESJARDINS, A. U.: The radiosensitiveness of cells and tissues and some medical implications. *Arch. Surg., 26:* 926–942, 1932.

ELLINGER, F.: *Biologic Fundamentals of Radiation Therapy,* New York, Elsevier, 1941.

FURTH, J. AND UPTON, A. C.: Vertebrate radiobiology: Histopathology and carcinogenesis, *Ann. Rev. Nuc. Science, 3:* 303–338, 1953.

HOLLAENDER, A. (Editor): High Energy Radiation, Parts 1 and 2, pp. 1265. In: *Radiation Biology,* Vol. I. New York: McGraw-Hill, 1954.

LEA, D. E.: Actions of Radiations on Living Cells, Second Edition, pp. 416, Cambridge, 1955.

Medical Research Council: *The Hazards to Man of Nuclear and Allied Radiations.* London: Her Majesty's Stationery Office, 1956.

MOON, V. H., KORNBLUM, K., AND MORGAN, D. R.: The nature and pathology of radiation sickness, *J. A. M. A. 116:* 489–493, 1941.

PACKARD, C.: Biologic effects of roentgen rays and radium, Chapter XVIII in: *Science of Radiology,* Springfield, Ill.: Thomas, 1933.

ROLLESTON, H.: Critical review, harmful effects of irradiation (X-rays and radium), *Quart J. Med., 24:* 101–131, 1930.

WARREN. S., *et al.*: Effects of radiation on normal tissues, a series of articles in: *Arch. Path., 34:* 1942, and *35:* 1943.

WARREN, S.: Histopathology of radiation lesions, *Physiol. Rev., 24:* 225-238, 1944.

Japanese:

BECK, J. S. P. AND MEISSNER, W. A.: Radiation effects of the atomic bomb among the natives of Nagasaki, Kyushu. *Am. J. Clin. Path., 16:* 586–592, 1946.

DeCOURSEY, ELBERT: Human pathologic anatomy of ionizing radiation effects of the atomic bomb explosions, *Mil. Surgeon, 102:* 427–432, June 1948.

LeROY, G. V.: The medical sequelae of the atomic bomb explosion, *J. A. M. A., 134:* 1143–1148, 2 Aug. 1947.

LIEBOW, AVERILL A., WARREN, SHIELDS, AND DeCOURSEY, ELBERT: Pathology of atomic bomb casualties, *Am. J. Path., 25:* 853–1027, 1949.

OUGHTERSON, A. W. AND WARREN, S. (Editors): Medical Effects of the Atomic Bomb in Japan. Division VIII, Vol. 8, 477 pp. National Nuclear Energy Series. New York: McGraw-Hill, 1956.

TSUZUKI, MASAO: Report on the medical studies of the effects of the atomic bomb, Appendix No. 9 in General Report of the Atomic Bomb Casualty Commission, National Research Council, Washington, D. C., 1947.

United States Strategic Bombing Survey, Medical Division: The Effects of Atomic Bombs on Health and Medical Services in Hiroshima and Nagasaki, Washington, D. C., U. S. Government Printing Office, 1947.

United States Strategic Bombing Survey, Source material on file at the National Archives, Washington, D. C.

WARREN, SHIELDS: The Pathologic Effects of an Instantaneous Dose of Radiation, *Cancer Res., 6:* 449–453, 1946.

Experimental, Atomic Bomb:

TULLIS, JOHN L., LAMSON, B. G., AND MADDEN, S. C.: Pathology of swine exposed to total body gamma radiation from an atomic bomb source, *Am. J. Path., 31:* 41–71, 1955.

TULLIS, JOHN L., AND WARREN, SHIELDS: Gross autopsy observations in the animals exposed at Bikini, *J. A. M. A., 134:* 1155–1158, 2 Aug. 1947.

TULLIS, JOHN L.: Radioresistant cells in certain radiosensitive tissues of swine exposed to atomic bomb radiation, *Arch. Path., 48:* 171–177, 1949.

TULLIS, JOHN L.: The response of tissues to total body irradiation, *Am. J. Path., 25:* 829–852, September 1949.

Experimental, General:

ALLEN, J. G., AND JACOBSEN, L. O.: Hyperheparinemia: cause of the hemorrhagic syndrome associated with total body exposure to ionizing radiation, *Science, 105:* 388–389, Apr. 1947

ALLEN, J G., SANDERSON, M., KIRSCHON. A., AND JACOBSON, L. O.: Hyperheparinemia (?): An anticoagulant in the blood of dogs with hemorrhagic tendency after total body exposure to roentgen rays, *J. Exper. Med., 87:* 71–86, Jan. 1948.

BLOOM, WILLIAM: *Histopathology of Irradiation from External and Internal Sources,* New York, McGraw-Hill, 1948.

BRECHER, G., ENDICOTT, K. M., GUMP, H., AND BRAWNER, H. P.: Effects of X-ray on lymphoid and hematopoietic tissues of albino mice, *Blood, 3:* 1259–1274, 1948.

DE BRUYN, P. P. H.: The effect of X-rays on the lymphatic nodule, with reference to the dose and relative sensitivities of different species, *Anat. Rec., 101:* 373–405, 1948.

HENSHAW, P. S. · Experimental roentgen injury I, II, III, *J. Nat. Cancer Inst.*, *4:* 477–512, Apr. 1944.

HICKS, S. P., WRIGHT, K. A., AND LEIGH, K. E.: Time-intensity factors in radiation response. 1. The acute effects of megavolt electrons (cathode rays) and high- and low-energy x-rays with special reference to the brain, *Arch. of Path.*, *61:* 226–238, 1956.

TESSMER, C. F., AND TULLIS, JOHN L.: The gross and histopathologic changes in swine exposed to 1000 kv x-irradiation, Project NM 007 039, unpublished data, Nav. Med. Res. Inst.

TULLIS, JOHN L., TESSMER, C. F., CRONKITE, E. P., AND CHAMBERS. F. W., JR.: The lethal dose of total body x-ray irradiation in swine, *Radiology, 52:* 396–400, March 1949.

TULLIS, JOHN L.: The sequence of pathologic changes in swine exposed to the LD100/30 of total body super-voltage X-radiation,. *Mil Surg.*, *109:* 271–280, Oct. 1951.

TULLIS, JOHN L., CHAMBERS, F. W., JR., MORGAN, J. E., AND ZELLER, JOHN H.: Mortality in swine and dose distribution studies in phantoms exposed to super-voltage roentgen radiation, *Am. J. Roentgenol.*, *67:* 620–627, April 1952.

ZIRKLE, R. E., *et al.*: The Plutonium Project (a series of articles comprising a symposium), *Radiology, 49:* 269–365, Sep. 1947.

Fallout in the Marshall Islands:

CRONKITE, E. P., BOND, V. P., CONRAD, R. A., SHULMAN, N. R., FARR, R. S., COHN, S. H., DUNHAM, C. L., AND BROWNING, L. E.: Response of human beings accidentally exposed to significant fall-out radiation. *J. A. M. A.*, *159:* 430–434, 1955.

CRONKITE, E. P., BOND, V. P., AND DUNHAM, C. L. (Editors): Some effects of ionizing radiation on human beings, TID 5358, U. S. Atomic Energy Commission, 1956.

Delayed Effects

AUB, J. C., EVANS, R. D., HEMPLEMANN, L. H., AND MARTLAND, H. S.: The late effects of internally-deposited radioactive materials in man, *Medicine, 31:* 221–329, 1952.

BRUES, A. M.: Ionizing Radiations and Cancer. Edited by J. P. Greenstein and A. Haddow, In *Advances in Cancer Research, 2:* 177–95. New York: Acad. Press, 1954.

FINKEL, M. P. AND HIRSCH, G. M. Progress Report: The incidence of malignant bone tumors in the long-term toxicity experiments with uranium, plutonium, and radium. Argonne Nat. Lab. ANL-4794, pp. 71–81, 1952.

FURTH, J. AND TULLIS, JOHN L.: Carcinogenesis by radioactive substances, *Cancer Res.*, *16:* 5–21, 1956.

FURTH, J. AND LORENZ, E.: Carcinogenesis by ionizing radiations. Edited by A. Hollaender, In: *Radiation Biology, 1:* 1145–1201. New York: McGraw-Hill, 1954.

FURTH, J., UPTON, A. C., CHRISTENBERRY, K. W., BENEDICT, W. H., AND MOSHMAN, J.: Some late effects in mice of ionizing radiation from an experimental nuclear detonation, *Radiology, 63:* 562–70, 1954.

LANGE, R. D., MOLONEY, W. C., AND YAMAWAKI, T.: Leukemia in atomic bomb survivors. I. General Observations, *Blood, 9:* 574–85, 1954.

LOONEY, W. B., COLODZIN, M., HURSCH, J. B., STEDMAN, L. T., ARNOLD, J. S., AND RUNDO, J.; Thorotrast Administration—A quarter century review, In preparation.

LOONEY, W. B. AND WOODRUFF, L. A.: Investigation of radium deposition in human skeleton by gross and detailed autoradiography, *Arch. Path.*, *56:* 1–12, 1953.

LORENZ, E.: Radioactivity and lung cancer; a critical review of lung cancer in the miners of Schneeberg and Joachimsthal, *J. Nat. Cancer Inst.*, *5:* 1–15, 1944.

LORENZ, E.: Some biologic effects of long continued irradiation, *Am. J. Roentgenol.*, *63:* 176–85, 1950.

MARTLAND, H. S.: The occurrence of malignancy in radio-active persons, *Am. J. Cancer*, *15:* 2435–2516, 1931.

MOLONEY, W. C. AND LANGE, R. D.: Leukemia in atomic bomb survivors. II. Observations on early phases of leukemia, *Blood*, *9:* 663–85, 1954.

TULLIS, JOHN L.: Long-range follow-up study in man of the harmful effects of medical and occupational exposures to ionizing radiations, Arch. Path., In press.

WARREN, S. (Chairman): Report of the Committee on Pathologic Effects of Atomic Radiation, Publication 452, Nat'l Acad. Sciences, Nat'l Res. Council, 1956.

9 ▸

The Hematology of Ionizing Radiation

EUGENE P. CRONKITE, M.D., V. P. BOND, M.D., Ph.D. AND
R. A. CONARD, M.D.

9.1 Scope and Status

The advent of the atomic era has been a great stimulus to research in
the field of hematology. This is quite understandable because changes in
the blood and blood-forming organs, imperfect indices though they may
be, still remain the most sensitive biological evidences for excessive exposure
to penetrating ionizing radiations. Within this chapter will be considered
the more common changes that are induced within blood and blood-forming
organs by acute and chronic exposure to ionizing radiations.

9.1.1 *Early Reports.* These changes have been studied extensively since
the early part of this century. Despite this, a diverse mass of data exists
in the literature, arising primarily from the inability of the early investigators to describe and measure adequately the dosage of ionizing radiation;
accordingly, there are many conflicting reports. However, the original
reports of Heinecke, 1903–5, remain qualitatively correct as does the
excellent report on blood changes in patients undergoing therapeutic irradiation (Minot and Spurling). An excellent analytic review up to 1942 is that
of Dunlap in Warren's general review. Since then there have been various
general dissertations on the relation of hematopoiesis to the effects of ionizing radiation (Jacobson, Lawrence, et al., and Osgood).

9.2 Cause of Discrepancies in Data

In addition to the discrepancies in dosage measurements, the differences in species sensitivity and response were not appreciated until the
last two decades. Of particular importance is the fact that many investigators were not aware of the difference between the pictures produced by uniform total body exposure, unequal total body exposure, and that produced

by partial body exposure. Complete or partial shielding of a portion of the body will greatly increase the amount of radiation that can be tolerated. Many of the phenomena that have been described for irradiation of portions of the body can be produced only by amounts of radiation that are greatly in excess of the amount of radiation that will kill one hundred per cent of the animals. For example, many of the characteristic histologic lesions of the gastrointestinal tract produced by local irradiation do not develop with amounts of radiation that produce a 100% mortality when the entire body is uniformly and simultaneously irradiated. The response of the peripheral blood is particularly altered. In a general sense, 300 r in a single dose to the entire body will give the same hematologic response as more than 600 r to the skeletal areas when the abdomen is shielded. These preliminary remarks express the opinion of the authors in emphasizing the futility of comparing hematologic responses unless the dosage factors, location and volume of tissue injured are accurately known. Total absorption of radiation energy as measured by the gram/roentgen is not satisfactory either, because the distribution of the absorbed energy throughout the body, in part, determines the response to the total energy absorbed (see also Chapter 10). Therefore, the remarks in this chapter will be largely limited to the effects on the blood produced by evenly distributed, penetrating, ionizing radiations of the same type to the whole body of animals. This type of experiment can be readily duplicated. However, it must be appreciated that these conditions may not approximate the conditions of radiation during an atomic bomb explosion. For example, there may be considerable shielding of various portions of the body by concrete and structural steel after detonation of an atomic bomb over an urban area. Regardless of that fact, this type of laboratory study affords a starting point for study of radiation phenomena of the whole animal that will serve as a point from which one can begin to extrapolate to man. This discussion further will be generally limited to the sublethal and zero to 100 per cent lethal range.

Since the purpose of presenting this material is to provide a more complete background by which one might better understand and prophesy from animal data what changes may be anticipated in the blood of man after an atomic bomb explosion, it would be desirable if the radiation from atomic bombs were uniform and monochromatic. Unfortunately, diverse rays of various energies and unequal shielding by buildings, heavy machinery and miscellaneous intervening objects in an urban area will produce a shadowing effect and unequal depth doses in the body of man and give, in many instances, unequal total body exposure to the spectrum of ionizing radiation produced by an atomic explosion. In addition, the energy of the scattered radiation will be a function of the scattering medium.

9.3 Mechanism of Injury

The mechanism by which the cellular changes take place has been the source of considerable research. Changes in the hematopoietic system are obviously a response to the basic effects of ionizing radiation upon protoplasm in general. These effects are considered in separate chapters (see Chapters 7 and 8). The problem of radiosensitivity of blood cells in the peripheral blood in contrast to cells in the hematopoietic organs, particularly the stem cells, has been investigated at length. At the present time there is no good evidence that the mature cells in the peripheral blood are significantly affected by amounts of radiation in the sublethal and 0–100 per cent lethal range (roughly 0–1000 r will cover all mammalian species), with the probable exception of lymphocytes. All the evidence indicates that changes in the peripheral blood are the direct and indirect results of injury to the formative cells in the hematopoietic organs. In the higher dose ranges hematopoiesis is stopped, at least temporarily. From about the LD_{50} (that dose which kills 50 per cent within a given time limit) down hematopoiesis is impaired for a variable time.

9.3.1 *Direct and Abscopal Effects.* The problem of direct versus indirect injury of the hematopoietic organs has interested many workers and as yet has not been satisfactorily answered. Kornblum, Boerner and Henderson state that partial body radiation, as in therapy, has both a direct and an indirect effect upon the peripheral blood and organs of hematopoiesis. The indirect effect upon non-irradiated parts is presumably mediated through circulating toxic products. Similar indirect effects have been alluded to by many other workers. Osgood, by virtue of a bone marrow culture technique, concluded that there were no indirect effects. Barnes and Furth, using parabiotic animals, concluded that there was a slight but definite indirect effect on the non-irradiated rat of the parabiotic pair. Lawrence and associates, in a complete analysis of the problem, reviewed the existing literature and presented evidence, based on cross-circulation experiments, that led them to believe that there is no good evidence for the presence of circulating toxins that significantly affect the peripheral blood. It is the opinion of these writers that the subject is not settled but the weight of the evidence today strongly suggests that there is no circulating "leukotoxin" that acts in a destructive manner on the blood and organs of hematopoiesis or other tissues. The use of the term "indirect" by biologists has been questioned by Mole since chemists have priority on its use in a manner distinctly different from the way in which it has been used by biologists. Chemists use it to describe the effects of radiation mediated by the products of irradiation of water (the chemical effects of free radicals, peroxides, etc.). Accordingly, Mole has coined the term "abscopal" to describe effects taking place remotely from the site of irradiation. The problem of abscopal effects has been investigated by Raventos and Bond et al. The latter group concluded that abscopal effects, such as spleen, thymus and adrenal weight changes, develop only if and when the irradiation given imposed a severe stress on the animal as indicated by gross illness. Under such conditions, changes in spleen, thymus and adrenal weights are characteristic of the stress syndrome.

Edelman et al. have reported evidence for the existence of a radiotoxin in irradiated animals. Similar experiments were repeated by Campo et al. and no evidence was found for existence of a toxic effect in serum from irradiated animals as measured by mortality or splenic thymic weight decrease in animals transfused with serum obtained from irradiated animals. These experiments do not support the concept but negative experiments do not eliminate the possibility of a radiotoxin.

9.4 Rate of Change in Peripheral Counts

The rate of change of various elements in the peripheral blood is related to the usual life span of the blood cell. Hence the rate of change in the level of the particular cells in the peripheral blood following radiation injury, when production is impaired, or ceases, is the result of the balance between the rate of utilization and rate of production. In the case of the red blood cell of man, which has a life span of about 125 days—a much longer life span that all of the other formed elements—changes in the red blood cell level take place at a much slower rate than white cells or platelets. In man, if all red cell formation were to cease, there would be a daily deficit of about 0.83 per cent of the total red cell mass (Wintrobe). The turnover of platelets, granulocytes and lymphocytes is not known with certainty. Platelets are reported to have a life span of perhaps 4 to 5 days (Lawrence and Valentine). Granulocytes reputedly have a life span of 3 to 5 days (Adams, Saunders and Lawrence). Lymphocytes are extremely short lived, with a life measured in hours (Lawrence, Ervin and Wetrick). Hamilton and Osgood, however, report a life span for some lymphatic cells of the order of 100 days which is not widely accepted. Except in the high dose ranges, where all hematopoietic activity stops, the rate of disappearance or decrease in the number of white cells will be slower than the theoretic rate of utilization. This latter will be true only if the rate of utilization is normal after irradiation in the lethal range. Irradiation in the lethal range may either directly or indirectly increase the rate of utilization. For example, the animals become susceptible to infection, and the development of frank infections will definitely increase the rate of utilization. Thus the rates of utilization that are measured in an irradiated animal may at times give values that are greater than the normal utilization. In the case of platelets, this does not seem to be the case.

9.5 Sensitivity Factor

There is considerable difference in the radiosensitivity of the stem cells. Precursors of erythrocytes (Bloom and Bloom) and lymphocytes (Warren) are extremely sensitive to ionizing radiation. The precursors of the granulocytic series are apparently less radiosensitive. Megakaryocytes appear relatively undiminished in number in the bone marrow of dogs exposed to lethal amounts of radiation for a period of 3 to 4 days after irradiation. In fact, megakaryocytes are still seen on the third day in the bone marrow of dogs exposed to 3000 r of 2.0 mev total body x-ray, an amount of radiation that is about seven times the hundred per cent lethal dose for dogs. In general, the immature and proliferating blood cells are more sensitive to irradiation than the adult blood cells. However, the reticuloendothelial cell, the common ancestor for all blood cells, is remarkably radioresistant. In other words, radiosensitivity of the blood forming cell seems to go through a maximum in the course of maturation (fig. 1). Under normal conditions, the actively proliferating cells are the more radiosensitive. This last statement apparently does not hold for all conditions. Investigations by Jacobson et al. have shown that extremely hyperplastic erythroid tissue is markedly radioresistant. In addition, Tullis has presented histologic evidence that there are exceptions to the law of Bergonie and Tribondeau. It seems that the radioresistance of the reticuloendothelial cell and of

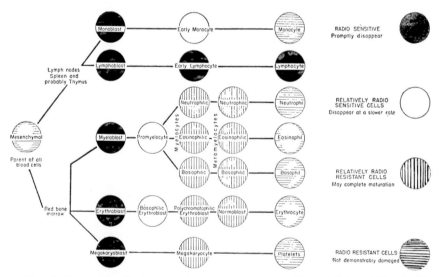

Fig. 1. Diagrammatic presentation of the relative radiosensitivity of blood cells and their precursors (based on animal data).

hyperplastic erythroid tissue challenges in part the classical law of Bergonie and Tribondeau. This law states, "The biological action of roentgen rays is greater the higher the reproductive activity of the cell, the longer the period of its mitosis, and the less the degree of differentiation of the cell in respect to its morphology and function."

Recovery of the stem cells, their reproductive rate, the release from the marrow and the rate of destruction determine the reappearance rate of the peripheral elements. It may take many months for the number of cells in the peripheral blood to return to pre-irradiation levels (figs. 2 and 3). Why the peripheral level of leukocytes is sometimes set at a lower level for a long period is not known. Perhaps the release mechanism is altered. In this respect, Brecher et al. and Cronkite et al. have shown that the level of blood cells in the peripheral blood of the mouse recovering from radiation injury is not a good index of the activity of the hematopoietic organs. For example, there may be extremely active hematopoiesis with persistent low levels of leukocytes in the peripheral blood. Residual injury of the formative cells may be manifested by the late appearance of blood dyscrasias. Similar delay in recovery was seen in the Marshallese (see par. **9.6.5**).

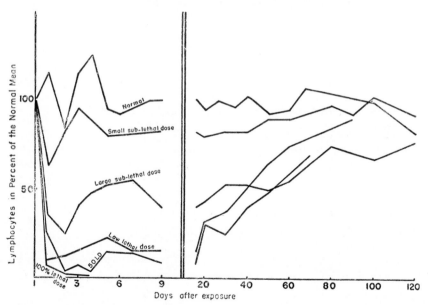

FIG. 2. Diagrammatic presentation of the rate of change in peripheral lymphocytes following various doses of penetrating ionizing radiation. (50 LD is the dose that kills 50 per cent within 30 days; 100 per cent lethal doses kill 100 per cent usually within 10 days.)

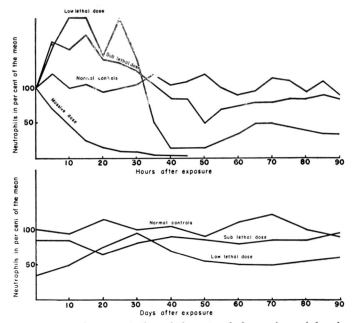

FIG. 3. Diagrammatic presentation of the rate of change in peripheral granulo-cytes following various doses of penetrating ionizing radiation. Sublethal and low lethal dose changes are based on rabbit work of Jacobson. Massive dose (100 per cent fatal within 72 hours) is based on Bikini animal data. Upper graph shows changes during the first 90 hours. Lower graph shows subsequent recovery period in days.

9.6 Variations in Number and Morphology of Blood Cells

Specific changes in the morphology and number of cells in the peripheral blood have been extensively studied. Particular attention has been paid to the relationship of dosage to the magnitude and rate of changes in the blood. The changes that take place after a single exposure to ionizing radiation will be considered first. Jacobson and associates have studied extensively the effect of single doses of different magnitude upon the blood of rabbits. All mammals seem to follow the same general pattern, except for some differences in the rate of change.

LeRoy has described the hematologic changes that were observed in the Japanese casualties at Hiroshima and Nagasaki. These changes will not be discussed in detail because the dosage factors and the general health of the Japanese are unknown factors. However, the general responses of the Japanese in respect to blood are comparable to that which has been seen in laboratory animals in most respects, with the exception that the tem-poral relationships appear different. It seems that it look a longer time for the Japanese casualties to reach the minimum leukocyte levels than it does in laboratory animals. The reader is referred to this excellent critical study of the hematology of atomic bomb casualties by LeRoy and to the report of the hematological findings in the Marshallese exposed to fallout radiation (Bond et al.).

9.6.1 *Lymphocytes.* Lymphocytes are particularly sensitive to radiation. *In vitro* studies by Schrek show that there is an increased rate of destruction of normal lymphocytes after exposure to as little as 50 r. One of five suspensions of lymphocytic leukemic cells was relatively insensitive to x-ray. Schrek, in further studies, decided that, "x-rays accelerate a normal metabolic process in lymphocytes. The degeneration of irradiated and non-irradiated cells results from the development of single or multiple focal intranuclear areas of hydration."

The lymphocyte levels in the blood begin to decrease immediately after exposure. The magnitude and the rate of change are closely related to the amount of radiation received, particularly in the sub-lethal dose range. In the higher dose ranges the rate of disappearance of lymphocytes probably approaches the rate of utilization because production has been completely stopped; or disappearance may exceed the normal rate of utilization because the diffuse cellular injury may increase the demand for lymphocytes and their metabolic end products. Thus it is easy to understand why changes in the lymphocyte levels can only be used in estimating sub-lethal exposure. Once all hematopoietic activity is stopped, changes become in part a function of normal utilization except when the dosage is so great that the cells are destroyed directly in the peripheral circulation. In rabbits (Jacobson et al.) a maximum decrease of about 25% in the lymphocyte count is detected 24 hours after exposure to 25 r. Recovery appears within two days. The greater the dosage, the greater the depression in the lymphocytes. At 800 r, a depression of 90% occurs in the first 24 hours. At a dosage of 800 r ($LD_{50/30}$) (that dose which kills 50 per cent of the animals within 30 days) recovery in the rabbit takes about 50 days from the time of the exposure. Between the 3rd and the 5th days after exposure, there is a temporary tendency for the lymphocytes to increase in number. This is followed by a decrease to almost the maximum depression that was present 24 to 72 hours after exposure (fig. 2). This type of recovery followed by a wave of destruction, is, in general, characteristic of all blood cells and tissues (Jacobson et al., Bloom). Similar changes were observed in swine exposed to 1000 kvp x-ray in various dosages, and in dogs after 2000 kvp x-ray (Cronkite et al.).

9.6.2 *Granulocytes.* *In vitro* studies on granulocytes have demonstrated that both the normal granulocytes and myelogenous leukemic cells are resistant to x-ray after doses of 1000 r (Schrek).

Changes in the number of granulocytes in the peripheral blood follow a different course (fig. 3). In general, all animals respond with a period of granulocytosis predominantly neutrophilic or heterophilic (rabbits) during the first 24 to 48 hours after exposure to amounts of radiation in the sub-lethal and lethal range. This granulocytosis appears as two peaks in the rabbit at about 12 and 18 hours after exposure. The first peak may represent mobilization of granulocytes throughout the body. The second peak may be due to accelerated liberation of cells from the bone marrow. The granulo-cytosis usually does not last for more than 24 hours but may last longer in some species and under certain conditions. Granulocytic responses have not been observed in the dog throughout the entire lethal dose range and after supra-lethal amounts of radiation. A definite granulocytosis, however, appears during the first 24 hours but the biphasic response of the rabbit was not observed. Generally, the maximum depression of the granulocytes is attained by 72 to 96 hours after exposure. Recovery of the granulocyte levels begins by 10 to 15 days after exposure, or sooner with small doses. In general, if granulocyte levels do not increase or remain constant, even though at a low level, by the 15th day, death usually ensues (Cronkite). As a rule, there are one or more abortive rises in the granulocytes that appear between the third and 12th days after exposure, depending on the animal species and the dose of radiation. This abortive rise is fairly con-sistent and apparently has little prognostic value. It may last for only 24 hours. The cause of this abortive rise in leukocytes is not well understood. It may be comparable to the waves of regeneration and destruction that have been described for other organs (Bloom). It has not been seen above LD_{80} in dogs and swine. Various explanations have been offered. Somatic mutations of precursors that result in abnormal progeny have been con-sidered (Bloom and Jacobson). These progeny or their precursors may have shorter life spans. There is no satisfactory explanation to date for this phenomenon.

9.6.3 *Erythrocytes.* Changes in the level of the red blood cells are much less striking in the early period after irradiation in the mid-lethal dose range. There is little increase during the first few days. In animals that survive radiation in the 0 to 100% lethal range there is a definite decrease in the levels of the red cell count, hematocrit readings and hemoglobins between the 10th and 30th days after exposure. The maximum degree of anemia is usually reached around the 15th to 20th days in the survivors. In the animals which do not survive, there is usually a marked decrease in the red cell levels a day or so before death. The decrease in the red cells are due to three factors: (1) decrease or cessation of production of red cells; (2) increased destruction; (3) hemorrhage (Warren; Jacobson et al.; Cronkite, Schwarz et al.; Davies et al.). The occasional macrocytosis that is seen in swine and other animals about 10 to 20 days after exposure to a low lethal dose is due to a concomitant reticulocytosis occurring as a result of regeneration of the bone marrow with release of large numbers of reticulocytes in the peripheral blood (Cronkite).

An increase in the number of the red cells is uncommon except in the high dose range, as was seen at Bikini during the atomic bomb test. There were some animals that developed a marked hemoconcentration within a few days of the exposure (fig. 4). The hematocrit of one goat attained a value of almost 80%. This hemoconcentration is due to dehydration resulting from anorexia, diarrhea, etc.

Nucleated red blood cells appeared in large numbers in the goats and swine about 13 to 17 days after exposure to the atomic bomb radiation at Bikini (Cronkite). Comparable observations have been made on other animals (Warren; Jacobson et al.; Kromeker).

Reticulocyte disappearance is a very sensitive index of a single intense exposure to radiation in the lethal range (fig. 5). In view of the observations of Bloom of the great radiosensitivity of erythroblasts one might logically expect the reticulocytes to disappear promptly. This they do within a period of about 48 hours following a single intense exposure to

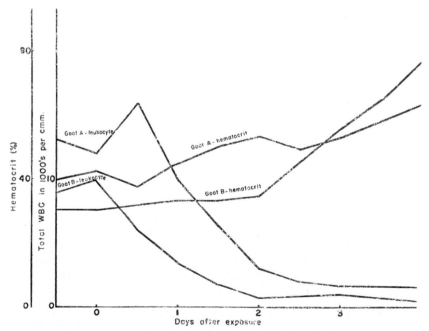

Fig. 4. Hematocrit and leukocyte changes in two goats exposed to massive amounts of atomic bomb radiation. Bikini, July 1946. (Note the extreme hemoconcentration.)

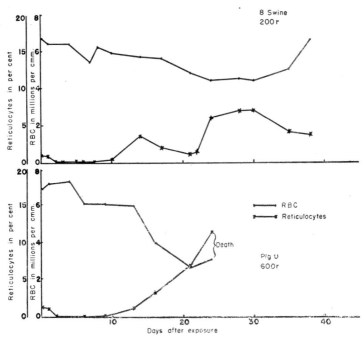

FIG. 5. Red blood count and reticulocyte changes in swine demonstrating the disappearance of reticulocytes within 48 hours and the reticulocytosis that usually indicates recovery but sometimes is followed by death.

radiation in the lethal range (Jacobson et al; Cronkite). However, the disappearance of reticulocytes, at least in the rabbit, does not occur at as low a dose as does the reduction in the number of lymphocytes. In swine (fig. 5) and in the Japanese exposed to the atomic bomb explosion at Hiroshima and Nagasaki, a return of the reticulocytes was a good prognostic sign for recovery but did not invariably indicate a favorable outcome (LeRoy, Cronkite, Tullis and Tessmer).

Most recently Stohlman, Brecher, Schneiderman, and Cronkite demonstrated that ionizing radiations produce intravascular red cell damage and shorten red cell life span. This injury is indirect as well as progressive, i.e., it is more pronounced the longer the red cells remain in the irradiated animal although they need not be present at the time of radiation. The red cell injury is slight and in the earliest stages can only be detected by superimposing a second minimal insult such as tagging of cells with chromium which in itself does not shorten red cell life span. It is of considerable academic and practical interest that the widely-used chromium label for determination of red cell life span is not necessarily innocuous, and after irradiation either the more heavily tagged cells or the label itself is lost at an accelerated rate. The effect is probably due to the chromium metal and not to its radioactivity. During the thrombocytopenic phase of radiation injury when many red cells are extravasated and return to the general circulation via the lymphatics, this passage through an extravascular cycle adds further damage to the red cell resulting in readily measurable shortening of red cell life span.

9.6.5 *Hematological Findings in the Marshallese Exposed to Fallout Radiations.* In March 1954, groups of Marshallese and Americans were accidentally exposed to fallout gamma and beta radiations from a megaton device. The groups were observed carefully after the exposure, and details of clinical and laboratory findings have been published (Cronkite, Bond and Dunham). The most heavily exposed group was composed of 64 Marshallese located on Rongelap atoll at the time of the accident, and the findings in this group will be dealt with most extensively here. None of those exposed died as a result of the irradiation. The Rongelap people received an estimated dose of 175 r of gamma radiation (air dose), sufficient beta radiation dose from adherent material to result in lesions in some exposed areas of skin (chapter by Conard et al.), and minimal internal contamination with radionuclides (chapter by Robertson and Cohn). Considerable uncertainty exists in the magnitude of doses received; however, the Rongelap group can be considered to represent the high sublethal exposure range. Hematological depression was considered to have resulted from the gamma exposure with little or no contribution from the surface beta or internal emitters.

Serial hematological determinations including total white count, differential, platelet count and hematocrit were made on each exposed individual over the initial observation period of 72 days, and repeat determinations have been made at 6 months, and then at yearly intervals following the exposure (Conard et al.). Details of methods and initial findings have been reported (Bond et al.). Unexposed groups for comparison were observed initially and at the times of follow-up studies; however, variations in findings in control groups have presented difficulties in precise interpretation, as in the Japanese exposed at Hiroshima and Nagasaki.

The average leukocyte and platelet counts are shown graphically in figures 6, 7 and 8. The first counts on the Rongelap group were done on post-exposure day 3, at which time a drop in total white count was evident (the exposed Americans showed a rise in total white count in the first 48 hours, as has been reported previously). The count then fluctuated, perhaps as a result of the beta lesions, with no severe depression over the first four weeks. A marked depression then occurred, reaching minimum levels at 6 weeks. The counts approached the levels of the unexposed populations by 2 years. The time course of neutrophil count changes followed closely that

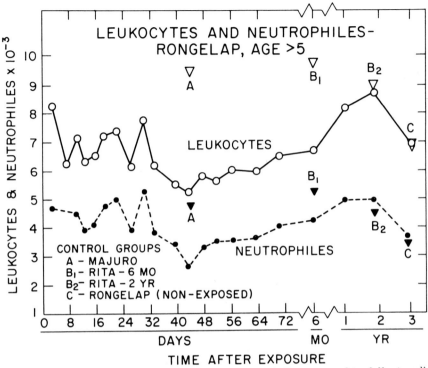

FIG. 6: Leukocyte and neutrophile counts in Marshallese exposed to fallout radiations.

of the total white count. Lymphocyte depression was early and profound (fig. 7) with gradual return toward normal. The counts remained below that of the unexposed groups at 3 years. The platelet count reached a low at approximately 4 weeks (fig. 8) with fairly rapid initial recovery followed by a secondary depression and slow return towards normal. At three years the mean platelet counts were still slightly below the mean of the unexposed population. The hematocrits at no time were remarkably different from the unexposed levels.

At the times of peak depression, some individuals had neutrophil counts below 1000/mm³ and platelet counts below 75,000/mm³. No infections attributable to the neutropenia were observed, however, and an epidemic of upper respiratory infection at approximately the time of maximum neutrophil depression was equally severe in the heavily and mildly exposed groups. No hemorrhagic phenomena could be attributed to the platelet depression. All individuals were ambulatory throughout, and no therapy (other than for the skin lesions) beyond that routinely required for any large groups of individuals was necessary or administered because of the radiation exposure.

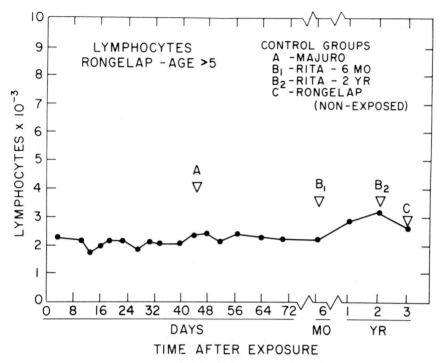

FIG. 7: Lymphocyte counts in Marshallese exposed to fallout radiations.

The findings allow accurate documentation of the response of the human being to total-body gamma exposure in the high *sublethal* range, not possible in the Japanese exposed at Hiroshima and Nagasaki. The time course differs in important aspects from that seen in most laboratory animals. The total white count shows an early rise, with only minimal lowering until maximum depression occurs at approximately 6 weeks. A similar trend is seen with the neutrophil count. The drop in lymphocytes is early and severe. The platelet count falls in a regular fashion, reaching a low at approximately 30 days. The rate of recovery is considerably slower than would be anticipated from laboratory animal data and is incomplete at 3 years. These findings are consistent with the incomplete data available on the Japanese exposed at Hiroshima and Nagasaki, and with the findings on the human beings exposed in reactor accidents (see Bond et al.). They are also consistent with later findings in patients exposed therapeutically either to total-body x-radiation (Miller, Fletcher and Gerstner; Nickson and Bane), or to internally-administered radionuclides (Wolins).

9.6.6 *Splenic, Thymic Weight Decrease.* Carter et al. had previously demonstrated a very close correlation between the dose of radiation and the

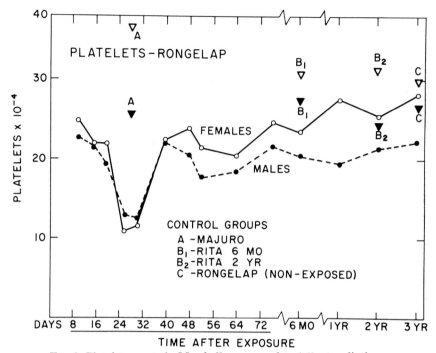

FIG. 8: Platelet counts in Marshallese exposed to fallout radiations.

decrease in the splenic and thymic weights on the 5th day after exposure to radiation. These observations made it possible to use the decrease in splenic thymic weight for mammalian dosimetry and in studying the effects of substances that may primarily neutralize the effect of radiation. This type of study has been extended by Kallman and Kohn. In their studies the time of minimum weight and dose response did not follow a simple relationship. The data behave as if there are two independent cell populations with different sensitivities. However, thymic weight 5 days after irradiation was a linear function of the logarithm of the radiation dose, as shown by Carter et al. earlier. In their hands the system was very useful as a biological dosimeter. Another careful mathematical analysis of the weight loss of the thymus and spleen was that of Stroud et al. who are essentially in agreement with Carter, Kallman and Kohn on the basic relationship and the usefulness of the procedures.

9.6.4 *Platelets*. Platelets decreased at a rate between that of the red cells and the granular leukocytes. Perhaps platelets are as sensitive an index to exposure to acute irradiation as the granulocytes in the rabbit (Jacobson et al.). In swine, goats and dogs, the decrease in platelets is definitely less rapid than that of the granular leukocytes (Cronkite; Lawrence, Morton

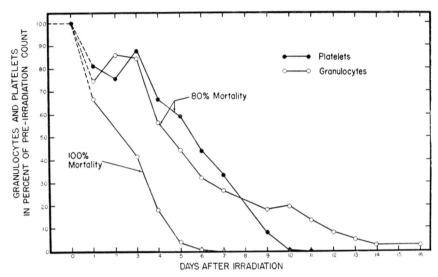

FIG. 9. Mean granulocyte and platelet count on 10 dogs exposed to atomic bomb gamma radiation that produced 10% mortality.

and Cronkite). Frequently the platelets trend upwards for 4–5 days after irradiation following which there is a decrease until platelets disappear or become constant at a lower level. Above doses of radiation that produce a 90% mortality the response of the platelets is maximal with platelets disappearing from the circulation by the 11th day. With lesser doses of radiation the platelets do not completely disappear but become constant at a lower level. This level is apparently a function of the dose of radiation received. This new, relatively constant level may be maintained for 2-3 weeks.

The relative response of granulocytes and platelets at different per cent mortalities is illustrated in figures 9 and 10. With a 10% mortality the platelets approach zero but are maintained constant at about 5% of the normal range. At this dose the granulocytopenia is only moderate and infections were not prominent clinically. In contrast to this at 80% and 100% mortality the platelets and the granulocytes reach zero and infections and hemorrhage are obviously present before death.

The foregoing statements cover the general picture of what occurs to the peripheral blood elements after a single intense exposure to ionizing radiation. However, this does not give a sufficiently complete picture of various facts and observations about the response of the blood to total body or to rather large segmental exposure as seen in therapeutic irradiation of some malignancies, or to what might be anticipated following exposure to mixed radiations of different penetrabilities.

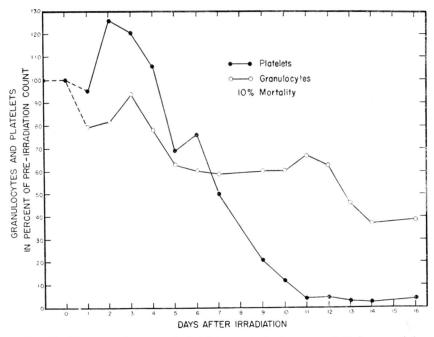

Fig. 10. Mean granulocyte and platelet counts in 2 groups of 10 dogs receiving atomic bomb gamma radiation that produced 80 and 100% mortality. Platelet response in 80% and 100% groups were identical.

9.6.7 *Miscellaneous Studies.* Warren has emphasized the great instability of the bone marrow in some people who have been exposed to small amounts of radiation (less than 50 r). Ellinger, Henshaw, Goodfellow and Warren have all remarked upon the great differences in strain, species, and individual in response to approximately the same dose. Lorenz has demonstrated the greater sensitivity and the more uniform response of the inbred animals to chronic exposure to radiation. Goodfellow has shown that humans under treatment for cancer with radium, in such a manner that a large volume of tissue is exposed, respond with an initial leukocytosis. His graphs demonstrate the phenomenon called "coasting" in which the white blood count continues to recede after therapy is discontinued. Mayneord and Piney have shown that repeated small exposures to x-ray may cause more complete and long-lasting damage to the bone marrow than a single exposure.

The changes induced by chronic low intensity exposure to ionizing radiation will be considered in the section on the detection of exposure to ionizing radiation.

9.6.8 *Morphology of Blood Cells.* Morphologic changes in the leukocytes are varied. Degenerating lymphocytes are seen in the circulation. Lympho-cytic nuclei may be fragmented, pyknotic, clover-shaped or only the usual nuclear pattern may be altered. Nucleoli may become very prominent, pre-senting the picture of "owl's eye nucleoli" (Warren). Large phagocytic mononuclear cells may be seen containing nuclear masses and occasional red cells. The cytoplasm of the mononuclears may be excessively basophilic. Vacuoles may appear. Immature cells may be present. Degenerating granu-locytes may be seen in the peripheral blood. Toxic granulation, vacuoles and basophilia may be observed. Platelets show some changes along with a reduction in number. Giant hyperchromatic platelets are usually present. Megakaryocytes have been reported as appearing in the blood, but were not seen in the blood smears of the Bikini animals. Supravital stains with Janus green and neutral red are reported as demonstrating alterations in the mitochondria and neutral red bodies. Dickie and Hempelmann have shown that there is an increase in the number of refractile neutral red bodies of the lymphocytes of persons acutely and chronically exposed to ionizing radiation. These bodies are seen only in supravital preparation, are not specific for radiation and were also seen in the lymphocytes of persons working with toxic chemicals. Bilobed lymphocytes have been reported in the blood of human beings chronically exposed to radiation and of hu-man beings working around cyclotrons (Ingram). Hypersegmented neu-trophils have also been seen.

9.7 Late Effects—Leukemia

The prolonged and late effects of exposure to ionizing radiation are of great and practical importance. Some men and animals who have had a single exposure or have been chronically exposed to ionizing radiation develop a persistent leukopenia. However, this does not, at least in some cases, prevent the organism from responding to infections and stresses with a marked, transitory leukocytosis, following which the individuals may return to their previous leukopenic level (Cronkite). Bloom and Jacobson described an apparent hyperplasia of the bone marrow in some rabbits that recovered from an $LD_{50/30}$ exposure. This "over compensation" was seen about two months after exposure. This type of response leads one to specu-late about the possible development of leukemia, following a single acute exposure to ionizing radiation. That leukemia will develop in animals, and probably in man, particularly lymphatic leukemia, following chronic or re-peated exposure seems well established from a statistical standpoint.

9.7.1 *Development of Leukemias after Chronic Exposure.* Krebs et al. found that the incidence of leukemia in irradiated mice was 3.5 per thousand mice as compared to 0.6 per thousand in the control mice. Hueper demon-strated a 74% incidence of leukemia in mice that had received 480 r over a period of six weeks. The spontaneous incidence in control animals was not stated. Furth and Furth used a single and repeated doses of 200–400 r in mice and reported an eight-fold increase in myelosis and a seven-fold increase in lymphomatosis. Weitz described the development of a case of myeloid leukemia in an x-ray technician that culminated in death. The blood was normal before exposure. Lymphocytosis, eosinophilia and mono-cytosis preceded the positive diagnosis of leukemia. Henshaw and Hawkins reported in 1944 that the incidence of leukemia in physicians was 1.7 times as great as in the male population. March statistically analyzed the incidence of leukemia in radiologists and found it to be ten-fold greater in radiologists than non-radiologists. Henshaw, in a long series of experiments in mice, demonstrated an increased incidence of leukemia in mice that were chronically exposed to small doses of radiation. Lorenz and associates have shown that over 0.11 r per day will, in general, increase the incidence of malignancies in mice, including leukemic processes. The foregoing data on the statistical relationship of leukemia to chronic exposure to ionizing radiation are not conclusive proof that leukemia can be caused by ionizing radiation in man, but there is such a strong correlation that it would be foolhardy indeed to ignore the probable relationship and not to take advantage of every conceivable means to reduce the exposure of all humans to a minimum, and in addition, actively support and operate protective and investigative projects to prevent excessive exposure to ionizing radiation.

9.7.2 *Leukemia after Single or a Few Repeated Doses of Radiation.* Heretofore, with the exception of the relationship of chronic exposure to leukemia induction discussed in the previous section, there had been little work on the influence of single or repeated doses of radiation on leukemogenesis. However, survivors from the atomic bombs at Hiroshima and Nagasaki who were close enough to the hypocenter to have received radiation in the potentially lethal range show a significantly greater incidence of leukemia than did survivors in the group outside the range of gamma radiation (Moloney). Those who had severe, acute radiation illness have shown the highest incidence of leukemia. The leukemia has been predominantly myeloid and, to a lesser extent, monocytic. This is in contrast to radiation-induced leukemia of animals, which usually has been lymphoid. In the pre-clinical state of human leukemia, a low alkaline phosphatase of separated leukocytes was found along with a neutrophilic leukocytosis and the presence of increased numbers of basophiles. Moloney and associates suggest that radiation-induced chronic myelogenous leukemia is attributable to a loss of growth-regulating factors. In addition to the appearance of leukemia in the atom bomb survivors, leukemia has now been shown to occur following radioiodine treatment of thyroid carcinoma (Blom et al.). Furthermore, Court-Brown has observed a significant increase in leukemia in human beings who have been treated for arthritis of the spine with x-ray.

The pathogenesis of leukemia induction by radiation has been extensively studied. It has been ably reviewed by Furth and Upton. All types of ionizing radiation are leukemogenic. Single and repeated exposures can produce leukemia. Repeated properly spaced exposures result in a more rapid induction and a higher incidence. The induction rate increases with the dose. Physiologic and genetic factors markedly influence the induction of leukemia in mice. Androgens and cortisone inhibit, and estrogens enhance, the induction of lymphoid leukemia. Cortisone, however, does not inhibit the production of myeloid leukemia. Shielding of the normal spleen, which contains all types of hematopoietic tissue in the mouse, protects against lymphoma induction in some strains of mice as do injections of bone marrow suspensions (Lorenz, Congdon, Kaplan and Brown, reviewed by Cronkite and Bond).

Kaplan has carried on an extensive series of studies on lymphoma induction in mice. These classical studies have shown that a particular fractionation increases the induction of lymphoma. Local thymic irradiation is ineffective in producing the tumors. Removal of the thymus prevents the lymphoma induction. Subsequently they showed that thigh shielding and injections of marrow suspensions accelerates the regeneration of thymic tissue and concomitantly thymic lymphoid tumors are inhibited. Recent studies have shown that lymphoid tumors develop in non-irradiated thymic tissue grafted into thymectomized irradiated mice. This observation would appear to establish the development of a cancer in a tissue not exposed to the carcinogenic agent. However, a cocarcinogenic effect of trauma and necrosis in the graft may have a contributory effect, and cell migration to the transplanted tissue cannot be ruled out absolutely. Recently Kaplan and associates have shown a definite time dependence for protection against induction of leukemia in mice by injections of homologous bone marrow. Lymphoid tumor induction is maximally inhibited when injections are made one and one-half hours after the last x-ray dose. After 16 days, the ability to inhibit the induction of tumors was lost. This group studied ribonucleic acid (RNA) and desoxyribonucleic acid (DNA) in thymic cells of thigh shielded and nonshielded irradiated mice. It was found that the DNA levels per thymic cell do not vary with age or treatment group and that RNA remains constant with time in the control group, but RNA increases 1 to 5 days after irradiation with a prompt return to normal in the thigh shielded group. The RNA per cell and RNA/DNA ratio remain markedly elevated over the entire course of treatment in the unshielded irradiated group. These authors suggest that the sustained elevation of RNA may be related to tumor induction, since shielding prevents induction and results in a rapid return of RNA to normal.

It is quite evident that leukemogenesis by ionizing radiation and the interactions between normal and irradiated hemopoietic tissues and endocrines, which are proved to influence induction, are most intricate. On the basis of the reports to date, it is not possible to determine whether the non-irradiated hemopoietic tissues supply a cellular or humoral factor that inhibits the induction. There is evidence for both views. It is also conceivable that the normal tissues may be capable of neutralizing a factor liberated from the irradiated tissues. The nature of the interactions between irradiated and normal tissues and the influence of endocrines on irradiated tissues remain obscure, but the existence of these physiological interactions that influence leukemogenesis is unquestioned.

The unquestioned, harmful late effects of ionizing radiation on hematopoiesis logically leads to a discussion on the value of a study of the blood in protecting against excessive exposure to ionizing radiation.

9.8 Factors Influencing the Effect of Ionizing Radiation.

Protective factors are discussed in detail in Chapter 10, section 10.7. Although preprotective agents may protect all cellular systems into which the chemical substances can penetrate, the most striking effects are seen in the blood-producing organs.

9.9 The Detection of Radiation Injury by Hematologic Procedures

The detection of radiation injury logically falls into two categories, the detection of the brief, intense exposure and the detection of cumulative small exposures. By hematologic standards, the detection of the brief intense exposure is fairly satisfactory in animals. However, the early hematologic changes in man after single intense total body exposure to various dosages are not well known. It is regrettable that few blood studies were performed on the Japanese casualties during the first week after the atomic bomb explosions. Therefore, it is necessary at this time to attempt, for the most part, to extrapolate to man from animal data. However, the Marshallese data help considerably.

9.9.1 *Effects of Acute Exposure.* Beginning shortly after the acute exposure one can anticipate a prompt decrease in the total lymphocyte count. The decrease will roughly be proportionate to the dosage in the sub-lethal range (fig. 2). The maximum depression will appear within 24 to 72 hours. The greater part of the fall takes place within 24 hours. Concomitant with a lymphopenia, a neutrophilic leukocytosis (fig. 3) can be expected. The number of refractile neutral red bodies in the lymphocytes will probably increase. From a practical standpoint the following conclusions can be drawn:

1. If there is no significant decrease in the total lymphocyte count during the first 24 hours, the exposure has probably been less than 25 r of total body ionizing radiation.

2. If a lymphopenia of minor degree appears with very mild or with no symptoms, the exposure is probably less than 100 r.

3. If the depression in lymphocytes approximates 90% of the usual lymphocyte count of man, and symptoms are present during the first 24 hours one can conclude that the exposure has been quite heavy, in excess of 100 r.

Needless to say the detection of minor degrees of lymphopenia necessitates a knowledge of normal lymphocyte levels of the person concerned. Under conditions of an atomic catastrophe this information will probably not be available, nor will it be feasible with present techniques to perform intensive blood studies. Other means of detecting exposure to ionizing radiation are:

a. the symptomatology
b. personnel radiation dosimeters and
c. the distance from the exploding bomb

These will be discussed in Chapter 11 on Diagnosis and Therapy.

The satisfactory development of good electronic blood-counting devices greatly simplifies the logistics of performing enormous numbers of blood counts in a catastrophe.

9.9.2 *Effects of Repeated Small Exposure.* The detection of repeated small cumulative exposures by hematologic studies poses an entirely different problem and logically becomes part of a broad health protection program. Observations on the blood of man chronically exposed to radiation are legion. Leukocytosis, lymphocytosis, leukemoid reactions, leukocytic leukemias, erythrocytosis, reticulocytosis, leukopenia, thrombopenic purpura, aplastic anemia, leukopenic leukemia, refractive neutral red bodies in the lymphocytes and changes in the blood coagulation have been described as occurring after chronic exposure to ionizing radiations. From a review of the literature, the following hematologic observations can be considered as presumptive criteria of excessive exposure to ionizing radiation or other toxic agent:

1. Persistent leukopenia (WBC below 4000/c.mm.).

2. Persistent leukocytosis with an absolute lymphocytosis (WBC above 15,000).

3. A macrocytosis (mean corpuscular volume increased, a shift to the right in the Price-Jones curve, or an increased mean corpuscular diameter).

4. Reticulocytosis (reticulocytes above 2 per cent).

5. Erythrocytosis (RBC over 5.6 million per c.mm. or hemoglobin over 18.0 gm./100 cc. blood).

Williams has analyzed the value of blood studies and protection against radiation injury and has concluded that numerous routine counts are unnecessary where good control of all circumstances is maintained. However, in radiation areas, more highly controlled hematologic studies are needed in order to obtain more information on the threshold and permissible values. Helde and Wahlberg have analyzed the lowering of the leukocyte count in human beings produced by minute amounts of whole-body radiation. They have utilized a statistical analysis. Although the mean leukocyte count is unchanged, the dispersion around the mean is considerably decreased by low exposure to irradiation, thus making it possible to use this statistical parameter as an indication of irradiation exposure.

A complicating observation is that of Wald et al. who has observed in the control population in Japan that was not exposed to radiation of the atomic bombs that there has been a progressive decrease in the leukocyte count over a period of the last ten years. The reasons for this change are obscure but obviously complicate the analysis of chronically exposed populations.

9.10 Evaluation of Blood Changes

The above criteria result from either a depression of or an increased lability of hematopoiesis. The establishment of the presence of these criteria can be greatly assisted by performing parallel studies on comparable groups of humans who are known not to be exposed to radiation or any other toxic agent. Statistical comparison of the potentially exposed control group will help to determine if a significant change has taken place. In a similar manner the pre-exposure counts of the suspected group or individual can be compared to the post-exposure counts. If there is a significant change in the latter one can state with some certainty that there has been excessive exposure to some toxic agent. A good criterion of excessive exposure of a group to radiation is a significant decrease in the group average leukocyte count below the pre-exposure level or below the average of the control group. As soon as any of the above criteria have been demonstrated, the individuals must be removed from any possible contact with radiation and the following studies should be performed in order to determine if radiation injury is the cause of the abnormality. In principle, the use of a group as its own pre-exposure control sounds secure, but admittedly the observations of Wald et al. indicate the potential unreliability of this approach. Accordingly, whenever possible, a comparable population of unexposed people should also be followed.

1. Endeavor to eliminate all other causes of temporary hematologic ab-

normalities, such as infectious mononucleosis, infectious lymphocytosis, infectious hepatitis, virus diseases, benzol and heavy metal poisoning.

2. Study the excreta and expired air for the possible presence of ionizing radiation to help determine the type and degree of internal exposure to radioactive isotopes.

3. Study the blood at weekly intervals to detect further changes and to search for the presence of refractive, neutral red bodies in the lymphocytes.

In this discussion of the role of hematology in the detection of chronic radiation injury, it is appropriate to state the changes discussed appear generally after the damage has been sustained. The main protection against ionizing radiation injury must be an accurate physical control of the radiation intensities to which personnel are exposed.

In concluding this section the reader is referred to the work of Knowlton and Carter in which a group of ten individuals was carefully followed over a long period of time while they were being chronically exposed to radiation. The hematologic studies suggest that definite changes were induced. The article demonstrates the difficulties and the potentialities of this type of analysis.

9.11 The Hemorrhagic Syndrome of Radiation Illness

In previous editions of this book, a long detailed discussion of the various facets believed to contribute to hemorrhage were discussed. Much of the controversy has been resolved. Historically (Fernau, Schramek and Zarzycki; Fabricius-Moller; Lacassagne, Lattes and Lavedan; Shouse; Warren and Whipple) observed hemorrhage. The most critical observations on pathogenesis were made by Fabricius-Moller who correlated platelet levels with bleeding and noted that lead shielding of a leg during irradiation prevented later bleeding and the thrombopenia was much less marked. (See Chapter 10 for detailed discussion of shielding.) Allen and associates claimed that heparinemia was a major cuase of bleeding in addition to the thrombopenia in irradiated dogs, and that the thrombopenia actually sensitizes to heparin. Of the latter there is little doubt. The concept of increased amounts of circulating heparin was readily accepted, probably because positive treatment by antiheparin could, in large part, control the bleeding. Such has not proved to be the case and the heparinemia concept has, in general, been refuted (Jackson et al.). The pros and cons are discussed in previous editions of this book and in a review by Cronkite and Brecher.

The following defects in hemostasis that lead to bleeding seem to be well documented. A progressive thrombopenia develops that is time- and dose-dependent. The thrombopenia leads to a quantitative deficiency in clot retraction, prothrombin utilization and capillary integrity. Lastly, at very low platelet levels with virtually no prothrombin conversion, the whole blood-clotting time becomes remarkably prolonged. Ulcerations, trauma and infections increase the bleeding tendency (Cronkite; Cronkite and Brecher, Jackson et al., and LeRoy).

The most direct evidence on the role of the platelet has been the proof that platelet transfusions will prevent bleeding or stop bleeding that has already commenced (Cronkite et al., Woods et al., and Allen). The control of the bleeding did not increase the survival rate at the LD_{80} level or above.

The platelet level at which bleeding may occur spontaneously was studied by Lamerton et al. in rats. At platelet levels above $40,000/mm^3$, bleeding and anemia did not occur. Similarly in human beings exposed to fallout with platelet counts as low as $35,000/mm^3$, bleeding was not observed (see section 8.6.6). Lastly, there is a real species difference in the rate of fall of platelets in man and other mammals (see section 8.6.6).

9.12 Value of Hematologic Studies in Acute Radiation Injury

From the serial studies of the blood that have been discussed it becomes apparent that there are certain hematologic signs that can be used as prognostic guides. None of these prognostic guides is absolute. The value of hematologic studies in radiation injury may be summarized as follows:

a. A favorable prognosis is suggested by an early reticulocytosis, a return of platelets, a granulocyte count greater than 1500 per cubic mm. and an early return of the lymphocyte.

b. An unfavorable prognosis is suggested by a complete disappearance of the lymphocytes, granulocytes and platelets, and an increase in the clotting time with the development of purpura and particularly when accompanied by fever. In animals, at least, if the favorable prognostic signs listed above do not appear by the 15th to 20th day after exposure, death is usual. The experiences of the Japanese physicians parallel the above observations, except that recovery occurred more slowly. Poor nutrition may have altered the natural course of the disease in the Japanese. Unfortunately, exceptions occur and it is impossible to prognosticate accurately the outcome of radiation illness on the basis of hematologic signs.

9.13 Relationship of the Hematopoietic System to Survival in Radiation Injury

This subject is extensively discussed in Chapter 10, section 10. Suffice it to say here that all post-radiation protective measures studied in animals appear to either accelerate the regeneration of hematopoietic tissues or to increase the survival time (antibiotics) by control of infection to give more time for the spontaneous regeneration of the injured hemopoietic tissues.

REFERENCES

ADAMS, W. S., SAUNDERS, R. H., AND LAWRENCE, J. S.: Output of lymphocytes in cats, including studies on thoracic duct lymph and peripheral blood. *Am. J. Physiol., 144:* 297–304, 1945.

ALLEN, J. G., ET AL.: Heparinemia—an anticoagulant in the blood of dogs with hemorrhagic tendency after total body exposure to roentgen rays. *J. Exper. Med., 87:* 71–85, 1948.

ALLEN, J. G.: Pathogenesis of Irradiation Hemorrhage, 5th Annual Conference on Blood Coagulation and Allied Subjects. Transactions of Josiah Macy Foundation, N. Y., 1952.

BARNES, W. A. AND FURTH, O. B.: Studies on indirect effect of roentgen rays in single and parabiotic mice. *Am. J. Roentgenol., 49:* 662–681, 1943.

BLOOM, W.: Radiosensitivity of erythroblasts. *J. Lab. & Clin. Med., 32:* 654–659, 1947.

BLOOM, W.: Plutonium project histological changes following radiation exposures. *Radiology, 49:* 344–348, 1947.

BLOOM, W., AND JACOBSON, L. O.: Some hematologic effects of irradiation. *Blood, 3:* 586–592, 1948.

BLOM, P. S., QUERIDO, A., AND LEEKSMA, C. H. W.: Acute leukemia following x-ray and radioiodine treatment of thyroid carcinoma. *Brit. J. Radiol., 28:* 165–166, 1955.

BOND, V. P., SWIFT, M. N., TAKETA, S. T., WELCH, B. P., AND TOBIAS, C. A.: Indirect effects of localized deuteron irradiation of the rat. *Amer. J. Physiol., 174:* 2, 1953.

BOND, V. P., ET AL.: Chapter 4 in: "Some Effects of Ionizing Radiation on Human Beings," edited by Cronkite, E. P., Bond, V. P., and Dunham, C. L. U. S. Gov't. Printing Office *TID* 5358, July 1956.

BOND, V. P. AND CRONKITE, E. P.: Effects of radiation on mammals. *Ann. Rev. Physiol., 19:* 299–328, 1957.

BRECHER, G., ENDICOTT, K. M., GUMP, H., AND BRAWNER, H. P.: The effects of x-ray on lymph node and hemopoietic tissue of albino mice. *Blood, 3:* 1259–1274, 1948.

BRECHER, G., AND CRONKITE, E. P.: Post-radiation parabiosis and survival in rats. *Proc. Soc. Exp. Biol. Med., 77:* 292–294, 1951.

CAMPO, R., BOND, V. P., CRONKITE, E. P.: Studies on suspected circulating "radiotoxins" in adrenalectomized irradiated rats. *Fed. Proc. 16:* 18–..., 1957.

CARTER, R. E., HARRIS, P. S., AND BRENNAN, J. T.: The effect of acute doses of x-irradiation on the splenic and thymic weight of CF-1, female mice. U. S. Atomic Energy Commission Document LA-1075, dated March 7, 1950.

CONARD, R. A., CANNON, B., HUGGINS, C. E., RICHARDS, J. B., AND LOWERY, A.: Medical survey of Marshallese two years after exposure to fallout radiation. Brookhaven National Laboratory Report, BNL 412 (T-80), 1956.

CONARD, R. A., LOWERY, A., MEYER, L., RALL, J. E., CANNON, B., BACH, S. A., CARTER, E. L., HECHTER, H., AND EICHER, M.: Medical survey of Marshallese three years after exposure to fallout radiation. Brookhaven National Laboratory Report, to be published.

COURT-BROWN, W. M. AND DOLL, R.: The incidence of leukemia among the survivors of the atomic bomb explosions at Hiroshima and Nagasaki. Medical Research Council report on "Hazards to Man of Nuclear and Allied Radiations," London, England, Her Majesty's Stationery Office (1956).

CRONKITE, E. P. AND BOND, V. P.: Effects of radiation on mammals. *Ann. Rev. Physiol., 18:* 483–526, 1956.

CRONKITE, E. P., BOND, V. P., AND DUNHAM, C. L.: Some effects of ionizing radiation on human beings. U. S. Gov't. Printing Office TID 5358, July 1956.

CRONKITE, E. P.: Clinical manifestations of acute ionizing radiation illness in goats exposed to an atomic bomb explosion, with comments on therapy, Bikini, 1946. U. S. Nav. M. Bull., 49: 199–215, 1949.

CRONKITE, E. P.: Diagnosis of ionizing radiation injury by physical examination and clinical laboratory procedures. J.A.M.A., 139: 366–369, 1949.

CRONKITE, E. P.: The hemorrhagic syndrome of acute ionizing radiation illness produced in goats and swine by exposure to the atomic bomb explosions at Bikini, 1946. Blood, 5: 32–45, 1950.

CRONKITE, E. P., TULLIS, J. L., AND TESSMER, C. F.: The response of the peripheral blood of swine to whole body x-ray radiation in the lethal range. Project NM 007 039, Report #21, Nav. Med. Res. Inst., Bethesda, Md., 7 April 1949.

CRONKITE, E. P., JACOBS, G., BRECHER, G., AND DILLARD, G. H. L.: The hemorrhagic phase of the acute radiation syndrome due to exposure of the whole body to penetrating ionizing radiation. Am. J. Roentgenol., 67: 796–803, 1952.

CRONKITE, E. P. AND BRECHER, G.: Defects in hemostasis produced by whole body irradiation. 5th Annual Conference on Blood Coagulation and Allied Subjects. Trans. of Josiah Macy Foundation, New York, 1952.

DAVIS, R. W., DOLE, N., IZZO, M. J., AND YOUNG, L. E.: The hemolytic effect of radiation. U. S. Atomic Energy Commission Report, UR-99, University of Rochester, 1949.

DICKIE, A., AND HEMPLEMAN, L. H.: Morphologic changes in leukocytes, persons exposed to ionizing radiation. J. Lab. & Clin. Med., 32: 1045–1059, 1947.

DUNLAP, C. E.: Effects of radiation on the blood and the hemopoietic tissues, in-cluding the spleen, thymus, and lymph nodes. In: S. WARREN: "Effects of radiation on normal tissues." Arch. Path., 34: 562–608, 1942.

EDELMAN, A.: New Evidence for a Toxic Substance Elaborated after Irradiation. Fed. Proc., 14: 42, 1955.

FABRICIUS-MOLLER, J.: Experimental Studies of the Hemorrhagic Diathesis from X-ray Sickness. Monograph. Copenhagen: Levin and Munksgaards Forlag, 1922.

FERNAU, SCHRAMEK AND ZARZYCKI: Ueber die Wirkung von induziertar Radioakt-witaet (Vorlaeufige, Mitteilung). Wien. klin. Wchnschr., 26: 94, 1913.

FURTH, J. AND FURTH, O. B.: Neoplastic diseases produced in mice by general irra-diation with x-rays; incidence and types of neoplasms. Am. J. Cancer, 28: 54–65, 1936.

FURTH, J. AND UPTON, A. C.: Leukemogenesis by ionizing radiation. Acta Radiol., Supplement 116, 469–476, 1956.

GOODFELLOW, D. R.: Radium in human leukocytes. Acta Radiol., 17: 1–50, 1936.

GOODFELLOW, D. R.: Leukocytic variations in radium workers. Brit. J. Radiol., 8: 669–752, 1935.

HAMILTON, L.: Control of lymphocyte production. Brookhaven National Laboratory, Symposia in Biology, No. 10, 1957.

HEINEKE, H.: Experimentelle Untersuchungen ueber die Einwirkung der Roentgen-strahlen auf das Knochermark, nebst einigen Bemerkungen ueber die Roent-gentherapie der Leukaemie and Pseudoleukaemie und des Sarkoms. Deutsch ztschr. J. Chir., 78: 196–230, 1905.

HEINEKE, H.: Ueber die Einwirkung der Roentgenstrahlen auf inners Organe. Muench. med. Wchnschr., 51: 785, 1904.

HEINEKE, H.: Ueber die Einwirkung der Roentgenstrahlen auf Tiere. Muench. med. Wchnschr., 1: 2090–2092, 1903.

HELDE, M. AND WAHLBERG, T.: Some observations on the relation between radiation dose measures and blood changes. *Acta Radiol., 40:* 435–442, 1953.

HENSHAW, P. S.: Experimental roentgen injury, tissue and cellular changes brought about with single massive doses of radiation. *J. Nat. Cancer Inst., 4:* 503–512, 1944.

HENSHAW, P. S.: Experimental roentgen injury, changes produced with intermediate range doses and comparison of relative susceptibility of different kinds of animals. *J. Nat. Cancer Inst., 4:* 485–501, 1944.

HENSHAW, P. S.: Experimental roentgen injury and effects on tissues and blood of C3H mice produced with single small whole-body exposures. *J. Nat. Cancer Inst., 4:* 477–484, 1944.

HENSHAW, P. S.: Experimental roentgen injury, effects of repeated small doses of x-ray on the blood picture, tissue, morphology, life span of mice. *J. Nat. Cancer Inst., 4:* 513–552, 1944.

HENSHAW, P. S., AND HAWKINS, J. W.: Incidences of leukemia in physicians. *J. Nat. Cancer Inst., 4:* 339–346, 1944.

INGRAM, M.: Health hazards in radiation work. *Science, 111:* 103–109, 1950.

JACOBSON, L. O., MARKS, E. K., AND SIMMONS, E. L.: The effect of total body x-irritation on a pre-existing induced anemia in rabbits. The response of animals with a phenylhydrazine induced anemia. MDDC-261, U. S. Atomic Energy Commission, University of Chicago Contract Number W-7401 ENG-37, 1946.

JACOBSON, L. O., ET AL.: Effects of x-rays on rabbits: The hematologic effect of total body x-irradiation in the rabbit. MDDC-1174, U. S. Atomic Energy Commission, 1946.

JACOBSON, L. O., SIMMONS, E. L., MARKS, E. K., ROBSON, M. J., BETHARD, W. F., AND GASTON, E. O.: The role of the spleen in radiation injury and recovery. *J. Lab. & Clin. Med., 35:* 746–770, 1950.

JACKSON, D. P., CRONKITE, E. P., LeROY, G. V., AND HALPERN, B.: Further studies on the nature of the hemorrhagic phase of radiation injury. *J. Lab. Clin. Med., 39:* 449–461, 1952.

JACKSON, D. P., CRONKITE, E. P., JACOBS, G., AND BEHRENS, C. F.: Prothrombin utilization in fatal radiation injury. *Am. J. Physiol., 169:* 208–217, 1952.

KALLMAN, R. F. AND KOHN, H. F.: Reaction of mouse thymus to x-rays. *Radiation Res., 2:* 280–293, 1955. *Ibid,* Reactions of mouse spleen to x-rays. *Radiation Res., 3:* 77–87, 1955.

KAPLAN, H. S., ET AL.: Indirect induction of lymphomas in irradiated mice. *Cancer Res., 16:* 422–425, 1956. *Ibid, Cancer Res., 16:* 426–428, 1956.

KNOWLTON, N. P.: Value of blood counts in individuals exposed to ionizing radiation. U. S. Atomic Energy Commission, Unclassified Report #397, Los Alamos Scientific Laboratory, 1949.

KORNBLUM, K., BOERNER, F., AND HENDERSON, S. G.: Effects of radiation on the normal blood cells as determined by blood count. *Am. J. Roentgenol., 39:* 235, 1938.

KREBS, K., RASK-NIELSEN, H. C., AND WAGNER, A.: Origin of lymphosarcomatosis and its relation to other forms of leucosis in white mice. *Acta radiol., suppl. 10:* 1–53, 1930.

KROMEKE, F.: Ueber die Einwirkung der Roentgenstrahlen auf die roten Blutkoerperchen. *Strahlentherapie, 22:* 608, 1926.

LACASSAGNE, A., LATTES, J., AND LAVEDAN, J.: Etude experimentale des effets biologiques du polonium introduit dans l'organisme. *J. Radiol. et d'Electrologie, 9:* 1–14, 1925.

LAWRENCE, J. S. AND VALENTINE, W. N.: The rate of utilization of cross-circulated platelets in the thrombopenic cat. U. S. Atomic Energy Commission, MDDC-217, 1947.

LAWRENCE, J. S., ERVIN, D. M., AND WETRICH, R. M.: Life cycle of white blood cells; rate of disappearance of leukocytes from peripheral blood of leukopenic cats. *Am. J. Physiol.*, *144:* 284, 1945.

LAWRENCE, J. S., VALENTINE, W. N., AND ADAMS, W. S.: Thrombopenic purpura; the failure of direct blood transfusions to raise the platelet level. *J. Lab. & Clin. Med.*, *33:* 1077–81, 1948.

LAWRENCE, J. S., VALENTINE, W. N., AND DOWDY, A. H.: The effect of radiation on hemopoiesis. Is there an indirect effect? *Blood, 3:* 593–611, 1948.

LEROY, G. V.: Medical sequelae of atomic bomb explosion. *J.A.M.A., 134:* 1143–1148, 1947.

LEROY, G. V.: Hematology of atomic bomb casualties. *Arch. Int. Med., 86:* 691–710, 1950.

LORENZ, E., ET AL.: Plutonium project; biological studies in tolerance range. *Radiology, 49:* 274–285, 1947.

MARCH, H. C.: Leukemia in radiologists. *Radiology, 43:* 275–278, 1944.

MAYNEORD, W. V.: Some effects of x-radiation on blood; measurement and distribution of radiation. *Brit. J. Radiol., 1:* 257–262, 1928.

Medical Report of Joint Commission for the Investigation of the Effects of the Atomic Bomb in Japan, 1947.

MILLER, L. S., FLETCHER, G. H., AND GERSTNER, H. B.: Systemic and clinical effects induced in 263 cancer patients by whole-body x-irradiation with nominal air doses of 15 to 200 r. Air University, School of Aviation Medicine, Randolph AFB, Texas, 1957.

MINOT, G. R., AND SPURLING, R. G.: The effect on the blood of irradiation especially short wave roentgen ray therapy. *Am. J. M. Sci., 16:* 215–240, 1924.

MOLE, R. H.: Whole body radiation—radiobiology or medicine. *Brit. J. Radiol., 26:* 234–241, 1953.

MOLONEY, W. C. AND KASTENBAUM, M. A.: Leukemogenic effects of ionizing radiation on atomic bomb survivors. *Science, 121:* 308–309, 1955.

NICKSON, J. AND BANE, H.: Personal communication.

OSGOOD, E. E.: Is action of roentgen rays direct or indirect? Investigation of this question by method of human marrow culture. *Am. J. Roentgenol., 48:* 214–219, 1942.

OSGOOD, E. E.: Control of peripheral concentration of leucocytes. Brookhaven National Laboratory Symposia in Biology, No. 10, 1957.

RAVENTOS, A.: An abscopal effect of x-ray upon mouse spleen weight. *Radiation Research, 1:* 381–387, 1954.

SCHREK, R.: Primary and secondary vacuoles in thymic cells exposed *in vitro* to x-rays. *J. Cell. & Comp. Physiol., 30:* 203–224, 1947.

SHREK, R.: Radiosensitivity of lymphocytes and granulocytes *in vitro* according to method of unstained cell counts. *Proc. Soc. Exper. Biol. & Med., 58:* 285–286, 1945.

SCHWARTZ, S., ET AL.: Studies of the hemolytic effect of radiation. MDDC-1342, U. S. Atomic Energy Commission, 1946.

SHOUSE, S. S., WARREN, S. L., AND WHIPPLE, G. H.: Aplasia of marrow and fatal intoxication in dogs produced by roentgen radiation of all bones. *J. Exper. Med., 53:* 421–435, 1931.

Stohlman, F., Jr., Brecher, G., Schneiderman, M., and Cronkite, E. P.: The hemolytic effect of ionizing radiations and its relationship to the hemorrhagic phase of radiation injury. *J. Hematology*, to be published 1957.

Stroud, A., Gurian, J. M., Brues, A. M., and Summers, M. M.: Organ weight analysis in mice given fractionated irradiation. *Radiation Res., 2:* 267–279, 1955.

Tullis, J. L., and Warren, S.: Gross autopsy observations in animals exposed at Bikini; preliminary report. *J.A.M.A., 134:* 1155–1158, 1947.

Wald, N., Truex, W. E., Sears, M. E., Suzuki, and Yamamoto, T.: Hematological findings in Hiroshima and Nagasaki atomic bomb survivors—a 10-year review. Atomic Bomb Casualty Comm. Report. National Research Council, Washington, D. C.

Warren, S.: Blood findings in cyclotron workers. *Radiology, 39:* 194–199, 1942.

Warren, S.: Effects of radiation on normal tissues. *Arch. Path., 34:* 443; 562; 749; 917; 1070, 1942.

Weitz, W.: Uber einen von Anfang an beobachteten Fall von Nyeloischer Leukamie bei einer Rontgenlaborantin. *Klin. Wchnschr., 17:* 1579–1580, 1938.

Wintrobe, M. M.: *Clinical Hematology*. Philadelphia: Lea, 1946.

Williams, E. K.: The white cell count in relation to occupational radiation dosage. *Acta radiol., 41:* 21–29, 1954.

Wolins, W.: Delayed hematological effects of internally administered Ga⁷². *Radiation Res., 3:* 358–359, 1955.

Woods, M. C., Gamble, F. N., Furth, J., and Bigelow: Control of the post-irradiation hemorrhagic state by platelet transfusions. *Blood, 8:* 545–553, 1953.

10 ▸

Acute Whole-Body Radiation Injury: Pathogenesis, Pre- and Post-Radiation Protection

V. P. Bond, M.D., ph.D., E. P. Cronkite, M.D., and R. A. Conard, M.D.

"False facts are highly injurious to the progress of science for they often endure long; but false views, if supported by some evidence, do little harm for everyone takes a salutory pleasure in proving their falseness."

Charles Darwin

10.1 General Notes

The opening quotation is particularly appropriate to the fields of clinical radiology and radiobiology for there have been numerous false views supported by some evidence. Many have fallen by the wayside and more are yet to fall. The pleasure of the assailants must be slight for the supporters of fallen and discarded views though still present are singularly quiet. The bywords in evaluating new developments in this field are caution and patience for the interested. Were the investigators endowed with similar caution and patience less confusion would result.

The release of atomic energy by military intention or industrial accident produces large amounts of ionizing radiations, some extremely penetrating, some not so penetrating. Exposure of the body to these radiations produces ionization in the tissues. There is disagreement as to the initial biological effect therefrom and the sequence of subsequent effects is not well understood. At the present time it is not possible to bridge the gaps between the effects of radiation on pure chemical systems, the single cell, and the integrated mammal. Accordingly little is precisely known about the mechanism of the action of ionizing radiation at the mammalian level. Of necessity the end result has been studied and is rather well characterized today.

Radiation illness in its broad sense can be produced by all types of ionizing radiation. However, the dose required varies with the kind, the rate of administration and the penetrability of the rays. Furthermore,

190

there may be situations in which the injuries are produced by a combination of different radiations, some of which are highly penetrating and some of which may be absorbed completely by the surface layers of the body.

Much confusion has arisen because of the inadequate means of measuring the response to radiation and the standardization of a physical unit that is adaptable for all sizes of animals and all types of radiation. The roentgen, or "r," a measure of the ionization in air, does not necessarily measure the dose absorbed by the tissue. At recent meetings (1950 to 1956) of the International Commission of Radiological Units, it has been recommended "that the dose be expressed in terms of the quantity of energy absorbed per unit mass (ergs per gram) of irradiated material at the place of interest." This quantity is not readily determined; however, tables for its estimation are provided in the 1956 report of the commission. The Commission further recommends that the roentgen be retained as the unit of measurement of x- and gamma rays. The conditions under which the exposure dose is measured should be designated as free in air, at skin surface, or at x-centimeters depth, and the data such as scatter, half-value layer, target-to-skin distance, and KVP should be included. In commenting on the Commission's recommendations, Failla stated that "no physical unit can fulfill the ideal requirements of making all biological effects of ionizing radiation appear independent of wave length or more generally, independent of specific ionization," and that "in the present state of our knowledge no chemical or biological unit can fulfill the ideal requirement either." For the purposes of correlating dose with effects on the whole body, depth dose and distribution of the absorbed energy becomes of great importance, as shown by Tullis et al. and Bond et al. Further, no single physical unit can satisfactorily characterize the total dose because of differences in relative absorption by different tissues.

It is essential to attempt quantification of the biological response, as well as the physically measured dose, when trying to correlate effect with dose. The biological measure may include the LD_{50} and the slope of the dose mortality curve, as in all toxicological studies. Other biologic measurements of dose are splenic-thymic weight decrease (Carter et al.), body weight (Chapman and Jerome), gut weight (Conard), the hematological response, survival time, iron uptake by erythrocytes (Hennessey et al.) and histologic changes. Quantitative measures of biological effect useful in mammalian radiology have been reviewed by Storer et al.

10.2 Classification of Radiation Injuries

Radiation injuries can be divided into two general categories, the acute and chronic injuries. The acute type results from brief intense exposure; the chronic type from prolonged exposures of lower intensity. The chronic type may also appear as late effects in survivors of more acute exposures. The following is an outline of the two categories, only the first of which is dealt with extensively in this chapter:

10.2.1. *The Acute Injuries Produced by Brief Exposure to Large Doses of Radiation.*

10.2.1.1 *Injuries from penetrating radiation.*

1. Total-body exposure: The acute illness produced by total-body radiation may occur in man from exposure to gamma and/or neutron radiations from a detonating atomic bomb, gamma exposure from close-in fallout from atomic bombs or from accidents with radioactive materials as nuclear power sources. Exposure of animals to such whole-body radiation under experimental conditions results in this type of illness.

2. Partial-body exposure: Acute illness may result from partial-body exposure to penetrating radiations as is commonly seen in therapeutic radiation as for cancer.

10.2.1.2 *Injuries from poorly penetrating radiations.* Acute injury of the skin or other body integuments may result from beta ray exposures of the skin as is seen with fallout radiation or from accidents involving handling of radioactive materials. This type of injury is discussed in the chapter on skin.

10.2.1.3 *Injuries from absorption of radioactive materials.* Absorption of radioactive materials may occur from inhalation, ingestion or entrance into the body from open wounds of fallout from atomic bombs or of radioactive materials in laboratory accidents. Such a hazard is much more likely to result in chronic long-term effects than in acute effects. This type of hazard is discussed in the chapter on internal effects.

10.2.2 *Chronic Radiation Injury*

10.2.2.1 *Injuries from penetrating radiation.* Total-body or partial-body exposure may result in chronic effects, some of which are listed below.

1. Blood dyscrasias such as anemia, purpura, leukemia.
2. Increase in degenerative diseases.
3. Increased aging and shortening of life span.
4. Increase in incidence of cancer.
5. Retardation of growth and development in children.
6. Increased incidence of cataracts.
7. Impaired fertility.
8. Genetic effects.

Such chronic effects are not discussed in detail in this book but are covered elsewhere (National Academy of Sciences report on Pathological and Genetic Effects of Radiation). Basic considerations are presented in Chapter 14.

10.2.2.2 *Injuries from poorly penetrating radiation.* Beta radiation injury may result in chronic effects on the skin in the form of chronic radiation dermatitis and cancer of the skin. Such effects on the skin are discussed in Chapter 13.

10.2.2.3 *Injuries from absorption of radioactive materials.* Absorption of radioactive materials include long-term effects such as leukemia and cancer of the bone. Such effects are discussed in the chapter by Robertson and Cohn (12).

10.3 Acute Illness from Total-Body Exposure to Penetrating Radiations.

This illness may be produced by exposure to a single type or a combination of different types of radiation (x-ray, gamma rays or fast neutrons). It will be a rare occurrence in civil life and for practical purposes will not be seen short of industrial accidents and atomic warfare. The syndrome in fulminating form was observed in the Japanese (appropriately termed "atombombendisease" by them) following the atomic bombings of Hiroshima and Nagasaki in August 1945, and was seen also, in mild form, in the Marshallese exposed to fallout radiations in 1954. In Japan, accurate clinical observations and laboratory studies were scanty during the first three weeks after the bombings. In the fallout accident involving the Marshallese, extensive clinical and laboratory observations were made; however, the dose range was below lethal. Patients have been exposed to total-body radiation (Miller, Fletcher and Gerstner); however, again the dose range is, of course, sublethal and the influence of the underlying disease is difficult to evaluate. Thus many inferences on dose response, survival time, mortality rate and symptomatology in man are based on animal experimentation. It is, therefore, well to point out the great differences in response that exist among species of mammals.

Representative $LD_{50}/30$ day values for a number of species are given in Table I (Bond and Robertson). The absorbed dose in rads is the significant parameter that determines the degree of biological response. All mortality data in the table refer to conditions of exposure such that dose distribution throughout the body is essentially uniform. The dose at midcenter has no particular significance except that it is convenient and represents the approximate dose that all tissues received (no single parameter is adequate to characterize an exposure under conditions of nonuniform dose distribution through the tissues). It can be seen at once from the table that the LD_{50} values show no consistent pattern as air dose. Expressed as absorbed dose, however, the LD_{50} values for large animals are considerably smaller than for small species, and the degree of variation among species is less with large animals.

The distribution of deaths as a function of time after irradiation varies

TABLE I

| SPECIES | TYPE OF RADIATION | LD$_{50}$/30 DAY | |
		Air exposure dose in r	Absorbed dose in rads at midcenter
Mouse	250 KVP X-ray	443	638
Rat	200 KVP X-ray	640	796
Guinea pig	200 KVP X-ray	337	400
Rabbit	250 KVP X-ray	805	751
Monkey	250 KVP X-ray	760	546
Dog	250 KVP X-ray	281	244
Swine	1000 KVP X-ray	510	247
Sheep	Gamma Approx. 0.7 Mev.	524	205
Goat	200 KVP X-ray	350	237
Burro	Gamma Approx. 1.1 Mev.	651	256

with the dose of radiation and with species. For example, with the dog in the lethal range, the mean survival time is approximately 12 days, with deaths occurring 6–26 days after exposure. With doses of 600–1500 r, some deaths occur earlier (3rd and 4th days) and the toxic symptoms of vomiting, anorexia, and diarrhea become more prominent. With doses of 1500–6000 r, all dogs die on the 3rd and 4th day. Severe diarrhea is present. With the mouse, the distribution of deaths after irradiation with doses less than an LD$_{50}$ is essentially unimodal with peak of deaths occurring 11 days after exposure (Cronkite, Bond, Chapman and Lee). In the LD$_{50}$ range the deaths become bimodal with a peak at 4–6 days and another at 11 days. As the dose is increased above the LD$_{100}$ the first peak of deaths becomes progressively more prominent and the second peak fades out so that with doses of 1500–10,000 r the mean survival time is approximately 4 days. A similar phenomenon is seen with rats; however, the first peak is more prominent at lesser doses of radiation. As a result of the work of Bond et al., Quastler et al., Brecher and Cronkite, Cronkite and others, the first peak of deaths has been correlated with severe gastrointestinal injury and dysfunction. The relative sensitivities of the species differ, the rat GI tract being relatively more sensitive. The second peak of deaths is correlated with the sequelae of pancytopenia (infection, hemorrhage, and anemia). If the LD$_{50}$ of the species is low so that amounts of radiation are less than that needed to produce the severe GI injury and dysfunction, the species has essentially a unimodal distribution of deaths in the lethal range, with a mean survival time of approximately 10–15 days, e.g., the dog. If LD$_{50}$ is high, a bimodal distribution of deaths may appear, e.g., mouse, rat and rabbit. Where man fits into the above relative sensitivities of tissue is not yet known.

The early diarrhea (first four days) is correlated with direct radiation injury of the gastrointestinal tract; however, late diarrhea (7–24 days) occurs as a result of ulcerations and hemorrhage due to the pancytopenia. Studies strongly indicate that complete histologic recovery of the bowel occurs by 4–5 days, hence if the animals survive to the stage of late diarrhea, the bowel has been reconstituted. Histologic studies show typical hemorrhagic and agranulocytic lesions in a bowel that is otherwise approximately normal in appearance.

With the preceding animal experience and the known Japanese experience in mind, the following is formulated with regard to the probable response of man to penetrating radiation exposure. With small amounts of total-body radiation (under 100 r), there may be no symptoms or at most a transient nausea. Leukopenia, particularly the lymphocytopenia, will be mild and of short duration. With larger amounts of radiation, 100 to 1000 r, the characteristic clinical picture may develop. Within a few hours, pronounced nausea, vomiting, malaise, weakness, headache, dizziness, anorexia, tachycardia, irritability and insomnia will generally appear. Leukopenia, anemia and thrombocytopenia will develop at different rates (Cronkite; Lawrence, Dowdy and Valentine; Jacobson et al.; LeRoy). The symptoms will usually subside within 24 to 48 hours to appear again after a few days. The interval between the initial and the subsequent symptoms has been termed "the latent period." This latent period will become shorter with larger doses and may be absent if the dosage is sufficiently high. With termination of the latent period, infections and hemorrhages will become more prominent. In the Japanese, infections were particularly apparent three to five weeks after exposure and hemorrhagic phenomena four to six weeks after exposure (LeRoy). Details of the serial blood changes have been covered in a previous chapter. With large amounts of radiation (2000–30,000 r), the signs and symptoms appear in an intensified form with mean survival time of about 3–4 days. With doses in excess of 30,000 r sudden deaths occur in mice preceded by convulsions, central nervous system symptoms, or respiratory difficulty (Langham et al.).

10.4 Acute Illness from Partial Exposure to Penetrating Radiations

The acute illness that is produced by exposure of part of the body to penetrating radiations is seen characteristically in patients undergoing high voltage x-ray therapy for cancer. With respect to the initial so-called "toxic symptoms," they are similar to the syndrome produced by a single intense exposure of the whole body to penetrating radiation. Radiation of certain areas of the body will produce the illness with greater frequency, or with less radiation than for exposure of other parts of the body. Exposure of a single part of the body does not produce the severe pancytopenia that results from exposure of the whole body to the same amount and type of radiation. Irradiation of the thorax and abdomen, particularly the upper abdomen, produces a high incidence of nausea, vomiting, and anorexia. In contrast to this, irradiation of the head and extremities rarely produces these symptoms. Since the clinical course and handling of this type of reaction to penetrating irradiation have been amply covered in recent text books and reviews of clinical radiology, further discussion is not necessary. Following partial or surface exposure, the organism is able to react locally and generally to injury, in accordance with the concept of adaptation (Selye). Bond et al. have demonstrated that local irradiation of the abdomen and elsewhere in the body produces the alarm reaction as described by Selye. In contrast to this, exposure of the whole body to large amounts of penetrating radiation produces diffuse injury of varying degrees to all tissues and the organism may be less able or unable to react with the usual protective and adaptive mechanisms.

10.5 Pathogenesis of Radiation Injury

Numerous theories have been advanced to explain the biologic effects of ionizing radiations. Only those theories which may help to understand the pathogenesis of total body radiation and which may indicate a possible therapeutic approach will be considered in this chapter.

For the purposes of our discussion the syndrome of acute radiation illness may be considered as being initiated and continued by one or more of the following mechanisms:

1. Enzyme inhibition; activated radicals
2. Alterations in cell membrane permeability
3. Generalized protein denaturation
4. Inhibition of mitosis
5. Production and circulation of toxins
6. Precipitation of adrenal cortical insufficiency
7. Adaptation syndrome
8. Pancytopenia and its sequelae

The syndrome is obviously the result of disturbances in the homeostasis of the animal produced by cellular injury of varying degrees in different organ systems. The 4th to 8th mechanisms are attempts to explain the clinical syndrome at a mammalian level. The 8th mechanism will explain the gross clinical and pathologic observations seen in animals dying in the lethal range.

10.5.1 *Enzyme Inhibition; Activated Radicals.* The concept of enzyme inhibition has been carefully and extensively studied by Barron and associates. In the past, enzyme inhibition was not considered important because the doses necessary to inactivate enzyme solutions were 10 to 1000 times greater than those that seriously injure living tissues. The idea that enzyme solutions are insensitive was in part based on inadequate experimental methods. The present status of the enzyme inhibition concept may be summarized as follows:

As a result of the work of Fricke, 1934, and of Dale, 1943, and others, it has been shown that in dilute solutions the number of molecules brought into reaction is proportional to the number of ions produced in the solution, and is independent of the concentration of the solution. This led to the concept that the action of the radiation is not primarily on the dissolved substance, but on the solvent. This has been termed "activation of water," hence the "activated water" is apparently capable of reacting with substances dissolved in it. The activation of water consists of the production of highly reactive oxidizing substances (OH, H_2O_2 and other complexes) as the result of ionizing radiation. The active products presumably oxidize the sulfhydryl groups (SH) of many enzymes to the enzymatically inactive disulfide form. This inactivation is generally reversible in the lower dose range. With larger amounts of radiation, the enzyme inhibition is also produced by protein enzyme denaturation by direct rupture of chemical bonds. This type of denaturation is irreversible. Reversible enzyme inhibition may play a part in the initiation of the syndrome of radiation illness, particularly in the lethal range, but is probably not the only and may not be the most important initiating mechanism. These theoretical aspects and experimental data concerned with the effects of radiation on water and the possible importance of these products of ionization of water upon biological systems is very entrancing but to date there is no conclusive proof that the major portion of the effects of radiation are mediated through this mechanism in the mammal.

10.5.2 *Alterations in the Permeability of Cell Membranes* have been postulated. Absorption of water and vacuole formation can be observed within nuclei. This may result in alterations in the permeability of cell membranes or an increased intranuclear osmotic pressure (Failla).

10.5.3 *Denaturation of Proteins,* in general, in addition to the protein enzymes already considered, has been postulated as being responsible for some of the phenomena that are observed. Denaturation is known to occur particularly in the higher dose ranges. It is produced by direct rupture of the chemical bonds and is probably irreversible (Barron).

10.5.4 *Inhibition of Mitosis; Chromosome Changes.* Mitotic inhibition occurs at relatively low dose levels. Apparent recovery may result, or the process may result in cell enlargement without division, or in abnormal division. There is no doubt that chromosomal changes result in the well-known genetic effects of radiation; however, the role of chromosome changes, or "somatic mutations" in producing early and late effects in the irradiated individual is not clear.

10.5.5 *Circulating Toxins.* The production and/or absorption and circulation of toxic substances from irradiated tissues or absorption from the bowel whose selective permeability has been changed, have been considered by some as contributing to the development of radiation illness. Others doubt its importance. Bacterial pyrogenic substances, digestive enzymes, and "enterotoxins" from the bowel and histamine-like substances from tissue in general have been considered by various investigators as playing some role in the pathogenesis of radiation illness. To date, the available evidence in favor of indirect effects upon the blood-forming organs by circulating toxic substances has not been conclusive (Lawrence; Valentine and Dowdy; Campo, Bond and Cronkite).

The histamine theory of radiation illness has been advocated by Ellinger, who considers that many of the effects of radiation are due to the production of histamine-like substances. Other investigators have failed to demonstrate significantly increased amounts of histamine in the blood and in tissues. Weber and Steggerda have recently published information showing that there is a correlation between the increase in histamine levels of rat plasma and depression in the blood pressure following x-irradiation. Techniques for detecting histamine are difficult and failure of some investigators may have been due to technical difficulties. In addition, the presence of increased levels of histamine does not necessarily mean that histamine is the cause of the various phenomena that are seen after irradiation but may simply be a result of the fundamental defect produced by the effects of ionizing radiation on tissue. Conard has shown in a study of the motility, tonus and contraction of the bowel immediately after irradiation locally that the behavior of the bowel is not identical to that produced by histamine baths or injections. Other evidence which suggests that histamine may play an important part in the pathogenesis of radiation illness is the fact that conditions that increase the histamine content of tissues may also increase the lethality rate from x-rays. For example, induced hyperthyroidism increases the histamine content of tissues (Parrot) and increases the lethality of total body x-rays in mice (Blount and Smith). Adrenalectomy also increases the histamine content of tissues of the rat (Rose and Brown) and definitely increases the lethality of x-rays (Cronkite and Chapman; Kaplan; Edelman and Campo).

10.5.6 *The Role of the Adrenals in the Acute Radiation Syndrome.* The adrenals have been shown to play a role in the acute radiation syndrome;

however, the importance of this role has received widely different evaluations. Certain similarities between adrenal cortical insufficiency and acute radiation injury, such as changes in blood chlorides, water metabolism, blood cholesterol, fat deposit in the liver and blood sugar, have been claimed. There is no doubt that polydipsia and polyuria follow heavy exposure, and that there may be a redistribution of fluids as indicated by blood volume, plasma and hematocrit changes, and some edema. The changes in blood chemistry are small and apparently inconsistent. The fluid balance changes noted following acute total-body exposure can be explained on the basis of vomiting and/or diarrhea, with the resulting fluid and electrolyte losses, as well as the eventual failure to eat and drink. Many of the changes may be explained as resulting from the stress accompanying the disease. Patt and associates have described a series of characteristic changes in the adrenals of the rat exposed to various dosages of x-radiation, which were prevented by hypophysectomy. Evidence has since been presented that indicates radiation is not an exception to the general rule that adrenalectomy sensitizes to all stresses (Cronkite and Chapman; Kaplan). Nims and Sutton presented data on the rat which indicated that the polydipsia and decrease in adrenal cholesterol level following WBR were the result of increased activity of the pituitary-adrenal system, and that the initial fall in liver glycogen was principally the result of lowered food intake. Lasser and Stenstrom, in a clinical study of patients following pelvic area irradiation, found the degree and time course of "radiation sickness" to correlate with changes in the absolute peripheral eosinophile count, but not with the Thorn ACTH-eosinophile, 4-hours response test. They concluded that the adrenal cortex underwent definite changes in the course of irradiation, but that the changes probably were not related to clinical "radiation sickness." Santisteban et al. showed that cortisone replacement therapy progressively restored the resistance of irradiated-adrenalectomized mice. However, events causing death in the irradiated-intact animals differed from those in the x-irradiated adrenalectomized group despite cortisone treatment, indicating that cortisone may only partially restore resistance. Bond et al. obtained highly selective irradiation of various small portions of the rat with a "pencil" beam of 190 mev deuterons, and found that the thymus, spleen, and adrenal weights characteristic of pituitary-adrenal stimulation resulted only if and when the irradiation given imposed severe stress on the animal, as indicated by the gross symptoms of illness and body-weight loss. Such changes could not be elicited by irradiation of the adrenals alone, nor were they prevented by adrenal irradiation if additional radiation damage to other tissues sufficient to put the animal under "stress" were present. The isolated, perfused calf's adrenal gland was used to study the effects of gamma radiation on the secretion of adrenal cortical hormones (Rosenfeld et al.). Secretion was markedly reduced; however, it should be noted that the doses used were in excess of 2000 r (some five times the LD$_{50}$ and always supralethal), and that the isolated organ was removed from secretory stimuli that may be present in the intact animal following acute total-body irradiation. Thus, the author's conclusion that the adrenal cortex must be considered a radio-responsive tissue cannot be considered to characterize the role of the adrenal in acute total-body irradiation. French et al. have demonstrated early changes in plasma hydroxycorticosteroid levels, as well as changes in the peripheral neutrophile, lymphocyte, and eosinophile counts of monkeys given from 50 to 400 r total-body radiation. The changes were maximal at 4 to 8 hours, and values were again normal by 12 hours. Shielding of the head or adrenals did not modify these early changes, implying that they were not the result of a direct effect on the pituitary-adrenal axis. Brayer et al. found, after a supralethal dose of WBR (1000 r) in swine, that a marked increase in urinary excretion of total adrenal cortical steroids occurred, which was most pronounced in the first 24 hours. In the case of the irradiated animal in the lethal dose range where pancytopenia is followed by its common sequelae of infection and hemorrhage, there is a depletion of the adrenal lipid and by inference one might say that this represents the stage of exhaustion in the adaptation syndrome. The present writers are inclined to interpret this terminal state as being simply the reaction of the organism to an overwhelming infection and not primarily to the initial radiation injury.

In view of our present knowledge, it appears quite certain that the role of the adrenal cortex is secondary to the stress of radiation in the development of the acute radiation syndrome. The previously quoted biochemical changes, the complications of hemorrhage, anemia and infections, the biological complexities of various mammals, and the simultaneous operation of factors which may change electrolyte and water metabolism in opposite directions at the same time point out the hazards that are contingent upon drawing conclusions that adrenal insufficiency exists because some of these changes are observed. The recent review of Sayers on the adrenal cortex and homeostasis points out this problem in great clarity. The problem is also discussed by Mole.

10.5.7 *Pancytopenic Sequelae, Infection.* The sequelae of pancytopenia are infection, hemorrhage and anemia. The latter two are discussed in Chapter 9. Infection here will be discussed as it relates to the lethal range of exposure, i.e., the range where some, but not all, of those exposed will die within a period of several weeks and to the sublethal range.

Evidence that infection is of importance in the acute radiation syndrome falls into several categories: (a) Clinical observations on human beings exposed to large doses of radiation in the Japanese bombings and in reactor accidents and similar observations on large animals dying from radiation exposure. (b) Correlative studies on mortality rate, time of death, and incidence of positive blood cultures in animals. (c) Challenge of irradiated animals with virulent and normally nonvirulent organisms. (d) Studies on germ-free animals. (e) Studies of the effectiveness of antibiotics in reducing radiation mortality rate. (f) Studies on the effectiveness of agents that will augment or restore natural antimicrobial defenses on mortality rate in irradiated animals. A brief word on each of these lines of evidence is given below:

The Japanese dying of "atombombendisease" and human beings heavily exposed at the Los Alamos accident (Hempleman et al.) showed unmistakable evidence of infection. Signs and symptoms included high fever, Ludwig's Angina and other mucosal and cutaneous infections, cellulitis, pneumonia and septicemia. Autopsy findings bore out the clinical picture. Similarly with large animals, particularly dogs, the temperature begins to rise 3 to 4 days before death, and is usually quite high prior to death. Orocutaneous lesions are common. At autopsy, pneumonia is the rule, as well as other evidence of infection.

At doses of total-body radiation even in the high sublethal range, however, (Marshallese exposed to fallout gamma radiation, Cronkite et al.) no evidence of increased susceptibility to infection may be manifest. The Marshallese, in some of whom the neutrophile counts fell below $1000/mm^3$, showed no increase in the incidence of infectious diseases over control groups. Epidemics of upper respiratory infection, measles and chicken pox, that occurred were no more pronounced in extent or severity in the exposed population compared to unexposed Marshallese in whom similar epidemics occurred at the same time.

The time of peak incidence of bacteremia in irradiated animals has been correlated with the time of peak incidence of mortality in the extensive studies of C. P. Miller and his group. The organisms are chiefly enteric in origin, and apparently gain access to the blood stream through the bowel wall. A positive correlation, of course, does not prove cause and effect, and it has been stated that such organisms represent agonal invasion and thus may be "incidental." A cause and effect relationship seems highly probable, however, particularly in the light of evidence from antibiotic therapy studies outlined below. Total-body irradiation has been shown to activate infections that otherwise remained "latent" (Bond et al.).

Challenge of irradiated animals with virulent, or normally nonvirulent bacilli results in death at infective levels that produce no mortality in non-irradiated control animals. With virulent organisms, an appreciable increase in mortality rate is seen at x-radiation dose levels below those producing mortality in the absence of challenge (Shechmeister et al.). With normally

nonvirulent organisms, the mortality rate following exposure in the lethal
range is appreciably enhanced. Increased susceptability to viruses, Rickett-
sia, parasites such as *Trichinella spiralis*, and bacterial toxins in the irradiated animal have been reported. A synergistic effect of x-radiation and
cortisone in increasing susceptibility to administered bacteria and viruses
has been reported (Friedman et al.).

It is of importance to point out, however, that there is considerable variation in the degree of increased sensitivity to different microorganisms or
toxins, and in the degree of effects depending on the route of administration
(see under mechanisms of increased susceptibility below). Specifically, Hale
and Stoner have shown that although a marked increase in susceptibility to
pneumococci is evident in the irradiated mouse, no such increase is found
for mice challenged with a virulent influenza virus. With the virus innocu-
lation, the animals were protected against secondary bacterial invasion with
antibiotics. The degree to which the reported increased susceptibility to
viruses in irradiated individuals is due to secondary bacterial invasion is
not known. Neutrophiles play a large role in resistance against bacterial,
but not viral diseases (Wood). The peripheral neutrophile count is profoundly affected by irradiation, and thus a greater degree of altered immunity to bacterial, rather than viral infections might be expected. At any
rate, blanket statements relating to susceptibility of the irradiated host are
not warranted, and specific consideration in each instance must be given to
the infecting agent, the host, the physiological state of the host and the
degree of exposure to both radiation and the infectious agent.

Germ-free animals die following total-body exposure to x-radiation (Reyniers). The dose required to kill, however, is somewhat higher than for
"normal" animals, and the survival time is increased. These results can be
taken as indicating that infection may be responsible for death in the irradiated animals in certain dose ranges. At higher doses, animals die even
in the absence of infection. Extensive hemorrhage probably is a major cause
of death in such animals; however, undoubtedly other poorly understood
biochemical changes contribute.

Antibiotics administered following radiation exposure have been shown
definitely to enhance survival under some circumstances. The incidence of
spontaneous mortality has been shown to be reduced, and mortality in
x-irradiated mice subsequently challenged with virulent organisms has been
decreased.

Results have not been uniformly encouraging, however, and completely
negative results have been reported. Two human beings exposed in the Los
Alamos reactor accidents died despite vigorous antibiotic therapy. It is
possible that improved results would be obtained with a schedule of administration designed to avoid the development of resistant bacteria

(Coulter and Miller). Of significance in this regard is the recent report (Hammond et al.) showing that mice exposed to neutron radiation are protected from death by antibiotics during the first 10 days, but not in the 11- to 30-day period when most mice die following x- or gamma radiation. This would indicate that under some conditions, at least, infection alone does not account for the mortality observed.

Thus, there is no doubt that infection contributes greatly to the disease process, and mortality following exposure to total-body radiation. However, it is equally clear that acute radiation illness is not an infectious disease in the usual sense; rather infection is a complication of a serious debilitating underlying disease which specifically interferes with defense mechanisms against bacterial invasion. Death may occur in some individuals whether infection is present or not, at high dose levels. Thus antibiotics cannot be expected to be curative as with primarily infectious diseases, and dramatic cures cannot be expected from this type of therapy. However, as with any debilitating disease, antibiotics definitely will prevent death in a certain number who might otherwise die—prevent death until regeneration and restoration of functions allows normal defense mechanisms to again protect the exposed individual.

10.5.7.1 *Mechanisms of increased susceptibility to infection.* Nearly all known body defenses against bacterial invasion have been reportedly impaired by large doses of total-body radiation. Thus the skin and mucous membranes may show small eroded areas, frequently secondary to hemorrhage, that provide portals of entry for bacteria. It has been shown that the number of bacteria able to cross the intestinal barrier does not increase following irradiation; however, those that cross are able to multiply and produce a fatal bacteremia in the host whose defenses in general are lowered (Gordon et al.). The leukopenia and impaired antibody production contribute greatly to the increased susceptibility to infection, and a failure to adequately clear the blood stream of bacteria indicates functional impairment of the phagocytic cells. Radiation mortality correlates well with the degree of granulocytic leukopenia (Smith et al.).

10.6 Résumé of Acute Radiation Effects

To recapitulate and summarize, it is apparent that diffuse cellular injury of different degrees is sustained by all tissues at the time of exposure to radiation. The exact mechanism by which this injury is produced remains poorly understood. The degree of injury of various organs is the function of the amount of ionization produced within the organ and it is apparent, without extensive discussion, that clinical pictures will vary with the relative degree of injury to various organs. For example, epilation may be very prominent, if conditions are such that the skin absorbs more radiation than deeper structures. This may occur if a combination of penetrating and slightly penetrating radiations are simultaneously received. The protoplasmic injury itself, wherever the cells may be located, is probably produced by a combination of enzyme inhibition, alteration in cellular permeability, protein denaturation, mitotic inhibition and perhaps release of "toxic substances." Concomitant with or shortly after the diffuse cellular injury, "toxic" symptoms (nausea, vomiting, perhaps diarrhea, malaise, headache, anorexia, etc.) develop. These "toxic symptoms" subside within 24 to 48 hours, and during a variable latent period, depending on the dosage, only the hematologic signs are easily found. With higher doses of radiation following which there is a very short survival time, there is no latent period, no subsidence of the initial toxic reaction. The vomiting continues, diarrhea develops, prostration occurs and is followed by death within a few days. In this high dose range, in excess of the minimal amount that will kill 100 per cent of the animals, the death is well correlated symptomatically and histologically with severe gastrointestinal injury which is not reversed during the survival period. At lower doses, complete histologic recovery takes place within 4 to 5 days (Brecher and Cronkite; Tullis). During the latent period, a series of cellular and histologic phenomena are occurring. In the opinion of the authors, the main reason for recurrence of symptoms and ultimate death in the lethal range is the failure of adequate regeneration of hemopoiesis. There may be an adrenal component or other as yet unknown factors contributing to the lethality but all evidence to date points towards the importance of hemopoiesis and its regeneration in survival from potentially lethal radiation injury. At any rate, the latent period is terminated with the recrudescence of symptoms and signs. The latter are well known, and in the mechanism of development can be fairly well explained as follows:

The panleukopenia is severe and progressive. In the granulopenic state, necrotizing, nonpurulent reactions develop at the site of infections. Hemorrhagic manifestations appear and may progress. The hemorrhage is most likely due to a combination of many factors, however, thrombocytopenia with a concomitant poor clot retraction, poor hemostasis, impaired prothrombin utilization, and the prolonged clotting time, probably can adequately explain all the phenomena. It is not necessary to introduce the concept of release of anticoagulants by irradiation in order to explain the prolongation of the whole-blood clotting time. However, evidence has been presented in the past that indicates an anticoagulant may at times be present and some investigators have inferred that the anticoagulant has heparin-like properties (see Chapter 9).

The anemia develops slowly, results from a partial or complete cessation of blood formation, from hemorrhage and perhaps from increased blood destruction (Lawrence, Dowdy and Valentine; Cronkite, 1948; Young).

In the animals that ultimately die, a severe cachexia is usually apparent before death. The extensive necrosis, ulceration, and edema of the bowel which is apparently secondary to the pancytopenia and extensive hemorrhage into the bowel, may contribute significantly to malnutrition. As a general rule, animals that cease to eat, particularly the mouse, die within 48 hours. The food intake and weight of all animals decreases in the first few days after irradiation, the survivors regain some of their weight and may not have a secondary drop. Those animals which fail to start eating again or who have a secondary occurrence of anorexia lose weight rapidly and die (Chapman and Cronkite, Smith et al.).

10.7 Factors Modifying the Response to Whole-Body Irradiation

Various factors may favorably or unfavorably influence the lethality of total-body exposure to ionizing radiation or the sensitivity of various structures to ionizing radiation (see also Chapter 13). These factors may conveniently be grouped into pre-irradiation and post-irradiation factors.

Before taking up those factors which are specifically proved to modify or not to modify the response, the following generalities have been assumed true by most, though not necessarily proved.

10.7.1 *Age and Sex.* The very young appear to be more sensitive to radiation (Abrams, Kohn and Kallman). Some evidence for increased sensitivity of children was seen in the exposed Marshallese (Cronkite et al.). There seems to be little dependence of sensitivity on age in the mature animal (Kohn and Kallman); however, no reports on the very old have appeared. There is evidence that the female may be more resistant than the male (Cronkite et al., Carter et al.); however, the difference is small and is not found consistently, particularly with small populations.

10.7.2 *Environment.* There is some evidence that cold, trauma, hunger, muscular exertion and noise will increase the lethality of a given dose of radiation. Since a major cause of death following potentially lethal irradiation is infection, it is not unreasonable to expect that anything that would increase the susceptibility to infection would increase the mortality.

10.7.3 *Allergy, Immunity, Metabolic Disorders, and Dietary Deficiencies.* There is little known about the influence of these factors on the survival of man. However, mice with induced hyperthyroidism are more sensitive (Blount and Smith). Dietary deficiencies of vitamins and proteins generally seem to increase the incidence of radiation illness after x-ray therapy, particularly over the abdomen. However, the data that have been presented are not statistically conclusive.

10.7.4 *Pharmaceutical Agents Administered Prior to Irradiation.* Hektoen apparently was the first to report an apparent protection against radiation by the injection of foreign protein 10 days prior to radiation. Treadwell et al. and Patt et al. demonstrated protection by injection of estradiol 10 days before irradiation of mice, and this has been amply confirmed. A great deal of interest in pre-protective agents resulted from the considerable protection found to result from cysteine (Patt) and glutathione (Cronkite et al.) administration. Since these SH-containing compounds were found to be protective, a host of compounds of varied structure have been shown to be protective. These include thiourea, cysteamine, dithiopropanol (BAL), paraminopropriophenone (PAPP), sodium nitrite, methylene blue, zinc, cyanide, methylamine (a competitive anticholine oxidase), malonylnitrite, azide, diethylstilbesterol, cobalt, ethyl alcohol, butyl alcohol, megaphen, magnesium sulfate, carbon monoxide, chlorpromazine, chelating agents, morphine, anesthetic agents, 4-acylpyrogallol, atabrine, oxytocin, cholinergic blocking agents, linoleate, tryptamine, glucosamine, oxypolygelatin and certain vaccines. Reported protection by flavanones given prior to and after exposure (Rekers and Field; Field and Rekers; Clark et al.; Sokolof et al.) has not been confirmed by others (Kaplan et al.; Cronkite et al.; Patt et al.; Kohn et al.; Dauer and Coon; Buchanan et al.). The compound S2, B-amino-ethylisothiouronium $\cdot$ Br $\cdot$ HBr (AET) shows particular promise practically because of its high degree of effectiveness, relatively low toxicity and potency when administered orally. These compounds have been reviewed (Alexander and Bacq; Bond and Cronkite; Bond and Robertson) where original references may be found. Severe hypoxia during irradiation also confers protection (Limperos; Dowdy et al.), as does hypothermia. Irradiation under increased oxygen tension increases sensitivity, a fact that may have application in clinical radiotherapy. It is not clear to what degree chemical pre-protective agents act by direct competition for active radicals, through temporary induction of hypoxia or by other biological means. Indications that at least some act through hypoxia induction are seen in the work of Salerno, who found reduced oxygen tension in the tissues of animals given cysteine in protective amounts. He also found that very high oxygen tensions abolished the protective effects of cysteine, PAPP and cysteamine in rats.

10.7.5 *Shielding Effects* (also see section **10.8.2**). The prototype of shielding experiments was initiated by Chiari who in 1912 demonstrated that bone marrow of the rabbit when transplanted to the spleen would grow only if the spleen were shielded and the rest of the animal were irradiated. Fabricius-Moller clearly demonstrated that shielding of portions of the skeleton prevented the fall in blood platelets and hemorrhage from doses which uniformly killed his unshielded animals. Chrom (1935) reported a series of experiments on shielding portions of the abdomen and its influence on phagocytosis of bacteria. The technique of shielding has been elaborated and exploited by Jacobson et al. in a large series of articles in the past few years. Jacobson and his group have shown a very striking protection of mice to an approximate 100 per cent lethal dose of radiation when the mouse spleen* and the other organs are shielded with lead. Shielding of these organs resulted in a very marked increase in rate of hemopoietic regeneration.

Other shielding experiments have demonstrated protection; for example, shielding of the adrenals (Edelmann) and the head (Allen et al.). Bond et al. have shown that the time sequence, survival time and nature of death is different when the abdomen is shielded than when the skeleton is shielded. It requires a larger dose in r to kill when the abdomen is shielded and less when only the abdomen is exposed, and thus a good part of the skeleton is shielded. Abdomen-exposed animals die more quickly. Protection is conferred if one-half of the body only is exposed, followed in a matter of minutes by exposure of the remaining half with shielding of the previously exposed portion (Swift et al.).

10.7.6 *Parabiosis.* Parabiosis accomplished some time prior to irradiation (Huff et al.; Brecher and Cronkite; Finerty et al.) markedly decreased mortality of animals exposed to an otherwise fatal dose of radiation.

10.8 Post-Radiation Factors

The factors that modify the radiation response after irradiation can be divided into those that increase the mortality rate, and those that favorably influence the mortality rate and survival time. The former will be considered first.

10.8.1 *Unfavorable Post-Irradiation Factors.* Smith and Smith showed that moderate exercise only slightly decreased the survival rate of mice. Strenuous exercise in the form of forced swimming after irradiation increased the mortality rate strikingly in rats (Kimmeldorf; Newry). Smith and Smith presented evidence showing that induction and maintenance of a hypermetabolic state by the administration of dinitrophenol after irradiation for the full observation period increased mortality. Anti-thyroid therapy with thiouracil and propyl-thiouracil did not influence the mortality rate. Ellinger reports that testosterone proprionate administered in daily doses of 0.25 and 0.5 milligrams to mice after irradiation with an LD_{50} increases the mortality rate. Smith et al. concluded that ACTH and cortisone do not increase the survival rate and that ACTH after irradiation may be harmful. It appears that synkavit and other related compounds of

---

* The mouse spleen shows extensive myelopoiesis under normal conditions; hence the protective effect of splenic shielding in the mouse is not necessarily something that is unique to the splenic tissue *per se.*

the vitamin K group will increase the mortality of irradiated animals. The material tends to concentrate in some tumors following intravenous injection (Mitchell et al.).

10.8.2 *Post-Radiation Factors that Increase the Survival Rate.* In general, one can divide post-radiation modification of radiation injury into three general categories: (a) the striking and rapid restoration of severely damaged, hemopoietic tissues by shielding of bone marrow or spleen, parabiosis, injection of bone marrow, or splenic homogenate, etc., which are effective following usually lethal doses of irradiation from which spontaneous recovery is rare; (b) the less striking effect of post-radiation stimulation of myelopoiesis and erythropoiesis. Myelopoiesis can be stimulated by sterile inflammation (Cronkite and Brecher) in the mid-lethal or sublethal, but not in the absolute lethal zone. Erythropoiesis is stimulated by anoxic stimuli or by normal anemic plasma in the sublethal range only; (c) modification of the histologic and clinical picture by substitution (red cell, white cell, and platelet transfusion) without greatly increased survival rate or induced restoration of hemopoietic tissues. The last category simply represents substitution of elements that are no longer being produced. In the second category, one can imagine the mechanism as being due to the stimulation of precursor cells that are injured, but still capable of responding to physiologic stimuli (erythropoietin, leukocytosis promoting factor, etc.) that are known to exist, although not yet adequately characterized. Interest has centered mainly around the mechanism of the restorative effect in the first category, and this will be pursued in some detail here (for reviews of this subject, see Cronkite and Bond; Bond and Cronkite; Jacobson).

Studies on post-radiation restoration of tissues had their genesis in shielding experiments. (Restoration rather than regeneration has been adopted as the most appropriate term in this connection, following Latarjet and Gray.) After doses of radiation from which there is survival, spontaneous regeneration of most tissues occurs. However, it is possible to have permanent atrophy of some tissues that are not essential to life, or of portions of tissues that are essential to life. It is not clear what influence the restoration induced by shielding or injecting hematopoietic tissue has on ultimate longevity, genetic effects and tumor induction. Shielding apparently protects against lymphoma induction in mice (Kaplan et al.); however, shielding or parabiosis did not protect against induction of other types of tumors (Maisin; Brecher et al.; Court-Brown; Finerty). Early studies on shielding and restoration of irradiated tissues go back to Chiari (1912) and Fabricius-Möller (1921) (see Cronkite and Brecher). The later studies of Jacobson and his associates led to the concept that "humoral factors" were present in the shielded spleen of the irradiated mouse which induced rapid restoration of the irradiated hemopoietic tissues elsewhere in the body. Their work and concepts are summarized in reviews by Jacobson et al. As a result, investigations aimed at the proof of the existence and isolation of the "humoral factor" have been conducted by workers in a number of laboratories.

Parabiosis induced after irradiation has been shown to increase the survival rate of irradiated rats. The nature of this effect has been pursued by Finerty et al.; Schneider et al.; Binhammer et al.; and Metz et al. and it was concluded that the effect was not mediated through spleen, adrenals, or hypophysis (Finerty et al.; Schneider et al.). Swift et al. successively irradiated portions of the body, followed after varying time intervals with irradiation of the entire remaining portion of the body. This procedure significantly increased the survival rate. These studies indicated strongly that the protective factor circulates and can be quickly picked up by tissues that have been irradiated.

Cole and associates have been most productive in investigating the possible existence and subcellular location of the protective "spleen factor." Early in their work, it became evident that age, strain and species were factors that influenced the results. The effectiveness of several subcellular fractions of spleen homogenates prepared by the Schneider-Hogeboom techniques was then tested. The experiments conclusively showed that there was no restorative effect connected with the mitochondria, microsomes or soluble supernatant fractions. The restorative effect was found only with the cell nucleus fraction. Since relatively few intact cells were found on stained smears of the nucleus fraction, it was believed that their experiments strongly supported the concept that the restorative effect was noncellular and associated with the nucleoproteins. Further studies on the splenic homogenates have shown that DNAase and trypsin inactivate the material, as does distilled water extraction under various conditions. Since enzymes are believed not to attack living intact cells, these experiments were interpreted as indicating that the active principle is associated with DNA and not necessarily with living cells. These contentions argued strongly for the noncellular concept.

It was thought early that studies with heterologous marrow might provide the definitive answer. Lorenz and Congdon, and Congdon and Lorenz reported that homologous and heterologous ground bone favorably modify lethal radiation injury in the mouse. Transplanted homologous bone developed bone marrow, but heterologous bone transplants did not show bone marrow formation. The same investigators reported protection of some strains of mice by intravenous injections of rat bone marrow emulsion from certain strains of rats. They interpreted the bone and bone marrow transplant studies as evidence in favor of the existence of a humoral factor. Cole et al. protected mice with rat bone marrow. Late deaths after two weeks were common.

A British group (Barnes and Loutit) have made a series of contributions on the nature of the restorative action of splenic implants and homogenates. Initially, they confirmed the effectiveness of splenic homogenates. Next, they showed that immunization of one strain of mouse (CBA) by strain A material prevents protection; whereas, short-lived protection of CBA mice could be obtained by use of strain A material in nonimmune mice. Further, they were unable to confirm the heterologous protection experiments of Lorenz et al. In general, their experience was the same as Cole et al. in that freezing, thawing, irradiation, and formalin-treatment inactivated the principle. Their more recent studies showed that the restorative principle of intact CBA mice spleens can be preserved when the spleens are equilibrated with glycerol serum and stored at −70°C. for as long as 83 days.

Recently very significant studies, incontrovertible when considered together, have been reported independently by several different laboratories conclusively proving that cellular transplantation can and does take place. Lindsley et al. availed themselves of the blood type of certain strains of rats and proved that functional erythropoietic tissue of the donor animal was implanted in the irradiated host and was producing cells characteristic of the donor. As pointed out by Ford et al., this might be comparable to transduction in bacteria. Nowell et al. took advantage of the fact that rat leukocytes give a strong positive alkaline phosphatase and mouse leukocytes give a negative reaction. Irradiated mice were injected with rat bone marrow. This increased the survival rate. Phosphatase-positive white blood cells were found in the peripheral blood and the bone marrow showing that transplantation had in all probability occurred. However, these authors do not rule out that the phenomenon may have been induced in the host cells; a rather unlikely explanation. Ford et al. have, without doubt, proved that transplantation of donor hemopoietic cells has occurred. They used a distinctive "marker chromosome" that had been induced by a radiation reciprocal translocation of chromosomes yielding a small distinctive easily detected chromosome. When spleen homogenates were prepared from the spleens of mice possessing this distinctive chromosome, the proliferative hemopoietic tissue of recipient mice consisted predominantly of the marked cells. Makinodan by quantitative immunologic tests on red cells proved that irradiated mice heterologously protected by rat bone marrow eventually developed 100 per cent rat red cells and also confirmed Nowell et al. on the presence of rat granulocytes by the distinctive phosphatase reaction. It would appear that these four studies would have driven the last "coffin nail" into the "humoral theory of Jacobson"; however, proof of transplantation does not exclude a humoral contribution. In fact, Jaroslow and Taliaferro have apparently demonstrated that there is a noncellular factor associated with diverse materials such as spleen mice, HeLa cells, and yeast autolysate that restores the ability to produce antibodies. C. L. Miller has also demonstrated a heat labile serum factor that is necessary to retain the protective effect of cells of embryo spleen or liver in tissue cultures, although the fact is not necessary for viability of the culture.

In general then, one must accept that cellular transplantation is a proved fact. The evidence indicates that the protective cell is intermediate between the primitive mesenchymal cell and the actively proliferating differentiated cell since tissues rich in primitive mesenchymal cells do not protect. If this concept is true, one would postulate that factors concerned with active division and maturation for any lineage are abundant in the irradiated animal, but that the cells which can respond to the stimuli have been eradicated. There is good histologic evidence for this. The defect then might be an inability of the primitive mesenchymal cells to mature to the stage where they can respond to stimuli that are present.

The problem now comes back to answering the more general old hemopoietic problem on the *de novo* origin of myeloid metaplasia. Is it autochthonous or metastatic? If autochthonous, is it induced by circulating chemical factors? From all the experimental evidence today, it is proved that cell transplantation does occur but one cannot exclude humoral contributions of the recipient and possibly of donor material. The restorative effect is genetically specific and is associated with primitive myeloid cells. In conclusion, it appears probable that the basic defect in fatally irradiated animals is an absence of cells of sufficient maturity to respond to physiologic factors of growth and differentiation that are present or can be released by appropriate stimuli in the irradiated animal. The restorative effect can be produced by introduction of cells in the depleted area with this degree of maturity, or presumably by a chemical influence that initiates heteroplastic hemopoiesis. The cellular explanation is a reality with shielded spleens or bone marrow, and with injected myeloid suspensions. A chemical influence is still an attractive hypothesis, the relative importance of which in repairing radiated tissues remains obscure.

REFERENCES

ABRAMS, H. L. AND KAPLAN, H. S.: The effect of shielding on mortality following irradiation. *Stanford M. Bull.*, *9:* 165–167, 1951.

ABRAMS, H. L.: Influence of age, body weight and sex on susceptibility of mice to the lethal effects of x-radiation. *Proc. Soc. Exper. Biol. & Med., 76:* 729–732, 1951.

ALLEN, B. R., WARDELL, H. G., AND CLAY, M.: Post irradiaton protection of rabbitsi by injection of "Splenic" plasma. *Science, 123:* 1080–1081, 1956.

ALPEN, E. L. AND SHELINE, G. E.: The combined effects of thermal burns and whole body x-irradiation on survival time and mortality. *Ann. Surg., 140:* 113–118, 1954.

BARNES, D. W. H. AND LOUTIT, J. F.: Protective effects of implants of spleen. *Proc. Roy. Soc. Med., 46:* 251–252, 1953.

BARNES, D. W. H. AND LOUTIT, J. F.: What is the recovery factor in spleen? *Nucleonics*, *12:*

BARNES, D. W. H. AND LOUTIT, J. F.: Proc. Intern. Conf. Peaceful Uses Atomic Energy, pp. 291–296 (United Nations, New York, N. Y., 1956).

BARRON, E. S. G., DICKMAN, S., MUNTZ, J. A., AND SINGER, T. P.: Studies on the mechanism of action of ionizing radiations. I. Inhibition of enzymes by x-rays. *J. Gen. Physiol.*, *32:* 537–552, 1949.

BARRON, E. S. G. AND DICKMAN, S.: Studies on the mechanism of action of ionizing radiations. II. Inhibition of sulfhydryl enzymes by alpha, beta, and gamma rays. *J. Gen. Physiol.*, *32:* 595–605, 1949.

BARROW, J. AND TULLIS, J. L.: The sequence of cellular response to injury in mice exposed to 1100 r total body X-radiation. *A.M.A. Arch. Path.*, *53:* 391–407, 1952.

BAXTER, H., DRUMMOND, J. A., STEPHENS-NEWSHAMM, L. G., AND RANDALL, R. G.: Reductions of mortality in swine from combined total body radiation and thermal burns by streptomycin. *Ann. Surg.*, *137:* 450–455, 1953.

BINHAMMER, R. T., SCHNEIDER, M., AND FINERTY, J. C.: Time as a factor in post-irradiation protection by parabiosis. *Am. J. Physiol.*, *175:* 440–442, 1953.

BLOUNT, H. C., JR. AND SMITH, W. W.: The influence of thyroid and thiouracil on mice exposed to roentgen radiation. *Science, 109:* p. 83, 1949.

BOND, V. P., ET AL: Sensitivity of abdomen of rat to X-irradiation. *Am. J. Physiol.*, *161:* 323–330, 1950.

BOND V. P. SWIFT, M. N., TAKETA, S. T., AND TOBIAS, C. A.: Indirect effects of deuteron irradiation in rats. *Am. J. Physiol.*, *174:* 259–263, 1953.

BOND, V. P., SILVERMAN, M. S., AND CRONKITE, E. P.: Pathogenesis and pathology of post-irradiation infection. *Radiation Res.*, *1:* 389–400, 1954.

BOND, V. P., SHECHMEISTER, I. L., SWIFT, M. N., AND FISHLER, M. C.: The effects of X-irradiation on a naturally occurring endemic infection. *J. Infect. Dis.*, *91:* 26–32, 1952.

BOND, V. P. AND CRONKITE, E. P.: Effects of radiation on mammals. *Ann. Rev. Physiol.*, *19:* 299–328, 1956.

BOND, V. P. AND ROBERTSON, J. S.: Vertebrate radiobiology (Lethal actions and associated effects). *Ann. Rev. Nuc. Science, 7:*

BOND, V. P., CRONKITE, E. P., SANDHAUS, C. A., ROBERTSON, J. S., AND BORG, D. C.: Geometrical and energy factors influencing the effect of penetrating radiations on man. *Radiation Res.*, *6:* 554–572, 1957.

BOWERS, J. Z. AND SCOTT, K. G.: Distribution and excretion of electrolytes after acute whole body irradiation injury. I. Studies with radiopotassium. *Proc. Soc. Exper. Biol. & Med. 78:* 645–648, 1951.

BRAYER, F. T., GLASSER, S. R., AND DUFFY, B. J. JR.: Effect of X-irradiation on the adrenal cortical steroid excretion in urine. *Science, 120:* 112, 1954.

BRECHER, G. AND CRONKITE, E. P.: Lesions of the alimentary tract in dogs exposed to whole body irradiation of 300 to 3000 r. Presented before Am. Assoc. Path. and Bact., Cleveland, April 26, 1951.

BRECHER, G. AND CRONKITE, E. P.: Post-radiation parabiosis and survival in rats. *Proc. Soc. Exper. Biol. & Med.*, *77:* 292–294, 1951.

BUCHANAN, D. J., PEARSON, W. N., AMARISINGHAM, C., HUDSON, G. W., AND DARBY, W. J.: Citrovorum and irradiation injury. *Am. J. Physiol.*, *175:* 437–439, 1953.

CARTER, R. E., BOND, V. P., AND SEYMOUR, P. H.: The relative biological effectiveness of fast neutrons in mice. *Radiation Res.*, *4:* 413–423, 1956.

CHAPMAN, W. H. AND CRONKITE, E. P.: Further studies on the beneficial effect of glutathione on x-irradiated mice. *Proc. Soc. Exper. Biol. & Med., 75:* 308–322, 1950.

CHAPMAN, W. H. AND JEROME, E. A.: An analysis of the effects of total-body x-irradiation on the body weight of white Swiss mice. *Radiation Res., 4:* 519–531, 1956.

CHIARI, O. M.: Vorläufigen Mitteilung über Knochenmarkstransplantation. *München. med. Wchnschr. 59:* 2503, 1912.

CHRON, S. A.: Studies on the Effects of Roentgen Rays Upon the Intestinal Epithelium and Upon the Reticuloendothelial Cells of the liver and spleen. *Acta radiol., 16:* 641–650, 1935.

CLAPPER, W. E., ROBERTS, J. E., AND MEADE, G. H.: Radiation effects on pneumococcol infection produced by subcutaneous injections into white mice. *Proc. Soc. Exper. Biol. & Med., 86:* 420–422, 1954.

CLARK, W. G., UNCAPHER, R. P., AND JORDAN, M. L.: Effect of flavonoids (vitamin P) on mortality from total body roentgen irradiation. *Science, 108:* 629–630, 1948.

COLE, L. S., FISHLER, M. C., ELLIS, M. E., AND BOND, V. P.: Protection of mice against X-irradiation by spleen homogenates administered after exposure. *Proc. Soc. Exper. & Biol. Med. 80:* 112–117, 1952.

COLE, L. S., BOND, V. P., AND FISHLER, M. C.: Protection against radiation by sodium nitrite. U. S. N. Radiological Defense Laboratory Report, San Francisco, 1952.

COLE, L. J. AND ELLIS, M. E.: Age, strain and species factors in post-irradiation protection by spleen homogenates. *Am. J. Physiol., 173:* 487–494, 1953.

COLE, L. J., FISHLER, M. C., AND BOND, V. P.: Subcellular fractionation of mouse spleen radiation protection activity. *Proc. Nat. Acad. Sc., 39:* 759–772, 1953.

COLE, L. J. AND ELLIS, M. E.: Studies on the chemical nature of the radiation protective factor in mouse spleen. *Radiation Res. 1:* 347–357, 1954.

COLE, L. J., HABERMEYER, J. G., AND BOND, V. P.: Recovery from acute radiation injury in mice following administration of rat bone marrow. *J. Nat. Cancer Inst., 16:* 1–9, 1955.

COLE, L. J. AND ELLIS, M. E.: On the nature of the spleen-bone marrow radiation recovery factor, in: *Fundamentals of Radiobiology,* BACQ, Z. M., AND ALEXANDER, P., Eds. London, England, Butterworth Scientific Publications, 389 pp., 1955.

COLE, L. J., FISHLER, M. C., AND ELLIS, M. E.: Studies on the nature of the radiation protection factor in mouse spleen. *Radiology, 64:* 201–207, 1955.

CONARD, R. A.: Cholinesterase activity, weight, water content and pathology of small intestine of rats subjected to x-radiation. *Am. J. Physiol., 170:* 428–425, 1952.

CONARD, R. A.: Effect of X-irradiation on intestinal motility of the rat. *Am. J. Physiol.* 1951.

CONARD, R. A., CRONKITE, E. P., BRECHER, G., AND STROME, C. P. A.: Experimental therapy of the gastrointestinal syndrome produced by lethal doses of ionizing radiation.

CONARD, R. A.: Some effects of ionizing radiation on the physiology of the gastrointestinal tract. *Radiation Res., 5:* 167–188, 1956.

CONGDON, C. C. AND LORENZ, E.: Humoral factor in irradiating protection. Modification of lethal radiation injury in mice by injection of rat bone marrow. *Am. J. Physiol., 176:* 297–300, 1954.

CRADDOCK, C. G., JR., AND LAWRENCE, J. S.: The effect of roentgen irradiation on antibody formation in rabbits. *J. Immunol., 60:* 241–254, 1948.

CRONKITE, E. P.: The clinical manifestations of acute radiation illness produced in goats by exposure to an atomic bomb, Test Able, Bikini, 1946, with comments on therapy. U. S. Naval Medical Bulletin 49: 199–215, 1949.

CRONKITE, E. P. AND BRECHER, G.: The experimental therapy of the hemorrhagic phase of the radiation syndrome with platelet transfusions. Acta radiol. Suppl., 116: 376–380, 1954.

CRONKITE, E. P., BOND, V. P., CONARD, R. A., SHULMAN, N. R., FARR, R. S., COHN, S. H., DUNHAM, C. L., AND BROWNING, L. E.: Some effects of ionizing radiation on human beings. Atomic Energy Document TID 5358, 1956. Gov't. Printing Office, Washington 25, D. C. Shortened version in: J. A. M. A., 159: 430–434, 1955.

CRONKITE, E. P. AND CHAPMAN, W. H.: A critical analysis of the syndrome of acute total body irradiation illness, its role in atomic warfare and its influence in the future practice of military medicine. Mil. Surgeon, 104: 7–21, 1949.

CRONKITE, E. P., ET AL.: Failure of rutin to decrease mortality of acute ionizing radiation illness in mice. Proc. Soc. Exper. Biol. & Med., 70: 125–128, 1949.

CRONKITE, E. P. AND CHAPMAN, W. H.: The effect of adrenalectomy and glutathione on X-ray induced mortality in mice. Fed. Proc., 9: 329, 1950.

CRONKITE, E. P. AND CHAPMAN, W. H.: The effect of adrenalectomy on radiation-induced mortality of the mouse. Proc. Soc. Exper. Biol. & Med. 74: 337, 1950.

CRONKITE, E. P., CHAPMAN, W. H., AND CHAMBERS, F. W.: Failure of a flavonoid (Vitamin P) to reduce radiation mortality in mice. Proc. Soc. Exper. Biol. & Med., 76: 282–284, 1951.

CRONKITE, E. P., JACKSON, D. P., LEROY, G. V., AND LUNDY, A. R. T.: The present status of the hemorrhagic phase of radiation injury. Proceedings of the International Soc. of Hematology, May, 1951.

CRONKITE, E. P., HALPERN, B., JACKSON, D. P., AND LEROY, G. V.: A study of the hemorrhagic state in dogs after lethal dose of 2-million volt X-rays. Proc. of the Central Soc. for Clinical Research 23: 26, 1950.

CRONKITE, E. P. AND BRECHER, G.: The protective effect of granulocytes in radiation injury. Ann. New York Acad Sc., 59: 815–833, 1955.

CRONKITE, E. P., BRECHER, G., AND CHAPMAN, W. H.: Studies on the mechanism of the protective action of glutathione against radiation injury. Mil. Surgeon, 109: 296–307, 1951.

CRONKITE, E. P., JACOBS, G., BRECHER, G. AND DILLARD, G.: The hemorrhagic phase of the acute radiation syndrome due to exposure of the whole body to penetrating ionizing radiation. Am. J. Roentgenol., 67: 796–803, 1952.

CRONKITE, E. P. AND BRECHER, G.: Defects in hemostasis produced by whole body irradiation. 5th Annual Conference—Blood Coagulation and Allied Subjects. Trans. Josiah Macy Foundation, New York, 1952.

CRONKITE, E. P., BOND, V. P., CHAPMAN, W. H., AND LEE, R. H.: Biological effects of atomic-bomb gamma radiation. Science, 122: 148–150, 1955.

DALE, W. M.: Effect of X-rays on aqueous solutions of biologically active compounds. Brit. J. Radiol., 16: 171–172, 1943.

DAUER, M. AND COON, J. M.: Failure of rutin and related flavonoids to influence mortality following acute whole body X-irradiation. Proc. Soc. Exper. Biol. & Med., 79: 702–707, 1952.

DILLARD, G. H. L., BRECHER, G., AND CRONKITE, E. P.: Separation, concentration and transfusion of platelets. Proc. Soc. Exper. Biol. & Med., 78: 796–799, 1951.

DOUGHERTY, T. F. AND SCHNEEBELI, G. L.: Role of cortisone in regulation of inflammation. Proc. Soc. Exper. Biol. & Med., 75: 854–859, 1950.

DOWDY, A. H., BENNETT, L. R., AND CHASTAIN, S. M.: Protective effect of anoxic anoxia against total body roentgen irradiation of mammals. *Radiology, 55:* 879–885, 1950.

EDELMANN, A.: Adrenal cortex and survival of rats after X-irradiation. *Fed. Proc. 9:* 36, 1950.

EDELMANN, A.: Adrenal shielding and survival of rats after X-irradiation. *Am. J. Physiol., 165:* 57–60, 1951.

EDELMANN, A.: Survival of adrenalectomized rats with and without replacement therapy following X-irradiation. *Am. J. Physiol., 167:* 57–60, 1951.

The Effects of Nuclear Weapons, 1957. Gov't. Printing Office.

ELLINGER, F. P.: The influence of pharmacological agents on effects of irradiation. *Radiology, 50:* 234–243, 1948.

ELLINGER, F. P.: *Biologic Fundamentals of Radiation Therapy.* New York: Elsevier, 1941.

ELLINGER, F. P., ROSWIT, D. B., AND GLASSER, S.: The treatment of radiation sickness with adrenal cortical hormones (desoxycorticosterone acetate). *Am. J. Roentgenol., 61:* 381–396, 1949.

ELLINGER, F.: Some effects of testosterone propionate on mice irradiated with X-rays. *Proc. Soc. Exper. Biol. & Med., 74:* 616–619, 1950.

ELLINGER, F.: Pharmacologic studies on irradiated animals. Effect of cortisone on X-ray mortality of mice. *Proc. Soc. Exper. Biol. & Med., 80:* 214–220, 1952.

ELLINGER, F.: Effect of cell-free aqueous extracts from normal and irradiated spleens on X-ray induced mortality in mice; a preliminary report. *Radiol. Clin., 23:* 229–239, 1954.

ESPLIN, D. W., MARCUS, S., AND DONALDSON, D. M.: Effects of x-irradiation and adrenalectomy on phagocytic activity. *J. Immunol., 70:* 454–460, 1953.

FABRICIUS-MOLLER, J.: *Experimental studies of the hemorrhagic diathesis from X-ray sickness.* Copenhagen: Levin and Munksgaards Forlag, 1922.

FAILLA, G.: *Influence of wave length on biological action of radiation, in Symposium on Cancer.* Pages 78–90, Univ. of Wisconsin, 1938.

FAILLA, G.: A theory of the biological action of ionizing radiations. Occasional publications of American Association for the Advancement of Science, #4, 202–214, Supplement to Science *85:* June 1933.

FAILLA, G.: Comments on the report of the International Commission of Radiological Units, Sixth International Congress of Radiology. *Amer. J. Roent. 65:* 477–480, 1951.

FINERTY, J. C., BINHAMMER, R. T., AND SCHNEIDER, M.: Survival of irradiated rats in parabiosis with hypophysectomized partners. *Science, 118:* 654–655, 1953.

FORD, C. E., LAMERTON, J. L., BARNES, D. W. H., AND LOUTIT, J. F.: Cytological identification of radiation chimaeras. *Nature, 177:* 452–454, 1956.

FORSTER, F. M., ET AL.: Degenerative changes in cerebral arteries following administration of desoxycorticosterone acetate. *J. Clin. Endocrinology 6:* 77–87, 1946.

FRICKE, E.: *Symposium; Quantitative Biology, 2:* 241, 1934.

FRIEDMAN, J., WERDER, A. A., ROTH, F. J., GRAHAM, A. B., OVIDIO, J. M., AND SYVERTON, J. T.: The synergistic effects of roentgen radiation and cortisone upon susceptibility of mice to pathogenic microorganisms. *Am. J. Roentgenol., 71:* 509–517, 1954.

GOLDFEDER, A., ET AL.: Agents influencing experimental radiation injury, effects of folic acid and pyridoxine. *Proc. Soc. Exper. Biol. & Med. 67:* 272–278, 1948.

GORDON, L. E., RUML, D., HAHNE, H. J., AND MILLER, C. P.: Studies on the susceptibility of infection following ionizing radiation. IV. The pathogenesis of endogenous bacteremia in mice. *J. Exper. Med., 102:* 413–424, 1955.

GRAHAM, J. B., GRAHAM, R. M., AND GRAFFEO, A. J.: The influence of Adrenal Cortical Hormones on Sensitivity of Mice to Ionizing Radiation. *Endocrinology, 46:* No. 5, 434–440, 1950.

GRAHAM, J. B. AND GRAHAM, R. M.: The modification of resistance to ionizing radiation by humoral agents. *Cancer 3:* 709–717, 1950.

HALE, W. M. AND STONER, R. D.: The effect of cobalt-60 gamma radiation on passive immunity. *Yale J. Biol. & Med., 25:* 327–333, 1953.

HALEY, T. J., MANN, S., AND DOWDY, A. H.: A comparison of the responses of normal and hypothyroid mice to acute whole-body Roentgen Radiation. *Science 112:* 333–334, 1950.

HAMMOND, C. W., VOGEL, H. H., CLARK, J. W., COOPER, D. B., AND MILLER, C. P.: The effect of streptomycin therapy on mice irradiated with fast neutrons. *Radiation Res., 2:* 354–360, 1955.

HARRISON, H. E., AND DARROW, D. C.: Renal Function in Experimental Adrenal Insufficiency. *Am. J. Physiol., 125:* 631–643, 1939.

Hearings before a subcommittee of the committee on government operations, House of Representatives, Congressional Record, 1956.

HEKTOEN, L.: Further studies on the effects of the roentgen ray on antibody production. *J. Infect. Dis., 20:* 28–33, 1918.

HENNESSEY, T. G. AND HUFF, R. L.: Depression of tracer iron uptake curve in rat erythrocytes following total body x-irradiation. *Proc. Soc. Exper. Biol. & Med., 73:* 436–439, 1950.

HOLDEN, W. D., COLE, J. W., PORTMANN, A. F., AND STORAASLI, J. P.: Hypothromboplastinemia following total body irradiation. *Proc. Soc. Exper. Biol. & Med., 70:* 553–556, 1949.

HOLLINGSWORTH, J. W. AND FINCH, S. C.: Effect of cross-circulation with normal rats on experimental E. coli bacteremia in irradiated rats. *Clin. Res. Proc., 4:* 19, 1956.

HOWLAND, J. W., ET AL.: University of Rochester, U. S. Atomic Energy Commission Project, U. R. –94, 1949.

International Commission on Radiological Units and Measurements (ICRU), reports in Radiology *62:* 106–109, 1954, and in Handbook 62, National Bureau of Standards, 1957.

JACKSON, D. P., CRONKITE, E. P., AND JACOBS, G.: Prothrombin utilization in fatal radiation injury. *Am. J. Physiol., 169:* 208–217, 1952.

JACKSON, D. P., CRONKITE, E. P., LeRoy, G. V., AND HALPERN, B.: Further studies on the nature of the hemorrhagic phase of radiation injury. *J. Lab. & Clin. Med., 39:* 449–461, 1952.

JACOBSON, L. O., ROBSON, M. J., AND MARKS, E. K.: The effects of x-irradiation on antibody formation. *Proc. Soc. Exper. Biol. & Med., 75:* 145–152, 1950.

JACOBSON, L. O., ET AL.: The Role of the Spleen in Radiation Injury. *Proc. Soc. Exper. Biol. & Med., 70:* 740–742, 1949.

JACOBSON, L. O.: Recovery from Radiation Injury. *Blood, 6:* 769–770, 1951.

JACOBSON, L. O., SIMMONS, E. L., MARKS, E. K., GASTON, E. O., ROBSON, M. I., AND ELDREDGE, J. H.: Further studies on Recovery from Radiation injury. *J. Lab. & Clin. Med., 37:* 683–697, 1951.

JACOBSON, L. O., SIMMONS, E. L., MARKS, E. K., AND ELDREDGE, J. H.: Recovery from Radiation Injury. *Science, 113:* 510–511, 1951.

JACOBSON, L. O., MARKS, E. K., GASTON, E. O., SIMMONS, E. L., AND ROBSON, M. L. *Bull. New York Acad. Med., 30:* 675–692, 1954.

JACOBSON, L. O.: *Am. J. Roentgenol.* (Janeway Lecture), *72:* 543–555, 1954.

JAROSLOW, B. N. AND TALIAFERRO, W. H.: The restoration of hemolysin-forming capacity in X-irradiated rabbits by tissue and yeast preparations. *J. Infect. Dis. 98:* 75–81, 1956.

JENNINGS, F. L.: Effect of protein depletion upon susceptibility of rats to total body irradiation. *Proc. Soc. Exper. Biol. & Med., 72:* 487–491, 1949.

Joint Committee, Public hearings on the hazards of ionizing radiations. Congressional Record, 1957.

KAPLAN, H. S.: Influence of age on susceptibility of mice to the development of lymphoid tumors after radiation. *J. Nat. Cancer Inst., 9:* 55–56, 1948.

KAPLAN, H. S., BROWN, M. B., AND PAULL, J.: Influence of bone-marrow injections on involution and neoplasia of mouse thymus after systemic irradiation. *J. Nat. Cancer Inst., 14:* 303–316, 1953.

KIMELDORF, D. J. ET AL.: The effect of exercise upon the lethality of Roentgen Rays for Rats. *Science, 112:* 175–176, 1950.

KOHN, H. I.: Changes in blood plasma of guinea pig during acute radiation syndrome. *Am. J. Physiol., 162:* 703–708, 1950.

KOHN, H. I.: Effect of immaturity, hypophysectomy, and adrenalectomy upon changes in blood plasma of rat during acute radiation syndrome. *Am. J. Physiol., 165:* 43–56, 1951.

KOHN, H. I. AND KALLMAN, R. F.: Age, growth and the LD_{50} of x-rays. *Science, 124:* 1078, 1956.

LAMSON, B. G., AND TULLIS, J. L.: The progression of morphologic lesions in Swiss mice exposed to 625 r, 2000 KVP, total body X-radiation. *Mil. Surgeon, 109:* 281–293, 1951.

LANGHAM, W., WODDWARD, K. T., ROTHERMAL, S. M., HARRIS, P. S., LUSHBAUGH, C. C., AND STORER, J. B.: Studies on the effect of rapidly delivered, massive doses of gamma rays on mammals. *Radiation Res., 5:* 404–432, 1956.

LASSER, B. C. AND STENSTROM, K. W.: Radiation sickness. A study of its relation to adrenal cortical function and absolute eosinophile count. *Am. J. Roentgenol., 72:* 474–487, 1954.

LATARJET, R. AND GRAY, L. H.: Definition of the terms "Protection" and Restoration." *Acta radiol., 41:* 61–62, 1954.

LARKIN, J. C.: Effect of atropine on acute irradiation sickness in mice. *Amer. J. Roentgenology 62:* 547–549, 1949.

LAWRENCE, G. H.: The Effect of Total Body X-radiation 17-Ketosteroid Excretion in Dogs. *Endocrinology 45:* 383–388, 1949.

LAWRENCE, J. S., DOWDY, A. H., AND VALENTINE, W. N.: The effects of radiation on hemopoiesis. MDDC-853. *Radiology, 51:* 400–413, 1948.

LAWRENCE, J. S., VALENTINE, W. N., AND DOWDY, A. H.: The effect of radiation on hemopoiesis. Is there an indirect effect? *Blood, 3:* 593–611, 1948.

LEA, D. E.: Actions of radiations on living cells. Cambridge Univ. Press, 1944.

LEROY, G. V.: The medical sequelae of the Atomic Bomb Explosion. *J.A.M.A., 134:* 1143–1148, 1947.

LIEBOW, A. A., WARREN, S., DE COURSEY, E.: Pathology of atomic bomb casualties. *Am. J. Path., 25:* 853–1028, 1949.

LIMPEROS, G.: Effect of varying tension on mortality of X-rayed mice. *J. Franklin Inst., 249:* 513–514, 1950.

LIMPEROS, G. AND MOSHER, W. A.: Protection of mice against x-radiation by Thiourea. *Science, 112:* 86–87, 1950.

LINDSLEY, D. L., ODELL, T. T., JR., AND TAUSCHE, F. G.: Implantation of functional erythropoietic elements following total-body irradiation. *Proc. Soc. Exper. Biol. & Med., 90:* 512–515, 1955.

LORENZ, E. AND CONGDON, C. C.: Modification of lethal irradiation injury in mice by injection of homologous or heterologous bone. *J. Nat. Cancer Inst.*, *14:* 955–964, 1954.

LORENZ, E., CONGDON, C., AND UPHOFF, D.: Modifications of acute irradiation injury in mice and guinea pigs. *Radiology*, 1952.

LYON, G. M.: Radiological Aspects of Civil Defense. *J.A.M.A.* 146: 465–471, 1951.

MAISIN, J., MAISIN, H., DUNJIC, A., AND MALDAGUE, P., Proc. Intern. Conf. Peaceful Uses Atomic Energy, pp. 315–29 (United Nations, New York, N. Y., 402 pp., 1956.

MAKINODAN, T.: Circulating rat cells in lethally irradiated mice protected with rat bone marrow. *Proc. Soc. Exper. Biol. & Med.*, *92:* 174–179, 1956.

MARCUS, S. AND DONALDSON, D. M.: Suppression of normal bactericidal action of rabbit serum following whole body x-irradiation. *Proc. Soc. Exper. Biol. & Med.*, *83:* 184–187, 1953.

METZ, G., BINHAMMER, R. T., SCHNEIDER, M., AND FINERTY, J. C.: Hematologic changes in rats protected from lethal X-radiation by post-irradiation parabiosis. *Radiation Res.*, *2:* 159–165, 1955.

MILLER, C. P., HAMMOND, C. W., AND TOMPKINS, M.: The Incidence of Bacteremia in Mice Subjected to Total Body X-Radiation. *Science, 111:* 540–541, 1950.

MILLER, C. P., HAMMOND, C. W., AND TOMPKINS, M.: Reduction of Mortality from X-Radiation by Treatment with Antibiotics. *Science, 111:* 719–720, 1950.

MILLER, C. P., HAMMOND, C. W., AND TOMPKINS, M.: The role of infection in radiation injury. *J. Lab. & Clin. Med.*, *38:* 331–343, 1951.

MILLER, C. P., HAMMOND, C. W. TOMPKINS, M., AND SHORTER, G.: The treatment of postirradiation infection with antibiotics, an experimental study on mice. *J. Lab. & Clin. Med.*, *39:* 462–479, 1952.

MILLER, C. L.: Recovery from irradiation following the administration of cultured tissues. *Nature, 178:* 142, 1956.

MILLER, L. S., FLETCHER, G. H., AND GERSTNER, H. B.: Systemic and clinical effects induced in 263 cancer patients by whole-body x-irradiation with nominal air doses of 15 to 200 r. School of Aviation Medicine, USAF, Report 57–92, 1957.

MOLE, R. H., PHILPOT, J. ST. L., AND HODGES, G. R. V.: Reduction in lethal effect of x-radiation by pretreatment with thiourea or sodium ethane dithiophosphonate. *Nature, 166:* 515, 1950.

MOLE, R. H.: Whole body irradiation and the idea of stress. *Brit. J. Exper. Path. 37:* 528–531, 1956.

NIMS, L. F. AND SUTTON, E.: Adrenal cholesterol, liver glycogen and water consumption of fasting and X-irradiated rats. *Am. J. Physiol.*, *177:* 51–54, 1954.

NOWELL, P. C., COLE, L. J., HABERMEYER, J. G., AND ROAN, P. L.: Growth and continued function of rat marrow cells in X-irradiated mice. *Cancer Res.*, *16:* 258–261, 1956.

PAINTER, E. E. AND COOLEY, M. A.: Fluid Volume Studies in Gut, Muscle, and Skin of Rats after Total Body X-radiation. *Fed. Proc. 10:* 100, 1951.

PARKER, D. B.: Engineers in Atomic Offense and Defense. *Military Engineer 42:* 257–259, 1950.

PATT, H. M., SWIFT, M. N., AND TYREE, E. B.: Progress report in physiology. AECD-2024-G, U. S. Atomic Energy Commission, 1947.

PATT, H. M., ET AL.: X-irradiation of the hypophysectomized rat. *Science, 108:* 475–476, 1948.

PATT, H. M., ET AL.: Adrenal Response to total body x-radiation. *Am. J. Physiol.*, *150:* 480–487, 1947.

Patt, H. M., Smith, D. E., and Jackson, E.: The effect of cysteine on the peripheral blood of irradiated rat. *Blood, 5:* 758–763, 1950.

Patt, H. M., Tyree, E. B., Straube, R. L., and Smith, D. E.: Cysteine protection against x-irradiation. *Science, 110:* 213–214, 1949.

Pearse, H. E. and Payne, J. L.: Medical progress, mechanical and thermal injury from atomic bomb. *New England J. Med. 241:* 647–653, 1949.

Pillemer, L., Blum, L., Lepow, I. H., Ross, O. A., Todd, E. W., and Wardlaw, A. C.: The properdin system and immunity: I. Demonstration and isolation of a new serum protein, properdin, and its role in immune phoenomena. *Science, 120:* 279–285, 1954.

Prosser, C. L., et al.: Plutonium project—The clinical sequence of physiological effects of ionizing radiation in animals. *Radiology, 49:* 299–313, 1947.

Quastler, H., Lanzl, E. F., Keller, M. E. and Osborne, J. W.: Acute intestinal radiation death. Studies on roentgen death in mice III. *Am. J. Physiol., 164:* 546–556, 1951.

Reid, J. D., Brooks, J. W., Ham, W. T., and Evans, E. I.: The influence of X-radiation on mortality following thermal flash burns: the site of tissue injury as a factor of determining the type of invading bacteria. *Ann. Surg., 142:* 844–850, 1955.

Raper, J. R.: Effects of total surface beta irradiation. *Radiology, 49:* 314–324, 1947.

Rekers, P. E., and Field, J. B.: Control of hemorrhagic syndrome and reduction in x-irradiation mortality with a flavonone. *Science, 107:* 16–17, 1948.

Rekers, P. E.: Univ. of Rochester Atomic Energy Project Report UR-104, 1951.

Rekers, P. E., Coulter, M. P., and Warren, S. L.: Effect of transplantation of bone marrow into irradiated animals. *Arch. Surg., 60:* 635–667, 1950.

Reyniers, J. A., In: LOBUND-ONR-AEC Report III. Lobund study on comparative effects of total-body radiation. Nov. 16, 1953.

Robbins, L. L., et al.: Superficial "Burns" of skin and eyes from scattered cathode rays. *Radiology, 46:* 1–23, 1946.

Rose, B. and Browne, J. S. L.: Effect of adrenalectomy on histamine content of tissues of rat. *Am. J. Physiol., 131:* 589, 1941.

Rosenfeld, G., Ungar, F., Dorfman, R. I., and Pincus, G.: Irradiation and adrenal steroidogenesis. Steroid transformation by irradiated isolated perfused calf adrenals. *Endocrinology, 56:* 24–29, 30–36, 1955.

Rosenthal, R. L. and Benedek, A. L.: Blood coagulation and hemorrhage following total body x-irradiation in the rabbit. *Am. J. Physiol., 161:* 505–515, 1950.

Ross, M. H. and Ely, J. O.: *Effects of Large Doses of Neutrons on Dogs, in Neutron Effects on Animals.* Baltimore: Williams & Wilkins, 1947.

Salisbury, P. F. et al.: Effect of Early Cross-Transfusion on X-irradiation Disease, *Science, 113:* 6–7, 1951.

Sargeant, J. C.: Civil Defense Organization and Medical and Health Services in Civil Defense. *J.A.M.A., 145:* 897–900, 1951.

Santistaban, G. A., Bowers, J. Z., and Dougherty, T. F.: Influence of cortisone on the mortality of X-irradiated adrenalectomized mice. *Endocrinology, 55:* 794–807, 1954.

Savitsky, J. P.: Control of radiation hemorrhage with splenic extracts. *Blood, 10:* 52–61, 1955.

Sayers, George: The Adrenal Cortex and Homeostasis. *Physiol., Rev. 30:* 241–320, 1950.

Schade, F. F.: Medical Defense Plan of a Metropolitan Area. *J.A.M.A. 145:* 457–460, 1951.

SCHNEIDER, M., WYBOURN, R. C., BINHAMMER, R., AND FINERTY, J. C.: Protection of irradiated rats by parabiosis with adrenalectomized or splenectomized partners. *Radiology, 62:* 234–240, 1954.

SELYE, H.: The general adaptation syndrome and the diseases of adaptation. *J. Clin. Endocrinol., 6:* 117–230, 1946.

SHECHMEISTER, I. L., BOND, V. P., AND SWIFT, M. N.: The susceptibility of irradiated mice to infection as a function of post-irradiation time. *J. Immunol., 68:* 87–95, 1952.

SHECHMEISTER, I. L.: Susceptibility of irradiated animals to infection. *Radiation Res., 1:* 401–410, 1954.

SINAIKO, E. S. AND NECHELES, H.: Liver damage by desoxycorticosterone. *Science, 109:* 37–39, 1949.

SMITH, D. E., PATT, H. M., TYREE, E. B., AND STRAUBE, R. L.: Quantitative aspects of the protective action of cysteine against x-irradiation. *Proc. Soc. Exper. Biol. & Med., 73:* 198–200, 1950.

SMITH, FALCONER AND SMITH, WILLIE W.: Exercise effects on tolerance to radiation. *Am. J. Physiol., 165:* 662–666, 1951.

SMITH, F., SMITH, W. W., ANDREWS, H. L., AND GRENAN, M. M.: Effect of parenteral injections of particulate matter on survival of X-irradiated animals. *Am. J. Physiol., 182:* 396–399, 1955.

SMITH, W. W., DOOLEY, R., AND THOMPSON, E. C.: Simulated High altitude following whole body radiation of mice. *J. Aviation Med., 19:* 227–237, 1948.

SMITH, W. W. AND SMITH, F.: Effects of Thyroid and Radiation on Sensitivity to hypoxia, Basal Rate of Oxygen Consumption and Tolerance to exercise. *Am. J. Physiol., 165:* 639–650, 1951.

SMITH, W. W., GONSHERY, L., ALDEMAN, I., AND CORNFIELD, J.: Effect of granulocyte count and litter survival of irradiated mice. *Am. J. Physiol., 178:* 474–476, 1954.

SMITH, W. W., ALDERMAN, I., AND RUTH, H. J.: Functional studies of the hyperplastic spleen of mice recovering from radiation damage. *Am. J. Physiol., 182:* 403–406, 1955.

SMITH, F. AND GRENAN, M. M.: Effect of hibernation upon survival time following whole body irradiation in the marmot (marmota monax). *Science, 113:* 686–688, 1951.

SMITH, W. W., SMITH, F., AND THOMPSON, E. C.: Failure of cortisone or ACTH to reduce mortality in irradiated mice. *Proc. Soc. Exper. Biol. & Med., 73:* 529–531, 1950.

SOKOLOFF, B., REDD, J. B., AND DUTCHER, R.: Capillary fragility and vitamin P protective actions against radiation. *Proc. Soc. Exper. Biol. & Med., 75:* 6–9, 1950.

STORER, J. B., HARRIS, P. S., FURCHNER, J. E., AND LANGHAM, W. H.: The relative biological effectiveness of various ionizing radiations in mammalian systems. *Radiation Res., 6:* 188–288, 1957.

STOREY, R. H., WISH, L., AND FURTH, J.: Changes in cell and plasma volumes produced by total body X-radiation. *Proc. Soc. Exper. Biol. & Med., 74:* 242–244, 1950.

STRAUBE, R. L., PATT, H. M., TYREE, E. B., AND SMITH, D. E.: Influence of level of adrenal cortical steroids on sensitivity of mice to X-irradiation. *Proc. Soc. Exper. Biol. & Med., 71:* 539–541, 1949.

SWIFT, M. N., TAKETA, S. T., AND BOND, V. P.: Regionally fractionated X-irradiation equivalent in dose to total-body exposure. *Radiation Res., 1:* 241–252, 1954.

SWINGLE, W. W. AND REMINGTON, J. W.: The Role of Adrenal Cortex in Physiological Processes. *Physiol. Rev. 24:* 89–127, 1944.

SWINGLE, W. W., ET AL.: The influence of adrenal cortical hormone upon electrolyte and fluid distribution in adrenalectomized dogs maintained on a sodium and chloride free diet. *Am. J. Physiol. 119:* 684–691, 1937.

SWINGLE, W. W., ET AL.: Relation of serum sodium and chloride levels to alterations of body water in the intact and adrenalectomized dog and the influence of adrenal cortical hormone upon fluid distribution. *Am. J. Physiol. 116:* 438–445, 1936.

TALBOT, J. M. AND PINSON, E. A.: The experimental use of bone marrow in acute radiation injury. *Mil. Surgeon, 108:* 412, 1951.

TREADWELL, A. DEG., GARDNER, W. U., AND LAWRENCE, J. H.: The effect of combining estrogens with lethal doses of roentgen-ray in Swiss mice. *Endocrinology, 32:* 161–164, 1943.

TULLIS, JOHN L., CHAMBERS, F. W., JR., MORGAN, J. E., AND ZELLER, J. H.: Mortality in swine and dose distribution studies in phantoms exposed to supervoltage roentgen radiation. *Am. J. Roentgenol., 67:* 620–627, 1951.

TULLIS, J. L.: The sequence of pathologic changes in swine exposed to the $LD_{100/30}$ of total body super-voltage X-radiation. *Mil. Surgeon, 109:* 271–280, 1951.

Effects of Atomic Weapons. U. S. Atomic Energy Commission. Superintendent of Documents. U. S. Government Printing Office, Washington 25, D. C., 1950.

VANDYKE, D. C. AND HUFF, R. L.: Epilation in the Non-irradiated Member of Parabiotically United Rats, *Proc. Soc. Exper. Biol. & Med., 72:* 266–270, 1949.

WARREN, S.: Effects of radiation on normal tissue. *Arch. Path., 34:* 443, 501, 562, 749, 917, 1070, 1942.

WARREN, S. L. AND WHIPPLE, G. H.: Roentgen ray intoxication. *Exper. Med., 35:* 1922, and *38:* 1923.

WEBER, R. P. AND STEGGERDA, F. R.: Histamine in rat plasma; correlation with blood pressure changes following x-irradiation. *Proc. Soc. Exper. Biol. & Med., 70:* 261–263, 1949.

WORKS, L. ET AL.: Effect of BAL on Radiation Mortality Rate in Mice. Quarterly Bulletin, Northwestern Univ. Med. Sch., Chicago, *24:* No. 4, P. 295, 1950.

WOOD, W. B.: *Harvey Lect.*, pages 72–98, 1951–1952. New York: Acad. Press, 271 pp.

VOLKIN, E. AND KOHN, H. I.: A factor in the plasma of the irradiated rat which changes the A/G ratio. *Arch. Biochem., 30:* 326–332, 1951.

11 ▶

Diagnosis and Therapy of Acute Radiation Injury

E. P. Cronkite, M.D., V. P. Bond, M.D., and R. A. Conard, M.D.

11.1 Introduction

In this chapter the practical aspects of the diagnosis and treatment of acute total-body radiation injury are presented. The pathogenesis of this disease, on the basis of which recommendations relating to rational diagnosis and therapy are made, has been outlined in Chapter 10. The reader is referred also to Chapter 10 for references on experimental protective and therapeutic procedures. Recommendations on the diagnosis and therapy of beta lesions and of internal radiation injury are given in Chapters 13 and 12, respectively.

The acute total-body radiation syndrome will not be seen to an appreciable extent short of atomic warfare, although a small number of individuals have been, and undoubtedly will be, severely exposed in laboratory accidents involving nuclear devices. Acute total-body radiation injury, of course, is but one of the medical problems encountered in atomic warfare, and its relative importance in terms of numbers of casualties will vary greatly with the type of nuclear device and the circumstances surrounding its detonation. Under some circumstances, essentially all potential radiation victims may succumb first to blast or thermal injury. All gradations may exist, to the fallout field circumstances in which a "pure" radiological situation with only radiation casualties may exist. The circumstances, of course, cannot be predicted, and thus radiation must be kept high in importance in medical thinking and planning. The most important aspects of medical planning for the defensive aspects of atomic warfare are those of logistics and supply in the face of mass destruction. It should be realized that while a number of undertakings such as evaluation of initial and residual radiation levels, degree of destruction, degree of shielding afforded, etc., are of great importance, the acute problems will be concerned mainly with sick human beings and their immediate fate. This is a problem for physicians only, and the physician primarily, not the physicist, health physicist or engineer will be sought out and looked to for aid. The complex problems involved can be met only if there is adequate planning prior to attack, and it is the responsibility of the physician to be prepared.

A number of individual articles and symposia on the subjects of atomic warfare and civil defense have appeared. However, the reader is referred to the extensive and well-documented 1956 Hearings in the House of Representatives, and to the 1957 Joint Committee Public Hearings. Material on all aspects of atomic warfare can be found in these authoritative documents. It is encouraging that, even though the size of weapons has increased enormously, the attitude of authors writing on these subjects has changed from the defeatism of 1945–1946 to one of constructive planning in preparation for atomic warfare if forced upon the democratic world.

11.2 Diagnosis of Radiation Injury

Since exposures of human beings after detonation of an atomic bomb will not necessarily be identical to the homogeneous whole body exposure that is attained in the laboratory, it is considered desirable to base all diagnostic and prognostic endeavors on the experiences of the Japanese physicians and the Joint Commission following the explosion of the bombs at Hiroshima and Nagasaki.

11.2.1 *Clinical Criteria.* An analysis of the Japanese clinical data demonstrates that the exposed population may be arbitrarily divided into three categories based on their likelihood of survival. (This classification differs from that of LeRoy, the Joint Commission, and Liebow et al. The LeRoy, Joint Commission and Dunham classifications are based solely on the severity of clinical symptoms. The Liebow et al. classification is based on the pathological picture. All classifications have their own merit and objective.) These three groups may be defined as:

Group   I. Survival from radiation injury is *improbable.*
Group   II. Survival from radiation injury is *possible.*
Group III. Survival from radiation injury is *probable.*

The segregation of an exposed population into the three groups defined above may be attempted by three criteria.

(1) Distance from the explosion.
(2) By personnel radiation dosimeters.
(3) By symptomatology as was observed in the Japanese.

The three procedures have various disadvantages:

The disadvantages of utilizing distance alone are:

(a) Shielding adequately is not known.

(b) The size, yield, and height of bomb are not known immediately.

(c) A uniform radial distribution of radiation is not assured because of intervening terrain, building, etc.

The disadvantages of personnel casualty dosimeters are:

(a) Not yet available in large numbers.

(b) Not independent of energy.

(c) The lethal range of radiation is not established for man and may vary from 200 to more than 600 r.

(d) The absolute sensitivity for any given individual can never be ascertained.

(e) The possibility of the dosimeter being shielded or exposed directly is always present.

The symptomatic approach is not perfect, but has the following attributes:

(a) The relationship of symptoms and the tempo of the illness to probable death, possible survival, and probable survival is well known on the basis of published Japanese data.

(b) Symptoms as observed in the Japanese are dependent on a wide dose range rather than a specific dose.

(c) No equipment is needed except good clinical observation and judgment.

By and large, in the light of our present knowledge, it is believed that the simplest approach to the diagnosis and prognosis of the relative degrees of radiation injury is the symptomatic approach. Utilizing these symptoms and the tempo of the illness the arbitrary groups are characterized as follows:

Group I casualties, in which survival from radiation injury is *improbable*, will present the following picture:

(a) Vomiting will occur within a few hours of the bombing.

(b) The vomiting will progress into prostration, diarrhea, anorexia, fever and early death.

(c) A profound depression in the white blood cell count will be apparent within 48 hours, survival time will be only a few days.

Group II casualties, in which survival from radiation injury is *possible*, will present the following picture;

(a) Vomiting will likewise probably occur on the day of bombing, but will subside within a matter of hours.

(b) Following the vomiting, there will be an asymptomatic latent period of one to three weeks.

(c) The latent period will be terminated by the recrudescence of the illness, presenting all or some of the following: purpura, epilation, oral and cutaneous lesions, infections of wounds, or burns that were otherwise healing well, and bloody diarrhea.

The untreated mortality of this group will be high.

Group III casualties, in which survival from radiation injury is *probable*, will be contrasted with Groups I and II by:

(a) There will be no vomiting on the day of the bombing. Transient nausea may occur.

(b) The late symptomatology, if any develops, will be similar to Group II.

(c) Without the development of late symptoms, this group could be detected only by serial studies of the leukocytes, by personnel radiation dosimeters or by location when the bomb exploded.

(d) Mortality will be low if uncomplicated by burns, trauma and intercurrent epidemics.

Recent work by Evans et al., Alpen et al., has demonstrated the probable additive effect of sub-lethal amounts of radiation and sub-lethal thermal burns in dogs.

In summary, "vomiting followed in quick order by fever, diarrhea, and leukopenia indicates a probable fatal outcome within two weeks. Vomiting followed by an asymptomatic period of one to two weeks before recrudescence of the illness indicates a serious exposure but recovery is *possible*. No vomiting on the day of the bombing suggests that exposure has probably been sub-lethal. If there is no leukopenia by the tenth day after the bombing, sub-lethal exposure is probable." (Cronkite).

It is possible that vomiting may not be limited only to people exposed to radiation. Vomiting may conceivably occur as the result of psychological factors, thus unnecessarily placing some individuals in the seriously exposed radiation group. The segregation of these individuals from the seriously exposed will be difficult but the distance from the exploding bomb and measurements by personnel dosimeters will be helpful. If it is feasible to do serial leukocyte counts under the conditions that exist, this will also aid in separating psychic vomiting from radiation vomiting.

11.2.2 *Laboratory Criteria.* Laboratory procedures, of course, are a most valuable aid in clinical diagnosis. It must be realized clearly, however, that laboratory aid may be minimal or non-existent because of the shortage of personnel and equipment. The following remarks are made with this in mind.

If the "typical" sequence of clinical events described above occur, laboratory tests will add little in terms of making the diagnosis and will be confirmatory only. Laboratory tests will be most valuable in the relatively less exposed groups, in which few or no early symptoms may appear. They are also of great value in distinguishing between radiation exposure and infectious or psychic disease that may simulate acute radiation exposure. Practically, the peripheral blood count provides the only useful index of the degree of exposure, and here considerable caution must be exercised. The neutrophile, lymphocyte and platelet counts are most useful, and each has advantages and disadvantages (see Bond et al., report of the exposed Marshallese).

For early diagnosis, the lymphocyte count is most indicative and changes occur within a matter of hours. Relatively small doses produce severe depression, however. In general, depression below 1000 cells/mm³ within 24 hours indicates severe exposure that may require later treatment.

The neutrophile count is not as sensitive as the lymphocyte count, and the rate of depression is slower. Since the count may rise in the first 24 to 48 hours before going below normal, an early neutrophile (or total white) count alone may be dangerously misleading. A normal total white or neutrophile count may be obtained in a lethally-exposed individual during this early time. In the lethal range, the neutrophile count falls after the initial rise, reaching a low in the second or third week, depending on degree of exposure. In the sublethal range, however, the count apparently can respond to stimuli such as infection, and thus a "normal" count may be obtained. The time of maximum depression is late, five to six weeks, and it is at this time that careful observation is required. Interpretation of the neutrophile count thus is subject to many pitfalls. The platelet count in the sublethal range falls late, in a regular fashion, beginning about 2 weeks after exposure. It apparently is relatively insensitive to other stimuli, and reaches a low at about 30 days. It thus is a more reliable indicator of the degree of exposure than is the neutrophile count. The neutrophile and platelet counts return towards normal within days of maximum depression; however, full recovery may require months or years. The return of lymphocyte levels to normal is markedly delayed.

11.3 Therapy of Acute Radiation Injury

Therapeutic problems concerned with this illness constitute a great challenge to the medical profession, both from a scientific standpoint and in terms of provision of adequate medical care and supplies in the cases of atomic warfare. The latter are under extensive study at the present time by the Office of Civilian Defense, the National Security and and Resources Board and the National Defense Establishment. In due course of time, definitive recommendations and action will be taken by these authoritative groups to provide medical care of atomic bomb casualties, to stockpile various valuable agents, drugs and dressings. It must be borne in mind that all statements made hereafter are the personal ones of the author and do not necessarily reflect the present policy or the future decisions of the above authoritative governmental groups.

11.3.1 *Analysis of Therapeutic Problems.* In the development of the syndrome that is contingent upon the initial effects of ionizing radiation on cells, one is confronted with the following therapeutic problems:

1. Prostration resulting from the profound dehydration and toxemia resulting from nausea, vomiting, diarrhea characteristic of absolutely fatal doses of radiation and only occasionally seen in the lower dose ranges
2. Maintenance of water, electrolyte and acid-base equilibria
3. Prophylaxis and treatment of:
   (a) infections in the presence of granulocytopenia
   (b) anemia
4. Treatment of the hemorrhagic manifestations

Therapy of the early shock-like syndromes which develop with the prostration following profound nausea, vomiting and diarrhea, is probably hopeless because the type of reaction is usually seen in the dose ranges (above 1000 r) that are uniformly fatal to 100 % of the animals within 10 days. The underlying therapeutic principles and the laboratory guides for adequate fluids and electrolyte therapy are now common knowledge and need not be elaborated upon in this chapter.

11.3.2 *Therapy of Infection.* Infections in the presence of granulocytopenia have always been difficult to handle, regardless of the cause. No agent prior to penicillin was of consistent value. On this ground alone, in general clinical experience, it is felt that penicillin administration should be seriously considered during the period when there is a significant granulocytopenia (neutrophils less than 1000 per cu. millimeter). Other antibiotics will definitely be indicated. Aureomycin, chloromycetin, terramycin and other newer antibiotics with a low degree of toxicity may make it possible to combat the entire spectrum of bacteria that may invade. The time to institute antibiotics, the preferable antibiotics, and the dosage are rather difficult to outline. The bacteria that reside within the body normally have a strong tendency to develop resistance to the antibiotics; it may therefore be undesirable to institute antibiotics prophylactically at too early a date. As a general rule, it would probably be preferable to give antibiotics prophylactically and refrain from parenteral use until there are definite clinical evidence of infection.

11.3.3 *Treatment of Anemia.* The causes of the anemia are well understood. It was previously stated by the author and others that maintenance of a relatively normal hemoglobin by transfusions of red cells, approximately equal to what would be lost per day, would be beneficial and indicated. The work of Allen et al. has demonstrated that the maintenance of hemoglobin levels by repeated transfusions in dogs does not increase the survival rate. On the basis of this work it would appear that routine red blood cell transfusions are not indicated. However, severe anemia must still be treated by blood transfusions. The author has repeatedly seen dogs so anemic that they are unable to rise from their cages and eat. These dogs following transfusions of whole blood sufficient to bring their hemoglobin up to levels that would permit adequate oxygen transport, would arise and start eating again. It is apparent that transfusions will still have a valuable role but it is equally apparent that routine transfusions would probably be a waste of a very valuable agent at a time when it will be also a critical agent in short supply and needed for many other clinical conditions.

11.3.4 *Therapy of the Hemorrhagic State.* The treatment of the hemorrhagic state in animals is not at all satisfactory. The maintenance of capillary integrity by rutin has been suggested; however the bulk of the evidence now demonstrates that rutin and other flavonones are of no value in the treatment of radiation injury. Since the heparinemia concept of Allen has not been confirmed, the use of protamine sulfate and toluidine blue would seem to have no rational basis. As discussed in the chapter on the hematology, it appears that one of the primary causes of radiation hemorrhage is the deficiency of platelets (Jackson et al., Cronkite). With the developments of methods for the separation and transfusions of platelets by Dillard et al., it has now been shown that platelet transfusions completely prevent bleeding in the irradiated animal and that the clotting defects are largely corrected. Unfortunately, replacement of platelets by transfusion remains an experimental tool and is not yet, and perhaps never will be feasible clinically on a large scale.

11.3.5 *Medicinal Agents.* Various agents, reported to be of value, or of no value, in the therapy of total-body radiation illness in animals, have been listed above in section 10.5.1.4. Most of these agents must be given parenterally. One agent, S,B-amino-ethylisothiouronium, appears to be effective orally. It is pointed out also that these agents must be given prior to exposure and none has as yet been shown to be of practical value in man. Only the antibiotics are of practical value when given after exposure. Bone marrow preparations are now being tried clinically in pancytopenic states; however, this approach would at present be impractical under disaster conditions.

11.3.6 *General Outline Therapy.* In the light of our present knowledge, the following therapeutic outline is suggested for the practical care of radiation injury as it might occur on small scale. There is no question that there will have to be practical considerations where large numbers of casualties are involved and that one would have to reduce the desirable care to a bare minimum that is consistent with the conditions that may exist following detonation of atomic bombs over large metropolitan areas.

General:

1. Complete physical and mental rest with mild sedation if necessary. Lavatory privileges will be determined by the severity of the reaction.

2. Diet should be bland and low in residue in order to protect the bowel. In the early stages, the diet should meet the basal requirements. As soon as it can be tolerated, the protein intake should be increased to a maximum.

3. Nursing care must be of the highest order. Particular attention should be paid to the hygiene of the mouth, teeth and skin in order to minimize lesions which may act as portals of bacterial entry.

Specific:

1. Antibiotics. The experience with the Marshallese indicated clearly that prophylactic antibiotics are not necessary in the sublethal range, even though the blood counts may reach relatively low levels. Thus, if the blood counts can be followed and the patients observed carefully, prophylactic use of antibiotics would be contraindicated unless the neutrophil count went below approximately 1000 cells/mm^3. If the patient cannot be followed closely, however, the criteria for use of prophylactic antibiotics might have to be relaxed considerably; however, considerations of probable short supply will also bear heavily on the decision to use antibiotics prophylactically. Antibiotics should be used vigorously if signs of infection appear in the heavily exposed individual. Even here, however, it is considered desirable to postpone the institution of antibiotics so as to minimize the chance of bacteria becoming resistant to the antibiotics at the time when they will be desperately needed, for example, when the granulocytes are at extremely low levels. It is the author's opinion that antibiotics should not be started until 5 to 7 days after exposure to radiation, unless there are specific clinical indications for their use, such as elevated temperature, oral or cutaneous ulcers or other clinical evidence of infection. The choice of antibiotics for prophylactic use is not simple. The spectrum of bacteria that may cause infection in the granulopenic state of man is wide and no single antibiotic is effective against all bacteria. Antibiotics are of proved value in other pancytopenic states and it only seems logical to expect them to be beneficial in the temporarily radiation induced pancytopenia. There is no easy answer at the present time to the prophylactic use of antibiotics in radiation injury as might be seen in man. It is believed that penicillin and aureomycin should both be used orally, commencing 5 to 7 days after irradiation. Penicillin tablets, 100,000 units, every four hours, and aureomycin, 250 milligrams every six hours, are

suggested. The above schedule is predicated on the stockpiling of sufficient antibiotics so that it will be feasible to use these on a very large scale. When it comes to the specific treatment of infections that develop in the granulopenic state, it is believed that parenteral antibiotics should be administered and for this purpose procaine-penicillin suspensions will probably be the most useful. Three hundred thousand units per day should be a good dose. If there is no response in the infectious process, or if organisms become resistant to the penicillin, other antibiotics should be instituted both orally and parenterally and the doses of all should be increased.

2. Transfusions of blood should be administered only when indicated for severe anemia. The actual amount of blood, and the interval between administrations will have to be determined by the clinical indications. Most decisions on the use of blood in a catastrophe will be dependent on clinical judgment because it will not be feasible to do laboratory determinations of hemoglobin.

3. Fluids and electrolytes should be given in amounts sufficient to maintain an adequate urinary output and proper acid-base equilibrium. The type and amount will be determined by appropriate laboratory and clinical studies. It should be apparent that following a major disaster the basis for the use of fluids and electrolytes will have to be clinical observations and good judgment, because it will not be feasible to perform large numbers of laboratory tests.

4. Plasma, albumin, and parenteral amino acids may be helpful in maintaining nutrition during the anorexic phase. Salt poor albumin may be of help if available in order to minimize the sodium chloride intake and thus decrease the opportunity of precipitating edema. The actual needs per patient cannot be foreseen. Each case that survives a matter of weeks will be a metabolic problem of its own, the needs of which will be determined by appropriate clinical and laboratory studies.

5. In the previous edition of this book it was considered that anti-heparin agents might have a role in the treatment of the hemorrhagic tendency. At the present time the evidence for heparinemia as stated in chapter 9 is negligible. At the present writing, the use of protamine sulfate and toluidine blue is considered to be of no value.

11.4 Summary

In summary, certain measures can be strongly advised on the basis of well-proved clinical therapeutic principles: rest, superb nursing care, strict asepsis, the use of transfusions and prophylactic antibiotics, the maintenance of proper fluid, electrolyte and acid-base balance, and maintenance of nutrition. The post-radiation use of various drugs, hormones and vitamins remains equivocal as based on present animal experimentation, and it is apparent that the simultaneous care of thousands of casualties along the lines outlined would be totally impractical. For those casualties following an atomic bomb explosion that have received supralethal doses of radiation, little more can be done in the light of our present knowledge other than palliation and maintenance of water and electrolyte equilibrium. The current limited supply of blood, antibiotics and medical personnel must be conserved by wise and careful use on those potential survivors, for whom we can do the most in terms of the therapeutic principles and knowledge that exists today.

In concluding this chapter, it is worth while to emphasize the uniform opinion of all American medical observers in Japan. All were certain that many more casualties would have survived if prompt adequate care for wounds had been possible and if ample amounts of penicillin and other antibiotics and whole blood had been available for intensive therapy. It is probable that these observers were thinking of the extensive trauma and infections in addition to radiation injury. At the present time there is evidence that the survival rate or survival time of animals or man following moderate exposure of the whole body to lethal amounts of radiation can be improved; however, the possibility of significantly improving the survival rate of those exposed to massive doses of radiation appears unlikely in the immediate future.

REFERENCES

Brown, B., et al.: Surgical treatment of radiation burns. *Surg. Gynec. & Obst. 88:* 609–622, 1949.

Cronkite, E. P. and Chapman, W. H.: A critical analysis of the syndrome of acute total body irradiation illness, its role in atomic warfare and its influence in the future practice of military medicine. *Mil. Surgeon 104:* 7–21, 1949.

Cronkite, E. P.: The diagnosis of ionizing radiation injury by physical examination and clinical laboratory procedure. *J. A. M. A. 139:* 366–369, 1949.

Cronkite, E. P. and Brecher, G.: The experimental therapy of the hemorrhagic phase of the radiation syndrome with platelet transfusions. *Acta. radiol. Suppl. 116:* 376–380, 1954.

Cronkite, E. P., Bond, V. P., Conard, R. A., Shulman, N. R., Farr, R. S., Cohn, S. H., Dunham, C. L., and Browning, L. E.: Some effects of ionizing radiation on human beings. Atomic Energy Document TID 5358, 1956, Gov't. Printing Office, Washington, D. C. Shortened version in *J. A. M. A. 159:* 430–434, 1955.

Cronkite, E. P.: The diagnosis, prognosis, and treatment of radiation injuries produced by atomic bombs. *Radiology 56:* 661–669, 1951.

Dunham, C. L., Cronkite, E. P., LeRoy, G. V., and Warren, S.: Atomic bomb injury—radiation. *J. A. M. A. 147:* 50–54, 1951.

Effects of Nuclear Weapons. Gov't. Printing Office, 1957.

Evans, E. I. and Brooks, J.: Symposium on burns. National Research Council, Washington, D. C., 1950.

Evans, E. I.: Atomic burn injury. *J. A. M. A. 145:* 1342–1345, 1951.

Guskova, A. K. and Baisogolov, G. D.: Two cases of acute radiation disease in man.

Presented at International Conference on the Peaceful Uses of Atomic Energy, Geneva, July 1955, (Russian Accident).

HASTERLIK, R. S.: Clinical report of four individuals accidentally exposed to gamma radiation and neutrons. Proceedings International Conference on Peaceful Uses of Atomic Energy. United Nations, N. Y., 402 pp., 1956.

Hearings before a Subcommittee of the Committee on Government Operations, House of Representatives. Congressional Record, 1956.

Hearings before the Joint Committee on Atomic Energy, Congress of the United States. Congressional Record, 1957.

HEMPLEMAN, L. H., LISCO, H., AND HOFFMAN, J. G.: The acute radiation syndrome: A study of nine cases and a review of the problem. *Ann. Int. Med. 36:* 279, 1952.

KIKUCHI, T., ET AL.: Studies on the atomic bomb injuries in Hiroshima City. Report to the Special Research Committee on the Atomic Bomb. Disasters Japan, 13 February 1950.

KIKUCHI, T. AND WAKISAKA, G.: Hematological investigations of the atomic bomb sufferers in Hiroshima and Nagasaki. *Acta scholae med. univ. Kioto 30:* 1–33, 1952.

LEROY, G. V.: The medical sequelae of the atomic bomb explosion. *J. A. M. A. 134:* 1143–1148, 1947.

OUGHTERSEN, A. W. AND WARREN, S.: *Medical Effects of the Atomic Bomb in Japan.* New York: McGraw-Hill, 1956.

TSUZUKI, M.: Radioactive damage of Japanese fisherman caused by Bikini ashes. *München med. Wchnschr. 97:* 988–994, 1956.

WARREN, S.: (Chairman) Report on the Pathologic Effects of Atomic Radiation on Man. National Academy of Sciences, NAS-NRC 452 Washington, D. C.

12▸

Radiotoxicity of Internally Deposited Radioactive Material[1]

JAMES S. ROBERTSON, M.D., PH.D. AND STANTON H. COHN, PH.D.

12.1 Introduction

The hazard of radiation from radioactive materials located within the body differs in several important respects from the hazard of radiation from external sources. The systemic effects of external radiation are associated chiefly with gamma rays, whereas with internally deposited radioactive materials, beta and alpha rays are more important. Internal radiation presents a more insidious problem than does external radiation. Because of the intimate contact of an internally deposited isotope with the tissue which it irradiates, minute quantities, often not detectable by external counting methods, can produce serious effects. Also, the effects from internal irradiation may appear years after exposure to the source of radioactive material. The following reasons are cited by the U. S. National Subcommittee on Permissible Internal Dose (1) as the basis for regarding internally deposited radioactive sources as being more hazardous than external sources of radiation:

1. They irradiate the body continuously until they are eliminated.

2. The biological transfer rates are very slow for some radioisotopes, and in most cases it is difficult, if not impossible, to increase appreciably the elimination rate from the body.

3. Sources inside the body are in intimate contact with the body tissue. This enables alpha and low-energy beta radiation (which, because of limited range, do not present an external hazard) to reach radiosensitive tissue inside the body and to dissipate all their energy in a small volume of tissue inside a critical body organ.

[1] Research supported in part by the U. S. Atomic Energy Commission.

4. It is very difficult to measure the amount and distribution of a radioisotope in the body, and even if such information is obtained, it is impossible to assess the hazard accurately. Methods of urine and fecal analysis have been developed for some radioisotopes, but most of these analyses are very tedious, time consuming, and expensive.

Only those internally distributed materials which are subject to metabolism within the body will be considered in this chapter. This restriction excludes consideration of radium, cobalt or other sources when introduced as needles, pellets or threads in brachytherapy. The hazard from radioactive materials which enter the body inadvertently, as by ingestion or inhalation of the fallout products from a nuclear detonation, will be emphasized. The beneficial applications of internally distributed isotopes in diagnosis and therapy are discussed in other chapters; only the harmful effects will be discussed here.

12.2 Extent of the Problem

Prior to the advent of artificially produced isotopes, particularly those produced as fission products, "radium poisoning" was the only important internal radiation hazard. Much of our present knowledge of the effects of internally-deposited radioactive material in man is based upon the experience gained from studies of people exposed to radium and mesothorium in connection with occupational exposures or from medical administration of these materials during the period from 1915 to 1930 when their use was popular.

The hazard from fission products in man is, providentially, still more anticipated rather than experienced. Very few serious exposures of human beings to these radioactive materials have occurred and our knowledge of their biological effects is largely derived from experiments with animals. Experience with man as the subject is limited to a few exposures in reactor and laboratory accidents, a small group of Marshallese people accidentally exposed to radiation from local fallout from the thermonuclear test on March 1, 1954 and from clinical experience with therapeutic trials of artificial radioisotopes.

The threat of world-wide contamination with fallout from atomic bomb tests is under intense scrutiny, particularly with respect to the hazard from strontium-90 (2, 3). At present, however, the average world contamination contributes a negligible amount of radiation relative to the unavoidable radiation exposure from cosmic rays, potassium-40 and other natural radiation sources and from medical and dental uses of X-rays. It is, of course, prudent to regard all ionizing radiation as being deleterious and any addition to our radiation exposure must be justified in terms of other benefits.

12.3 Physical and Biological Factors

Among the important physical and chemical factors upon which the effects of internally deposited radioactive materials depend are the nature and composition of the material, the amount of activity, the half-time for radioactive decay, and the kind and energy of the particles or rays emitted.

In contrast with the problem of external irradiation which will occur as a consequence of proximity to nuclear detonation in weapon testing and in accidents (reactors getting out of control, atomic ships or planes crashing, etc.), the problem of internal radiation (outside of laboratories) is primarily associated with the general problem of contamination of the world-wide atmosphere (and consequently plant and animal life) through the dispersal of fission products and unconsumed portions of atomic material, and through the disposal of radioactive wastes. While it is possible, theoretically, to avoid radiation from external sources with proper precautions, it is much more difficult to avoid the internal radiation hazard associated with the accumulation of very small amounts of radioactivity that appear in the air, or that may be incorporated into our food and water.

The characteristics of the radioactive particles from a nuclear detonation and their distribution in the atmosphere are determined by many physical factors, such as type of detonation, altitude, and meteorological conditions. Detonations of sufficient power may result in the transport of radioactive particles into the stratosphere with resulting world-wide distribution. Small particles do not fall back into our atmosphere until months or years later.

Internal radiation is of primary concern in the production of long term effects produced by (1) internally deposited isotopes with long radioactive and biological half-lives; (2) accumulated doses of short-lived as well as long-lived isotopes; and (3) high doses to individual tissues resulting from selective localization of isotopes.

The two most important routes of admission of radioactive materials into the body are via the respiratory system and the gastrointestinal tract. They may also enter via cuts in the skin. Radioactive materials entering the body through ingestion and inhalation are deposited in vital organs, (such as bone and thyroid), where they bombard radiosensitive cells until the material is removed from the body by natural processes (biological decay) or rendered harmless by radioactive decay.

Uranium, plutonium and the radioelements formed in nuclear fission have, in general, a limited solubility in body fluids. However, the amount which can produce injurious effects when deposited within the body is minute because of the intimate contact of the isotope with the tissue it irradiates.

The inhalation hazard is associated with both the immediate exposure to fallout or a radioactive aerosol and the later exposure to residual surface deposited contamination which may become resuspended. Following inhalation there is damage to lung tissue and, in addition, damage may occur in the G.I. mucosa due to passage of material moved up from the tracheobronchial tract and the nasopharyngeal region. In addition, there is a radiation hazard to organs and tissues which selectively concentrate the material that gets into the systemic circulation. The kinetics of the uptake and retention of the inhaled radioactive aerosol are very complex and depend on a number of factors, such as particle size and solubility (4, 5, 6, 7).

Radioactive isotopes follow the same metabolic processes in the body as the naturally occurring inactive isotopes of the same element and of chemically similar elements. One of the fission products of greatest potential hazard is radiostrontium, which is analogous to calcium, and thus becomes fixed in the calcifying tissue of bone. This element and certain other heavy metals are known as "bone-seekers," and have, in general, long radiological half lives and slow biological turnover characteristics. They cause greater damage to bone and to the radiosensitive bone marrow than to other tissues, but through damage to the blood forming tissue, they also affect the entire body. Thus, the internal radiation problem is characterized by its chronic nature, as opposed to the more generally acute nature of external radiation.

Calculation of the radiation dose from internally deposited radioactive material may be very difficult. A major difficulty is that uniform distribution cannot be assumed, even within the tissue of maximal localization. For example, radioautographic studies of radium in bone reveal that the radium is found in small areas of high focal concentration irregularly distributed in both compact and cancellous bone (8). (A lower intensity, more uniform distribution is found with longer exposures.) Therefore, the average dose as calculated by the usual methods (9) may give a very misleading estimate of the hazard involved. From a knowledge of the metabolic path of the material involved, however, an estimate of the radiation dose delivered to various tissues, particularly the lungs and gastrointestinal tract can be calculated, if the length of time spent at each site can be estimated.

The final question as to whether the radiation delivered will produce biological effects depends also upon the sensitivity of the tissue irradiated to radiation, the balance between the dose rate and the tissue's recovery rate, and to the degree of damage to the tissue which is necessary for detection. There is considerable variation of response among individuals of a species.

12.4 Biological Effects of Internal Emitters

Some of the best documented data on the effects of small amounts of internally deposited radioactive material in human beings have been obtained from studies of radium poisoning, particularly of the watch dial painters of New Jersey (10–14) and of patients administered radium salts therapeutically (8, 15). The metabolism and biological effects of a number of fission products have been studied in laboratory animals (16, 17). At certain points the animal data have been correlated with the cases of accidental exposure or poisoning of humans by radiation. A comprehensive study of the biological effects of radiation was recently made by the National Academy of Science (2).

12.5 Radium Poisoning

The term "radium poisoning" is used to include the effects attributed to mesothorium (Ra^{228}) as well as those from radium (Ra^{226}). Although it is not obvious from the nomenclature used for these substances, radium and mesothorium are isotopic. Their metabolism and distribution in the body may therefore be regarded as being identical. Their half-lives, energies and disintegration schemes, however, are different, and variations in effects due to differences in the metabolism of the disintegration products may appear.

The experimental data on radium metabolism have been thoroughly reviewed in the book edited by Fink (18). In rats given radium chloride intravenously, radium is found to be deposited mainly in the inorganic part of the skeleton, with small amounts concentrating in the intestinal tract, the muscles, skin and kidneys. By the 10th day after injection the soft tissues have lost almost all of their radioactivity. In the rat, the soft-tissue radium is excreted in the urine and feces in roughly equal amounts, with a small amount going to the skeleton as evidenced by a slight rise seen in the skeletal radium during the first 10 days. Within the skeleton the highest concentration was found in the trabecular and epiphyseal bone, with the lowest concentrations in the metaphyses, skull and vertebrae on the 10th postinjection day. The portions of bone which take up radium the fastest also tend to lose it the fastest, so that at 275 days postinjection the teeth and metaphyses have retained the largest percentage of their 10th day Ra content.

In man, the metabolism of radium is similar to that in the rat but there are quantitative differences. Excretion of radium in human subjects is mainly in the feces rather than equally in the urine and feces as in the rat (10, 19). After the initial rapid excretion of radium, a much lower steady level of excretion is attained. The most complete long-range data on radium metabolism was published by Norris et al. (19A). They found that after 22 years 0.6% of radium administered intravenously is retained. About 70% of the radon produced by the retained radium is exhaled. Looney (8, 19) found that most of ingested radium is eliminated in the 1st week and that within months 90–99.9 % is eliminated. After 10 years the coefficient of elimination is 0.002–0.009 % of the remaining body content/day (8) figures which are in agreement with those reported by other workers (10, 11). Radium elimination may be regarded as occurring in three phases (8): (1) early and rapid elimination from soft tissues; (2) elimination from the more accessible parts of the skeleton, that is, those with the more rapid turnover rates; and (3) after the 1st year the elimination from the more inaccessible parts of the skeleton is predominant. In bones from the patients studied (8, 20) years after the ingestion of radium, radium was found in small areas of high focal concentration irregularly distributed in both compact and cancellous bone. The small, highly concentrated areas may have been areas in which bone formation was taking place at the time of administration or redistribution of the radium. It is conjectured that the more uniform and less dense distribution seen may be the result of inorganic ion exchange. (8)

No attempt will be made here to describe the acute effects of radium poisoning because they resemble in many respects the acute effects seen with other modes of whole body irradiation with injury to the blood forming tissues being a conspicuous feature, and because few cases of acute radium poisoning have occurred since 1930. In the subacute form of illness seen in luminous dial painters, jaw necrosis and severe anemia were characteristic features (12).

The late effects of radium poisoning in man have been described by Martland (13, 14), by Aub et al. (10) and by Looney (8, 15, 20). The long half-life of radium (1620 years) makes its contribution to the radiation dose relatively constant over a period of years, whereas for mesothorium (half-life 6.7 years) the contribution diminishes steadily. The clinical and physical evidence presented by Aub et al. (10), however, indicate that the irradiation delivered by the disintegration products of mesothorium were very important in producing the delayed effects observed in some of the patients.

The fundamental lesion observed as a late effect of internally-deposited radium occurs in the skeleton. Among the first clinical symptoms are loosening of individual teeth. Destructive changes in the teeth cause a reduction in their density which gives a pinkish hue to the teeth (8). Extraction of the loosened teeth may be followed by osteomyelitis.

The first abnormality of bone noted in roentgenograms is a coarsening of the trabeculae. Gradually expanding areas of rarefaction then develop in the trabecular portion of the long bones and in the skull. Later, this type of bone destruction can also be seen in the cortical portion of the bones. A lesion regarded as being characteristic of chronic radium poisoning (10) occurs primarily near the ends of long bones when, as bone rarefaction becomes evident one can also observe small areas of increased density which may become confluent and then impart a mottled appearance to the bone. In older patients with severe and long standing radium poisoning, extreme destruction and collapse of a weight-bearing portion of a long bone or vertebra sometimes occurred.

Another form of delayed tissue damage is the production of malignancy. Eight malignancies, of which four arose from bone, were noted in the series reported by Aub et al. (10). Three were osteogenic sarcomas and one a giant cell tumor. The other tumors were a fibrosarcoma of the knee joint capsule and three epidermoid carcinomas arising in the nasal accessory sinuses or near the temporal bone. Malignancy was responsible for 7 of the 10 deaths in the series reported (10).

In contrast to the prominent bone lesions, injury to the blood forming tissues was absent or not serious in the patients with late effects studied. Eight cases of mild anemia were observed. It is doubted whether the one patient who allegedly died of leukemia did have a true leukemia (10).

12.6 The Strontium-90 Hazard

On the basis of our present knowledge of the nature, distribution and metabolism of fission products, strontium-90 appears to be the critical isotope in considerations of long term effects from internally deposited radioactive sources originating from weapons tests. Strontium-90 is important in old fission products from any source. The degree to which strontium-90 contamination of the atmosphere already constitutes a health hazard has aroused considerable controversy in both the scientific and the popular literature, and the problem of world-wide contamination from fallout is being investigated most thoroughly.

Strontium-90 is produced in considerable quantity in nuclear detonations (approximately 1 gm Sr^{90}/KT of fission yield) and has a radioactive half-life of 28 years. It decays by β^- emission to yttrium-90, which also decays by β^- emission, with a 64-hour half-life. Sr^{90} is readily absorbed into the body where it is firmly fixed in the skeleton. On the other hand, because of the immense dilution in the atmosphere of fission products, the possibility of world-wide inhalation or ingestion of significant amounts of fallout from nuclear test detonations is, at present, very small. The amount of activity which has been added to the atmosphere is but a fraction of the natural radioactive content, except in the immediate vicinity of nuclear detonations (2, 3, 21, 22, 23).

In evaluating the importance of the world-wide contamination by fallout, the food chain is a most important factor to be considered. Radioactive material settling down on the earth and in reservoirs and lakes is transported through plant and animal material to man himself. In particular, the uptake of fallout by forage plants, the consumption of these contaminated plants by grazing cattle, and the subsequent incorporation of fallout into dairy products, provides a most important source of radioactive fallout material to man.

The quantitative aspects of the soil-plant relationships for the uptake of fission products are not completely understood. It is known, however, that the uptake of Sr^{90} by plants is inversely correlated with the amount of "exchangeable" calcium in the soil (24, 25).

The absorption of strontium depends on the physiological state of the animal (such as its calcium requirements in skeletal growth) as well as on the chemical and physical form of the element. Twenty per cent of the strontium administered is absorbed from the gastrointestinal tract in man. The main pathway of excretion is via the urine and only 10% of the absorbed Sr is excreted via the intestinal tract. Of a single dose of parenterally administered Sr^{90} 50–75% will be excreted in 2 weeks and about 95% excreted in a year. The 5% Sr^{90} remaining in the body may be considered fixed in the bones (26, 27). The body burden of radiostrontium following chronic ingestion of contaminated food is governed first by the Sr^{90}/Ca ratio of the food, and secondly by the differentiation between the metabolism of strontium and calcium by the body. Fortunately for man, the body discriminates against strontium in favor of calcium, primarily by different rates of absorption and excretion (28). Although strontium follows calcium rather closely in its metabolism, it is also discriminated against in every step of the ecological chain. For example, the Sr^{90}/Ca ratio in feed and milk of cows under equilibrium conditions were 1.0 and 0.13, respectively (29). These data indicate an eightfold lowering of the Sr^{90} content of the milk relative to the feed, which tends to minimize the ingestion of radioactive strontium by human beings.

The localization of Sr in the skeleton is also of importance in determining the biological effects of internally deposited radiostrontium. The Sr^{85}/Ca ratio in the various bones of a human subject has been shown to vary widely following a single administration of Sr^{85} (23). Further, Sr has been shown to localize in active building sites in bone producing what has been referred to as "hot spots" (30, 31, 32). These "hot spots" result in a greatly increased radiation dose to a small localized area (5–10 times) but have not been correlated with the subsequent carcinogenic effect of the internal emitter. Yttrium-90 has been shown to remain in equilibrium with and at the same site as bone deposited Sr^{90} (33).

Strontium-90 has never been found in human beings in dangerous amounts. The biological effects of this isotope are, therefore, inferred by correlating the biological effects of radium^{226} in animals and in human beings, comparing these with the effects produced by the administration of Sr^{89} and Sr^{90} to animals, and extrapolating the results to man.

On the basis of the carcinogenic effects produced by a sustained human body burden of 1 μg (1 μc) of Ra^{226}, the stated maximum permissible concentration (MPC) for a whole body burden has been set at 0.1 of this amount, that is, a sustained level of 0.1 μc of radium in the body (1, 34).

Experiments with Sr^{89} and Ra^{226} in mice have established a relative toxicity ratio on a curie-for-curie basis of 1:10 (35). As the energy absorbed from internally deposited radium by human beings is about twice that absorbed by mice (primarily because of the exhalation of differing amounts of radon), the MPC for Sr^{89} based on radium data should be 1:20. However, since Sr^{90} has approximately twice the energy released in its decay scheme as Sr^{89}, the ratio becomes 1:10 for strontium^{90}/radium^{226} in human beings. The MPC for Sr^{90} is therefore set at 1.0 μc in the body (1, 34). This level of 1 μc Sr^{90}/1,000 gm of calcium (average amount of calcium in the body of man) has been designated as 1 "MPC unit" of Sr^{90}. The MPC value of 1.0 μc in the body will, if a uniform distribution of the Sr^{90} is assumed, result in a dose rate of less than 2.5 rad/yr to the skeletal system.

The Sr^{90} MPC is based on a single experimentally obtained Sr^{89}/Ra^{226} ratio in mice and the extrapolation to man is based on meager clinical data of Ra effects in adult man. Thus, the stated maximum permissible value for Sr^{90} is only an approximation based on the best available information and can serve only as a guide in any particular situation.

The toxic effects of Sr^{90} have been studied in a number of laboratory animals. The LD_{50}/30 days for Sr^{90} is reported to be 6 μc/gm in the mouse (35, 36), 2.5–3.0 μc/gm in the rat (37, 38), and 0.15 μc/gm for dogs (39). A single injection of 0.2 μc/gm was fatal to monkeys (40).

Since the metabolic behavior of Sr^{90} is very similar to that of radium^{226} (particularly with respect to concentration in the skeleton), the important pathological change to be anticipated is chiefly the production of bone sarcoma (41). The threshold level of Sr^{90} in human beings required to produce carcinogenic effects can be estimated. Since 0.5–1μc of radium^{226} has been shown to produce bone damage in human beings (15), 5–10 μc of Sr^{90} would be expected to produce the same changes. Another estimate of the minimal level of Sr^{90} required to produce bone damage in man can be derived from animal experimentation.

Early bone changes preceeding long term carcinogenic effects have been noted in animals receiving acute doses of Sr^{90} (17, 37, 38). The injury to the bone is to the growing trabecular bone adjacent to the epiphyseal cartilage plate. In the rat, injected dose levels of Sr^{90} ranging from 2.5 to 3.0 μc/gm body weight, (LD_{50}/50 days) resulted in such histological bone changes as the disruption of the epiphyseal line, osteosclerosis, aseptic necrosis of the trabecular bone and depression of the myeloid elements.

The few data on the chronic toxicity effects of Sr^{90} in dogs are available from studies conducted at the Argonne National Laboratory. No gross bone damage in dogs injected with 0.01 μc/gm of Sr^{90} was found in an 8 year period (42).

While the above threshold levels apply to the production of bone sarcoma, other biological effects may be produced by lower levels of Sr^{90}. The earliest effect observed following injection of low levels of Sr^{90} is the damage to the bone marrow. Following injection of 5 μc/gm body weight there is almost complete loss of hematopoietic activity in mice and rats. Doses as low as 0.1 μc/gm of Sr^{90} in mice produce a transient depression of the blood platelet level, starting at 3–7 days after injection. In rats, injection of 0.1 μc/gm resulted in a small decrease in marrow cellular content. Studies of acute Sr^{90} toxicity in dogs have indicated that hematological damage occurs at injected levels of 0.15 μc/gm body weight. This depletion of hematopoietic activity is related to the fact that Sr^{90} deposits in the mineral structure of actively growing bone adjacent to the marrow spaces, subjecting them to β^- radiation. Since the range of the energetic β^- particles in tissue is of the order of millimeters, the difference in Sr^{90} toxicity in small and large animals may be due to the differences in radiation exposure geometry.

Lewis (43) has recently estimated that an increase from 5 to 10% in the spontaneous incidence of myelogenous leukemia would occur if the population were to reach and maintain a body level of Sr^{90} amounting to 0.1 of the stated maximum permissible concentration. Although leukemia has not been observed as a late effect of radium poisoning, this absence of effect may be due to the inability of alpha particles emitted from radium to penetrate in quantity to the soft tissue of the bone marrow. In this respect the high energy β^- particles from Sr^{90} and its daughter product Y^{90} may be expected to be somewhat more hazardous. Objections to Lewis's conclusions may be raised, however, on the grounds that the relationship between radiation and leukemia in humans has not been determined quantitatively, particularly at the low doses involved. The literature on this subject has been reviewed by Furth and Upton (44). Data are available only for relatively high doses of radiation. Since there may be a threshold for the leukemogenic effect, extrapolation to low doses is not justified by the existing data. The possibility that chronic irradiation from Sr^{90} will produce leukemia must be kept in mind, but much more experimental data are required before the Sr^{90} hazard can be evaluated accurately enough to predict the increase in leukemia which may result from a given Sr^{90} body burden.

The principal biological effects of low levels of Sr^{90} can be summarized as transient hematopoietic depression and radiation injury to growing bone followed at a long interval by osteogenic sarcoma, and possibly by leukemia.

12.7 Other Isotopes: Maximum Permissible Concentration of Radioisotopes in the Human Body

Although many isotopes have been used in tracer studies in human beings, only a few, notably Na^{24}, P^{32}, Cl^{38}, Ga^{72}, I^{131} and Au^{198} have been used in therapeutic doses, i.e., in quantities sufficient to produce acute effects. Because of their short effective half-lives, however, repeated administrations of these isotopes would be required to produce chronic effects.

The maximum permissible concentrations which have been agreed upon are based upon comparisons with X-ray, γ-ray damage, and radium damage, the knowledge from studies of the naturally occurring background (radium, carbon-14, K^{40}, cosmic rays), and animal experimentation. The established recommendations are discussed in two publications, the report of the U. S. National Committee on Radiation Protection and the International Commission's Recommendations (34). It should be emphasized that the figures given in both of these publications are for chronic exposures over many (30 or more) years. Although higher concentrations may be considered permissible for acute exposures, no official standards have been established for acute exposures, except for the general recommendations covering maximum permissible radiation doses (45). Table I is abstracted from tables in references (1) and (34). These sources should be consulted for references to the data supporting the choice of figures given.

12.8 Internal Radiation Hazard in Human Beings Exposed to Radioactive Fallout

The first instance in which a large group of people received a significant amount of internal radioactive contamination together with a large but sublethal dose of external radiation occurred as a consequence of the nuclear detonation of March 1, 1954 (46). At this time 239 Marshallese and 28 Americans were accidentally contaminated by fallout material. The radioactive fallout spread out over an area thousands of square miles beyond the range of thermal and blast effects. The Marshall Islands involved in this accidental exposure were contaminated to the extent that evacuation of the inhabitants was necessary.

Under the sponsorship and with the cooperation of the U. S. Navy and the Atomic Energy Commission, a medical team was quickly dispatched to provide treatment for all persons affected. A detailed study of the clinical, hematological and pathological effects of the radiation on the exposed human population, as well as an estimate of their internal radioactive contamination was made. At the same time, an investigation was made of the contamination of the animals, plants, soil and water of the exposed atolls. The findings on the internal radiation hazard which are detailed below are

TABLE I
Maximum Permissible Internal Concentrations of Radioisotopes

RADIOISOTOPE AND TYPE OF DECAY	EFFECTIVE ENERGY	EFFECTIVE HALF-LIFE	CRITICAL ORGAN	FRACTION REACHING CRITICAL ORGAN		MAXIMUM PERMISSIBLE TOTAL BODY BURDEN
	Mev	$days$		By ingestion	By inhalation	$\mu c.$
H^3(HTO) β^-	0.006	19	Total body	1.0	0.75	10^4
Be^7 K, γ	0.009	48	Bone	3.5×10^{-3}	0.09	725
$C^{14}(CO_2)$ β^-	0.053	35	Fat	0.5	0.36	260
F^{13} β^+	0.24	0.078	Bone	0.1	7.5×10^{-2}	5
Na^{24} β^-, γ	2.7	0.60	Total body	0.95	0.73	15
P^{32} β^-	0.68	14	Bone	0.2	0.2	10
S^{35} β^-	0.055	18	Skin	0.08	0.074	300
Cl^{36} β^-	0.26	19	Total body	0.95	0.73	230
A^{41} β^-	1.78		Total body			33
K^{42} β^-, γ	1.59	0.51	Muscle	0.7	0.53	21
Ca^{45} β^-	0.085	151	Bone	0.25	0.41	14
Sc^{46} β^-, γ	0.5	13	Spleen	1.5×10^{-5}	7.5×10^{-3}	6
			Liver			5
Sc^{47} β^-		2.8	Spleen			15
		2.8	Liver			11
Sc^{48} β^-, γ		1.6	Spleen			5
		1.6	Liver			3
V^{48} K, β^+, γ	0.54	12	Bone	5×10^{-4}	.025	10
Cr^{51} K, γ	0.01	22	Kidneys	0.0007	0.004	600
Mn^{56} β^-, γ	1.1	0.104	Kidneys	0.004	2.2×10^{-2}	25
		0.106	Liver	0.01	0.09	8
Fe^{55} K	0.006	61	Blood	0.8	0.65	10^3
Fe^{59} β^-, γ	0.54	27	Blood	0.8	0.65	13
Co^{60} β^-, γ	0.72	8.4	Liver	0.004	0.007	3
Ni^{59} K	0.05	8	Liver	0.004	0.007	42
Cu^{64} K, β^-, β^+, γ	0.11	0.53	Liver	0.09	0.13	120

Zn^{65}	K, β^+, γ	0.085	21	Bone	1.5×10^{-2}	4.5×10^{-2}	400
Ga^{72}	β^-, γ	0.8	0.59	Bone	0.0004	0.1	3
Ge^{71}	K	0.01	3.9	Kidneys	2×10^{-3}	5×10^{-3}	72
As^{76}	β^-, γ	1.1	1.09	Kidneys	0.0003	2.7×10^{-3}	11
Rb^{86}	β^-, γ	0.73	7.8	Muscle	0.42	0.33	64
Sr^{89}	β^-	0.55	52	Bone	0.25	0.22	2
$Sr^{90} + Y^{90}$	β^-	1.0	2.7×10^{3}	Bone	0.25	0.22	1
Y^{91}	β^-	0.57	51	Bone	2.8×10^{-4}	0.14	3
$Zr^{95} + Nb^{95}$	β^-, γ	0.154	48	Bone	0.13	0.12	10
Nb^{95}	β^-, γ	0.22	21	Bone	0.0002	1.8×10^{-4}	44
Mo^{99}	β^-, γ	0.49	2.8	Bone	2.5×10^{-3}	2.5×10^{-3}	17
Tc^{96}	K, γ	1.4	2.1	Kidneys	2×10^{-5}	0.01	5
$Ru^{106} + Rh^{106}$	β^-, γ	0.33	19	Kidneys	0.01	1.7×10^{-2}	4
Rh^{105}	β^-, γ	0.074	1.5	Kidneys	0.02	3.5×10^{-2}	9
$Pd^{103} + Rh^{103}$	K, e^-	0.74	4.4	Kidneys	1.2×10^{-4}	1.6×10^{-3}	7
Ag^{105}	K, γ	0.37	2.8	Liver	1.2×10^{-4}	1.6×10^{-3}	19
Ag^{111}	β^-	0.04	2.1	Liver	1.9×10^{-3}	0.19	39
$Cd^{109} + Ag^{109}$	K, γ	0.087	77	Liver	0.0026	0.076	45
Sn^{113}	K, γ	0.28	44	Bone	0.0007	0.02	84
Te^{127}	β^-, γ	0.89	13	Kidneys	0.0007	0.02	4
Te^{129}	β^-, γ	0.22	10	Kidneys	0.2	0.15	1.4
I^{131}	β^-, γ	0.183	8	Thyroid			0.6
Xe^{133}	β^-, γ	0.562	0.38	Total body			320
Xe^{135}	β^-, γ	0.57		Total body			100
$Cs^{137} + Ba^{137}$	β^-, γ	1.06	17	Muscle	0.48	0.36	98
$Ba^{140} + La^{140}$	β^-, γ	0.76	12	Bone	0.07	0.2	1
La^{140}	β^-, γ	1.29	1.6	Bone	1.2×10^{-3}	0.1	1
$Ce^{144} + Pr^{144}$	β^-	0.31	180	Bone	2×10^{-4}	0.10	6
Pr^{143}	β^-	0.067	11	Bone	1.3×10^{-3}	0.063	25
Pm^{147}	β^-	0.02	140	Bone	1.7×10^{-4}	0.09	90
Sm^{151}	β^-		3.9×10^{4}	Bone	2.8×10^{-5}	0.05	

< page number>246</>

TABLE I—*Continued*

RADIOISOTOPE AND TYPE OF DECAY	EFFECTIVE ENERGY	EFFECTIVE HALF-LIFE	CRITICAL ORGAN	FRACTION REACHING CRITICAL ORGAN		MAXIMUM PERMISSIBLE TOTAL BODY BURDEN
				By ingestion	By inhalation	
	Mev	*days*				*μc.*
Eu^{154}	β^-, γ	0.366	8.2×10^2	Bone	1.7×10^{-4}	0.09	7
Ho^{166}	β^-, γ	0.65	1.1	Bone	0.0001	0.07	4
Tm^{170}	β^-, γ	0.32	59	Bone	3.5×10^{-4}	0.18	4
Lu^{177}	β^-, γ	0.14	3.2	Bone	0.5×10^{-4}	0.075	18
Ta^{182}	β^-, γ		60	Liver			6
W^{181}	K, γ, e$^-$		4.8	Bone			24
Re^{183}	K, γ	0.09	0.5	Thyroid	1.3×10^{-3}	1.3×10^{-3}	37
		0.003	5	Skin	0.12	0.12	650
Ir^{190}	β^-, γ	0.07	7.3	Kidneys	0.01	1.75×10^{-2}	23
			10	Spleen			21
Ir^{192}	β^-, γ	0.46	17	Kidneys	0.01	1.75×10^{-2}	3
			45	Spleen			3
Pt^{191}	β^-, γ		2.9	Kidneys			2
Pt^{193}	K, γ, e$^-$		4.0	Kidneys			3
Au^{196}	K, β^-, γ		5	Liver			8
			5	Kidneys			32
Au^{198}	K, β^-, γ	0.40	2.6	Liver	0.024	0.072	3
			2.6	Kidneys			10
Au^{199}	β^-, γ	0.14	3.1	Liver	0.024	0.072	9
			3.1	Kidneys			30
Tl^{200}	K, γ, e$^-$		1.06	Muscle			40
Tl^{201}	K, γ		2.6	Muscle			310
Tl^{202}	K, γ, e$^-$		6.9	Muscle			230

Tl^{204}	β^-	0.12	16.7	Muscle	4.5×10^{-2}	9.8×10^{-2}	200
Pb^{203}	K, γ		2.16	Bone			61
Pb^{210} + dr	α, β^-, γ		6.76×10^2	Bone			0.2
Po^{210} (sol)	α, γ	5.3 α	40	Spleen	0.0003	0.004	0.04
Po^{210} (insol)			31	Lungs		0.12	0.02
At^{211}	K, α	6.8 α	0.31	Thyroid	0.07	0.05	10^{-3}
Rn^{220} + dr	α, β, γ	19.5 α		Body			
				Lungs			
Rn^{222} + dr	α, β, γ			Body			
				Lungs			
Ra^{226} + 55% dr	α, β, γ	14.5 α	1.6×10^4	Bone	0.015	0.026	0.1
Ac^{227} + dr	α, β, γ		10^3	Bone			0.01
Th-natural	α, β, γ		4.3×10^4	Bone			0.01
Th-natural (insol)	α, β, γ						2×10^{-3}
Th^{234} + Pa^{234}	β^-, γ		24.1	Bone			2
U-natural (sol)	α, β^-, γ	4.43 α	30	Kidneys	0.0002	0.08	0.04
U-natural (insol)	α, β^-, γ		120	Lungs		0.12	0.01
U^{233} (sol)	α, γ	4.9 α	300	Bone	10^{-4}	0.05	0.04
U^{233} (insol)	α, γ		120	Lungs		0.12	0.016
Pu^{239} (sol)	α, γ	5.16 α	4.3×10^4	Bone	0.0001	0.18	0.04
Pu^{239} (insol)	α, γ		360	Lungs		0.12	0.02
Am^{241}	α, γ	5.45 α	890	Bone	1.3×10^{-4}	0.063	0.06
Cm^{242}	α	6.08 α	120	Bone	1.25×10^{-4}	0.063	0.06

indicative of the nature, although not necessarily of the degree of the effects which may occur in a nuclear accident.

Radiochemical analysis of urine from the exposed persons showed that the degree of internal absorption of radioactive materials was roughly proportional to the calculated external dose and, therefore, to the concentration of airborne fission products. The degree of internal radiation hazard was too low to have contributed significantly to the acute radiation syndrome observed. The concentration and type of internal radioactive contaminants minimized the possibility of the occurrence of any significant long term effects from the internal radiation.

The evidence accumulated from this study and from controlled laboratory experiments with animals points to the conclusion that the internal radiation hazard following an acute exposure to fallout is very small in comparison with the hazard from the external dose. This conclusion, of course, applies to the inhalation hazard immediately following exposure to fallout from a nuclear detonation, and does not apply to the effects produced by acute exposure to large amounts of long-lived radioisotopes, or to chronic exposure to very small amounts of long-lived fission products.

A large number of animals exposed to fallout from the Pacific nuclear detonation were collected and brought back alive for study. These animals were the source of much valuable data, as they were exposed to radioactive fallout for fairly long periods of time, and so received significantly high doses. Detailed studies were made of the uptake, distribution and retention of the various fission products. The major portion of the internally deposited activity was found in the skeleton. The autoradiograph, Figure 1, illustrates the sites of deposition within the growing region of a tibia taken from a pig exposed to fallout.

Although a large number of fission products were present in the environment, relatively few gained entry into the body. These included strontium[89-90], barium[140], iodine[131] and some of the rare earth elements. The elements which entered the body were characterized chiefly by their high solubility. Biological and radioactive decay reduced the level of the radioactivity in the animals rapidly, so that at 6 months after the detonation the radioactivity in the animals was barely detectable. To date, these animals have shown no sign of delayed radiation effect.

Surveys of the fallout contaminated areas were also made at 1 and 2 years following the accident. These data form the basis for an estimate of the long term radiation hazard associated with chronic exposure to residual contamination, and thus lead to an assessment of the habitability of fallout contaminated areas.

The levels of radioactivity in the environment and in the plants and animals of the Marshall Islands at 2 years were only a small fraction of the

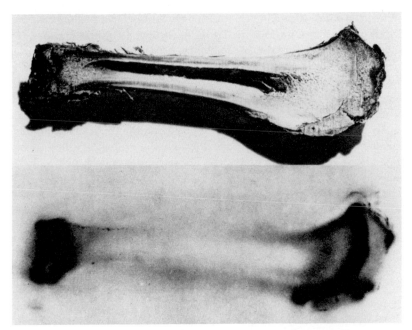

Fig. 1. Autoradiograph of tibia of a pig exposed to fallout

levels originally found after the accident (47, 48). At two years the activity in biological specimens on the islands was contributed primarily by cesium[137], and smaller amounts of ruthenium[106], strontium[90] and rare earth elements. The marine specimens from the lagoon contained primarily zinc[65] and cobalt[60]. The plants and animals acted as concentrators of radioisotopes and thus had concentrations of specific radionuclides manyfold greater than were found in their environment.

Aside from the early transitory depression of the blood cell level, there have been no pathological or histological changes observed in these animals which could be ascribed to radiation. It is therefore necessary to express the potential radiation hazard in terms of the concentration of fission products retained by the animals. Since strontium[90] is clearly the critical element responsible for long term radiation effects, an estimate of the potential internal radiation hazard to man in this situation was derived from the concentration of Sr[90] found in animals which lived on these islands during the 2-year period, assuming the diet of the animals and man to be the same. The Sr[90] concentration (in terms of the Sr[90]/calcium ratio) of several animals collected on the Island at 2 years was approximately one-half of the currently accepted maximum permissible concentration for man (1000 $\mu\mu c$ Sr[90]/8 Ca).

While the data collected in this study of a Pacific Island Community give an indication of the internal radiation hazard resulting from exposure to fallout, quantitative differences might be expected in different situations. For example, the physical and chemical properties of the fallout material as well as meteorological conditions and properties of the biosphere will influence strongly the uptake and retention of fission products in man via the soil-plant-animal cycle and thus will determine the internal radiation hazard to man. For these reasons further information on the transport of low levels of fission products (especially Sr^{90}) through the ecological cycle in other communities is required to assess the internal radiation hazard to human beings living in fallout contaminated areas.

As part of the third annual medical examination of the Rongelap people (50) several Marshallese were studied by the whole-body gamma spectroscopy method at the Argonne National Laboratory (51). The levels of cesium-137 and zinc-65 were higher in the Marshallese than in Americans, but did not approach tolerance levels.

12.9 Reactor Accidents

A few power reactors are in operation, a number are under construction, and many more are being designed. There is every reason to expect that within a few decades reactors will be important sources of power throughout the world. Although a reactor cannot produce an A-bomb type of explosion, the possibility does exist that accidental release of the accumulated fission products from a large reactor could contaminate many square miles with radioactive material, with resultant internal deposition of fission products in human beings. Such release could conceivably come about not only from loss of control of a reactor, but from external catastrophic events such as bombing, earthquakes and floods. If reactors are also to be used for propulsion of ships and aircraft, the possible causes of accidents and the probability of their occurrence increase greatly, as do the problems of controlling dissemination of the radioactive material released. To date there has been no case of an accident involving a power reactor and the probability of such an accident at the present state of development is extremely small.

The nuclear accidents which have occurred to date have involved research or experimental reactors. Internally deposited radiation has not been an important feature of the few cases of injury which have been reported. Hempelmann, Lisco and Hoffman (52) report studies on nine patients exposed to neutrons and gamma rays from temporarily uncontrolled fission reactions in two accidents. The induced activity, particularly sodium-24 in the blood serum, was sufficiently high to provide a good basis for calculating the neutron flux, and hence the radiation dose, but the contribution from induced activity to the total body dose of radiation was negligible (52, 53).

Activity in a gold filling in the teeth of one of the patients apparently did produce local radiation effects. Neither in these accidents nor in two others which have been reported (54, 55) was there any internal deposition of fission products.

In the Chalk River accident (56, 57) a complex concurrence of mechanical defects in the shut-off-rod system coupled with operating errors produced a power surge during preparations for experiments at low power. The cooling arrangements in operation were adequate only for low power operation and the metals separating the fuel elements from the cooling system melted. Some 10,000 curies of fission products were released into the cooling water and an intensely radioactive cloud of fission products was released into the atmosphere, resulting in deposition of radioactive materials on downwind fields and buildings. No one was injured, but the incident points up the possibility of such an occurrence. Research reactors, with their more frequent variations in operating conditions are perhaps more susceptible to accidents than the steady-operating power reactors, but power reactors will contain much larger quantities of fission products.

In recognition of the necessity for evaluating the theoretical hazard from power reactors, a report outlining the possible consequences of a disaster involving a large reactor (58) was prepared for the Atomic Energy Commission. The following data are abstracted from the reactor safety report. For a 500,000 kilowatt reactor, after 180 days of operation, the fission product inventory is approximately 4×10^8 curies, when measured 24 hours after shutdown. Some components of significance in consideration of the hazard from internal distribution are:

Strontium[90]	3.8×10^5 curies
Strontium[89]	1.7×10^7 curies
Cerium[144]	8×10^6 curies
Plutonium[239]	3.8×10^3 curies
Iodines	5×10^7 curies
Noble Gases	3.4×10^7 curies
Total volatile fission products	8.4×10^7 curies

The amount of strontium[90] listed is equal to that produced by a nuclear detonation of 3.8 megatons total yield (fission).

For calculation of the relative radiation dose from the different isotopes and at different distances, doses are expressed in terms of the acceptable emergency dose (AED), taken to be 25 r of whole body gamma radiation in an acute exposure, or 50 r in 3 months. In AED units, the relative radiation dose for exposure for 1 second in a cloud containing 1 curie per cubic meter is estimated as indicated in Table II. In the first column, designated "full fission product release," it is assumed that a sizable fraction of all the fission products contained in the reactor are dispersed. In the column headed

TABLE II
Relative Radiation Dose from a Radioactive Cloud for 1 C-sec/m³ of Exposure

	FULL FISSION PRODUCT RELEASE	VOLATILE F.P. RELEASE
External γ dose	0.0112 AED	0.0505 AED
Lung β dose	.0096	.0072
Bone dose from Sr⁹⁰	.02	.001
Bone dose from Sr⁸⁹	.0116	.00058
Bone dose from Ce¹⁴⁴ + Pr¹⁴⁴	.021	0
Lung dose from Pu	.0012	0
Thyroid dose	.01	.049
G.I. tract dose	.0112	0

TABLE III
Estimates of Exposure Required for Biological Effects

EQUIVALENT WHOLE BODY GAMMA RADIATION	50% FULL F.P. RELEASE	VOLATILE F.P. RELEASE
	C-sec/m³	C-sec/m³
450 r Lethal	400	350
100–450 r Illness likely	90–400	80–350
25–100 r Injury unlikely	10–90	10–80
25 r No injury	10	10
Urgent evacuation (within 12 hr.) necessary	0.2	0.1
Evacuation necessary	0.01	0.1
Possible temporary evacuation, restrictions on outdoor work	.001–0.01	0.01–0.1

"volatile FP release" it is assumed that the reactor fuel melts and that only the volatile fission products, principally noble gases and halogens, with about 1 % of the strontium, are liberated.

Assuming that the bone doses are additive, the figures given in Table III were adopted as estimates of the intensity of exposure expected to produce the effects or require the action listed.

The relationship of the figures in Table III to an accident involving a 500-megawatt reactor requires the adoption of many more assumptions: the fraction of the fission products released, the temperature condition of the release, particle size, meteorological conditions, population density, etc. Several hypothetical situations are considered in detail in the Brookhaven report. Assuming one of the worst possible situations, with 50 % of the gross fission products released on a rainy night and with particle sizes of a median diameter of 1 micron, lethal exposures could be expected up to 15.5 miles away and urgent evacuation would be required at distances up to 100 miles.

It must be re-emphasized that the figures quoted from the reactor safety report represent a barely credible situation and even the most pessimistic guesses assign extremely low probabilities to a reactor accident of proportions sufficient to injure working personnel or the public.

12.10 Diagnosis and Treatment of Radioactive Poisoning

Internally deposited radioisotopes continue to irradiate the tissues adjacent to their site of deposition until they are removed from the body by the normal biological processes of turnover and elimination, or until they are rendered inactive through radioactive decay.

12.10.1 *Diagnosis.* Because acute effects may be lacking, and because small amounts of radioactive materials may produce serious late effects, it is important to obtain a good history when radioactive poisoning is suspected. The diagnosis and treatment are dependent upon the understanding of the radiobiology of the radioactive material in question. For example, radium, strontium and plutonium are deposited primarily in bone, while thorium is deposited in the liver, spleen and the bone marrow. The following outline of diagnostic procedures follows that given by Looney (8).

1. *History.* The typical patient suffering from late effects usually has been in apparent good health for many years after exposure. In one patient who did not remember receiving radium, diagnoses of osteoid osteoma, osteomyelitis, Ewing's tumor, giant cell tumor, and multiple myeloma were entertained in a 2-year period before the patient died with osteogenic sarcoma attributed to radium poisoning (8). In acute cases it is important to establish precisely which elements are involved.

2. *Skeletal roentgenographic changes.* In the case of radium poisoning, and presumably for other bone-seekers, depending upon their degree of similarity to radium, the skeletal lesions described above in the section on radium poisoning are characteristic and may be diagnostic.

3. Collection of breath samples and determination of radon in the expired air, assuming a certain ratio of radon to total body radium. About 0.02 μg of radium can be detected. This method is now used for routine monitoring by industrial users of luminous paints.

4. Radiochemical analysis of excreta (59).

5. External measurement of γ activity using scintillation counters. In conjunction with gamma spectrum analysis this method not only gives the total body burden but makes it possible to distinguish different isotopes. The Argonne National Laboratory group uses an 8-inch diameter by 4 inches thick NaI crystal, a 256 channel gamma spectrum analyzer, and a special 52-ton "portable" iron room which serves as a gamma shield (60, 61, 62). Another type of whole body counter using a liquid scintillator is in use at the Los Alamos Scientific Laboratory (63).

6. Radiochemical analysis of bone biopsies.

12.10.2 *Treatment*. Since it is not possible at the present time to reverse the effects of ionizing radiation on living tissue, the treatment of radioactive poisoning at early times takes the form of interfering with the deposition of the radioactive material in the tissues. Once the material becomes fixed in the skeleton, the approach to the problem becomes one of releasing the fixed material and eliminating it from the body (64–66).

In general, no single treatment is effective for the many radioactive poisons. There are such a variety of radioactive materials extant today, that the likelihood of a single approach is extremely small. Thus, one must take into account first of all the chemical nature of the poison, just as one does with non-radioactive poisons. Other factors that are of importance in determining the type of treatment to be used are the route of entry, age and health of the patient, and time elapsed after the exposure.

A. *Early Treatment*. The chances of reducing the body content of a radioisotope are highest in the early stages after exposure. During the first hours it is generally found that most of the material is in the soft tissues and blood stream, and is not yet fixed by the skeleton. Deposition of the radioisotopes in the body tissues can be retarded by minimization of absorption from the G.I. tract with the use of precipitating agents (such spinach and rhubarb, which contain oxalates); and by the use of emetics and cathartics.

Experiments with rats have also indicated that the maintenance of high level of calcium in the diet decreases the absorption of strontium from the gastrointestinal tract (67).

B. *Treatment after Radioisotopes are Absorbed into the Body*. 1. *Decalcification therapy*. Administration of NH_4Cl, parathormone, or the use of a low calcium diet, all designed to increase bone resorption, enhance only slightly the elimination of radium and strontium in acute and chronic poisoning. Such therapy is not practical, as the treatment can be maintained for very limited periods, so that the net depletion of the body content of the radioisotope is not significant. Decalcification therapy has no effect on the retention or excretion of non-alkaline earths such as plutonium and the rare earth elements.

2. *Complexing or chelating agents*. A promising new approach to the problem of increasing the elimination of isotopes lies in the use of chelating agents. These agents are effective with plutonium and the rare earth elements, but are ineffective for radium and strontium. The complexing agent combines *in situ* (particularly in the soft tissue) with the toxic metal, thus preventing it from combining with cellular constituents. The complex is subsequently eliminated from the body. Ethylenediamine tetraacetic acid (EDTA) is the most effective agent of this kind found to date (64–67).

3. *Use of colloidal ion exchange carriers*. Another promising chemical

agent is zirconium citrate, which has some degree of effect on nearly all the fission products (67). The mechanism of action of the zirconium has been postulated to be a colloidal ion exchange carrier. The zirconium salt decomposes in the blood, forming colloidal particles of the metal hydroxide. These adsorb the fission products in the blood stream and are excreted from the body. Zirconium citrate is effective only when administered within hours of an exposure. The combined use of zirconium citrate and EDTA appears to be more effective than use of either agent singly.

While several technics are available for the treatment of radioactive poisoning, their effectiveness is small, particularly in the case of radiostrontium poisoning. The normal excretion rate is an extremely small fraction of the material in the body, once it becomes fixed. Thus, even if one induces a 10-fold increase in the rate of elimination, the actual amounts retained in the body remain essentially unchanged. In order to reduce appreciably the deposits in the body, treatment for chronic cases would have to be maintained for a period of several years.

REFERENCES

1. *Maximum permissible amounts of radioisotopes in the human body and maximum permissible concentrations in air and water.* National Bureau of Standards Handbook 52, U. S. Government Printing Office, Washington, 1953. 45 p.
2. *Pathological effects of atomic radiation.* National Academy of Sciences, Publication 452, U. S. Government Printing Office, Washington, 1956. 200 pp.
3. EISENBUD, M.: Global distribution of strontium-90 from nuclear detonations. *Scient. Month. 84:* 237–244, 1957.
4. MARINELLI, L. D., NORRIS, W. P., GUSTAFSON, P. F. AND SPECKMAN, T. W.: Transport of radium sulfate from the lung and its elimination from the human body following single accidental exposures. *Radiology 61:* 903–913, 1953.
5. ABRAMS, R., SEIBERT, H. C., POTTS, A. H., LOHR, W. AND POSTEL, S.: Inhalation of inhaled fission product aerosols, U. S. Atomic Energy Commission Document MDDC-248, 1946. 114 p.
6. SCOTT, K. G., AXELROD, D., CROWLEY, J. AND HAMILTON, J. G.: Deposition and fate of plutonium, uranium and their fission products inhaled as aerosols by rats and man. *Arch. Path. 48:* 31–54, 1949.
7. COHN, S. H., LANE, W. B., GONG, J. K., FULLER, R. K. AND MILNE, W. L.: Radiotoxicity resulting from exposure to a fallout simulant, II. The metabolism of an inhaled and ingested simulant of fallout produced by a land-based nuclear detonation. USNRDL-TR-118, 24 p., 1957.
8. LOONEY, W. B., Late effects (25 to 40 years) of the early medical and industrial use of radioactive materials. *J. Bone & Joint Surg. 37A:* 1169–1187, 1955; *38A:* 175–218 and 392–406, 1956.
9. HINE, G. J. AND BROWNELL, G. L., (editors): *Radiation Dosimetry.* New York: Acad. Press, 932 p., 1956.
10. AUB, J. C., EVANS, R. D., HEMPELMANN, L. H. AND MARTLAND, H. S.: The late effects of internally-deposited radioactive materials in man. *Medicine 31:* 221–329, 1952.

11. Evans, R. D.: Protection of radium dial workers and radiologists from injury by radium. *J. Ind. Hyg. & Toxicol. 25:* 253–269, 1943.

12. Martland, H. S.: Occupational poisoning in manufacture of luminous watch dials. *J. A. M. A. 92:* 466–473, 1929.

13. Martland, H. S.: The occurrence of malignancy in radioactive persons. *Am. J. Cancer 15:* 2435–2516, 1931.

14. Martland, H. S.: Occupational tumors of bones. *Encl. Health and Hygiene,* Geneva, 1939.

15. Looney, W. B., Hasterlik, R. J., Brues, A. M. and Skirmont, E.: A clinical investigation of the chronic effects of radium salts administered therapeutically (1915–1931). *Am. J. Roentgenol. 73:* 1006–1037, 1955.

16. Hamilton, J. G.: The metabolism of the fission products and the heaviest elements. *Radiology 49:* 325–343, 1947.

17. Bloom, W. (ed), Histopathology of irradiation from external and internal sources, 1st Edition, McGraw-Hill Book Co., Inc., New York, 1948. 808 p.

18. Fink, R. M. (ed): *Biological Studies with Polonium, Radium and Plutonium, National Nuclear Energy Series, Division VI.* New York: McGraw-Hill, 411 p., 1950.

19. Looney, W. B., and Archer, V. E.: Radium inhalation accident and radium excretion study. *Am. J. Roentgenol. 75:* 548–558, 1956.

19A. Norris, W. P., Speckman, T. W. and Gustafson, P. F.: Studies of the metabolism of radium in man. *Am. J. Roentgenol. 73:* 785–802, 1955.

20. Looney, W. B.: Late skeletal roentgenographic histopathological, autoradiographic and radiochemical findings following radium deposition. *Am. J. Roentgenol. 75:* 559–572, 1956.

21. Libby, W. F.: Radioactive strontium fallout. *Proc. Nat. Acad. Sc. 42:* 365–390, 1956.

22. Andrews, H. L.: Radioactive fallout from bomb clouds. *Science 122:* 453–456, 1955.

23. Kulp, J. L., Eckelman, W. R. and Schulert, A. R.: Strontium[90] in man. *Science 125:* 219–225, 1957.

24. Fuller, W. H. and Flocker, W. J.: Tech. Bull. No. 130, Uptake of Radiostrontium by certain crops from calcareous soils. Arizona Agriculture Experiment Station, Univ. of Arizona, Tucson, Arizona. 1955, 32 p.

25. Menzel, R. G. and Brown, I. C.: Leaching of fallout and plant uptake of fallout. Report from U. S. Dept. of Agriculture, March–April, 1953.

26. Spencer, H., Lazlo, D. and Brothers, M.: Sr[85] and Ca[45] metabolism in man. *J. Clin. Invest. 36:* 680–688, 1957.

27. Cowan, F. P., Farabee, L. B. and Love, R. A.: Health physics and medical aspects of a Sr[90] inhalation incident. *Am. J. Roentgenol. 67:* 805–809, 1952.

28. Comar, C. L., Wasserman, R. W. and Nold, M. N.: Strontium-calcium discrimination factors in rat. *Proc. Soc. Exper. Biol. & Med. 92:* 859–863, 1956.

29. Comar, C. L. and Wasserman, R. W.: Radioisotopes in the study of mineral metabolism. *Progress in Nuclear Energy,* Vol. 5, London: Pergamon Press Ltd., 481 p., 1955.

30. Jowsey, J., Owen, M. and Vaughn, J.: Microradiographs and autoradiographs of cortical bone from monkeys injected with Sr[90]. *Brit. J. Exper. Path. 34:* 661–667, 1953.

31. Arnold, J. S.: Metabolism of bone as studied by the autoradiographic distribution of calcium, plutonium and radium. *Am. J. Physiol. 167:* 765, 1951.

32. ARNOLD, J. S. AND JEE, W. S. S.: Haversian system growth and formation in rabbits. *Anat. Rec. 115:* 276, 1953.

33. ARNOLD, J. S., STOVER, B. J. AND VAN DILLA, M. A.: Failure of Y-90 to escape from skeletally-fixed Sr-90. *Proc. Soc. Exper. Biol. & Med. 90:* 260–263, 1955.

34. Recommendations of the International Commission on Radiological Protection, *Brit. J. Radiol.*, Supp. No. 6, 1955, 92 p.

35. FINKEL, M.: Relative biological effectiveness of internal emitters. *Radiology 67:* 665–672, 1956.

36. COHN, S. H. AND MILNE, W. L.: Effects of combined administration of Strontium-90 and external radiation. USNRDL-TR-89, 1956. 15 p.

37. ANDERSON, W. A. D., ZANDERS, G. E. AND KUZMA, J. F.: A study of the toxic doses of Strontium-90 in the adult rat. *Arch. Path. 62:* 433–440, 1956.

38. RAY, R. D., THOMSON, D. W., WOLFF, N. K. AND LaVIOLETTE, C. D.: Bone metabolism, II. Toxicity and metabolism of radioactive strontium (Sr^{90}) in rats, *J. Bone & Joint Surg. 38:* 160–174, 1956.

39. FINKEL, M. P. AND BRUES, A. M.: Sequelae of radiostrontium administration to dogs. *Radiation Res. 3:* 224–225, 1955.

40. EDINGTON, G. M., JUDD, J. M. AND WARD, A. H.: Delayed toxicity of radio-strontium in monkeys. *Nature 175:* 33, 1955.

41. LISCO, H., FINKEL, M. P. AND BRUES, A. M.: Carcinogenic properties of radioactive fission products and of plutonium, *Radiology 49:* 361–363, 1947.

42. FINKEL, M. P., LESTINA, J., SCRIBNER, G. M., LISCO, H., FLYNN, R. J. AND BRUES, A. M.: Toxicity of radiostrontium in dogs: current status of long-term experiments, ANL-5426, 33–37, 1955.

43. LEWIS, E. B.: Leukemia and ionizing radiation. *Science 125:* 965–972, 1957.

44. FURTH, J. AND UPTON, A. C.: Leukemogenesis by ionizing radiation. *Acta radiol.* Suppl. 116, 469–476, 1954.

45. TAYLOR, L. S.: Maximum permissible radiation exposures to man. *Radiation Res. 6:* 513–516, 1957; *Radiology 68:* 260–261, 1957.

46. COHN, S. H., RINEHART, R. W., GONG, J. K., ROBERTSON, J. S., MILNE, W. L., BOND, V. P. AND CRONKITE, E. P.: Internal deposition of radionuclides in human beings and animals. In: Some effects of ionizing radiation on human beings; a report on the Marshallese and Americans accidentally exposed to radiation from fallout and a discussion of radiation injury in the human being, U. S. Atomic Energy Commission TID 5358, U. S. Government Printing Office, 1956. 106 p.

47. RINEHART, R. L., COHN, S. H., SEILER, J. A., SHIPMAN, W. H. AND GONG, J. K.: Residual contamination of plants, animals soil and water of the Marshall Islands one year following Operation CASTLE Fallout, USNRDL-454, 1955. 29 p.

48. WEISS, H. L., COHN, S. H., SHIPMAN, W. H. AND GONG, J. K.: Residual contamination of plants, animals, soil and water of the Marshall Islands two years following Operation CASTLE Fallout, USNRDL-455, 1956. 52 p.

48A. COHN, S. H., WEISS, H. L., SHIPMAN, W. H. AND GONG, J. K.: Extent of internal radioactive contamination of Pacific Island communities exposed to local fallout. AIBS meeting, Symposium on Ecological Aspects of Fallout, Stanford, August 1957.

49. CONARD, R. A. ET AL.: Medical survey of the Marshallese two years after exposure to fallout radiation, Brookhaven Nat. Lab. BNL 412, 1956. 18 p.

50. CONARD, R. A. ET AL.: March 1957 Medical Survey of Rongelap and Utirik Peo-

ple Three Years after Exposure to Radioactive Fallout, Brookhaven Nat. Lab. BNL 501, 1958, 26 p.

51. MILLER, C. E. AND STEINGRABER, O. J.: Measurements on Some Residents of the Marshall Islands, ANL-5755, 53–57, 1957.

52. HEMPELMANN, L. H., LISCO, H. AND HOFFMAN, J. C.: The acute radiation syndrome: A study of nine cases and a review of the problem. *Ann. Int. Med. 36:* 279–510, 1952.

53. HOFFMAN, J. G. AND HEMPELMANN, L. H.: Estimation of whole-body radiation doses in accidental fission bursts. *Am. J. Roentgenol.* 77: 144–160, 1957.

54. HASTERLIK, R. J. AND MARINELLI, L. D.: Physical Dosimetry and Clinical Observations on Four Human Beings Involved in Accidental Critical Assembly Excursion, pp. 25–34 in: *Biological Effects of Radiation*, Vol. 11, Proceedings of the International Conference on the Peaceful Uses of Atomic Energy, United Nations, New York, 1956.

55. GUSKOVA, A. K. AND BAISOGOLOV, C. D.: Two Cases of Acute Radiation Disease in Man, pp. 35–44 in: *Biological Effects of Radiation*, Vol. 11, Proceedings of the International Conference on the Peaceful Uses of Atomic Energy, United Nations, New York, 1956.

56. LEWIS, W. B.: The accident to the NRX Reactor on 12 December 1952, Chalk River Report DR-32, AECL-232, July 13, 1953. 14 p.

57. HURST, D. G.: The Accident to the NRX Reactor, Chalk River Report, GPI-14 AECL-233, October 23, 1953. 33 p.

58. Theoretical Possibilities and Consequences of Major Accidents in Large Nuclear Power Plants, WASH-740, Dec. 1957.

59. LANGHAM, W.: Determination of internally deposited radioactive isotopes from excretion analyses, *Am. Indust. Hyg. Assoc. Quart.* 17: 305–318, 1956.

60. MARINELLI, L. D., MILLER, C. F., GUSTAFSON, R. F. AND ROWLAND, R. E.: The quantitative determination of gamma ray emitting elements in living persons, *Am. J. Roentgenol.* 73: 661–671, 1955.

61. MARINELLI, L. D., ET AL.: Radium Toxicity, Argonne National Lab. Semiannual report, ANL-5456, 107–123, 1955.

62. MILLER, C. E., Measurements of gamma rays *in vivo*, Argonne National Lab. Semiannual report, ANL 5596, 26–33, 1956.

63. ANDERSON, E. C., SCHUCK, R. L., PERRINGS, J. D. AND LANGHAM, W. H.: A whole body gamma counter for human subjects, Los Alamos Scientific Laboratory report LA-1717, 1955. 43p.

64. ROSENTHAL, M. W. (editor): Therapy of radioelement poisoning. Transcript of a meeting on "Experimental and Clinical Approaches to the Treatment of Poisoning by Radioactive Substances," Argonne Natl. Lab., ANL-5584, Aug. 1956.

65. SCHUBERT, J.: Removal of radioelements from the mammalian body. *Ann. Rev. Nuc. Sc. 5:* 369–412, 1955.

66. COHN, S. H., GONG, J. K. AND MILNE, W. L.: Experimental treatment of poisoning from fission products. *Arch. Indust. Health 14:* 533–538, 1956.

67. Division of Biology and Medicine Report, No. 100A, U. S. Atomic Energy Commission, July 1954.

13▸

Fallout Radiation: Effects on the Skin

ROBERT A. CONARD, M.D., EUGENE P. CRONKITE, M.D.,
AND VICTOR P. BOND, M.D., PH.D.

13.1 Introduction

Until recently it has been generally assumed that injury to the skin from ionizing radiation was not a serious hazard associated with the detonation of nuclear devices. However, in 1954 the importance of this hazard became apparent when widespread radiation lesions of the skin developed in a large group of people accidentally exposed to fallout radiation in the Marshall Islands following the experimental detonation of a large nuclear device. In addition to exposure of some 239 Marshallese people and 28 Americans, there were 23 Japanese fishermen exposed on their fishing boat. The radiation effects and skin lesions in this latter group have been described by Koyama *et al.* and others. Prior to that time, a limited number of skin lesions on the backs of cattle (Bird; Paysinger *et al.*) and horses (Atomic Energy Commission Report) has been noted from fallout following experimental detonations. In addition, exposure of the hands of several individuals who had carelessly handled fission product samples from a detonation resulted in the development of severe lesions (Knowlton *et al.*). Other cases of beta lesions in human beings of accidental or experimental nature have been described by Robbins *et al.*; Crawford; Low-Beer; Wirth and Raper; Conard and Tessmer; Kepp; Griffith *et al.* and Kepp, Miller and Reich; Nodle; and Witten *et al.* Some of the rather numerous studies on the effects of beta radiation on animal skin are reported by Henshaw; Raper and Barnes; Snider and Raper; Lushbaugh; Moritz and Henriques; Paysinger *et al.*; Brues; Cloudman *et al.*; Glucksmann; Kharchenko and Venolurov; Koletsky *et al.*; Minisov; Passonneau and Hamilton; Shubik *et al.* and Ungar *et al.*

The recent accident in the Marshall Islands affords the first example of large numbers of lesions of the skin in human beings from fallout. Studies of these lesions in the Marshallese and Americans exposed have been documented (Conard et al.) and will be referred to frequently in this chapter.

Lesions of the skin induced by fallout are primarily due to the beta radiation from the fission products adhering to the fallout material and are, therefore, frequently referred to as beta burns. So-called beta burns of the skin may also result from accidental exposure to, or contamination with, radioisotopes used in science and industry. The possibility of such accidents must be considered seriously in view of the increasingly widespread use of radioisotopes.

13.2 Fallout Situations Resulting in Skin Damage

With detonation of nuclear devices, serious radiation injury to the skin is only associated with fallout situations where the radioactive material is sufficiently concentrated. Such concentrations are most likely to occur with close-in fallout, i.e., fallout that occurs within several hundred miles of the detonation. It seems probable that the fallout will be visible if serious acute skin damage is to result; however, this cannot be stated with certainty. In the Marshall Island accident, the extent and severity of the skin lesions were directly correlated with the amount of visible fallout. On the most distant of the contaminated islands, some 200 miles from the site of detonation, the fallout was not visible and no beta lesions of the skin developed among the inhabitants.

The world-wide deposit of fallout which occurs slowly from the troposphere or stratosphere does not result in skin injury since in this situation the fallout material is greatly diluted and reduced in amount.

Damage to the skin such as that seen with beta radiation does not result from the immediate penetrating gamma or neutron radiation associated with detonation of nuclear devices since the dose of such radiations necessary to severely damage the skin results in early deaths from damage to the bone marrow and the deep organs. Thus the skin burns observed in the Japanese casualties from the Hiroshima and Nagasaki bombs were not the result of ionizing radiation and were caused chiefly by thermal radiation. Fallout radiation associated with these bursts was insignificant.

13.3 Characteristics of Fallout Material

The chemical and physical make-up of fallout will vary according to the type of terrain or soil over which the detonation occurs. All fallout is particulate in nature, but the size of the particles will depend to some extent on the physical and chemical characteristics of the soil. The fallout associated with the Castle detonation, March 1, 1954, was a white, powdery material largely composed of incinerated coral. Aside from the radioactive component, the calcium oxide of the material was in itself irritating to the skin due to its caustic nature. Moreover, it was probably partly dissolved in the perspiration on the skin, thus increasing its irritating action. This also may have enhanced the radiation to the skin by bringing the radioactive materials in closer contact with the skin. The presence of irritating chemicals on the skin is known to enhance the radiation effect (MacKee, Cipollaro and Montgomery). Fallout produced from other types of soil, not predominantly coral, might vary considerably in chemical and physical make-up and ability to irritate the skin. Color and particle size would also vary. For instance, siliceous type soils would probably form much less irritating fallout.

The particulate nature of the material results in a spotty distribution of lesions on the body. The Marshallese claimed that the material adhered closely to the skin and was difficult to brush off. This was borne out by the difficulties encountered in decontaminating the skin of the exposed individuals.

13.4 Sources of Radiation from Fallout

Figure 1 is a rough diagrammatic sketch showing the relatively uniform distribution of fallout on the ground, buildings, trees and personnel. The penetrating gamma radiation which is represented by the wavy, shaded areas penetrates many yards in air before it is attenuated appreciably, while the beta radiation represented by the stippling is completely attenu-

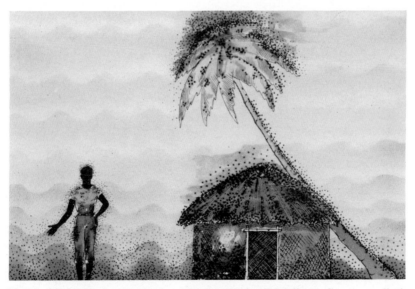

FIG. 1. Diagramatic sketch showing distribution of fallout. Gamma radiation represented by wavy shaded areas, beta radiation by stippling.

ated in several feet. Damage to the skin results largely from the beta component of the fallout in view of the fact that all of the beta radiation entering the skin is absorbed in the skin and because of the high beta to gamma ratio. Estimates of this ratio vary widely up to 150/1, depending on the exposure conditions. The skin does receive some radiation from penetrating and soft gamma radiation, but by far the greater part of the dose is contributed by the beta radiation. Alpha emitters are usually not present in fallout to any great extent and due to their very weak penetrating ability, they are not likely to add significantly to the skin damage.

The skin dose results from two sources of beta radiation: the fallout material in direct contact with the skin (contact hazard) contributes by far the largest part of the dose to the skin, and the material on the ground (beta bath hazard) contributes a much smaller amount. The fallout in contact with the skin will usually be spotty in distribution and due to the particulate nature will result in multiple point sources of radiation on the skin. Though radiation from these sources is largely from the skin surface, it is possible that some deeper radiation may result from percutaneous absorption as well as penetration into the dermal region via hair shafts, sebaceous and sweat glands. Some of the fission products are water soluble, and it is possible that some are lipid soluble, which would enhance this effect. Witten *et al.* have shown that thorium-x applied to the skin results in some percutaneous absorption and entry into the hair shafts and glands.

Beta dose to the skin from fallout on the ground will be largely confined to the lower parts of the body, particularly the feet and legs, since the beta particles are completely stopped in approximately 2 meters of air.

13.5 Estimation of Skin Dose

Measurement of beta doses to the skin from fallout is an exceedingly difficult problem due to the complicated spectrum of different energy beta emitters present, the non-uniform distribution on the skin, and the fact that practical dose meters have not yet been perfected which will adequately discriminate between the beta radiation and the contaminating gamma component.

The penetration of beta particles into the skin depends, of course, on the beta energies of the component isotopes. Each radioisotope has its own characteristic spectrum of beta energies up to a maximum energy. Relatively few particles are of the maximum energy, however, and the average energy (roughly one-third of the maximum energy) and the 50 per cent attenuation thickness of tissue are more meaningful in estimating skin effects. Thus an isotope emitting low energy radiation, confined largely to the dead, horny layer of skin, would be relatively ineffective; more energetic radiation, penetrating through the epidermis could result in transepidermal necrosis;

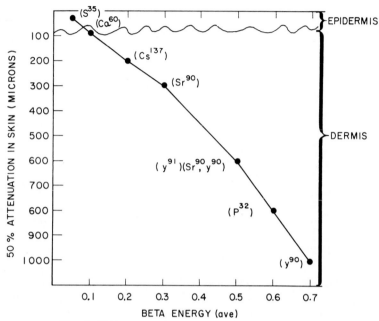

Fig. 2. 50% attenuation in skin, of various isotopes

and deeper penetration into the dermis could result in more severe ulcerating lesions. Figure 2 shows roughly the tissue depth necessary to produce 50 per cent attenuation of the beta particles from several isotopes.

In Table I data from animal studies from several investigators show the

TABLE I

Surface Doses Required to Produce Recognizeable Epidermal Injury

INVESTIGATOR	ANIMAL	ISOTOPE	AVE. ENERGY	SURFACE DOSE
			mev	*rep*
Henshaw, et al.	Rats	P^{32}	0.5	1,500–4000
Snider and Raper	Mice	P^{32}	0.5	2,500
Raper and Barnes	Rabbits	P^{32}	0.5	5,000
Lushbaugh	Sheep	S^{90}	0.3	2,500–5000
Moritz and Henriques	Pigs	S^{35}	0.05	20,000–30,000
Moritz and Henriques	Pigs	Ca^{60}	0.1	4,000–5,000
Moritz and Henriques	Pigs	Cs^{137}	0.2	2,000–3,000
Moritz and Henriques	Pigs	Sr^{90}	0.3	1,500–2,000
Moritz and Henriques	Pigs	Y^{91}	0.5	1,500–2,000
Moritz and Henriques	Pigs	Y^{90}	0.7	1,500–2,000

(Courtesy Brookhaven Nat. Lab.)

TABLE II

Human Exposure to Beta Radiation

INVESTIGATOR	RADIATION	EST. DOSE	REACTION
		rep	
Wirth and Raper	P^{32}	635	1st degree (threshold)
Wirth and Raper	P^{32}	1180	2nd degree (threshold)
Low-Beer	P^{32}	143*	1st degree (threshold)
Low-Beer	P^{32}	7–17,000	2nd degree
Robbins et al.	Cathode rays (1200 kv)	1–2000	3rd degree
Knowlton et al.	Fission products (1 mev ave. energy)	3–4000	2nd degree
Knowlton et al.	Fission products (1 mev ave. energy)	5–10,000	3rd degree
Knowlton et al.	Fission products (1 mev ave. energy)	5–10,000	3rd degree
Knowlton et al.	Fission products (1 mev ave. energy)	8–16,000	3rd degree

* Estimated dose in 1st mm. layer.

(Courtesy of Brookhaven Nat. Lab.)

energy dependence of beta particles from various isotopes in producing recognizable skin reactions. Note that the surface doses for threshold reaction (erythema, epidermal atrophy) are fairly dependent on the energy of the beta particles of the various isotopes. Thus it takes 20,000–30,000 rep from S^{35} (ave. energy 0.05 mev) to produce a reaction, while it takes only 1500–2000 rep of Sr^{90} or Y^{90} (ave. evergy 0.3, 0.7 mev) to produce the same reaction.

The degree of skin damage therefore is dependent on the absorbed dose at a certain critical depth in the skin. Moritz and Henriques found that the dose at 0.09 mm. depth of the pig skin (estimated to be the epidermal thickness) was constant within several hundred rep to produce transepidermal injury. Wilhelmy has also noted that it takes roughly the same dose of electrons and soft x-rays at the level of the subpapillary layer to produce erythema. On this basis, Parker has advocated the use of beta-detecting instruments with chamber walls corresponding in milligrams per square centimeter to the thickness of the relatively inert epidermal layer. Thus in expressing skin dosage, it is probably more informative to use the depth dose at a level corresponding to the basal cell layer of the epidermis.

Table I also indicates the species difference in skin sensitivity to beta radiation. Rabbits and sheep required larger doses than mice to produce the same effect with roughly the same energy beta. Porcine skin, which is reputedly more like human skin than other animals, apparently is more sensitive than the rabbit or sheep skin. Some of these differences, aside from species differences, may be due to variation in thickness of the epidermis of different species and differences in techniques used.

Table II shows beta dosage data from some human experiments and accidents found to produce various effects on the skin. These data must be interpreted with great caution due to differences in experimental techniques and dosimetry. The authors have taken the liberty of interpreting the severity of the skin reactions given by these investigators in degrees. A first degree reaction implies erythema and/or dry desquamation; a second degree, transepidermal necrosis with ulceration; and third degree, lesions which show deeper dermal involvement with breakdown and the development of chronic radiation dermatitis. It can be seen that there is a considerable variation in dose reported to produce the various reactions.

In the Marshallese the dose to the skin could not be calculated with any degree of accuracy due to the aforementioned reasons. The majority of the beta radiation was of low energy (ave. 0.1 mev, Sondhaus et al.) and accounted for the fact that most of the lesions were superficial in nature. However, there was sufficient penetration of more energetic components at the level of the hair follicles to result in temporary epilation. Due to the rapid attenuation of beta particles in tissue, the skin surface dose may have been quite high. The contribution of beta radiation to the skin of the Marshallese from the ground has been estimated by Sondhaus et al. to have been about 2000 rep to the feet, 600 rep at hip level and 300 rep to the head. These doses were insufficient in themselves to produce detectable lesions, though they probably contributed significantly to the severity of the foot lesions that occurred.

13.6 Effects of Fallout Radiation on the Skin

13.6.1 *Acute Effects.* In general beta radiation effects on the skin are similar to effects produced by more penetrating radiation such as gamma or x-radiation (Low-Beer; MacKee, Cipollaro and Montgomery; Warren; Nodl; and Walbach). However, the less penetrating beta radiation produces more superficial lesions with less damage to the dermis. The lesions are more like those produced by grenz-rays and ultra-violet rays (MacKee, Cipollaro and Montgomery; Ellinger). Consequently, they are usually less painful and heal more rapidly. The time sequence of beta lesions varies considerably with the dose to the skin. A general description of the sequence of changes is presented below.

13.6.1.1 *Early Effects.* During the first 24–48 hours after exposure, itching, burning, or tingling sensations of the skin are usually experienced. These symptoms may also involve the eyes with accompanying lachrymation. As pointed out earlier, fallout of an alkaline nature may contribute to this symptomatology. The above symptoms occurred in many of the Marshallese. In more severely damaged skin, erythema, edema and areas of blanching may be noted. Erythema was not observed in the Marshallese, perhaps due to the dark color of the skin.

13.6.1.2 *Latent Period.* The early signs and symptoms usually disappear within a few days and a relatively asymptomatic latent period ensues. The length of this latent period may vary from a few days to several weeks and is related to the dose to the skin; the higher the dose, the shorter the latent period. In the Marshallese, the more heavily exposed group developed lesions about 2 weeks after exposure, a week earlier than the less heavily exposed groups.

13.6.1.3 *Development of Gross Lesions.* Following the latent period the evidence of skin damage becomes apparent with intensification of signs and symptoms. A secondary wave of erythema may be seen along with gross

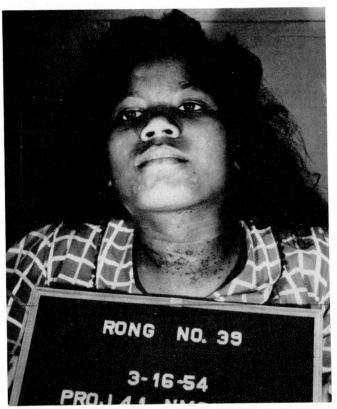

Fig. 3. Early hyperpigmented maculopapular neck lesions at 15 days. Case 39, age 15, F.

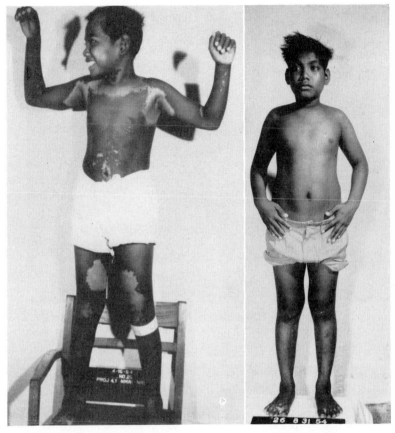

FIG. 4   FIG. 5

FIG. 4. Extensive lesions in 13-year old boy at 46 days post exposure. Case 26
FIG. 5. Same case as in fig. 4 six months after exposure showing healed lesions and
regrowth of hair.

changes in the skin. Such changes may be in the form of simple tanning or more marked pigmentation with the formation of macules, papules, or raised plaques of thickened pigmented skin. Mild lesions may cause only slight itching and burning and superficial desquamation from the center of the lesion outward, leaving depigmented thinned areas of epidermis which gradually repigment and heal the following week or so. In the more heavily exposed Marshallese group of 64 people, about 90 per cent developed multiple, spotty, pigmented lesions on exposed parts of the body. Most of these lesions were superficial in nature (see Figs. 3, 4 and 5). More severe exposure to the skin results in vesiculation and ulceration. Such lesions may be quite

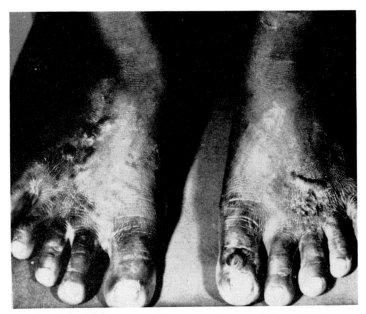

Fig. 6. Hyperpigmented raised plaques and bullae on dorsum of feet at 28 days after exposure: one lesion on left foot shows deeper involvement. Feet were painful at this time.

painful and secondary infection may occur. They require longer to heal and may result in some degree of atrophy and scarring of the skin. Repigmentation may be long delayed or may never be complete. Only about 20 per cent of the Marshallese group referred to developed ulcerating lesions and secondary infection occurred in a few cases. Lesions on the dorsum of the feet were generally the most severe, showing bullae formation followed by ulceration (Fig. 6). At three years after exposure some of these lesions continue to show incomplete repigmentation of the skin with atrophy or scarring in some cases (see Fig. 7).

Epilation may occur along with the development of the skin lesions. The head region is more sensitive to epilation than the axillary, pubic, or eyebrow regions. If the radiation dose to the follicles has not been too high, regrowth of hair commences in several months. Permanent epilation may result if the skin dose is high. Usually by 5 or 6 months, regrowth of hair is complete. In the Marshallese group, spotty epilation of varying degrees occurred in 90 per cent of the children and about 30 per cent of the adults (Fig. 8). Regrowth of hair commenced in all cases about 3 months post-exposure and by 6 months, hair was of normal color, texture and abundance (Fig. 9). Though change of color of hair from black to gray has been fre-

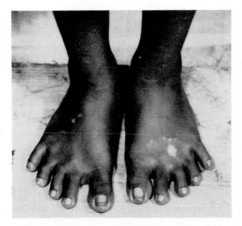

FIG. 7. Same case as in fig. 6 six months later. Foot lesions have healed with repigmentation, except depigmented spots persist in small areas where deeper lesions were.

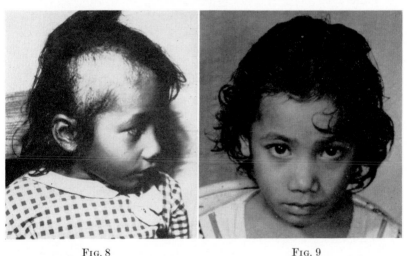

FIG. 8	FIG. 9

FIG. 8. Epilation in 7-year old girl at 28 days after exposure. Case 72
FIG. 9. Same girl as in fig. 8 six months after exposure showing complete regrowth of normal hair.

quently observed in animals (Hance and Murphy; Chase), regrowth is usually of normal color in the human being. However, Conard and Tessmer have reported a case in which regrowth of the hair of the eyebrows (previously black) regrew white in a lesion presumably due to fission product contamination.

13.6.2 *Chronic Effects, Carcinogenesis.* Following large doses of beta radiation, imperfect healing may result. Damage to the vessels of the dermis may result in sufficient impairment of circulation to cause cycles of breakdown and repair of the epidermis or chronic, indolent ulcers may result. Also commonly seen are atrophy, scarring, keratosis and telangiectatic vessels. The hair follicles, sweat and sebaceous glands may be injured sufficiently to result in permanent epilation and dryness of the skin. Such lesions are fertile ground for the later development of malignant change. Lesions of the skin resulting from beta radiation are less likely to result in chronic radiation dermatitis than are the lesions produced by more penetrating radiation such as are sometimes seen following x-ray or radium therapy.

Malignant changes in the skin have been reported in animals following beta radiation (Raper *et al.*, Brues, Glucksman, Kolotsky, Shubik), but so far as the authors are aware, such changes have not been reported in the human being. Though malignancy usually develops at the site of chronic radiation dermatitis, as a result of repeated exposures to radiation, it may develop as a sequel to mild exposures with little chronic changes in the skin. It has been reported to occur in animals following a single exposure to beta radiation with little or no chronic change in the skin (Raper *et al.*).

In view of the superficial nature of most of the Marshallese lesions and the low evidence of chronic effects in the skin, the likelihood of skin cancer in this group seems diminished.

13.6.3 *Histopathology of Beta Lesions.* By and large, the histopathological changes in the skin produced by beta radiation are much the same as those produced by gamma or x-rays. Since histological changes induced by the latter radiations have been well documented (MacKee, Cipollaro and Montgomery; Warren; Bloom and Bloom; and Walbach, etc.), a detailed description of the changes induced by beta radiation will not be presented. A limited number of studies of the histological changes in the skin of animals (Snider and Raper; Moritz and Henriques) and in man (Low-Beer) from beta radiation have been reported.

In general the changes produced by beta radiation are more superficial than those produced by more penetrating radiations with relatively much greater damage to the epidermis than to the dermis. With fallout radiation the damage is spotty in character with areas of damage surrounded by relatively normal tissue.

The histopathological changes induced in the skin by fallout in the Marshallese lesions were studied in sections of a number of biopsies taken during the first 7 weeks, at 6 months and at 2 years. Details of these changes can be found elsewhere (Conard *et al.*). Some of the major changes seen are summarized below. During the early, acute period of the lesions, the epidermis showed marked damage characterized by atrophy and flattening of the rete pegs with disorganization of malpighian and basal layers and marked cellular changes (pleomorphic nuclei, pyknosis and cytoplasmic halos). Additional features were atrophy or absence of the stratum granulosum, imperfect keratinization, and loose fibrillation and hyperkeratosis of the stratum corneum. Cells laden with pigment were frequently present throughout the epidermis. In the dermis the changes were largely confined to the upper part with edema, telangiectasis of vessels with perivascular infiltration of lymphocytes. Chromatophores filled with melanin were prominent. Fig. 10 shows some of these changes in a pigmented lesion biopsied 3 weeks after exposure.

By 6 months there was considerable improvement in the histological appearance of the lesions. The following changes were found to persist in varying degrees: focal atrophy of the stratum granulosum, slight focal pigmentary disturbances in cells of the basal layer, and slight distrubances in polarity of the epithelial cells in basal papillary projections. In the dermis, telangiectasis of slight to moderate degree persisted.

At 2 years, biopsies at sites of persistent gross abnormalities revealed that none of the lesions were neoplastic or showed alterations suggestive

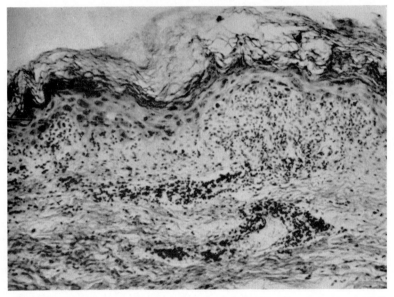

FIG. 10. Section from beta lesion of neck at 3 weeks after exposure to fallout. (× 100) Epidermis: extensive transepidermal damage (with slightly less involved zones on either side). Loose lamination of stratum corneum, absence of stratum granulosum. Parakeratinization with exfoliation of pigment containing cells. Disorganization of the malpighian layer. Dermis: mild edema of pars papillaris with indistinct capillary loops. Perivascular cellular infiltrate (lymphocytes and mononuclear phogocytes), in superficial corium with telangiectasis. Case 26.

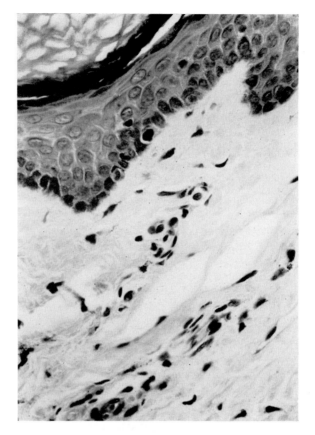

Fig. 11. Section (333 ✕) from lesion on back of neck at 2 years after exposure to fallout. Lesion showed mottled pigmentation and depigmentation grossly. Section shows some loss of pigment in the basal layers of the epidermis and telangiectasis in the dermis. Case 39.

of a precancerous condition. In some sections, acanthosis, absence of pigment in the basal layer and atrophy and benign dyskeratosis were noted in the malpighian layer of the epidermis. In the dermis degenerative changes in the collagen were noted frequently, and capillary dilation persisted. Some of these features may be seen in Fig. 11, which is a section taken at two years of a lesion on the back of the neck which showed gross pigment changes.

13.7 Therapy of Beta Lesions

The treatment of beta lesions during the acute stage is very similar to the treatment of thermal burns. Mild lesions will only require daily cleansing and application of bland antipruritic lotions and ointments. Calamine lotion with 1 per cent phenol is soothing. Analgesic and anesthetic ointments are helpful in allaying more painful symptoms and in keeping the skin soft in lesions that are dry and thickened. Antibiotics applied locally and/or parenterally should be used if secondary infection occurs, or prophylactically if the lesion is associated with severe leukopoenia from whole body radiation. The above treatment proved quite adequate with the Marshallese lesions.

In severe lesions with the development of necrotic tissue, surgical debridement should be carried out. Use of pressure dressings, splinting and elevation of affected parts may be necessary. Early skin grafting should be considered in cases developing painful or progressive chronic radiation dermatitis (Brown *et al.*). For more detailed therapy of radiation lesions, the reader is referred to standard textbooks on the subject such as that of MacKee, Cipollaro and Montgomery.

Several agents have been reported in recent years to be beneficial in the treatment of radiation lesions of the skin. Among these are preparations of the Aloe Vera plant (Lushbough; MacKee, Cipollaro and Montgomery). The use of vitamins such as A and D are advocated by some investigators in the acute stages. The use of triiodothyronine preparations in such lesions appears to be beneficial from results of preliminary work (Nickson). Prednisone injections have been reported to reduce post-irradiation inflammation (Matthewson). Further clinical experience with these agents is necessary before they can be recommended for general use in the treatment of beta burns.

13.8 Factors Influencing Severity of Skin Lesions from Fallout

13.8.1 *Physical Factors.* Usually fallout material must be in contact with the bare skin to result in significant skin damage. Most of the lesions in the Marshallese occurred on exposed parts of the body, and protection was afforded by clothing, even a single layer of cotton material. Since clothing would probably not result in more than about 25 per cent attenuation of the beta particles, additional protection must have been afforded by the fact that the loosely-fitted clothing tended to hold the radioactive material away from the skin. Avoidance of skin contamination by taking shelter offers almost complete protection. No lesions developed in those Marshallese who remained in their houses during the fallout.

The ultimate dose to the skin depends on the radiation characteristics of the fallout material, the time after detonation that the fallout occurs, and the length of time that the material is in contact with the skin before decontamination is accomplished. Due to the process of radioactive decay which is quite fast during the first few hours, the earlier the time of the fallout, the greater is the dose rate from a given sample. This fact emphasizes the importance of early decontamination of the skin, particularly if contamination takes place during the first day after detonation. The fact that thorough decontamination of the Marshallese was not accomplished until their evacuation some two days after the accident, resulted in an appreciable increase of their skin dose. Those individuals that bathed or went swimming during the early period developed few lesions.

13.8.2 *Biological Factors.* There are certain *biological factors* known to influence the sensitivity of the skin to radiation. In addition to species differences referred to, it is known that the skin of certain parts of the body is more sensitive to radiation than that of others. In general, the thinner-skinned flexor surfaces of the body are more sensitive than the thicker-skinned extensor surfaces (MacKee, Cipollaro and Montgomery). This was found to be true in the Marshallese. Lesions were more prevalent on the front and sides of the neck, axilla and antecubital fossae. Another factor is associated with pigmentation of the skin. Darker-skinned people, brunettes, are known to be less sensitive to radiation than blondes or people with ruddy complexions, and Negro skin is the most resistant (MacKee, Cipollaro and Montgomery; Bloom and Bloom).

Areas of the body where perspiration is more profuse, such as the folds of the neck, axillae, and antecubital fossae tend to cause the fallout to stick and collect. It was found that skin lesions in these areas were more abundant in the Marshallese. This effect is increased in a warm, humid climate, such as in the Marshall Islands.

13.9 Concluding Remarks

As a result of the Marshallese accident, the potentialities of serious injury to the skin from fallout associated with the detonation of large nuclear devices are apparent. Of concern also is the occurrence of similar radiation injuries to the skin from accidental exposure to radioisotopes which are being used increasingly.

The skin hazards associated with fallout can be greatly reduced by taking simple precautionary measures. Much was learned from the Marshallese experience in this regard. This group of people was not aware of the hazards of fallout and only minimal, if any, efforts were made to protect themselves. This situation represents an extreme example, and the extensiveness of the skin effects could have been greatly reduced had proper measures been taken. Based on the experiences of these people during the critical fallout period and the skin lesions that developed on an individual basis, the following facts emerge:

1. Avoidance of contact of fallout material on the skin by taking shelter

or covering the body with clothing virtually eliminates the possibility of skin effects.

2. Prompt, thorough decontamination of the skin and hair is of utmost importance. Repeated scrubbing with soap or detergent and water may be necessary. If contamination of the hair is severe, it may be advisable to clip the hair close or shave the head.

3. Areas of the body where perspiration is more profuse tend to cause the fallout material to collect. Such areas should be carefully checked for contamination. A warm, humid climate will naturally aggravate this effect.

4. Moderately severe beta lesions of the skin and epilation may result from fallout situations in which the whole body penetrating dose of radiation is sublethal. With such doses, the skin lesions do not appear to complicate the radiation syndrome.

5. In situations where skin lesions are associated with larger doses of whole body radiation with marked leukopoenia, such lesions might become secondarily infected more easily and afford portals of entry leading to bacteremia or septicemia.

6. Severe skin irradiation with minimal whole body irradiation might result in fallout situations where prompt evacuation from the contaminated area occurred, but skin decontamination was delayed.

7. Early skin and eye symptoms might be mildly disabling during the first day or two after exposure to fallout and later symptoms associated with full-blown lesions might be quite disabling. Late effects on the skin in the form of chronic radiation dermatitis and malignancy are possible complications.

REFERENCES

BIRD, J. M.: The Effects of Irradiation from Atomic Bomb Fallout upon a Group of Hereford Cattle. Tenn. University, College of Agriculture, 1952, 78P AECU, 2695. On Microcard.

BLOOM, W. AND BLOOM, M. A.: *Radiation Biology*, Vol. 1, Part II, p. 1119, New York: McGraw-Hill, 1954.

BROWN, J. B., McDOWELL, F. AND FRYER, M. P.: Radiation burns, including vocational and atomic exposures. Treatment and surgical prevention of chronic lesions. *Ann. Surg. 130:* 593, 1949.

BRUES, A. M.: Carcinogenic effects of radiation. *Advances in Biology and Medical Physics 2:* 178–9, 1951.

CHASE, H. B.: Greying of hair. 1. Effects produced by single doses of X-rays on mice. *J. Morphol. 84:* 57, 1949.

CLOUDMAN, A. M., HAMILTON, K. A., CLAYTON, R. S. AND BRUES, A. M.: Effects of combined local treatment with radioactive and chemical carcinogens. *J. Nat. Cancer Inst. 15:* 1077–1083, 1955.

CONARD, R. A. AND TESSMER, C. F.: Beta radiation lesion of the skin. *Arch. Dermatol. 74:* 663–666, 1957.

CONARD, R. A., CANNON, BRADFORD, HUGGINS, C. E., RICHARDS, J. B. AND LOWERY, Austin: Medical survey of Marshallese two years after exposure to fallout radiation. *J.A.M.A. 164:* 1192, 1957.

CONARD, R. A., SHULMAN, N. R., WOOD, D. A., DUNHAM, C. L., ALPEN, E. L., BROWNING, L. E., BOND, U. P. AND CRONKITE, E. P.: Chapter III in: Some Effects of Ionizing Radiation on Human Beings. Edited by CRONKITE, E. P., BOND, V. P. AND DUNHAM, C. L. Government Printing Office, TID 5358, July, 1956.

CRAWFORD, STANLEY: Leonard or cathode "ray" dermatitis. *Arch. Dermat. u. Syph. 27:* 579–583, 1933.

ELLINGER, F.: *The Biologic Fundamentals of Radiation Therapy.* New York: Elsevier, Chap. XXII, 1941.

GLUCKSMANN, A.: The histogenesis of radiation-induced and of benzpyrene-induced epidermal tumours in the mouse. *J. Pathol. Bacteriol. 63:* 176–177, 1951.

GRIFFITH, H. D., PHILIP, J. F. AND SEINDELL, G. E.: Skin reaction to protracted beta irradiation. *Brit. J. Radiol. 27:* 107–112, 1954.

HANCE, R. T. AND MURPHY, J. B.: Studies on X-ray effects, XV. The prevention of pigment formation in the hair follicles of colored mice with high voltage X-ray, *J. Exper. Med. 44:* 339, 1926.

HENSHAW, P. S., SNIDER, R. S. AND RILEY, E. F.: Aberrant tissue developments in rats exposed to beta rays. *Radiology 52:* 401–415, 1949.

KEPP, R. K.: The effects of irradiation of the human skin with high speed electrons. *Strahlentherapie 81:* 201–214, 1952.

KEPP, R. K., MULLER, K. AND REICH, H.: The Time Factor in Beta Radiation of the Human Skin, *Strahlentherapie 84:* 224–244, 1951.

KHARCHENKO, A. M. AND VENOLUROV, I. N.: Functional and histomorphological changes in the skin of rabbits after application or radioactive phosphorous, Vestnik, Venerol, Dermatol. No. 5, 14–8 (Sept.–Oct. 1955) CLML 29: no. 43987.

KNOWLTON, N. P., LEIFER, E., HOGNESS, J. R., HEMPLEMANN, LOUIS H., BLANEY, LOREN F., GILL, DAN C., OAKES, WILLIAM R. AND SHAFER, CHARLES L.: Beta ray burns of human skin, *J.A.M.A. 141:* 239–246, 1949.

KOLETSKY, S., BONTE, F. J. AND FREEDELL, H. L.: Production of malignant tumors in rats with radioactive phosphorus. *Cancer Res. 10:* 129–138, 1950.

KOYAMA, Y. ET AL.: Iryo (Published by Iryo Dokokai, Medical Affairs Bureau, Ministry of Health and Welfare, Tokyo, Japan) *9:* no. 1, 5–45, Jan. 1955.

LOW-BEER, B. V. A.: External therapeutic use of radio phosphorous. 1. Erythema studies. *Radiology 47:* 213, 1946.

LUSHBAUGH, C. E., SPALDING, J. F. AND HALE, D. B.: Report on Sheep Losses Adjacent to the Nevada Proving Grounds, AEC Report Jan. 6, 1954.

LUSHBAUGH, C. E. AND HALE, D. B.: Experimental acute radio-dermatitis following beta radiation. V. Histo-pathological study at the mode of action of therapy with aloe vera. *Cancer 6:* (4) 690, 1953.

MATHEWSON, J. B.: Post radiation inflammation reduced by prednisone. *New York J. Med. 56:* 3903–3906, 1956.

MACKEE, G. M., CIPOLLARO, A. C. AND MONTGOMERY, H. M.: *X-ray and Radium Treatment of Diseases of the Skin* (4th ed.). Philadelphia: Lea, 1947.

Major Activities in Atomic Energy Programs, July–December 1953, U. S. Atomic Energy Comm., 15th Semiannual Report, Jan. 1954, p. 50.

MINISOV, V. S.: Effect of Radioactive Phosphorous in the Skin in Rabbit, Preliminary Communication, Vestinik, Ventrol, Dermatol. No. 1, 16–20, April 1953, Ca 47, p. 7000A.

MORITZ, A. R. AND HENRIQUES, F. W.: Effect of beta rays on the skin as a function of the energy, intensity, and duration of the radiation. *J. Lab. Invest. 1:* 167, 1952.

NICKSON, J. J.: Memorial Hospital, New York City, Personal Communication.

NODL, F.: Tissue changes of the human skin after action of fast electrons, *Strahlentherapie 92:* 576–589, 1953. (Article with the same title also in *Arch. Dermat. u. Syph. 200:* 136–137, 1955.) CLML *29:* No. 1207.

PARKER, H. M.: Some Physiological Aspects of the Effects of Beta Radiation on Tissue, AECD 2859.

PASSONNEAU, J. V. AND HAMILTON, K.: Beta-irradiation Effects from Diffuse and Point Sources of Sr. 90. In Argonne Nat. Lab., Div. of Biology and Medical Research, Quarterly Report August, September, and October, 1950, p. 23–25, ANL 4531.

PAYSINGER, J., PLUMLEO, M. P., SIKES, D., WEST, J. L., COMAR, C. L., HANSARD, S. L., HOBBS, C. S. AND HOOD, S. L.: Fission Product Retention and Pathology of Alamorgordo Cattle, AEC Report UT-AEC-1, 1954.

RAPER, J. R. AND BARNES, K. K.: *Biological Effects of External Beta Radiation* (1st. ed.). New York: McGraw-Hill, 1951, Chap. 4.

ROBBINS, LAWRENCE L., AUB, JOSEPH C., COPE, OLIVER, COGAN, DAVID G., LANGOHR, JOHN L., CLOUD, R. W. AND MERRILL, OLIVER E.: Superficial "burns" of skin and eyes from scattered cathode rays. *Radiology 64:* 1–23, 1946.

SHUBIK, P., GOLDFARB, A. R. AND RITCHIE, A. C.: Latent carcinogenic action of beta-irradiation on mouse epidermis. *Nature 171:* 934–935, 1953.

SNIDER, R. S. AND RAPER, J. R.: *Biological Effects of External Beta Radiation* (1st ed.). New York: McGraw-Hill, 1951, Chap. 9.

SONDHAUS, C. A. ET AL.: Chapter I, Some effects of Ionizing Radiation on Human Beings, edited by E. P. CRONKITE, V. P. BOND, AND C. L. DUNHAM, Government Printing Office, TID 5358, July, 1956.

SULZBERGER, M. B., BAER, R. L. AND BOROTA, A.: Skin Changes Induced by Low Voltage Roentgen Radiation, AEC Report AECU-161, n.d.

UNGAR, G. E., DAMGAARD, E. AND WILLIAMS F.: Protection by spleen homogenate in beta-irradiated skin. *Proc. Soc. Exper. Biol. & Med. 87:* 383–386, 1954.

WALBACH, S. B.: The pathologic histology of chronic X-ray dermatitis and early X-ray carcinoma. *J. Med. Res. 16:* 415, 1909.

WARREN, SHIELDS: The histopathology of radiation lesions. *Physiol. Rev. 24:* 225–237, 1944.

WARREN, SHIELDS: Effects of radiation on normal tissue. *Arch. Path. 35:* 304–353, 1943.

WILHELMY, ERNST: Ueber die Reaktion der Haut auf Langwellige Roentgenstrahlen und Kathodenstraklen, *Strahlentherapie 55:* 498–523, 1936.

WIRTH, J. E. AND RAPER, J. R.: *Biological Effects of External Beta Radiation* (1st. ed). New York: McGraw-Hill, 1951, Chap. 12.

WITTEN, V. H., ROSS, M. S., OSHRY, E. AND HOLMSTROM, V.: Studies of thorium X applied to human skin. *J. Invest. Dermat. 20:* 93, 1953.

WITTEN, V. H., ET AL.: Erythema effects of a pure beta emitter (strontium 90) on human skin. *J. Invest. Dermat. 23:* 271–285, 1954, NSA *9*, No. 836.

WITTEN, V. H. ET AL.: Studies of thorium X applied to human skin. III. The relative effects of alpha and beta-gamma irradiation in the production of erythema. *J. Invest. Dermat. 21:* 249–257, 1953, NSA 8, No. 986. Other parts not pertinent.

14 ▶

Permissible Dosage and Risk Factors of Ionizing Radiation

CHARLES F. BEHRENS, M.D.

14.1 Nature of Problem

With the advent of newer developments in the field of ionizing radiation, the dosage and risk factors involved come to embrace a variety of problems related both to the more familiar occupational hazards from small dosages over long periods, and also to the hazards of larger dosages which may be entailed in use of nuclear reactors, or by resort to atomic weapons.

The cumulative and remote effects are naturally related to standard exposure limits, and accordingly in large measure to the more insidious hazards which have, in years gone by, ambushed so many unwary workers. Dangerous amounts of radiation may be received without the occurrence of anything obviously alarming to alert the individual to his peril. Radiation can well prove to be a subtle agent of mischief and also an assassin. As such, it demands serious concern and grave respect. On the other hand, it calls for neither dread nor panic. The answers to the problems involved lie in a proper perspective that is best and most adequately derived from knowledge of the facts; and this knowledge now becomes of greater and greater importance as the number of nuclear reactors increases, the use of radioactive isotopes spreads rapidly, cyclotron and high energy apparatus sprout up everywhere, and the general use of x-ray increases all the time.

As regards isotopes, it has often been pointed out that their great and increasing availability for research, diagnosis and therapy forms an intensely interesting and comforting bright spot in this atomic era, compensating in some degree for the stultifying and revolting applications of science to mass slaughter. It is, however, well to point out that these gorgeous prospects may well be marred by a few mourning bands for those who in enthusiastic use neglect precautions. The use of isotopes involves

278

different technics and problems than those many of us are familiar with in the clinical and industrial uses of x-rays and radium. There is far greater danger of spillage and general contamination of the individual as well as the environment; moreover, use in therapy and with experimental animals will often entail special provision for safe disposal of radioactive excretions. These matters will be considered elsewhere in detail.

14.2 General Nature of Effects

In keeping with the sensitivity scale, actively dividing types of cells are most vulnerable and this holds for chronic and late effects as well as acute. Accordingly, we find ourselves concerned most intensely with (1) embryonal blood cells of all types, (2) gonads and (3) the skin and its appendages, also the mucous membranes.

However, no tissues are immune, and in addition to primary effects there may be devastating secondary effects and inadequate repair. Various internal structures may also be affected by absorbed radioactive substances and in regard to this category we become concerned with local areas of lodgment, chiefly the bones and lungs. Once more the blood comes in for consideration because of the location of many embryonal blood cells in bony structures. It is to be noted also that blood vessels are adversely affected and connective tissue hyalinized so that seriously damaged tissue will often suffer eventually from poor blood supply.

14.3 Skin Effects

Effects on the skin are readily observed and were among the first to be noted, so that it is convenient to start with a detailed consideration of these.

14.3.1 *Historical Background.* History presents the subject in a dramatic fashion and it is most instructive to dip into it a bit. The discovery of the x-ray by Wilhelm Conrad Roentgen in 1895, followed closely by the discovery of natural radioactivity by Henri Becquerel, created an enormous stir in the closing years of the last century and early years of the present one. It may not have been quite as big a stir as that made in our own time by the atomic bomb, but x-rays and radioactivity formed the great wonder of the day.

In the early days there was some little apprehension concerning the newly found and mysterious x-ray and "Becquerel" rays but unfortunately fears were largely absurd and misdirected. A few people did envision the energy possibilities of radioactivity, and thus Henry Adams, in his classic *Education of Henry Adams*, mentioned this matter, noting the great increase in the number of scientists working on the problems of radioactivity and speculating on the heavy responsibilities entailed by the virtually unlimited power which some day might be gained from this source. Again, Einstein in 1905 suggested that radioactivity would probably yield the basis for proving his amazing equation relating mass to energy as equivalents ($e = mc^2$). Scarcely anyone seemed to realize that there might be biologic dangers. Instead, the public was treated to imbecilities. Thus, the *Pall Mall Gazette* considered fluoroscopy revolting and indecent, and suggested it would be best to execute the discoverer and dump the fluorescible compound (calcium tungstate) in the ocean. It opined that observing each other's bones should be left to the fish. A New Jersey congressman introduced a bill prohibiting the use of x-rays in opera glasses, and in London, x-ray-proof underwear was advertised. *Punch*, in a satirical poem, advised Roentgen to keep his radiographs for his epitaph and go to work on spooks.

These silly objections came to nothing but, on the other hand, there was no sensible caution either. The enthusiasm and zeal with which people delved into the field of radiation were not tempered with any large measure of caution, either reasonable or unreasonable, and it must be admitted too that the early workers were most unreceptive to what should have been obvious danger signals. There were only a few exceptions. Roentgen himself escaped, by careful shielding of his tubes, although it appears that he was chiefly concerned with the prevention of photographic fogging. For the most part there was a sublime disregard of consequences. It would seem that nearly all of us, scientists or not, dislike to acknowledge unpleasant things about our favorite devices and inventions. At all events, the record shows that ill effects were first blamed on such things as ultraviolet from the Crooke tubes, platinum particles, cathode rays, electrostatic discharge and heat. Thus when erythema was seen involving the hands, arms and faces of people working with x-ray apparatus, it appears that this was considered of scarcely any more importance than erythema from sunlight, that is, plain sunburn. The result was that practices were common and persisted in, even after the occurrence of ill effects, that make us shudder today. Unrestricted fluoroscopy was performed without safeguards and it was common practice to test the cranky and uncertain apparatus of that day by fluoroscopy of one's own hand to determine if the tube was functioning well. Again, workers were prone to expose themselves to x-rays merely to reassure patients or for demonstration purposes at meetings and fairs. Before long a tragic list of disastrous consequences began to unroll and nearly all the early workers were victims, many of them fatally injured.

14.3.2 *Early X-ray Martyrs.* Mr. Hawks, a volunteer assistant to Professor Pupin at Columbia University, noted in 1896 that his skin had begun to dry and itch, and after a little longer exposure, that his hand developed inflammation lasting for about ten days, after which the skin peeled as in sunburn and the hair fell out. He also lost his finger nails several times. Mr.

Hawks learned his lesson at this point and avoided further exposure. Thirty-eight years later, he was able to state that his hand was in good shape except there were scarred effects and that the skin was thicker. Most of the other workers were not so fortunate, or rather they continued to be reckless.

Dr. Kassabian wrote of x-rays as an irritant in 1900 and described how the fingers, knuckles and dorsum of his left hand developed an erythematous condition which lasted about a month. Itching was intense, and the skin became tough, glossy, edematous and pigmented. His condition became

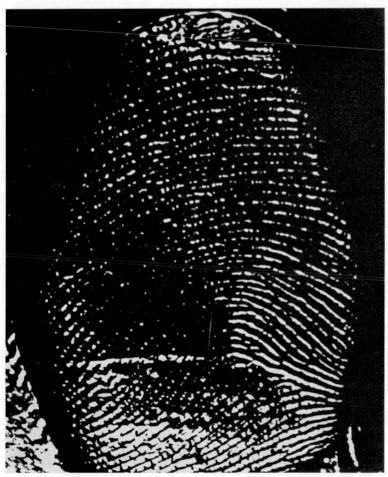

FIG. 1. Normal finger impression
(Courtesy of Roger A. Harvey, M.D.)
(From Atomic Energy Commission report MDDC-216)

worse and in 1903 he wrote that he had used every remedy mentioned in all the textbooks, without avail. In 1908 an area of ulceration showed malignant changes and in 1909, in spite of amputations, there were axillary metastases and death soon followed.

This story with minor variations can be repeated for Clarence Dally, one of Edison's assistants, Mrs. Ascheim, who sacrificed herself in fluoroscopic and radiographic work, much of it on Spanish-American Veterans,

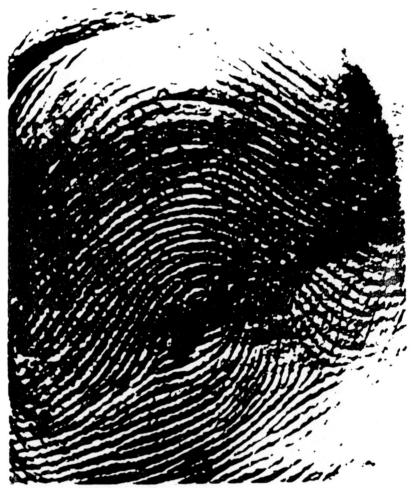

FIG. 2. Impressions submitted by a radiologist who had practiced five years with X-rays and radium. Early flattening and localized atrophy of ridges are demonstrated.

(Courtesy of Roger A. Harvey, M.D.)

(From Atomic Energy Commission report MDDC-216)

Dr. Early of Ohio, Dr. Leonard of Philadelphia, Dr. Dodd of Boston, Dr. Egelhof of Chicago, Dr. Caldwell, one of our great pioneers who tried to interest this country in photofluorography, Mr. Machlett, a pioneer in tube manufacturing, Dr. Baetjer, a pioneer in bone tumors, and others.

In 1907 Dr. Kassabian recorded 7 fatal cases. In 1908 Rowntree listed 20 American and 11 English victims, and other lists appeared. In 1911 Hesse reported 54 victims. Krause in 1930 listed 126 additional cases and we can be sure that there were many cases not reflected in these records.

14.3.3 *Details of Skin Damage.* Let us now look into the matter of skin changes in more detail. We have seen that when radiation dermatitis sets in there are inflammation, swelling, loss of hair, dryness of the skin and atrophy of finger nails. Histologically, there is replacement of normal

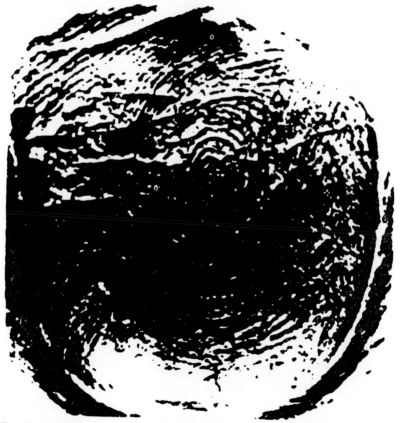

Fɪɢ. 3. Impressions submitted by a radiologist who had practiced fifteen years with X-rays. Generalized atrophy and atrophic fissures are present.

(Courtesy of Roger A. Harvey, M.D.)

(From Atomic Energy Commission report MDDC-216)

collagen by a dense hyaline type. Later there are obliterative changes in the blood vessels and atrophy of glandular structures with resultant dryness which further aggravates skin damage. Repair efforts are irregular and inadequate resulting in keratoses, warts and telangiectases. Inevitably, there ensues increased susceptibility to injury resulting in abrasions and ulcers which heal with great difficulty and, of course, frequent incidence of malignancy.

In this day we do not usually expect to see such extreme effects and we keep an eye open for early injuries. Nonetheless, let no one believe that those drastic changes are a thing of the past. Radiologists may become careless and in any event may be exposed over too many years; preoccupied and enthusiastic scientists take chances; orthopedists working with fluoroscopy tend to forget or disregard warnings and limitations; unscrupulous quacks and so-called beauticians occasionally use x-ray for permanent depilation—ignorant of and indifferent to the dangers. I have had to deal with one such victim myself within recent years. Finally, in connection with therapy there will be occasional unavoidable instances of severe skin damage, although here the advent of supervoltage apparatus has been a great boon.

Considering the milder injuries of the skin, the following may be observed:

1. Brittleness and ridging of the nails.
2. Increased susceptibility of the hands to chapping.
3. Blunting or leveling of the finger ridges.
4. Dryness and epilation.
5. Changes in the nail fold capillaries in the way of disordered pattern.

14.4 Ocular Effects

Regarding the eyes, it has been known for some time that extensive radiation therapy involving the eye is often productive of cataract and it appears that exposure to approximately an erythema dose may bring this about, after a latent period of several years. Surprisingly enough, however, cataract has been rare with radiation workers and it would appear that concentration of dosage is a great factor. This hardly warrants carelessness, as it may well be that a number of our early workers might have developed cataract if they had not died too soon of skin cancers. In addition, for many years, lead glass has invariably been used to cover fluoroscopic screens so that the eyes have often escaped, even when there was excessive exposure of the hands, and other parts of the body. However, it now appears that some scientists engaged in cyclotron work have developed cataracts from exposure to neutrons. About 10% of Japanese exposed to neutrons from the atomic bomb have developed cataracts.

14.5 Roentgen Unit

With this introduction to the harmful effects of radiation, it is well to pause and look more precisely into the physical factors involved and units of measurement, before proceeding further.

In the early days of radiology, and indeed for quite a few years thereafter, there were no precise means of measuring the amounts of radiation. Recourse was commonly had to estimating dosage on the basis of voltage applied to the tube, the milliamperes of current, distance and filtration. These were related to skin erythema. Unfortunately people vary much in regard to this effect and observers also differ in what they regard as erythema, so that this type of measurement has never been satisfactory. Photochemical detection in the form of "pastilles" of one type or another was also used without much satisfaction. Photographic methods were tried, but although they are now usable with good results they were not sufficiently precise in early days.

Eventually dosage came to be based on the ionization produced by x- and gamma rays, when it became possible to measure this accurately and without too much trouble. This method is the one now used in x-ray therapy. The standard unit employed is the roentgen or "r" and is based on the production by x-rays or gamma rays of 1 esu of charge in 1 cc. or 0.001293 gm. of air. In order to apply the figure to other types of radiation we resort to equivalence of ionization energy and biologic effects and use the terms "rep" and "rem." The "rep" signifies roentgen equivalent physical and is a unit proposed to apply to statements of dose of ionizing radiation not covered by the definition of the roentgen. It has been variously defined as the dose which produces energy absorption of 83 ergs per gram of air or 97 ergs per gram of tissue. The actual energy absorption in tissue per roentgen is a function of the tissue composition and of the wave length of the radiation, and ranges between 60 and 100 ergs per gram. The term "rem" stands for roentgen equivalent man and is defined as the dose of any ionizing radiation that will produce the same biologic effect as that produced by 1 roentgen of high-voltage x-radiation. A new term, the "rad" has been introduced and very conveniently is the amount of radiation which results in the absorbtion of 100 ergs/gram in the irradiated material. It is thus very nearly the same as the rep.

But we must remember that dosages, however measured, are not enough in and of themselves unless supplemented by knowledge of energies, wave length and associated penetrative effects as well as time factors.

14.6 X-ray and Gamma Ray Dosage Factors

The most important radiations are those in the electromagnetic sphere or category of photons, ranging from soft x-rays of 0.5 A to gamma of

0.01 A. The shorter the wave length, the greater the penetration and depth effects. The longer the wave length, the less the penetration and greater the skin effect. Naturally, the effects are greatest where most absorption takes place. The difference is considerable. Thus, 300–350 r of x-ray from sources of 80–100 kv will usually produce erythema. So-called Grenz rays (very soft x-ray) from 10 kv generators will produce erythema with about 100 r. About 600 r from 200 kv machines are needed for the same result and 1000 r or more for gamma and multimillion volt x-ray.

Relating this to formal permissible dosage levels, it has not been found feasible to set up different standards of permissible dosage for these various types as it would be complex, and since in practice, exposure to monochromatic beams is rare and variation in secondary and scattered radiation not sufficiently marked. However, one can gain an idea as to how excessive dosage is apt to show itself by having regard to the type of radiation and manner of exposure. A person exposed to general body radiation from high voltage and gamma is apt to show systemic effects, whereas a person working with low voltage fluoroscopes is in more danger of skin damage to hands and forearms. A person working with radioactive materials directly may endanger his fingers and hands, and also sustain systemic effects as well, depending on working conditions and materials employed. A person exposed to external radiation from an atomic explosion is most apt to show serious damage from the deep effects of hard gamma rays. However, a person exposed to fission products may receive damage from beta rays as well, both externally and internally after absorption.

14.7 Beta Dosage Factors

Considering skin effects from beta rays we find that the beta particles have ranges up to 13 meters in air and may penetrate 1 cm. or more in tissue so that they can readily reach the germinal layer of the skin to cause damage. The powerful beams of electrons from betatrons are equivalent to high energy beta rays and can cause serious burns in a few seconds, as some unhappy workers discovered to their sorrow. In one instance, 6 men received burns of the skin and eyes in a few seconds while adjusting a betatron. At Bikini, as described in the JAMA, several workers received very severe burns of the hands due to incautious handling of contaminated materials; these were due to beta rays. Chap 12 records skin damage in natives at Rongelap.

It appears that burns from beta rays appear sooner, heal a bit faster and may be somewhat less painful than those from x- or gamma rays. It is possible too that deep sclerosing effects on blood vessels may be less. Nevertheless, beta radiation must, in general, be considered very seriously in regard to skin effects.

14.8 Alpha Particle Dosage Factors

Alpha particles belong in a different category by reason of size, mass and charge (4 mass units and double positive charge). Penetration is so slight that merely a heavy piece of paper or 0.6 mm. Al will suffice to stop most of them, and range in tissue is usually 30 to 50 microns. Thus the horny layer of the skin usually affords good protection, so that alpha particles are of practically no consequence as an external hazard. In fact, the effects of alpha irradiation on ulcers is out of keeping with usual ionization effects. Thus, alpha radiation from radon in petrolatum appears to exert a healing effect on radiation ulcers, possibly, it has been suggested, because of changes in the petrolatum, or to trace amounts of elements from transmutation. At any rate, alpha emitters need to be absorbed and operate internally before they do significant damage. What they can do then is most vicious, as will be related later. Ionizing power is great and biologic effectiveness extremely great at short range—being estimated at 10–20 times greater in REM's when equivalent in REP.

14.9 Neutron Dosage Factors

When we come to neutrons, we have a peculiar story. They penetrate readily, and although they lack direct ionizing power nevertheless cause much dense ionization indirectly by ejecting protons from nuclei. In addition, there are other effects, as mentioned in the previous account of ionizing radiations. Thus when H nuclei capture neutrons to form deuterons, gamma rays are produced. Induced radioactivity and transmutations also occur and it is likely that changes in the atomic nuclei will produce chemical disturbances aside from those due to the ionization related to ejection of orbital electrons. Thus, there are good grounds for the disproportionate effects noted in fact. The equivalent of 1 r in neutron radiation (as determined in an ionization chamber by the indirect means of secondary ions liberated usually from boron by the neutrons) has double the energy production in tissue so that a unit designated as an "n" is occasionally used as being equivalent to 2 r. However, the discrepancy is still more marked biologically, and thus 200 REP of fast neutrons have been found to produce the same result as 1000 r of gamma in terms of erythema. Again, there is some reason to believe that genetically neutrons may be still more effective. Thus, the permissible limit for fast neutrons is usually placed at one-tenth the REP for x- or gamma rays and one-fifth for slow neutrons.

14.10 Proton Dosage Factors

Protons were noted as being ejected by neutrons and are given a biologic equivalence of four times that of gamma rays. Protons, like alpha particles, produce heavy dense ionization of columnar type. Protons are not of primary significance in natural radioactivity or in present-day radiologic practice. They are, however, significant in connection with cyclotrons. With extremely high voltage or energy they can penetrate and cause damaging effects and it is worth noting something of the depth effects. By applying the very high energy of 115 mev, a penetration of 10 cm. is possible with the curious fact that in the last centimeter, ionization is six times the surface value and in the last half centimeter, 16 times that value (Bragg ionization effect). This is because ionization increases as the velocity of the proton diminishes, very likely because it is a little slower in passing atoms and thus is able to exert an effect for a longer time. At any rate, this gives us theoretical hope of reaching deep tumors by high voltage "sharp shooting" of protons and with comparatively slight skin damage.* Naturally much study and research will be needed before clinical application can be made, aside from the fact that apparatus capable of emitting protons of such energy is apt to be prohibitively expensive for routine use.

14.11 Dosage Rate and Recovery Factors

Since we have little precise quantitative information regarding effects of small dosages over long periods, let us look into some indirect evidence. We know for instance that a single dose of about 600 r of conventional "deep therapy" radiation (200 kv with filtering out of soft component) will produce erythema. Now if we fractionate dosage and give 200 r daily, about 1500–2000 r may be given before erythema develops. It is thus apparent that recovery factors are present and so one can figure that when dealing with such amounts, there is 75 to 80 per cent recovery in 24 hours for the purpose of estimating the amount of radiation that may be given on the next day with equivalent skin effect. Thus, theoretically, one might start with 200 r the first day, give 150 r the next and 128 r the following and so on to a considerable dosage without more effect than from the original 200 r. This, of course, is not the case because there are residual cumulative effects leading to irreversible changes. Thus, even when dosage is fractionated, those of us who deal with radiation therapy have great concern for total accumulated dosage and possible late effects. Accordingly radiologists inquire into and procure records of any previous treatment as a routine practice. The upshot of the matter is that (1) since there are recovery factors, dosage concentrated in a short time is apt to prove more harmful than the same dosage spread over a long time; (2) on the other hand, since there are decided limits to recovery factors, even small dosage cannot be piled up indefinitely with impunity. It might be noted that in the matter of recovery complex factors are involved, and that functional restitution to normal may be less a matter of repair of actually damaged cells than of

* See 17.4.1.

undamaged cells assuming a greater share of the burden. Most tissues have a wide margin of safety in this regard. What may well be irreparable, however, are even slight changes in the chromatic pattern, since these involve the integrity of the genes and the behavior of chromosomes. Such changes tend to result in abnormal or even nonviable daughter cells and the hereditary pattern may persist. Hence the severe effects on all tissues in which there must be a constant renewal of cellular elements.

14.12 Permissible Dosage: Introductory Remarks

The general knowledge that exposure to ionizing radiation is harmful needs of course to be supplemented by quantitative data. The insidious nature of many harmful effects, the long time lag and the uncertainty as to the dosages involved have made it difficult to decide on permissible limits. In the occasional exposures usually involved in clinical work it was an early practice to establish limits on the basis of so many milliampere seconds of exposure, in order to avoid erythema or epilation. This method was of little avail for occupational exposure and efforts were soon made to effect more precise control.

14.13 Development of Exposure Standards

In 1902 a limit was suggested, based on plate fogging probably amounting to the very heavy dose of 10 r. Not much heed was paid to this suggestion. Efforts were made in 1914 to standardize x-ray and radiation protection without avail; and much harm, that should have been avoided, victimized x-ray workers in World War I. There were many instances of skin damage and it is also probable that more serious effects resulted. In 1920–1922 the American and British Roentgen societies proposed safety standards chiefly involving protective materials. Mutscheller in 1925 suggested permissible dosage figures based on 0.01 erythema dose per month which has been calculated to represent about 150 mr per day. In 1928, the r unit was established and an international congress recommended a limit of 0.2 per day. Failla in 1932 favored a limit equivalent to 0.001 of an erythema dose from radium as a monthly limit. This would correspond to about 60 mr/d. In 1931 the Bureau of Standards Advisory Committee on x-ray and radium protection recommended a 200 mr/day limit which in 1936 was reduced to 100 mr/d. On the European continent the 200 mr standard was then retained. The standard limit is now 0.3 r per week subject however to restrictions which in effect reduce it to about 0.1 r per week. (See 14.18)

14.14 Margin of Safety

We can thus see that although there is much minor variation, the figures fall within the same general order of magnitude and it is probable that we are somewhat near a proper figure with the present level. However, it was originally thought that we had a safety factor of about 25-fold, whereas it is probably not even twofold. Some experimental animals have shown notable and considerable damage at much less than a 25-fold increase in exposure level and also an increased death rate with corresponding reduction in life span from gradually accumulated dosage of over 1000 r. Again, female mice have shown an increased incidence of ovarian tumor when exposed to moderate amounts of radiation. On the other hand, it does not appear that the therapeutic use of radium and x-ray for metropathic hemorrhages at the menopause has determined an increased incidence of ovarian malignancies. Better clarification of the matter will probably come in time. Nevertheless, in view of these findings and also in view of possible genetic effects, we should consider sterilization of women by radiation as a permanent measure only. Temporary sterilization should not be attempted and so-called stimulating doses to the ovaries would appear open to question. Finally, there are genetic considerations which suggest that the permissible limits for cumulative dosage should be quite low. This is taken up later.

14.15 Hematologic Considerations

It has been recognized for years that lowered blood counts resulted from exposure to ionizing radiation and this has been the basis for periodic blood counts on people working where radiation hazards are involved. The leukocyte count is first affected but the red count soon follows, the difference being due not to lesser susceptibility but to the longer persistence of individual red cells in the blood stream. Red cells appear to last about 120 days, as compared to a few days for granulocytes and a matter of hours for lymphocytes.

Statistically, average changes are manifested early, but in the case of individuals early changes are difficult to evaluate because of the considerable variations between individuals and variations in the same individual, even from hour to hour. It is, therefore, well to establish a base line for each individual before work involving consistent exposure to radiation is started or before there has been a chance for significant exposure to accumulate. Several counts are needed for this purpose as well as a well-standardized and careful technic.

14.15.1 *Hematologic Standards.* Various ranges of permissible variations, and various limits calling for interdiction of exposure have been set up. However, these should ordinarily not be regarded as absolute; rather we might well regard them as levels at which serious evaluation of individual circumstances is in order. At present a liberal range of variations within which routine exposure might be considered permissible is about as follows:

```
WBC.............................................. 4000-12,000
RBC.............................................. 3.5-6.5 M
Lymphs........................................... 20-40 per cent
Granulocytes..................................... 55-80 per cent
```

There is some uncertainty as to precise normals and it appears that in addition to individual factors altitude, season and climate exert effects. Again, it is not unusual for lymphocytes in young men to reach 50 per cent. Thus in borderline cases, the absolute number of various cells should also be considered. Usual ranges in presumably normal people are about as follows:

```
Total WBC....................................... 4000-12,000
Granulocytes.................................... 1000-7000
Eosinophils..................................... 50-500
Monocytes....................................... 100-1000
Lymphocytes..................................... 1000-4000
```

	Hb (PER CENT)	RBC (MILLIONS)
Males........................	75-100	4-6
Females......................	70-100	3.75-5.50

14.15.2 *Hematologic Effects.* Typical effects of small dosages over lengthy periods are apt to manifest themselves by lower white counts (statistical), hypersegmentation, abnormal lymphocytes and a shift to the left. Certain abnormalities in lymphocytes can be well shown by supravital staining using the method of Dickie and Hempelmann. This involves a special staining technic by which, in cases exposed to radiation, a striking increase in the number of refractive neutral red bodies in the cytoplasm of circulating lymphocytes can be demonstrated—a change it must be noted that is also produced by toxic chemicals such as Pb. These changes begin to show almost at once and on a basis of exposure of from 0.3 to 0.5 r per month. Thus, very slight exposure will show effects by this staining method. The stain contains Janus green and neutral red and its use involves a difficult and meticulous technic.

Of considerable although remote concern is the relationship between leukemia and exposure to ionizing radiation. It has become evident in recent years that there is an increased incidence of leukemia in personnel consistently exposed to such radiation, although there are no precise figures relating this increase to the amount and derivation of exposure. This effect is probably on the same basis that operates to cause an increased incidence of skin cancer in people much exposed to wind and weather, namely, irritation. As is generally conceded, chronic irritation appears to be a frequent predisposing or precipitating factor in the development of malignancies and since ionizing radiation is fundamentally an injurious irritant as regards effects on primitive blood cells, it is not unreasonable to expect the increased incidence of leukemia. At all events, it is notable that physicians in general show a slightly increased incidence of leukemia attributable to radiation and that radiologists in particular show a mortality rate from leukemia about 9 times that of physicians in general, as well as a higher incidence of cancer.

However, in any individual case of leukemia it is usually impossible to say that ionizing radiation is responsible. One can only point out that there is an increase in statistical possibility, that without such exposure the patient might not have developed the disease so soon or possibly not at all. It would be an extremely small factor since the general incidence of the disease in exposed personnel is still very small. Nevertheless, although this places the matter in a twilight zone from a medicolegal aspect, it points up a fundamental lesson in radiologic safety and that is: regardless of being within "permissible limits," *always seek to minimize exposure.*

Not much stress has been placed on coagulation factors as an index of exposure, but there is some evidence to show that an increase in the prothrombin time results from radiation.

14.15.3 *Dosimetry Implications.* Concluding this consideration of hematologic effects, we can note that, in general, the blood furnishes a sensitive means of detecting exposure, but with the drawbacks that (1) supravital staining involves marked technical difficulties, and detects lesser amounts than we are much concerned about, and that (2) variations in the blood picture of a given individual are often difficult of evaluation and may not show a sufficient change until later than we might desire. Nevertheless, blood studies permit a ready index to prevent serious overexposure and to call for withdrawal from exposure to radiation hazards of individuals with blood abnormalities which might be aggravated by radiation or perhaps falsely blamed on radiation. Blood counts should supplement physical and photographic dosimetry as part of preemployment and periodical physical examinations.

14.16 Developmental and Genetic Effects

These are of serious and far reaching importance subject to much public discussion. They constitute a main feature of the 1956 report by the National Academy of Science on "The Biological Effects of Radiation".

Developmental defects and genetic damage are interrelated since genetic effects produce developmental changes. However, not all developmental defects are of genetic origin. The report mentioned above gives 4–5 per cent as the percentage of serious congenital diseases and malformations, and attributes perhaps 2 per cent to genetic causes. These are impressive figures, and it is essential to good judgment to remember that only part of the estimated 2 per cent of genetic defects can be laid at the door of radioactivity such as background radiation and, in this century, clinical and other radiation exposure.

14.16.1 *Developmental Effects*. These are well known and documented for dosages ranging into several hundred or more r units. Miscarriages, still births, early deaths, microcephalic idiocy, retarded mental and physical growth and various aberrations are on record. The work of the Drs. Russell at Oak Ridge on mice shows that for 200 r dosage at 250 kv, there are three main phases, dependant on the stage of gestation in which radiation is received: (1) In the earliest stage, that of *preimplantation*, radiation causes a high prenatal mortality but virtually no abnormalities in survivors; (2) The next phase, that of *organogenesis and limb bud formation* responds by a high neonatal death rate and many abnormalities at term; (3) Late stages show low levels of radiation effects.

Quantitatively as little as 50 r produced identifiable abnormalities and 25 r some changes.

The work of Dr. Hicks at Harvard University (Deaconess Hospital) indicates a special vulnerability of the primitive differentiating nerve cells. Irradiation with dosages of 100–400 r at various stages of gestation was performed and demonstrated that after an initial stage of no damage in surviving progeny, anencephaly and severe head defects developed from radiation on the 9th day. From thence on, effects ranged through a wide variety of damage to the central nervous system and other structures in decreasing measure until the neonatal period when cerebellar defects and occasional instances of stunted growth were noted.

Relating this to the human species, the most vulnerable stage extends from the second to the 6th or 7th week. Thus it includes a period of a week or more in which the possibility of pregnancy is present though not clinically manifest. Hence, the advice that pelvic irradiation should be avoided in the last two weeks of the menstrual cycle if the possibility of conception exists. Naturally, the same interdiction holds for the whole first trimester and to a decreasing extent throughout the period of gestation. Nevertheless, as will be shown later, urgent pelvic radiography need not involve more than minor dosage and there is no call for apprehension, let alone panic, if such becomes essential. Likewise, if radiographic pelvimetry is advisable, the dosages involved are not major, normally occur near term and in many thousands of cases, have entailed no developmental harm.

The more serious human exposures during pregnancy have resulted from therapy or from nuclear weapons. A review of clinical literature by the Russells emphasizes the time elements. The records show that all of 11 cases irradiated in the first and second months showed harm, 7 out of 11 exposed in the 3–5-month stage and 5 out of 13 exposed after the 6th month.

Japanese experience has been extensively studied and an ABCC report of 1953 indicated that in 11 survivors of serious prenatal exposure, there were 7 cases of microcephaly, 2 mongoloid idiots and 2 apparently normal infants. Yamazaki and the Wrights, reporting 30 cases of prenatal exposure, listed 7 fetal deaths and 6 neonatal and infant deaths. Of the survivors, one died of dysentery at age 2, four showed mental and physical retardation, and all showed significantly smaller growth and head circumference. Dosages in these cases were such that the mothers showed one or more major signs of radiation sickness, such as epilation, purpura and petechiae, and oropharyngeal lesions and so probably approximated 300 or more r.

As a final note on the subject, let us nor forget in our preoccupation with radiation that it is not the only demon in the picture of developmental damage and, in the ordinary course of events, far from the principal one. The evil effects of German measles in early pregnancy are well known. Again, some as yet unrecognized factors operating in early months cause mongolian idiocy. Serious virus infections of various types are subject to concern. Toxic materials of many types are detrimental and agents such as nitrogen mustard, triethylenemelamine, and aminopterin are well-known for detrimental effects in experimental animals. Cortisone and related hormones can cause defects; vitamin deficiencies likewise. Many interesting studies are under way on this important subject.

14.16.2 *Genetic Effects.* Recognition of the importance of harmful genetic effects from radiation is almost universal but evaluations are widely discrepant and final answers appear quite a way off. Nevertheless, present knowledge provides a firm basis for caution and conservatism; also, for skepticism regarding extravagant alarms.

A whole host of hereditary defects, anomalies and diseases are known involving complex modes of transmission related principally to defective genes which have undergone mutation. Genes are units of large molecular weight aligned in loci in the chromosomes in such manner as to form matching pairs, one from each parent. These govern the hereditary patterns of development. They almost always reproduce themselves precisely but are subject to spontaneous and induced changes known as mutations which are reflected eventually in altered characteristics of the progeny in succeeding generations. They are mostly harmful, rarely beneficial, often minor and in largest part recessive; that is, the mutant genes when not matched by ones similarly affected from the other parent produce little or no obvious effect. Exceptions occur in what are called *dominant mutations*, some of which are lethal, causing embryonic or neonatal death. Matching of recessives appears to follow statistical probabilities and so, hereditary defects from this cause are related to the large pool of detrimental recessive mutations carried along in the germ plasm of the human race. New mutations need not show in the first generation or any fixed one, but are virtually sure to do so eventually unless the individual dies without issue, or his line dies out before appearance.

Quantitative data are of particular concern and unfortunately, estimates of spontaneous mutation rates and of increments from radiation vary widely due to variables and lack of precise data. Thus, (a) susceptibility to mutations is not constant. Radiation induced lethals are strikingly dependent on the stage of oogenesis at which the radiation is received. Spermatogonia are more sensitive than their descendant cells. In general, cells are most vulnerable in the prophase of mitosis. (b) Genes differ widely in susceptibility. (c) Species differences exist. (d) Not all mutations can be recognized, and diseases and malformation of genetic origin cannot always be differentiated from those due to other detrimental effects. Due to such factors estimates vary roughly between 10^{-5} to 10^{-7} mutations per gene per generation with the number of genes variously estimated between 10,000 and 100,000. Quantitative estimates for the human race are largely extrapolations from studies involving specific unit characteristics in experimental animals and so truly call for the proverbial grain of salt.

Ionizing radiations operate by increasing gene mutations and in large doses causing various chromosome aberrations. It has thus become a convenient though possibly dubious expedient to assess damage in terms of the amount of radiation required to double the natural rate. Variations in such estimates have ranged from a few r to several hundred settling down lately to between 5 and 150 r with probability in the 30–80 r zone. N. A. S. consultants assigned the problem of estimating the number of mutations in 100 million children of parents who had received 10 r of gonadal exposure, produced figures clustering around 5 million—a 5 % figure. Uncertainty was estimated as a 10× factor.

Despite such inprecision it is obvious that substantial genetic harm results and moreover genetic radiation effects appear highly cumulative. Wherefore, and with good cause, there has developed more and more conservatism toward gonadal exposure, both in the interest of public health and prevention of individual tragedy, an attitude moreover fostered by radiological authorities and the A. M. A. There is, however, an obverse side to this situation in that direful predictions or rather conjectures featuring the worst and far transcending probability, conduce to unnecessary fears of sensible clinical radiology and extravagant antagonism to weapon testing and even power reactors. Let us remember that despite the harmful nature apparently characterizing most mutations and the increments to their number from the ceaseless background radiations, that upward evolution has taken place eventuating in more and more complex and higher forms of life when it would seem from quantitative data now at hand, that despite nature's weeding out processes, the odds should be overwhelmingly in favor of progressive degeneration. The complete story is far from being in, and, in the midst of caution, let's not be too hasty in envisioning the doom of the human race from modern use of clinical radiation, nuclear warfare, and reactor accidents.

At all events, genetic hazards provide the major limiting factor in maximum permissible exposures and these levels will be considered in **14.18**.

14.17 Other Considerations

There still remain a few long-range deleterious effects to consider. Of these one of the most important and widely discussed is the matter of carcinogenesis.

14.17.1 *Malignant Disease.* Skin cancer has already been mentioned as resulting from the chronic effects of overdosage; also leukemia in connection with the Japanese bombings and in radiologists. It is now suspected that a general increase in leukemia, noted in vital statistics, of from 42 cases per million in 1490 to 68 in 1954 may derive largely from radiation. Thymic irradiation in infancy has been found associated with an increased incidence of leukemia in a follow-up of 1400 children for 15 years: seven verified and one unverified cases developed whereas the normal incidence would be 0.6 for this number. Again, extensive therapy to the spine in cases of ankylosing (Marie-Strumpell) spondylitis has resulted in a 5–10 × increase in this disease for that group. Elaborate calculations based on all available data by Dr. E. B. Lewis of California Institute of Technology bespeak an increased incidence of from 0.7–6 × 10^{-6} per rad per year. The same author, considering the problem of Sr^{90} fallout effects, calculates that a constantly maintained concentration of 0.1 μc should result in 500–1000 additional cases of leukemia per year, an increase of 5–10 per cent. Now, a mathematical web can be thrown about any problem but does not necessarily connote accuracy and the validity of such figures remains uncertain. However there can be no doubt that a definite effect is indicated, and that the finger of caution undoubtedly points to conservatism and care. On the other hand individual probability of malignancy remains low and some increase in such hazards is definitely to be preferred to jeopardizing our national freedom and security; or on the scale of the individual, accepting unnecessary suffering and disability.

Another feature of irradiation in infancy relates to a subsequent increase in the incidence of thyroid carcinoma in cases where the thyroid was presumably included in the areas treated. However, it does not appear that treatment of hyperthyroidism by I[131] has occasioned an increased incidence of thyroid carcinoma.

Finally, as is well known, long-lived radioactive isotopes with affinity for the bones, are prone to cause bone malignancies and blood dyscrasias.

All this may seem discouraging at first glance but quantitative factors indicate that serious effects relate to serious cases where therapy enters the picture; and even here the risks are usually minor as compared to gains or may constitute the alternative to death or incapacitating disability. However, there can be no doubt either that the need for care, good judgment, and intelligent conservatism is again pointed up.

14.17.2 *Longevity.* The adverse effects of radiation in heavy dosage naturally reduce longevity averages in exposed groups due to incidence of leukemia, malignancies, and blood dyscrasia. However there appears to be some reduction in life-span aside from these and possibly relates to acceleration of the aging process. Interest, as always, centers on quantitative factors, and these are still far from adequate. The N.A.S. report cites a loss of about 5 years affecting radiologists but the statistical basis appears faulty and in any event satisfactory data on dosage are lacking.

Some light is afforded by experimental work although quantitative extrapolation to the human species is still uncertain. Studies on mice by J. W. Gowen of Iowa State College reveal significant effects from nuclear detonation radiation heavily filtered to increase neutron proportion. Little effect was manifest under 75 rep; then increasing dosages brought increasing mortality from acute effects and a reduced life span for survivors. Thus the 270 r exposure left 34 per cent survivors with a life span of 415 days compared to 652 for controls. For 100 kv X-ray in single doses, effects were minor below 160 r, the difference in results from nuclear radiation in rep being related to the greater effectiveness of neutrons. At 640 r there was a 27 per cent reduction in life span. Work at Oak Ridge on burros also reveals great reductions in longevity from large dosage and formulae expressing results have been worked up by various investigators. However, there is still a long way to go and for practical purposes the outcome is that we have still another reason for careful judgment but that serious concern relates largely to fairly high levels which are avoidable save in special therapeutic cases, accidents, and nuclear warfare.

It is interesting to note that from a genetic standpoint the work on mice resulted in reduced fertility but no abnormalities in the first generation.

14.17.3 *Dental Effects.* Harmful effects are well known from heavy therapeutic radiation for oral malignancies and are discussed in Chapter 23. They have not been a feature of dental radiography but fears have been expressed that devitalization and subsequent loss of teeth might result from too many "routine full mouth" examinations. Rather loosely used figures can lend color to this fear. If we estimate on the basis of the NAS figure of 5 r skin dosage per film we find that a conventional set of 14 views would entail a total of 70 r. Such a figure is subject to variation dependent on filtration and other technical features and, of course, additional occlusal or other films would entail an increase. In fact, newspaper accounts mentioned 250–300 r per set. These figures, however, are quite misleading in that no single tooth or skin area receives the total amount because the dozen or more exposures are spread about both sides as well as the anterior aspects of both upper and lower jaw. Only the teeth in the direct sharply coned beam receive a substantial part of the full skin dose of a given exposure. For other teeth dosage will diminish greatly. The studies of Baily at Buffalo, N. Y. gives dosages as follows for adults: center maxilla 8.5 r; center mandible 17 r; posterior maxilla 8.1 r; posterior mandible 11 r, (routine full mouth exam. with 14 films).

There is thus ample leeway for necessary work. At the same time all the general considerations of radiation effects counsel against extravagant resort to radiography in dentistry as well as all fields of work.

14.18 Standards

In order to avoid harm, maximum permissible exposure limits (M.P.E.) have long been in effect and have also been steadily reduced in view of better appreciation of hazards. The 0.3 r/week level has been in effect for some time and is still retained but with restrictions on the periods it may be accepted. The result is that over a period of several years the M.P.E. drops to 0.1 r/wk. As was mentioned in this chapter in the last edition 0.3 r/wk. permits of unduly large totals and this outcome is not surprising.

At present the N.A.S. report recommends that the general population should not average more than 10 r of gonadal exposure beyond natural background level by the age of 30; also that individuals should receive no more than 50 r by that age with an additional 50 r limitation for the next decade. These levels appear to represent prevailing scientific opinion and are largely followed by our N.B.S. in present revision of safety standards.

14.18.1 *Handbook 59 (Permissible Dose, etc.) Revision.* Preliminary version permits of 5 r/year with provision for temporary increases. The general formula is:

MPE for any given age $(N) = 5(N - 18)$ rems provided that no annual increment exceeds 15 rems. The various other provisos permit the following: 1 week 0.3 rem; 13 weeks 3.0 rem (more than 0.3 r/wk. may be received provided that the total for 13 weeks does not exceed 3.0 rem); 1 year 5 rem; age 30, 50 rem (but not over 15 rem in any given year); age 40, 100 r; age 50, 150 r and so on up to 250 rem limit for age 70. An emergency dose of 25 r once in a lifetime is not considered to affect tolerance status; medical exposures likewise. These MPE levels are for all critical organs except the skin for which the value is double.

Gonadal exposure for the entire population is limited to 14 million rems per million people for the period from conception to age 30, plus one-third that amount for each decade thereafter, averaging to be done for the population group in which cross breeding may be expected.

Such limits can be met readily for occupational exposure provided there is not gross negligence, indifference or ignorance. However, increments from clinical radiology have come into question not only from radiation therapy which involves special problems and evaluations, but from diagnostic procedures. Thus a discussion of this matter is essential.

14.18.2 *Dosages from Clinical Radiology.* The N.A.S. report estimates average gonadal dosage for the general population by age 30 as follows: Background 4.3 r, medical 3.0 r, nuclear tests 0.02–0.5 r; total 7.32–7.8 r with an increase to about 8.5–9 r at high altitudes from increased cosmic radiation. This is well within the 14 rems limit established by the N.B.S. but nevertheless the N.A.S. committee found the 3 r estimate for medical procedures disturbing. Now such a figure is subject to many uncertainties and enormous individual variations, and it appears of greater value to review figures from recent studies of actual exposures.

Radiologists have long been alert to hazards as numerous studies attest and of which a few are of special interest. One by Ritter, Warren and Pendergrass of the University of Pennsylvania in 1952 is very comprehensive and another by Stafford and Vance in England is devoted to gonadal dosage as is a third by Billings et al. published in 1957.

The table given below is derived from these studies and shows some sharp differences dependent on technics. It is notable in this regard that the addition of 3 mm. Al filtration reduces skin dosage to about a fourth; 2 mm. Al to about a third. High voltage technics also reduce exposure and wherever practicable are advisable. They do not however always produce satisfactory results notably in chest and extremity work.

Sharp coning and the use of drapes serve to reduce gonadal dosage to a marked extent in much work.

In general it must be recognized that the figures presented here are likely to vary considerably from those derived from other installations. Nevertheless they furnish useful approximations. Fluoroscopy in particular is apt to show gross variations dependent not only on physical factors but the working habits and skills of the fluoroscopist; also eye accommodation to the low levels of fluoroscopic illumination.

The studies of the Billings' group also includes statistical analyses of much interest. These tend to indicate probability of average gonadal ex-

TABLE OF RADIOGRAPHIC DOSAGES SELECTED FROM VARIOUS SOURCES

DOSAGE TO SKIN IN ROENTGENS

SOURCE OF DATA	Skull, pa.	Chest, pa.	Lat. dorsal spine	Abdomen	Lat. lumbar spine	Pelvis, ap.	Pelvimetry lat.	NOTES
Ritter group (low kv; 1Al filt.)	4.1r	0.06r (24mas)	4.0r	1.0–1.3r	13.5r (450mas)	5.3r (420mas)	26.7r (780mas)	Fluoroscopy 17.7r/min (1.5Al) mas = milliamp. sec.
Billings group (low kv; 3Al filt.)	Not given	0.015 (13mas)	Not given	0.46	1.8r (200mas)	0.5r (100mas)	Not given	*
Billings group (120 kv; 3Al filt.)	Not given	0.003 (0.7mas)	Not given	0.21	1.5r (70mas)	0.35r (16mas)	2.05r (100mas)	

* Fig. for lat. lumbo-sacral area.

DOSAGE TO GONADS IN MILLIROENTGENS

SOURCE OF DATA	Skull, pa.		Chest, pa.		Lat. dorsal		Abdomen		Lat. lumbar		Pelvis		Pelvimetry lat.	NOTES
	Male	Fem.	Male	Fem.	Male	Fem.	Male	Fem.	Male	Fem.	Male	Fem.		
Ritter group (low kv; 1Al filt.)	Not given		Not given		Not given		Not given		Not given		Not given	600mr	3500mr	
Stafford & Vance (factors not given)	0.2mr	0.05	0.36mr	0.07	13mr	2.1	69mr	200	7mr	16mr	1100mr	210	840mr	800 for lat. lumbo-sacral
Billings group (low kv; 3Al filt.)	0	0	0	0	Not given		0	155mr	0	480 upper 80 lower	500mr	200	Not given	
Billings group (120 kv; 3Al filt.)	0	0	0	0	Not given		0	75mr	0	500 upper 100 lower	350mr	155	600mr*	See footnote

* Fig. for exposure to ovary in lat. lumbo-sacral.

posures of 0.73 r for males and 1.1 r for females by age 30 from radiography (fluoroscopy not included).

As regards the chest, recent figures from W. Ed. Chamberlain of Temple University show 0.25 mr. gonadal dosage for conventional 14 x 17 films, 5 mr. for fluorographs by usual techniques and 1.5 mr. with the new mirror lens equipment.

The above table indicates zero dosage for the Billings study due evidently to coning, barriers or drapes.

In general the figures furnish neither basis for alarm nor excuse for laxity. Clinical radiography and fluoroscopy appear reasonably safe if in competent hands. This includes pelvimetry also, although this should be reserved for special cases as is now the customary practice.

There is little justification in accepting any substantial risk to mother or unborn child to avoid a few r of exposure late in pregnancy. Nor are a few abdominal exposures early in pregnancy to be seriously feared though they should be deferred, if the situation permits, at least to the second trimester.

14.18.3 *Qualifications of People Using X-Ray.* The matter of competent supervision deserves earnest consideration: Only a small proportion of x-ray units are in the hands of trained radiologists. In 1953 a Public Health report listed 4100 radiologists, radiologic residents, and physicians who devoted most of their time to radiology as compared to 31,000 general practitioners and other specialists owning their equipment, 67,000 dentists, and 11,000 osteopaths and chiropractors. The amount of work done by qualified radiologists is certain to be well out of proportion to their numbers but nevertheless the situation involves obvious liabilities since it is not to be expected that many out of these latter groups will be well versed in radiological hazards and safety requirements. In addition there are thousands of shoe-fitting fluoroscopes operated by shoe clerks! There are also numerous anti-theft and antisabotage units. Shoe-fitting fluoroscopy appears to be diminishing and subject to ever widening disapproval so that we can hope that before long this useless hazard will be a thing of the past. In regard to radiography by people with sketchy and rudimentary training, if any, continuous and well-publicized educational activities are needed and it is gratifying to note that the AMA for a long while has included articles and editorials bearing on the subject.

14.18.4 *Safety Measures in Clinical Radiology.* In regard to clinical radiography let us keep in mind a few salient points: (1) Careful conservative judgment in requesting x-ray studies; (2) inquiry, requests for records, and borrowing of films to reduce the number of repeats in chronic cases prone to change doctors, clinics and hospitals, either by choice or necessity; (3) regard for possible pregnancy in certain examinations, also genetic effects;

(4) in x-ray departments: Optimal technical factors, precise work, well selected views and care to obviate technical failures necessitating more exposures; (5) in fluoroscopy, regard for all physical factors and periodic review of working habits and practices with a view to economy of exposure; also avoidance of fluoroscopy for diagnosis of orthopedic conditions. This is very seldom advisable or adequate. Orthopedic fluoroscopy in reduction of fractures is, of course, in a different category but involves decided hazards. Therapy involves special problems and also many situations which justify serious risks. It should be remembered, in addition, that in nonmalignant cases, much good can often be accomplished by very modest doses, sharply limited to the areas concerned and of negligible remote concern.

14.18.5 *X-Ray Therapy in Sterility.* Of particular interest is x-ray therapy to remedy sterility. This has often been successful and the resultant offspring healthy. Thus it has usually been deemed innocuous by clinicians. However, it involves radiation to the ovaries, probably 25 rads or more, and certitude of some genetic mutations. Thus geneticists view the procedure with grave misgiving. Since the total for any individual is likely to remain below 50 rads it would seem that an absolute ban cannot be called for. Nevertheless the procedure should not be lightly adopted; it should be a last resort.

14.18.6 *Miscellaneous Notes.* Rheumatoid spondylitis has already been mentioned. Here too the risk of leukemia does not appear of such magnitude as to interdict radiation therapy for this highly disabling disease. At the same time, economy in dosage and special concern for repeated courses are surely in order.

Thymic irradiation except for malignancies is now largely a thing of the past. Thyroid exposure, when therapy to the ears or eustachian areas becomes advisable, should be largely preventable by shielding.

14.18.7 *Universal Dosimetry and Records.* The establishment of M.P.E.'s for gonadal exposure of entire populations entails the obvious conclusion that we should known what dosage each and everyone has received. We can approximate this by a history of exposures and use of tables, but obviously accuracy leaves much to be desired. It is now recommended in the N.A.S. report that we resort to universal personnel dosimetry. This sounds very plausible but would involve great expense and bother along with difficulties anent effective cooperation; and in return for all this effort the gains would be minor. It is not favored by the A.C.R.

A glance at the figures will indicate that the great bulk of clinical work produces very low gonadal dosage. A minority of chronic cases, and still fewer cases where therapy is called for are the only ones seriously concerned; and here special factors enter the picture. Thus it does not appear warranted to foist such a nuisance as universal dosimetry would prove, on a whole population. Moreover accuracy would still be questionable. The gonadal dosages given above often entailed special techniques not feasible under ordinary working conditions. Accordingly more pilot and exploratory studies appear advisable before we plunge into universal dosimetry.

Certain chronic and special cases call for record keeping of some sort and, of course, careful and elaborate records are already routinely kept in therapy cases. It would not be difficult for cases subject to the need for repeated radiography and fluoroscopy of the abdomen and pelvis to be provided with a brief record of exposures. This would be appropriate for those to whom genetic considerations apply and especially those who travel about or are prone to change doctors. However, the practical value of this, too, becomes minor where it is the policy to be conservative in ordering work and to look over past records and films, inquiring and borrowing as needed. In serious cases the work must be done anyway.

14.18.8 *Calculated Risk* (*Emergency Exposures*). The advent of the new and startling applications of nuclear energy brings in its wake increased possibilities that many people may be subjected to exposures in excess of those we are accustomed to regard as permissible.

Heavy exposure may be inescapable as in an atomic bomb burst or may involve rescue, escape or command decisions in the event of operations in a contaminated area. Until recently our main concerns in the matter of radiological safety have been related to the cumulative effects of small amounts of radiation in occupations where some degree of constant exposure is involved, and to the larger but more occasional exposures of patients in clinical radiology. To these we now find we must add concern for:

1. Immediate effects of an atomic bomb air burst.
2. Persistent effects from an atomic bomb due to contamination by fission products or resulting from induced radiation. This is likely to be important only when there is a subsurface or surface burst.
3. Exposures involved by purposeful contamination by radiological warfare agents. The use of these is conjectural and practical considerations would seem to make such employment dubious. Yet, under some circumstances, possible employment has to be reckoned with.
4. Exposures incidental to operation of nuclear reactors, more especially when and if accidents occur.

These newer categories of radiological hazards relate to single or occasional exposures over limited periods of time and may involve stern and inescapable necessities. Thus, the permissible limit of 0.3 r per week, devised to take care of customary working risks over long periods, has only limited application to this type of problem. The situation is more or less the same as in the case of radiation therapy where different standards apply and we consider first of all practical therapeutic necessities. In this perspective we must balance radiation hazards against the importance of objectives to be gained, and also consider the effectiveness of the personnel concerned.

Precise answers to the quantitative factors are lacking but we find some leads in the therapeutic use of general body radiation. Varying amounts have been given such as from 10–20 r daily to 50 r several times weekly up to totals of from several hundred to 500 r. These dosages have produced relatively mild symptoms. Those cases receiving 50 r three times weekly were noted as suffering from nausea, anorexia, and headache.

As we proceed to apply this type of knowledge to calculated risk probabilities, it is, of course, an inevitable and practical necessity that some general recommendations be made in terms of r units. However, it is important to recognize that in addition to considering the number of r units received, it is important to appraise each individual situation from the standpoint of the nature of the radiation and its energy, i.e., its kv or mev equivalence and rate of emission. We also have to think in terms of personnel who may be called on for the utmost of physical and mental exertion rather than in terms of patients who in general are recipients of great care and attention or of personnel free to rest and recuperate. Aside from these more or less tangible features, when groups of individuals are concerned, morale factors cannot be safely neglected. Finally, it must be remembered that there are great differences in individual susceptibility; also that at the time of exposure, individual circumstances, such as partial shielding, the orientation of the body as regards the incident rays, and possible use of protective devices or garments, may make a very great difference.

Thus the exposure levels mentioned in the forthcoming discussion should not be regarded as sharp dividing lines applying in all circumstances, but as outlining convenient zones which lack definite borders. These are subject to modification, as noted above, and moreover often involve considerable deductive analysis rather than any considerable body of directly applicable data. In other words, there is not a little extrapolation involved and when it comes to the practical handling of a situation involving radiation hazards, accurate information, alertness, knowledge, and good sense become all the more essential and cannot be replaced by any table.

With this in mind, it can be said that current thought on calculated risk levels runs about as follows:

A. 25 r and below: It is generally anticipated that no symptoms or detectable clinical findings are likely to develop, and that there would be no impairment of efficiency. However, it appears that some patients have voiced minor complaints after such dosage.

B. 50 r level: No particular trouble is anticipated here either. However, as related above, patients receiving this dosage thrice weekly had definite complaints and it should be anticipated that there are likely to be some instances of nausea, anorexia and malaise.

C. 100 r level: It appears expected that most people should be able to take this dosage pretty well in stride. Nevertheless, depending on circumstances and individual variation, it seems reasonable to anticipate that not a few individuals would experience some nausea and perhaps vomiting and that for several days after such an exposure a number of individuals might show lassitude and increased fatigability.

D. 200 r level, this is definitely in the zone of serious radiation illness, when the radiation is of high energy and received in a short or so-called "acute" exposure. Most people so exposed would show nausea, vomiting, and fatigue within a few hours, become definitely ineffective and constitute casualties.

E. Higher levels: Illness becomes more and more severe and fatalities increase as dosage goes beyond 200 r until, beyond the level of 600 r, recovery would be rare. It is also to be borne in mind that substantial doses of general body radiation are likely to render those affected more susceptible to fatigue, exposure and infection, and may gravely influence for the worse the outcome of burns and other injuries.

F. Repeated exposures: Missions involving exposure up to 25 r or thereabouts could probably be repeated a number of times at approximately weekly intervals without notable falling-off in efficiency. Just where a halt must be called to such repetition would depend on various factors, but in general it would appear that an accumulated total of about 200 r, received in comparatively large increments over a period of a few months should not be exceeded without the most compelling necessity. In any event, close medical surveillance and critical judgment should be applied to each individual case.

Table 11.57 of the "Effects of Nuclear Weapons gives much the same picture with details summarized below:

0–50   r:No obvious effects

80–120 r: Nausea and vomiting 1 day in 5–10%; fatigue.

130–170 r: 25% develop radiation sickness.

180–220 r: 50% radiation sickness

270–330 r: Nearly all sick; 20% mortality, convalescence 3 months.

400–500 r: LD_{50} within 1 month; convalescence of survivors 6 months.

550–750 r: Up to 100% mortality

1000 r   : Nausea and vomiting within 1–2 hours. Probably no sur-
             vivors.
5000 r   : Almost immediate incapacitation. Fatal within 1 week.

In general, the circumstances and background of calculated risk types of exposure should always be carefully scrutinized and careful planning and sincere effort should be used to minimize it and, when possible, avoid it. Shielding and protective garments should be given earnest consideration.

Compensating time out should be provided as early as possible and considering that concentration of dosage increases damage this time might well be increased beyond that calculated from the 0.3 r/wk standard.

14.19 Concluding Remarks

Dosage and risk factors now involve all creation in as much as there is some degree of man-made increase to natural background radiation. It is obviously very slight at present but possibilities of significant increase are unfortunately not lacking if worst comes to worst. The hazards of fallout and induced radiation have already been considered but it is of interest to note that the main dangers in nuclear warfare and reactor accidents are still related to external exposure—certainly the shorter range hazards. This is not to say that the internal hazards are negligible or that over the period of generations we can dismiss genetic concerns.

Evaluations have already been presented but it appears appropriate to note here that the tragedies of the radium dial painters and the fatuous optimism manifest in the unjudicious prescription of radium for various illnesses early in the century, show very dramatically the need for caution and vigilance, and the ease with which enthusiasm runs away with discretion. On the other hand fears, too, can be overemphasized and inflated. Let us remember that clinical radiology has played a substantial role in alleviating suffering and promoting the longevity we are now justly proud of. Sober reflection indicates that we have a goodly amount of leeway for well-controlled and conducted work in that field. Our main problem is to avoid profitless exposures resulting from uncritical judgment, general laxity, sales appeal as in shoe-fitting fluoroscopy, and technics or procedures productive of needlessly high dosage. Radiological procedures involving human exposure should be in the hands of those adequately qualified and it is hoped that the present clamor will help close the door, still far too wide open, to the utilization of radiological procedures by those lacking such qualification.

Economy of exposure to radiation needs to be the "Order of the Day" but let it be wise economy. Without thought, care and good judgment we may well find ourselves avoiding the penalties of *"too much"* by incurring the perils of *"too little"*.

REFERENCES

Amer. Coll. of Radiology: Comment on Report of the National Academy of Science on "The Biological Effects of Atomic Radiation", Summary of Reports and also Report to the Nation. Official Bulletin, Chicago 6, Ill. 20 N. Walker Drive. 1957.*

BAILY, NORMAN A.: Patient exposure to ionizing radiation in dental radiography. *Radiology, 69:* 42–45, 1957.

BEHRENS, C. F.: Fluoroscopic hazards. *Naval Med. Bull., 44:* 233–240, 1945.

BILLINGS, NORMAN AND GREENFIELD: Gonad dose during routine roentgenography. *Radiology, 69:* 37–41, 1957.

BLAIR, H. A.: A Formulation of the Relation between Radiation Dose and Shortening of Life Span. Proceedings of the International Conference on the Peaceful Uses of Atomic Energy, Geneva 1955. Vol. 11: Biological Effects of Radiation: 118–120. United Nations, N. Y., 1956. U. S. Sales Agent: International Document Service, Columbia Univ. Press, 2960 Broadway, New York 27, N. Y.

BROWN, P.: *American Martyrs to Science Through the Roentgen Ray.* Springfield, Ill.: C. C. Thomas, 1936.

BROWN, W. M., AND ABBOTT, J. D.: Incidence of leukemia in ankylosing spondylitis treated with x-rays. Preliminary report. *Lancet, 1:* 1283–1285; Abs. in Year Book of Radiol. pp. 395–396, 1956–1957.

BUGHER, J. C.: Biological effects of radiation. Peaceful Uses of Atomic Energy. Vol. 11, pp. 45–48. (Complete ref. under Blair, H. A.)

CARTER, T. C.: The genetic problem of irradiated human populations. Peaceful Uses, etc. Vol. 11, pp. 184–186. (Complete ref. under Blair, H. A.)

CLARK, D. E.: The association of irradiation with cancer of the thryoid in children and adolescents. Peaceful Uses, etc. Vol. 11, pp. 146–148 (Complete reference under Blair, H. A.).

CROW, J. F.: Genetic considerations in establishing maximum radiation doses. *Radiology, 69:* 18–29, 1957.

DUBLIN, L. I., AND SPIEGELMAN, F.: Mortality of medical specialists, 1938–1942. *J.A.M.A., 137:* 1519–1542, 1948.

DUNLAP, C. E.: Delayed effects of ionizing radiation. *Radiology, 69:* 12–17, 1957.

ELLINGER, F.: *Medical Radiation Biology.* Springfield, Ill.: C. C. Thomas, 1957.

FAILLA, G.: Considerations bearing on permissible accumulated radiation doses for occupational exposure. The aging process and cancerogenesis. *Radiology, 69:* 23–29, 1957.

GLASSER, O., AND CONRAD, W.: *Roentgen and the Early History of the Roentgen Rays.* Springfield, Ill.: C. C. Thomas, 1934.

GOWEN, J. W.: Effects of whole body exposure to nuclear or x-ray energy on life span and life efficiency. Peaceful Uses, etc. Vol. 11, pp. 105–109 (Complete reference under Blair, H. A.).

HARNEY, R. A.: *Effects of Radiations on Finger Nail Ridges.* Atomic Energy Commission, MDDC 218, 1946.

---

* Brochure on Medical and Dental Use of X-Ray with Control of Radiation Hazard issued in 1958 by the College, to all physicians.

HENSHAW, P. S.: Genetic transition as a determinant of physiologic and radiologic aging and other conditions. *Radiology, 69:* 30–36, 1957.

HICKS, S. P.: The effects of ionizing radiation, certain hormones, and radiomimetic drugs on the developing nervous system. *J. Cell. & Comp. Physiol., 43:* Suppl. 1, 151–178, 1954.

LEA, D. E.: *Actions of Radiation on Living Cells* (2nd ed.). Cambridge Univ. Press, 1955.

LEWIS, E. B.: Leukemia and ionizing radiation. *Science, 125 ℣* 3255: 965–972, 1957.

LOONEY, W. B. AND COLODZIN, M.: Late follow-up studies after internal deposition of radioactive materials. *J.A.M.A., 160:* 1–3, 1956.

MACHT, S. H. AND LAWRENCE, P. S.: Congenital malformations from exposure to roentgen radiation. *Am. J. Roentgenol. 73:* 442–466, 1955.

MARTIN, J. H.: Radiation doses to gonads in diagnostic radiology and their relations to long term hazard. *M. J. Australia 2:* 8–6–810, 1955; Abs. in: *Yr. Book of Radiol.* pp. 20–22, 1956–1957.

MARTLAND, H. S.: Occupational poisoning in manufacture of luminous watch dials; General Review of Hazard Caused by Ingestion of Luminous Paint, with Especial Reference to the New Jersey Cases. *J.A.M.A., 92:* 446–552, 1929.

MEWISSEN, D. J. ET AL.: A formula for chronic radiation dosage vs. shortening of life span: Application to a large mammal. *Radiation Res., 6:* 450–459, 1957.

MOELLER, TERRELL, AND INGRAHAM: Radiation exposure in the United States. *Pub. Health Rep. 68:* 57–65, 1953.

MULLER, H. J.: How radiation changes the genetic constitution. Peaceful Uses, etc. Vol. 11, pp. 387–399 (Complete reference under Blair, H. A.)

NATIONAL ACADEMY OF SCIENCE, N. R.C.: The Biological Effects of Radiation, Summary Reports; also, A Report to the Public. N.A.S. Publications Office, 2101 Constitution Ave., Washington, D. C.

NATIONAL BUREAU OF STANDARDS, U. S. DEPT. OF COMMERCE: Permissible Dose from External Sources of Ionizing Radiation. Handbook 59. Government Printing Office, Washington 25, D. C.

NEWELL, R. R.: Genetic Injuries. Editorial in *Radiology, 69:* 111–114. July 1957.

PERKINS, J. E.: Importance of chest x-rays in total radiation exposure. *Tuberculosis Abstracts, Nat. T.B. Assoc., XXX;*, Jan. 1, 1957.

RITTER, WARREN, AND PENDERGRASS: Roentgen doses during diagnostic procedures. *Radiology, 59:* 238–251, 1952; Abs. in *Yr. Book of Radiol.,* pp. 9–11, 1953–1954.

RITVO, D'ANGION AND RHODES: Radiation hazards to non-radiologists participating in x-ray examinations. *J.A.M.A., 160:* 4–10, 1956.

RUSSELL, L. B. AND W. L.: Hazards to the embryo and fetus from ionizing radiation. Peaceful Uses, etc. Vol. 11, pp. 175–178 (Complete reference under Blair, H. A.).

RUSSELL, L. B. AND W. L.: Pathways of radiation effects in the mother and embryo. *Cold Spring Harbor Symposia on Quantitative Biology,* Vol. XIS, 1954.

RUSSELL, L. B. AND W. L.: An analysis of the changing radiation response of the developing mouse embryo. Symposium on effects of radiation and other deleterious agents on embryonic development. *J. Cell. & Comp. Physiol., 43:* Suppl. 1, 103–149, 1954.

RUSSELL, L. B. AND W. L.: The Sensitivity of Different Stages in Oogenesis to Radiation Induction of Dominant Lethals and Other Changes in the Mouse. Proceedings of the 4th Internat. Conf. Rad., Cambridge, England, pp. 187–192. Ed. by MITCHELL, HOLMES, AND SMITH. London: Oliver & Boyd, 1956.

RUSSELL, W. L.: Comparison of x-ray induced mutation rates in drosophila and mice. *The American Naturalist* XC ℣80. Jan.–Feb, 1956.

STANFORD, R. W. AND VANCE, J.: Quantity of radiation received by reproductive organs of patients during routine diagnostic x-ray examinations. *Brit. J. Radiol.* *28:* 266–273, 1955; Abs. in *Yr. Book of Radiol.*, pp. 21–23, 1955–1956.

TAYLOR, L. S.: Current situation with regard to permissible exposure levels. *Radiology, 69:* 6–11. July 1, 1957.

TSUZUKI, M.: Late effects of radiation injury. Peaceful Uses, etc. pp. 130–131 (Complete reference under Blair, H. A.).

U. N. SCIENTIFIC COMMITTEE ON EFFECTS OF ATOMIC RADIATION: Responsibilities of the medical profession in use of x-ray and other ionizing radiation. *Radiology Res. 6:* 517–519, 1957.

WAGNER, R. P. AND MITCHELL, H. K.: *Genetics and Metabolism.* New York: Wiley; London: Chapman & Hall, Ltd., 1955.

YAMAZAKI, J. L. AND WRIGHT, S. W. AND P. M.: A study of the outcome of pregnancy in women exposed to the atomic bomb blast in Nagasaki. Symposium on effects of radiation and other deleterious agents on embryonic development. *J. Cell. & Comp. Physiol. 43:* Suppl. 1, 319–328, 1954.

15▸

Radiation Protection

O. SCHNEIDER, M.D.

Revised by Charles F. Behrens, M.D.*

---

15. Radiation Protection poses manifold problems in many fields, many of them of universal concern as is well elucidated in this book. This chapter is accordingly devoted to basic technical aspects. Many details pertinent to the general subject will also be found in Chapter 14 on Permissible Dosage etc., Chapter 6 on detection and measurement and Chapter 21 on laboratory operation. Numerous N.B.S. handbooks with a wealth of detailed data are available from the Government Printing Office and are listed in references. The new "Effects of Nuclear Weapons" also contains much helpful information.

15.1 Terminology and Quantitative Notes

It is desirable to commence by recalling that the Roentgen or r unit is based on ionization, the rep and rad on energy absorption, the rem on biological equivalence and the curie on disintegrations per second. (See **6.8** for definitions.)

Ionization produces ion pairs formed by electrons and positively charged atomic particles, 1 r causing 1 esu of charge per cc air. Since the electron charge is 4.8×10^{-10} esu this means the formation of 2.083×10^9 ion pairs per cc air.

Since an average of 32.5 electron volts (ev) of energy is required to produce one ion pair, $32.5 \times 2.08 \times 10^9 = 6.77 \times 10^{10}$ electron volts is the amount of energy absorbed by 1 cc of air from 1 r.

The ev is an energy unit equivalent to 1.6×10^{-12} ergs. Accordingly,

---

* Changes relate largely to new values and deletion of some overlapping material.

one gram of air with a density of 0.001293 absorbs from one r of x- or gamma-radiation:

$$\frac{6.77 \times 10^{10} \times 1.6 \times 10^{-12}}{.001293} = 83.8 \text{ ergs*}$$

The roentgen is thus equivalent to:

1 esu of ion pairs per cc air
2.083 $\times$ 10^9 ion pairs per cc air
1.6 $\times$ 10^{12} ion pairs per gram of air
6.77 $\times$ 10^4 mev (million electron volts) per cc of air
5.24 $\times$ 10^7 mev per gram of air
87   ergs absorbed per gram of air

15.1.2 *Rep* (roentgen equivalent physical) and Rad. The rep is defined as "that amount of any ionizing radiation from which tissue will absorb energy equivalent to 87 ergs per gram of air. Actually tissue will absorb approximately 93 ergs per gram per incident roentgen. The rep is then equivalent to:

$$\frac{93}{87} \times 5.24 \times 10^7 \text{ mev} = 5.61 \times 10^7 \text{ mev per gram soft tissue}$$

The rep is widely used for comparing the effects of different types of radiation. However, a new unit, the *rad*, has been adopted with a value of 100 ergs/gram. It is convenient to work with, and for practicable purposes of radiological safety the difference between the rad and rep is negligible.

15.1.3 *Rem* (roentgen equivalent man or mammal). One rem is the estimated amount of energy absorbed in tissue which is biologically equivalent in man to 1 r of gamma- or X-rays.

15.1.4 RBE (Relative Biological Effectiveness). These units still do not provide a sufficient basis for complete evaluation since the biological effectiveness of the various radiations varies widely from equivalence in reps or rads. Over short ranges the heavy alpha particles and protons produce disproportionate effects by reason of dense ionization. Neutrons, too, show disparate effects. Thus the term *Relative Biological Effectiveness, RBE,* is utilized widely and is very useful. Once again, however, this too falls short of precision because there are great variations in different tissues and with different energies. Thus the main value of RBE figures, is to serve as a convenient means of estimating potential hazards with a large margin of safety. In this regard it is well to recall that the value of 10 for fast neutron

---

* Varies with different qualities of x or γ rays. Present average value 87 ergs/ gram/r. (Ed.)

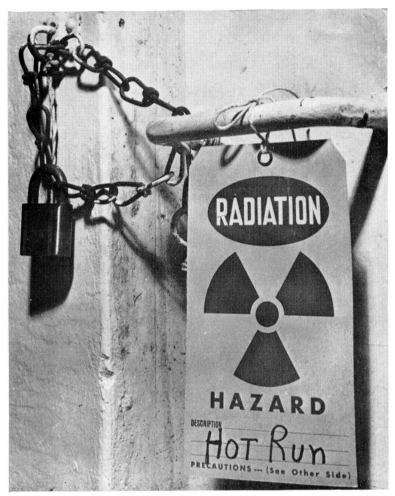

Fig. 1. Warning tag. Radiation symbol is magenta against a yellow background (Oak Ridge, Tenn.).

TABLE I

Radio-Biological Effectiveness of Radiations

TYPE OF RADIATION	RBE
X- or gamma (γ)	1
Beta (β)	1
Proton (p)	10
Alpha (α)	10
Fast neutron (n_f)	10
Slow neutron (n_s)	~ 5

TABLE I(a)

Specific Ionization as Related to RBE and LET*

AVERAGE SPECIFIC IONIZATION (IN ION PRS. PER μ WATER)	RBE (γ, X-RAY, ELECTRONS AND POSITRONS ASSIGNED VALUE OF 1)	LET (KEV PER μ WATER)
100 or less	1	3.5 or less
100–200	1–2	3.5–7
200–650	2–5	7.0–23
650–1500	5–10	23–53
1500–5000	10–20	53–175

* From Handbook 59, N.B.S.

RBE relates to slight cataract formation. The RBE for radiation sickness and possible lethal effects from fast neutrons is about 1.7.

15.1.5 *Specific Ionization and* LET. Somewhat more accurate approximations may be made when *specific ionization* is known. This is the relative ionization capacity in terms of the number of ion pairs produced per micron of water. It is related to the *linear transfer of energy* also which however is usually given as Kev of energy produced per micron of water. (See Table I (a).) However, most practical work deals in terms of r units, rads, rems, reps, and curies.

15.2 Electromagnetic Radiation

The electromagnetic spectrum includes, in the order of decreasing wavelength, the radiations shown in Table II.

The radiations are propagated in the form of quanta of energy, or photons. The energy of a photon is dependent upon the wave-length and the frequency of vibration of the ray as shown in the following relation:

$$E = h\nu = \frac{hc}{\lambda} \tag{15.1}$$

Where E is the energy of the photon, h is Planck's constant (6.62×10^{-27}

TABLE II*

Electromagnetic Radiations

RADIATION	WAVE RADIATIONS
Electric waves	∞–3×10^6 cm
Radio waves	$3 \times 10^6 - 0.3$
Infra-red	$0.3 - 7.6 \times 10^{-5}$
Visible light	$7.6 \times 10^{-5} - 4 \times 10^{-5}$
Ultra-violet	$4 \times 10^{-5} - 10^{-8}$
X-rays	$10^{-6} - 10^{-12}$
Gamma rays (γ)	$10^{-8} - 10^{-11}$

* From Lapp and Andrews, Nuclear Radiation Physics, Second Edition.

erg-seconds), ν is the frequency in vibrations, or cycles, per second, c is the speed of light (3×10^{10} cm/sec) and λ is the wave-length in cm.

EXAMPLE 15.1

What is the wave-length of an 80-megacycle radio wave?

$$\lambda = \frac{c}{\nu} = \frac{3 \times 10^{10} \text{ cm per sec}}{80 \times 10^{6} \text{ per sec}}$$

$$= 375 \text{ cm} = 3.75 \text{ meters}$$

EXAMPLE 15.2

What is the photon energy of a gamma-ray with a wave-length of 10^{-10} cm (.01 A)?

$$E = h\nu = \frac{hc}{\lambda} = \frac{6.6 \times 10^{-27} \text{ erg-sec} \times 3 \times 10^{10} \text{ cm/sec}}{10^{-10} \text{ cm}} =$$

$$2 \times 10^{-6} \text{ ergs} = 1.2 \text{ mev}$$

Gamma rays are produced by energy changes in the nucleus of an atom, usually following the emission of a β-particle, while x-rays are produced by energy changes in the inner electron shells of an atom usually as a result of bombardment by electrons.

15.3 Radioactivity

15.3.1 *Radioactive Decay.* An atom of an unstable element may undergo a spontaneous process of disintegration during which it emits a charged particle from the nucleus and becomes transformed into the isotope of an entirely different element. The charged particle emitted is either an alpha particle (helium nucleus) or a beta particle (usually an electron, occasionally a positron). Usually a radioactive transformation is followed closely by the emission from the new nucleus of one or more gamma ray photons. These processes may be illustrated by the following nuclear equations:

$$\alpha \text{ decay of } Rn^{222}: {}_{86}Ra^{222} \rightarrow {}_{84}Po^{218} + {}_{2}He_{4}$$

$$\beta^{-} \text{ decay of } Na^{24}: {}_{11}Na^{24} \rightarrow {}_{12}Mg^{24} + {}_{-1}e^{0} + \gamma$$

$$\beta^{+} \text{ decay of } Na^{22}: {}_{11}Na^{22} \rightarrow {}_{10}Ne^{22} + {}_{1}e^{0} + \gamma$$

Sometimes radioactive decay takes place by a process known as K-capture, wherein the nucleus captures one of its satellite K-electrons, with a loss of one positive nuclear charge, and the emission of one or more gamma photons. Occasionally an unstable nucleus has the choice of decaying by either K-capture or positron emission, as in the case of Cobalt-58:

$$\beta^+ \text{ em: } {}_{27}\text{Co}^{58} \rightarrow {}_{26}\text{Fe}^{58} + {}_{1}e^0 + \gamma \text{ (14.5\%)}$$

$$\text{K-cap: } {}_{27}\text{Co}^{58} + {}_{-1}e^0 \rightarrow {}_{26}\text{Fe}^{58} + \gamma \text{ (85.5\%)}$$

A great variety of radioactive decay schemes is possible and each takes place in accordance with statistical laws whereby, if a sufficiently large number of atoms are present, a certain proportion of them will decay in a given period of time. Decay takes place in accordance with the equation

$$N = N_0 e^{-\lambda t} \tag{15.2}$$

Where N is the number of radioactive atoms present at the end of any time interval t, N_0 is the number originally present (when $t = 0$). e is the base of natural logarithms, and λ is the number of atoms decaying in unit time.

By substituting $\dfrac{N_0}{2}$ for N, $T_{\frac{1}{2}}$(the time for $\frac{1}{2}$ of the atoms originally present to decay) for t and solving for $T_{\frac{1}{2}}$ we find that

$$T_{\frac{1}{2}} = \frac{0.693}{\lambda} \tag{15.3}$$

Where 0.693 is the natural logarithm of 2. By means of this formula, if we know the half-life, $T_{\frac{1}{2}}$, of an element, we can easily find the decay constant, λ.

15.3.2 The *specific activity* of a radioactive isotope is the number of radioactive disintegrations which it undergoes per gram in unit time, ordinarily taken as one second (9).

EXAMPLE 15.3

What is the specific activity of pure Na^{24} (half life 15 hours)?
The number of atoms per gram of Na^{24}, is Avogadro's number (6×10^{23}, approx.) divided by 24. Thus we have:

$$N_g = \frac{6 \times 10^{23}}{24} = 2.5 \times 10^{22}$$

$$\text{Sp. activity} = \lambda N_g = \frac{.69 N_g}{T_{\frac{1}{2}}}$$

$$= \frac{.69 \times 2.5 \times 10^{22}}{15 \times 3600}$$

$$= 3.2 \times 10^{17} \text{ disintegrations per sec per gm.}$$

This amounts to $\dfrac{3.2 \times 10^{17}}{3.7 \times 10^{10}} = 8.7 \times 10^6$ curies per gram!

It is hardly necessary to point out that the shorter the half-life, the greater the specific activity. The activity of any radio-isotope may be calculated by the method illustrated above, or by the following simplified formula.

$$\frac{\text{gms}}{\text{curie}} = 7.66 \times 10^{-9} A T_r \tag{15.4}$$

where A is the atomic weight and T_r is the radioactive half-life in days.

By referring to a chart or to a table of isotopes one sees that most of the radioactive nuclides are artificially produced. Of the relatively few naturally radioactive isotopes, the majority are at the heavy end of the periodic table, and are members of the four radioactive series. Several of the lighter elements have naturally radioactive isotopes. The most important of these biologically is potassium-40, which is accountable for much of the background radioactivity of the body. The exposure to the human body from this source will be calculated in a later example. Ages ago, when the earth was much younger, many more naturally radioactive isotopes must have existed. But those which had short half-lives disappeared unless they were members of a decay chain so that their abundance was maintained in spite of their rapid decay.

15.3.2.1. RADIOACTIVE EQUILIBRIUM. When a parent element decays into a series, the relative quantities of parents and daughters eventually reach an equilibrium so that the number of atoms of parent isotope to that of the daughter is in ratio with their half-lives. Thus

$$\frac{N_1}{N_2} = \frac{T_1}{T_2} \tag{15.5}$$

Where N_1 is the number of atoms present of parent element, N_2 the number of atoms present of any succeeding member of the chain, and T_1 and T_2 are their respective half-lives. For example, we find that, in 238 grams of natural uranium with an abundance of U^{238} of .993 there are:

$$\frac{226 \times 1620 \times .993}{4.51 \times 10^9} = 8.05 \times 10^{-5} \text{ gm Ra}^{226}$$

Conversely, if one is able to determine the number of atoms of parent and of daughter elements, the half-life of one can be calculated if the half-life of the other is known.

The decay rates of radio-isotopes of reasonably short life may be measured directly by plotting the activity of a sample for a sufficiently long period of time as in the case of a sample of P^{32} shown in Fig. 2.

15.4 Absorption of Radiation

15.4.1 *Alpha particles.* Alpha particles emitted by radioactive decay have ranges in air up to about 10 cm before they are completely stopped. In tissue, these ranges are of the order of about 0.005 mm. or 50 microns. For this reason, these particles cannot penetrate the epidermis, and are not an external hazard. But when an alpha-emitting element becomes lodged in the body, the heavy ionization which these particles produce can be very injurious locally. Further, it happens that some of the alpha emitters are bone-seekers, a few even becoming lodged in the trabeculae adjacent to the bone marrow, to which tissue the alpha particles can do serious damage.

Alpha particles can be accelerated by high-voltage apparatus to energies of 25 to 100 mev or more in which case a beam of such particles could penetrate the skin and produce local damage thereto, and even to the underlying tissues.

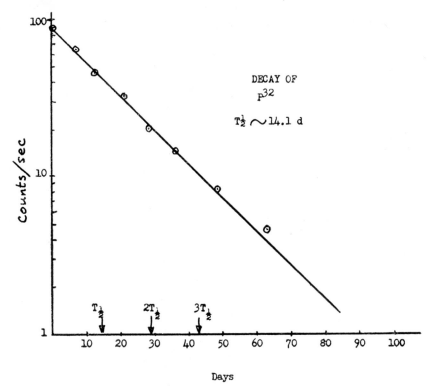

FIG. 2. Decay of P[32]

TABLE III*
Energy (E) of alpha particles in mev with corresponding Ranges (R) in cm of air

E	R	E	R	E	R
0.2	0.17	2.5	1.35	11.0	12.40
0.4	0.27	3.0	1.70	12.0	14.18
0.6	0.38	3.5	2.08	13.0	16.24
0.8	0.47	4.5	2.97	14.0	18.35
1.0	0.57	5.0	3.48	15.0	21.17
1.2	0.66	6.0	4.52	20.0	32.5
1.4	0.74	7.0	5.90	30.0	71.0
1.6	0.84	8.0	7.35	40.0	115.7
1.8	0.94	9.0	8.89	50.0	154†
2.0	1.05	10.0	10.55	100.0	494†

* From Pollard and Davidson, *Applied Nuclear Physics*, John Wiley & Sons, New York, 1946.
† Estimated.

TABLE IV*
Relative Stopping Powers as Compared to Air

ABSORBER	MICA	Al	Cu	Ag	Au
Mg/cm² = 1 cm air.................	1.4	1.62	2.26	2.86	3.96

* From R. E. Lapp and H. L. Andrews, *Nuclear Radiation Physics*, Prentice-Hall, Inc., New York, 1954.

It is sometimes desired to find the range in tissue of an alpha particle. This is difficult if not impossible to do exactly. But a practical approximation may be made by first finding the range in air, which is related to the energy of the alpha particle as shown in Table III.

The air equivalents of a few common absorbers are given in Table IV.

The range in air having been found by referring to Table III, the range in tissue may be determined by the following rough formula:

$$\text{Range in Air} \times \text{Density of Air} = \text{Range in Tissue} \times \text{Density of Tissue}$$

The density of tissue being about 1.0, the range in tissue is:

$$R_{\text{tissue}} \simeq 0.00129 \times R_{\text{air}} \qquad (15.6)$$
$$(\text{cm}) \qquad\qquad (\text{cm})$$

15.4.2 *Beta particles*, both negative electrons and positrons, are given off in a continuous energy spectrum ending with a characteristic maximum energy level, $E_{\max}$. Since the total energy released by each β-emission must be equal to $E_{\max}$, the energy difference between any other β particle, say E_i, and $E_{\max}$ was postulated by Pauli as being carried off from the nucleus by a different sort of particle, the neutrino. The emission of a neutrino, then, accompanies each beta transformation wherein the electron is of lesser energy than $E_{\max}$. The neutrino is a particle of no electric charge, and little if any mass, but having kinetic energy. If β^- particles are formed in the nucleus when a neutron decays to a proton, the reaction may be shown as follows:

$$_0n^1 \rightarrow {}_1p^1 + {}_{-1}e^0 + \nu$$

where ν is the neutrino. When a proton becomes a neutron with the emission of a positron the reaction is as follows:

$$_1p^1 \rightarrow {}_0n^1 + {}_1e^0 + \nu$$

The neutrino is of no inherent biological significance, since it is not absorbed.

Since beta particles are so much lighter than alpha particles, they are far more easily deflected. Therefore their ranges in air cannot be determined with any accuracy. But their ranges in solid absorbers such as metallic foils can be reliably measured. These ranges, usually given in terms of mg/cm^2 of aluminum, provide the maximum beta energy, which varies with different isotopes. From the maximum energy, one can determine the biologically significant energy, which is the average energy, E_{av}, using the approximate relation (13):

$$E_{av} \simeq \tfrac{1}{3}E_{\max} \qquad (15.7)$$

Values for $E_{\max}$ may be found in isotope charts and tables, but the methods of determining $E_{\max}$ are of interest to all workers with radioactive isotopes. Lack of space precludes a discussion of these methods, and the reader is referred to standard texts for the necessary explanation. For convenience, however, the following equations given by Glendenin and Coryell showing the relation between $E_{\max}$ and range of beta particles, are included:

$$E_{\max} = 1.85\, R_{\max} + 0.245 \qquad \text{for } R_{\max} > 0.3 \text{ gm/cm}^2 \quad (15.8)$$

$$R_{\max} = 0.542\, E_{\max} - 0.133 \qquad \text{for } E_{\max} > 0.8 \text{ mev} \qquad (15.9)$$

$$E_{\max} = 1.92\, R_{\max}{}^{0.725} \qquad \text{for } R_{\max} < 0.3 \text{ gm/cm}^2 \quad (15.10)$$

$$R_{\max} = 0.407\, E^{1.38} \qquad \text{for } E_{\max} < 0.8 \text{ mev} \qquad (15.11)$$

$R_{\max}$ is characteristic for a given β-emitter and can be used in its identification, as well as to compute the value of $E_{\max}$, the maximum beta energy. $R_{\max}$ may also be found in isotope tables, or determined experimentally.

Because β particles are so much lighter than alpha particles, and are therefore so much more easily scattered, and because they carry only one-half as much charge, they produce far less ionization per centimeter of path. Consequently they are not as injurious when emitted by isotopes taken into the body as are alpha particles. Their greater range in air and other materials, including skin and underlying tissues, makes the β-emitters external hazards when the body or a portion of it happens to be near enough to a sufficiently intense β source.

15.4.3 γ- *and x-rays.* As shown above, alpha and beta particles have limiting ranges for penetration of matter—given a sufficiently thick wall of material, all of them will be absorbed eventually. The same is not true in the case of electro-magnetic radiation which, theoretically, is never completely absorbed, no matter what the thickness or density of the material may be. Schematic absorption curves for alpha, beta, and gamma radiation are shown in Fig. 3. The ranges of alpha particles fall off abruptly until all are absorbed. Those of beta particles fall off gradually, but also to a

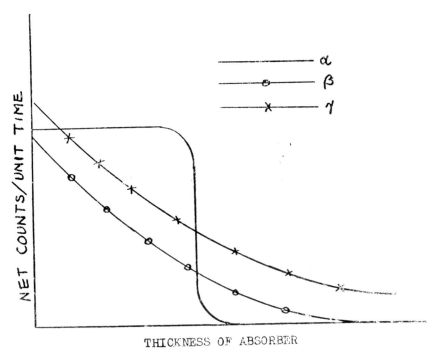

FIG. 3. Schematic absorption curves for α, β, and γ radiations

point of complete absorption. A small number of gamma photons, however, will escape absorption, no matter what the thickness of the absorber.

The absorption of gamma- and x-rays follows the exponential law

$$I = I_0 e^{-\mu x} \qquad (15.12)$$

where I is the intensity of the beam at a distance x in the absorber, I_0 the intensity at the point where the beam enters the absorber, μ the *linear absorption coefficient* of the absorber, and e the base of natural logarithms. By dividing the *linear absorption coefficient* μ by the density of the absorbing material, ρ, the result will be the *mass absorption coefficient* μ_m which is usually expressed in cm²/gm. The familiar unit gm/cm² is then the reciprocal of the mass absorption coefficient and is related to the linear absorption coefficient as follows:

$$\text{gm/cm}^2 = \frac{\rho}{\mu} \qquad (15.13)$$

A value for the *half-thickness*, $x_{\frac{1}{2}}$, or the thickness of absorber which will reduce the initial intensity by one-half, may be determined from Eq. (15.12) by setting $I/I_0 = \frac{1}{2}$ and solving:

$$x_{\frac{1}{2}} = \frac{0.693}{\mu} = \frac{0.693}{\mu_m \rho} \qquad (15.14)$$

Similarly the *tenth-value layer* or thickness of absorber which will reduce the initial beam intensity by a factor of 10 is

$$x_{1/10} = \frac{2.3}{\mu} = \frac{2.3}{\mu_m \rho} \qquad (15.15)$$

The relation between the half-thickness and the tenth-value layer may then be shown by simple proportion:

$$\frac{x_{\frac{1}{2}}}{x_{1/10}} = \frac{.69}{2.3} \qquad (15.16)$$

Units. In calculations involving equations (15.12) to (15.16) inclusive the following units are ordinarily used

I and I_0 = roentgens/hr or fractions and multiples thereof.

ρ = grams/cm³

μ = cm⁻¹ (decrease of intensity *per cm* thickness of absorber)

μ_m = cm²/gm

x = cm

The absorption of gamma- and x-radiation in matter takes place by the methods described in Ch. 5, viz., the photoelectric effect, Compton scattering, and pair production. The photon energies preferentially absorbed by these processes are about as follows

less than 0.1 mev: photoelectric effect

0.08—1.2 mev: Compton scattering

1.02 mev and over: Pair production predominates above 50 mev.

In tissue the absorption by pair production is not appreciable except in the case of photon energies of from 5–10 mev (12) and upwards;

For each of the three methods of absorption, however, there is a different absorption coefficient. Also the coefficient for each process will vary with the atomic composition of the absorber. As a result, it becomes necessary to take into account the energy of the gamma photon when making absorption calculations. Table V gives the linear absorption coefficients as well as half-value thicknesses for photons of different energies and for various absorbing materials. Tenth value layers may be found by applying the relation shown in Eq. (15.16).

It happens that in spite of these complexities, for energies of from 0.5 to 2 mev, the gamma ray absorption coefficient for soft tissue changes but little and may be taken as 0.07. If the radiation consists of photons of radically differing mono-energetic components, the total dose must be computed as the sum of the doses from all of the components. If there is no great difference in the energies of gamma components and if each is over

TABLE V*

Linear Absorption Coefficients (μ) for γ Rays (or X-Ray)

PHOTON ENERGY Mev	MATERIALS				
	Air	Water	Concrete	Iron	Lead
0.5	1.11×10^{-4}	0.097	0.22	0.66	1.7
1.0	0.81×10^{-4}	0.071	0.15	0.47	0.80
2.0	0.57×10^{-4}	0.049	0.11	0.33	0.52
3.0	0.46×10^{-4}	0.040	0.088	0.28	0.47
4.0	0.41×10^{-4}	0.034	0.078	0.26	0.47
5.0	0.35×10^{-4}	0.030	0.071	0.25	0.50
10.0	0.26×10^{-4}	0.022	0.060	0.23	0.61

* From Effects of Nuclear Weapons

0.1 mev, the absorption coefficients may be averaged, and the composite result will not be too greatly in error.*

The decay scheme will provide information needed to compute the energy absorption for the gamma radiation from each isotope. The differences caused by isomeric transition and internal conversion must be taken into account when indicated. In the latter case the gamma photon is consumed by its ejection of an electron from the K-shell, and lower energy x-rays result as the vacancy is filled and moves outward.

The fraction of the total number of gamma rays, whether from a source within the body or external to it, which is absorbed by the tissues as distinguished from the fraction which escape from the body, or pass through it, is a difficult point to decide. A rough procedure in the case of external radiation is to calculate the reduction in intensity which occurs when the radiation passes through the thickness of soft tissue involved, and neglect the rest.

EXAMPLE 15.4

If a narrow beam of 1 mev gamma rays of 1 r per hour intensity is incident upon the ventral surface of the body (thickness 30 cm), what portion will escape from the dorsal surface? Assume a uniform density through the body and use a μ of 0.07:

$$I_{\text{dorsal}} = I_{\text{ventral}} e^{-\mu x} = 1 \times e^{-0.07(30)} = e^{-2.1}$$
$$= 0.12 \text{ r/hr}$$

Under these assumptions 88% of the incident radiation is absorbed in passing through the body.

For gamma radiations emitted by radioactive substances taken into the body, the formula given below yields the approximate amount of energy per disintegration absorbed by the tissues.

$$E_{\text{eff}}/\text{dis} = E_{\gamma}[1 - e^{-(\mu - \sigma_s)x}] \tag{15.17}$$

* The following values, taken from ORNL-421, Supplement 2, prepared by W. S. Snyder and J. L. Powell, indicate the mass absorption coefficients in tissue for gamma rays of certain energies.

E_{γ} (Mev)	μ_m(cm²/gm)
0.1	.165
0.5	.093
1.0	.068
1.5	.055
2.0	.048
3.0	.038
4.0	.033
5.0	.029

Where E_γ is the photon energy in mev, μ and $\sigma_s{}^*$ the total absorption and Compton scattering coefficients respectively for a given photon in tissue, and x the thickness of the organ in cm. E_{eff}/dis has been calculated for a number of isotopes as shown in Table 1 of Chapt. 12.

phot. E (mev)	0.5	1	2	3	4	5
Pb	0.52	0.32	0.18	0.13	0.10	0.08
Tissue (calculated)	0.06	0.04	0.02	0.01	0.01	0.01

The Compton scattering coefficient σ_s is a function of the energy of the gamma ray quantum and of the number of electrons present in the absorber.

15.4.4 *Neutrons*, having no electrical charge, are incapable of producing ionization directly. Their energy of motion is lost by elastic collision with atomic nuclei. In this manner they are slowed down or "moderated" to thermal energies, of the order of 0.025 electron volts. (See Table VII.) The nuclei with which the neutrons have collided acquire a kinetic energy of their own and become capable of causing dense ionization over a limited range. The element principally involved in this mechanism is hydrogen. Fast neutrons are not easily captured by atomic nuclei, unless resonance capture peaks exist for a particular nucleus. But when the neutrons have been slowed to thermal energies they become easily absorbed by many nuclei, sometimes with the emission of a gamma ray. The new nuclei are often radioactive and also contribute to the ionization of tissue. Finally,

TABLE VI

Densities of Common Materials

SUBSTANCE	GM/CM³
Air	0.00129
Aluminum	2.7
Concrete	2.2
Glass	3.0
Graphite (theoretical)	2.25
Graphite (actual)	1.8
Lucite	1.2
Mica	3.0
Paper	1.0
Paraffin	0.9
Sea Water	1.025
Steel	7.8
Wood	0.7

* Values of $\sigma_s(cm^{-1})$.

TABLE VII*

Slowing a 1 mev Neutron to 0.025 ev

	ELEMENT					
	H	D	He	Be	C	O
At. wt.	1	2	4	9	12	16
Fraction of energy lost per collision	0.63	0.52	0.35	0.18	0.14	0.11
No. of collisions	18	25	42	90	114	150
Capture cross-section (barns) (n_s)	0.32	0.001	~ 0	0.01	0.005	0.002

* Adapted from Glasstone, S. Sourcebook on Atomic Energy.

it is theoretically possible for such few neutrons as escape capture and wander freely in the tissues to undergo radioactive decay (half-life 20 min) giving off a beta particle with a maximum energy of 0.78 mev, and leaving a proton as the daughter product. Both of these particles are capable of causing ionization. The equations representing these nuclear reactions are as follows:

$$\text{Absorption in H: } {}_1\text{H}^1 + {}_0n^1 \to {}_1\text{H}^2 + \gamma$$

$$\text{Absorption in N: } {}_7\text{N}^{14} + {}_0n^1 \to {}_6\text{C}^{14} + {}_1\text{H}^1$$

(In this reaction, the carbon atom recoils from its ejected proton and both particles produce a considerable amount of chemical derangement of organic molecules. In addition the C^{14} nucleus is radioactive.)

$$\text{Absorption in Na: } {}_{11}\text{Na}^{23} + {}_0n^1 \to {}_{11}\text{Na}^{24} + \gamma$$

$$\text{Decay of Neutron: } {}_0n^1 \to {}_1\text{H}^1 + {}_{-1}e^0 + {}_0\eta^0$$

The absorption of gamma rays in tissue results in the production of light charged particles (electrons) while the effect of moderation of neutrons produces heavy charged particles. The absorption of neutrons by atoms in the tissues follows the same general law as the absorption of neutrons in a cyclotron target or in a nuclear reactor:

$$A = \phi N V \sigma t \tag{15.18}$$

where A = no. of new nuclei produced

ϕ = neutron flux in neutrons/cm² per sec

N = target nuclei per cm³

V = volume of target in cm³

σ = neutron capture cross section in barns (1 barn = 10^{-24} cm²)

t = time of exposure of target to neutron flux, in seconds.

The factors N and V may be taken together as NV = no. of target nuclei.

TABLE VIII*

Attenuation of Various Types of Radiations in Air and Tissues

TYPE OF RADIATION	MAX. ENERGY CONSIDERED	RANGE IN AIR	RANGE IN TISSUE	HALF-THICKNESS IN AIR	HALF-THICKNESS IN TISSUE
	mev	*cm*	*cm*	*cm*	*cm*
α	5	3.48	0.0037	—	—
	1	0.57	0.0006	—	—
β	5	1900	2.2	$\sim$310	$\sim$0.4
	1	370	0.42	$\sim$30	$\sim$0.04
n	5	∞	∞	8,700	4.8
	1	∞	∞	6,300	1.7
γ	5	∞	∞	20,000	24
	1	∞	∞	8,500	10

* K. Z. Morgan (In U. S. A. E. C. Pub. TID-388, 1951).

A comparison of the degree of attenuation of various radiations in air and in tissues is provided in Table VIII.

EXAMPLE 15.7

What is the range in tissue of a plutonium-239 α particle?

From the Table of Isotopes Appendix I we find that a Pu^{239} α particle has an energy of 5.14 mev. From Table III we find that the range in air of a particle of this energy is about 3.6 cm. By Eq. 15.5:

$$R_{\text{tissue}} \simeq .00129 \times R_{\text{air}}$$

$$= 1.29 \times 10^{-3} \times 3.6$$

$$= 4.6 \times 10^{-3} \text{ cm} = 46 \text{ microns}$$

EXAMPLE 15.8

If the body were to be uniformly exposed to a flux of 10^{10} slow neutrons per cm^2 for 5 seconds how many deuterium atoms would be produced? Take the body content of H as 7000 gm.

$$A = \phi N V \sigma t = 10^{10} \times 7000 \times 6 \times 10^{23} \times .32 \times 10^{-24} \times 5$$

$$= 6.7 \times 10^{13} \text{ atoms of } H^2$$

EXAMPLE 15.9

If the RBE = 1 for the absorption of the γ ray produced in the (n, γ) H^2 reaction of Example 15.8, and the energy of the ray is 2.2 mev, what is the dosage to the tissues just from this source? (body wt = 7×10^4 gm).

$$\frac{2.2 \times 6.7 \times 10^{13}}{5.9 \times 10^7 \times 7 \times 10^4} = 36 \text{ rep or rem}$$

15.5 Summary of Biological Effects

These are amply presented in Chapter 14 as regards protection and are implicit in the chapters on radiation effects. It is only appropriate to state here that the basic considerations relate not only to keeping dosage below MPE limits but to reduce it as much as practicable without, on the other hand, resorting to a crippling perfectionism which would seriously handicap clinical radiology and jeopardize national security.

15.6 Maximum Permissible Exposures to Radiation

In the selection of criteria to be used in the establishment of a permissible dosage rate of ionizing radiation, considerations have ranged from the metaphysical to the statistical. Comparisons have been made between radiation exposures and the use of whiskey or tobacco, the danger of highway and other accidents, the risks of warfare, exposure to heat and cold, and other influences to which man is subjected during life. Rationalizations of this nature, while not necessarily justifiable, are at the same time not surprising in view of the lack of fundamental and exact knowledge concerning the radiobiological mechanism. The establishment of numerical exposure limits is, however, made on the basis of practical experience, and extrapolations from experimental work on genetics.

On the basis of these effects, and upon other considerations, including metabolism of various isotopes, energies and types of radiations, their absorption in tissue, and their relative biological effectiveness, the maximum permissible dosage rates are established by quasi-authoritative bodies such as the International Commission on Radiological Protection (ICRP) of the International Congress of Radiology, and the Advisory Committee on X-ray and Radium Protection, sponsored by the National Bureau of Standards (USA).

15.6.1 *External Radiation.* Limits have been given in 14.18 and it will only be noted here that although the limit for a single week remains at 0.3 r/wk.; that for general average exposure is 5 r/yr. or about one-third that amount. Individuals, however, are permitted up to 50 r by age 30 years plus 50 r for each decade thereafter. Average gonadal exposure for the entire population is limited to 14 r by the age 30 years plus one-third that amount for each decade thereafter.

For purposes of dosage computation the accepted figures are

8 hours per day

40 hours per week

50 weeks per year

70 years duration of "lifetime" for non-occupational exposure.

TABLE IX
Background Radiation and Non-Occupational Exposures

SOURCE	AMOUNT OF RATE
Cosmic rays, sea level	~0.1 mr/d
Cosmic rays, 15,000 ft alt	0.5 mr/d
Cosmic rays, 55,000 ft alt	7.5 mr/d
Cosmic rays, top of atmosphere	70 mr/d
Air, radon (incl. thoron)	~10^{-10} μc/cc
Natural "background"	0.01–0.1 mr/hr
Earth's outer crust:	
Uranium, by weight	6 ppm
Thorium, by weight	12 ppm
Radium, by weight	2 × 10^{-6} ppm
Sea water:	
K^{40}	0.33 μc/m^3
U	0.0015 mg/kg
Drinking water	10^{-16}–10^{-12} curies/cc
Cow's milk	10^{-14} curies/cc
C^{14} (isotopic abund. 1.6 × 10^{-12})	16 d/m per gm carbon
Human body, K^{40}, total	0.23 μc
Human body, C^{14}	0.0068 μc
Wrist watch dial, (~1 μg Ra)	~1 mr/hr, γ, wrist
Airplane instruments (10–100 μg Ra per dial):	
At face of each dial	5–10 mr/hr
At pilot's position	<1 mr/hr
Shoe fitting (20 sec exp)	av 10–15 r to feet
Diagnostic X-ray:*	
14 × 17 chest plate	0.05–0.25 r
Photofluorographic chest	0.7–1.2 r
Extremities	0.25–1.0 r
Skull	1.3 r
Abdomen	1.3 r
GI series	0.65 r/plate
Lumbar spine, lat	5.7 r
Pregnancy, lat	9.0 r
Fluoroscopy	0.28 r/sec
Dental	0.5 r/film
Spectacle lenses containing U	1–8 mr/hr β to eyes
Average background exposure	0.4 mrep/day

* There is apt to be considerable variation depending on filtration, distance and techniques. See par. **14.18.2**

15.6.2 *Exposure to Internal Radiation.* (See chapter 12.) Radioactive substances may gain entrance to the body by inhalation, ingestion or by absorption through the intact or broken skin. The maximum permissible exposure of an organ to radiation absorbed internally is the same as if the radiation were absorbed in the organ from an external source, but the determination of the quantities of various radioisotopes which would produce this much radiation in the organ is a very complex matter, requiring consideration of numerous factors, some of which are:

1. The mode of entry and initial body retention. This in turn depends upon the solubility of the substance in question. Some elements, such as plutonium, are poorly absorbed from the G.I. tract. In the case of soluble substances present as aerosols, it is assumed in the absence of specific information that 25 % of the amount inhaled reaches the lower respiratory tract and is absorbed into the blood stream, while 50 % is retained in the upper respiratory tract and swallowed, so that a portion of the latter amount is also absorbed. If the substance is insoluble, it is assumed that 12 % reaches the lower respiratory tract as the critical organ, while the rest is eliminated by exhalation and swallowing (10).

2. Fraction going from blood stream to critical organ or tissue.

3. Radiosensitivity of critical tissue.

4. Size of critical organ which affects the concentration of isotope in some instances (e.g. iodine in thyroid).

5. Essentialness of critical organ to proper functioning of body. (By "critical organ" is, of course, meant the *determining* organ with respect to maximum permissible levels.) The bone-marrow, liver, kidneys, for example, are more essential to the functioning of the body than the thyroid gland, and therefore the effect on the former vital organs must be considered first.

6. Biological half-life, or rate of elimination of the isotope. This varies considerably. Radium and plutonium are slowly excreted, while sodium is very rapidly eliminated. Ordinarily there is an initial unsteady, rapid rate of elimination. After the element has been transferred to the critical tissue the rate becomes exponential.

7. Radiological half-life. In general, the isotopes with very long half-lives are serious hazards only if they tend to become fixed in the critical organ. Those of very short half-life are less hazardous because they promptly decay to insignificant levels (less than 1 % after 7 half-lives). But those of intermediate half-life, say 5 to 50 years, constitute the greatest hazards.

8. Type and energy of radiation and RBE.

Taking these and other factors into consideration, calculations have been made giving for a number of isotopes of current interest the maximum body content to be permitted, as well as the maximum allowable concentrations in air and water. The values are listed in Table I of Chapter 12.

Emergency levels are as follows:

TABLE X

*Emergency Level for Beta-Gamma Activity in Food and Water**

DURATION OF CONSUMPTION	MICROCURIES PER CC	DISINTEGRATIONS PER MIN. PER CC
10 days	9×10^{-2}	3×10^3
1 month	3×10^{-2}	1×10^3

* From Effects of Nuclear Weapons, Table 12.101

The Subcommittee on Internal Dose further advises that as additional data become available, it may be necessary to revise some of these values. The recommendation is made that, owing to many uncertainties, every precaution should be taken to keep the intake of all radioactive substances down to the minimum consistent with reasonable effort and expense. In the event of exposure of the individual to more than one radioisotope, or to both internal and external radiation, the maximum permissible concentration of each isotope and the exposure to each external source should be weighted so that the total does not exceed limits.

A rough formula for computing the daily dosage rate to a tissue from a quantity of radioisotope which it contains is given by E. E. Anderson (In U.S.A.E.C. pub. TID–388, 1951) as:

$$r_t = 6.1 \times 10^7 \frac{ce}{w} \tag{15.19}$$

Where $r_t = $ rep/day $e = $ (effective) energy of radiation, mev

$c = $ curies $w = $ weight of tissue in grams

Internal dosimetry calculations often involve the use of the following approximations:

$$(\text{MPC})_{\text{air}} = \frac{q}{2 \times 10^7 f_a T_{\text{eff}}} \tag{15.20}$$

$$(\text{MPC})_{\text{water}} = \frac{q}{2.5 \times 10^3 f_w T_{\text{eff}}} \tag{15.21}$$

Where MPC = Maximum permissible concentration
in μc/cc

$q = $ body burden in μc

$f_a = $ fraction absorbed into critical organ from air

$f_w = $ fraction absorbed into critical organ from water (or food)

$T_{\text{eff}} = $ effective half-life in days

The daily consumption of air is 2×10^7 cc. That of water is 2.5×10^3 cc.

EXAMPLE 12.11

What should be the MPC of K⁴⁰ in drinking water?

By referring to Table IX we note that the body contains 0.23 μc of K^{40}. This is

$$0.23 \times 3.7 \times 10^4 \times 8.6 \times 10^4 = 7.3 \times 10^8 \text{ disint./day}$$

The effective energy per disintegration of K^{40} is 0.53 mev. Thus, the exposure of the body (muscles, 3×10^4 gm) to its own K^{40} is

$$\frac{7.3 \times 10^8 \times .53}{5.9 \times 10^7 \times 3 \times 10^4} = 2.2 \times 10^{-4} \text{ rep/day}$$

By proportion, q, the maximum body burden, based on 5 days' exposure per week, is given by

$$\frac{0.23\mu c}{2.2 \times 10^{-4} \text{ rep/day}} = \frac{q\mu c}{0.3/5 \text{ rep/day}}$$

$$q = \frac{0.23 \times .06}{2.2 \times 10^{-4}}$$

$$= 63\mu c$$

The effective half-life in the body of K^{40} is roughly 41 days.

Also for most soluble compounds the fraction absorbed into the critical organ from the GI tract is slightly less than 1.0. To be on the safe side let us use this figure. Then

$$(\text{MPC})_{\text{water}} = \frac{q}{2.5 \times 10^3 f_w T_{\text{eff}}}$$

$$= \frac{63}{2.5 \times 10^3 \times 1 \times 41}$$

$$= 6 \times 10^{-4} \mu c/cc \text{ (ans)}$$

15.6.3 *Emergency Dosage.* This is considered in 14.18. It is worth noting here however that a single exposure of 25 r need not be considered as reducing permissible dosage for a given individual.

15.7 Protection against External Radiation

The reduction of exposure to external radiation may be accomplished by each one or a combination of four rather obvious methods.

1. Decrease the intensity of the radiation field. It is desirable at all times to keep the strength of x-ray beams and the amount of radioactive material to a minimum, but operational needs will always dictate the quantity of radiation against which personnel must be protected.

2. Keep the exposure time as short as possible. This demands careful planning of work and painstaking rehearsal, without the radiation source, of each detail of the operation. It also demands foresight in physical

arrangement of equipment, and assurance that no mechanical failure will delay or disrupt any task. Where high-level sources are involved, it is sometimes necessary to execute a piece of work by sending operators into the radiation field in relays, so that none is excessively exposed.

3. Interpose a shielding material between the source and the operator. The common shielding materials used to absorb gamma radiation include lead, iron, concrete, and earth. For beta radiation light materials such as aluminum, glass and plastics are usually sufficient, but additional thicknesses of these materials or heavier materials are needed to attenuate the bremsstrahlung, which are electromagnetic radiations produced by the beta particle as it approaches the end of its path. Thermal neutrons are absorbed by substances with high capture cross-sections, such as boron, cadmium and bismuth. Fast neutrons must first be moderated to thermal energies and for this purpose the lightest elements are the best. For this reason hydrogen-containing materials, e.g., paraffin and other hydrocarbons, are useful. Beryllium is likewise used as a moderator. Sometimes elements of high cross-section are combined with lighter elements in a solution or mixture which will both moderate and absorb fast neutrons. Boron carbide is an example of a chemical compound which can function in this manner. In this connection it is well to remember that the absorption of neutrons by hydrogen, boron and cadmium results in the emission of gamma rays so that these materials should be backed by gamma-absorbers.

For gamma radiation from a point source there is a widely-employed unit known as the rhm, or roentgen-per-hour-at-one-meter. As the name of the unit suggests, this is the quantity of radioactive material which, unshielded, produces one r per hour of ionization at a distance of one meter (3). Thus if the same quantiy of material were enclosed in a shield such that the radiation intensity at one meter would be 0.1 r per hour then the effective strength of this source would be 0.1 rhm.

The source strength of one gram of radium, unshielded, but in equilibrium with its decay products has been calculated as 0.969 rhm. Measurements made with the radium enclosed in a filter of platinum show the values for one gm of Ra to be as follows:

0.25 mm Pt	0.88 rhm/gm Ra
0.5 mm Pt	0.816–0.847 rhm/gm Ra*
2.5 mm Pt	0.63 rhm/gm Ra
5.0 mm Pt	rh0.64/gm Ra

---

* Radium in equilibrium with its decay products, in a 0.5 mm platinum container will produce a gamma ray field given by

$$r/hr = \frac{8.4 \times mg \text{ of } Ra}{D^2}$$

for all distances greater than 20 times the greatest dimension of the source.

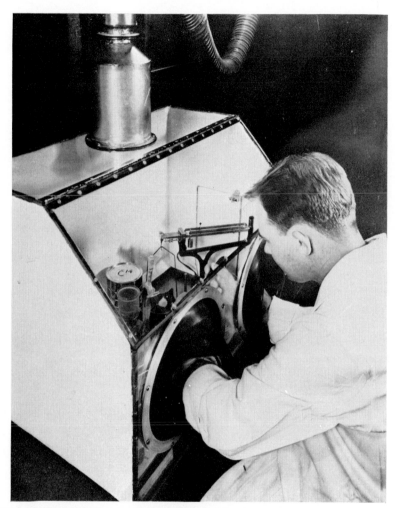

FIG. 4. Weighing radiobarium. Rubber gloves protect hands from β radiation (Argonne National Laboratory, Chicago).

Another convenient unit, in much use by laboratory workers, is the r/hour at 1 foot. Used for gamma photons of from 0.5 to 2.0 mev, this unit is given by the following relation (4):

$$1 \ rhf = 6 \ ce \qquad (15.22)$$

where c is the source strength in curies and e the energy per photon in mev.

EXAMPLE 15.12

What thickness of lead shielding is required to reduce the radiation at one foot from a 1-curie Co^{60} source to the maximum permissible exposure level (7.5 mr/hr for 40 hr week)?

Decay of Co^{60}:

$$\left.\begin{array}{l}\text{one 0.3 mev } \beta \text{ (neglect)}\\ \text{one 1.1 mev } \gamma\\ \text{one 1.3 mev } \gamma\end{array}\right\} \text{ per disintegration}$$

$$r/hr \text{ at } 1 \text{ ft} = 6 \, ce$$

$$= (6) \, (1) \, (1.1 + 1.3)$$

$$= 14.4 \text{ r/hr} = 14400 \text{ mr/hr}$$

μ for Pb for 1.3 mev $= 0.68 \text{ cm}^{-1}$

$$I_{Pb} = I_o e^{-\mu x}$$

$$\frac{I_{Pb}}{I_0} = \frac{7.5}{14400} = e^{-0.68x}$$

$$-0.68 \, x = \ln 7.5 - \ln 14400$$

$$= 2.02 - 9.58 = -7.56$$

$$x = 11.14 \text{ cm (ans)}$$

4. *The Inverse Square Law.* Increasing the distance between the body and a radiation source will also decrease the exposure. The intensity of radiation from a source decreases with the square of the distance as shown below.

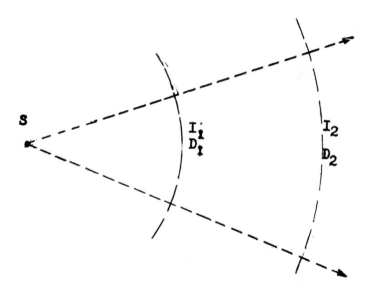

In the above sketch, the intensity of radiation I_1 from the source S at a distance D_1, is given by

$$I_1 = \frac{S}{4\pi D_1^2}$$

while that of I_2 at D_2 is given by

$$I_2 = \frac{S}{4\pi D_2^2}$$

Combining these two equations:

$$4\pi I_1 D_1^2 = 4\pi I_2 D_2^2$$

$$I_1 D_1^2 = I_2 D_2^2$$

or:

$$\frac{I_1}{I_2} = \frac{D_2^2}{D_1^2} \tag{15.23}$$

EXAMPLE 15.13

In the preceding example the rhf from an unshielded Co^{60} source was 14.4 r/hr. How far away (neglecting absorption in air) should a person stand so as not to receive more than 7.5 mr/hr?

$$\frac{D_1^2}{D_2^2} = \frac{I_2}{I_1} = \frac{7.5}{14400} = \frac{1}{D_2^2}$$

$$D_2 = \sqrt{\frac{14400}{7.5}} = 44 \text{ ft.}$$

Scattering of gamma radiation may account for about 1 % of the direct beam. Under some conditions this may produce a substantial exposure. Accordingly any shield which is designed for protection against the beam should be properly formed to reduce the scattering effect and should in addition be made thick enough to absorb an amount of direct radiation equivalent to the amount scattered.

The amount of shielding, expressed in gm/cm^2 needed to protect against beta radiation, may be determined by referring to Eqs. 15.7 and 15.8, remembering that

$$gm/cm^2 = \rho x \tag{15.24}$$

where x is the thickness of the absorbing material in cm and ρ is its density in gm/cm^3.

Fig. 5 shows the β-ray stopping characteristics of several materials.

15.8 Protection Against Internal Radiation

In principle, the prevention of radiation damage to the organs and tissues of the body is simply a matter of preventing the intake of radioactive materials, to be accomplished by good working methods, cleanliness and proper design of laboratories and workshops. In practice, however, the adoption of appropriate safety measures is often very difficult, requiring a thorough understanding of all phases of the work being undertaken, an adequate knowledge of the radiation properties of the material handled, the institution of a practical system of monitoring and almost endless forethought and planning to assure the safe execution of each detail. The magnitude of the operation is not necessarily a sound guide as to the extent of the needed protective measures, for even the smallest quantities of radioisotopes require safe transportation, storage, use, and disposal, in order to prevent their inhalation or ingestion.

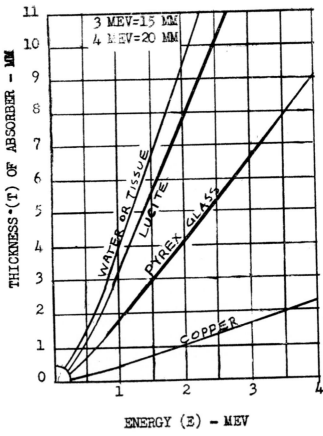

Fig. 5. Thickness, T mm, of typical materials required to stop completely beta-rays of maximum energy, E mev. (Additional shielding may be required for the Bremsstrahlung.) (From N.B.S. Handbook 42.)

In the event of spillage, or loss of control over quantities of radioactive materials, the spread of contamination will be hard to avoid unless careful preparation has been made to control this spread and to decontaminate the affected areas, equipment, or personnel.

The difficulties attending the establishment of a well-integrated radiation protection system should not, however, be regarded as an additional operational burden. Experience has shown that good safety practices, aside from their intrinsic value in preventing personal injury, almost invariably result in improved plant output as well. On this basis, the control of radiation hazards does not differ from the control of other hazards. Indeed, the radiation protection system may be regarded as a part of the over-all safety program of an organization.

That the hazards of working with radiation are no greater than dangers associated with many other industries has been shown by K. Z. Morgan who cites that in 1948, for all industries, the injury rate was 11.49 per million man hours, while in the same year, the rate for the Oak Ridge National Laboratory was 2.03.

Many excellent reports are available which set forth in detail the requirements for optimum protection of workers with radioactive materials. Handling equipment, laboratory fixtures and apparatus, ventilation systems, waste disposal, monitoring instruments and methods, medical supervision, decontamination methods, first aid, safety rules, and other features of radiation protection are adequately presented especially in the readily available National Bureau of Standards Handbooks. The more important titles will be found in the bibliography for this chapter. The expansion of knowledge and increased experience in the field of radiation protection has made it necessary to limit the present discussion to a description of general principles.

Since the prevention of internal radiation injury to the body is essentially a matter of keeping radioactive materials out of it, the art of safety in accomplishing this purpose depends on:

1. The prevention of contamination by the employment of careful workers observing thoroughly planned procedures in carrying out their tasks.

2. The prevention of ingestion of active substances by refraining from eating, drinking, smoking, and even using cosmetics, while at work. A good general rule is to avoid touching anything with the hands except objects directly concerned with the task.

3. The prevention of inhalation of excessive amounts of radioactive materials by assuring that these do not get into the air of the laboratory or work-room. Properly designed hoods or local exhaust ventilation arrangements should be used when necessary, and at times masks should be worn.

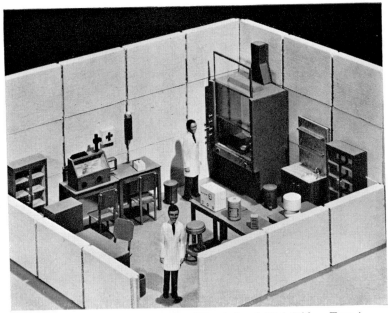

FIG. 6. Two-man laboratory, millicurie level (Oak Ridge, Tenn.)

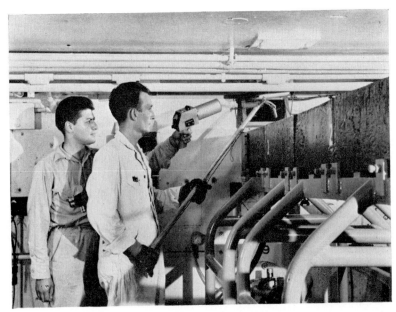

FIG. 7. Monitoring samples from pile (Oak Ridge, Tenn.)

It is well to remember that it is possible to produce an aerosol even by removing the stopper from a bottle.

4. The prevention of absorption of radioactive materials by way of the intact or broken skin. Those having any open lesion of the skin should not work with radioisotopes. Those whose skin is intact should take every precaution to avoid injuring themselves while at work. The use of organic solvents to cleanse the hands will increase the permeability of the skin.

5. Careful monitoring of the work area is needed to assure that contamination does not go un-noticed. Likewise, monitoring of the individual is a good practice, to guard against excessive exposure and contamination of the worker or his clothing.

6. The use of change-rooms and appropriate protective clothing is frequently demanded to prevent spread of contamination.

7. Training in first-aid and decontamination methods should be included in the radiation protection plan of every unit which uses radioactive materials.

8. Facilities for proper disposal of radioactive waste must be adequate and properly used.

9. The laboratory or shop must be kept clean.

10. Finally, all persons exposed to radiation sources should be under medical supervision at least to the extent of providing reasonable assurance that their work will not result in injury to their health. This will ordinarily

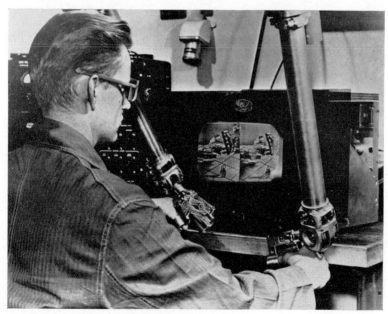

FIG. 8. Remote control operation (Argonne National Laboratory, Chicago)

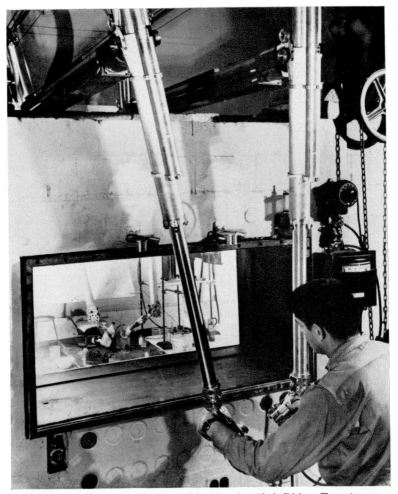

FIG. 9. Mechanical hands behind barrier (Oak Ridge, Tenn.)

require pre-employment and periodic follow-up examinations. These examinations should include laboratory examinations for possible deposits of radioactive materials in the body, when the individual concerned has been potentially exposed to their absorption. Medical and surgical assistance should be available if needed, for the care of persons who have been overexposed or seriously contaminated.

15.9 Monitoring Instruments and Methods*

The detection of nuclear radiations depends on their property of producing ionization. In the case of electrons, protons, and alpha particles, the

* See also Ch. 6.

ionization is produced by their electrical charge as well as their speed. In the case of gamma rays and neutrons, the ionization is the result of inelastic collision, whereby the photon or particle gives up all or part of its energy to separate an atom from one of its electrons.

If a single electron, a beta particle, with an energy of, for example, 1 mev, is travelling through a volume of gas, and if 32 ev are expended by it in producing an average ion pair, then the particle is capable of producing $10^6/32 = 31,000$ ion pairs before its energy is expended. Since each ion has a charge of 4.8×10^{-10} esu or 1.6×10^{-19} coulomb, the total charge resulting from the stoppage of the single electron is $3.1 \times 10^4 \times 1.6 \times 10^{-19}$ $= 5 \times 10^{-15}$ coulomb (or 5×10^{-15} ampere-seconds). With the exception of the electrometer, which could be made sufficiently sensitive to measure this small charge, there is no instrument which could approach this degree of sensitivity unaided. It becomes necessary, therefore, to use special instruments such as ionization chambers, scintillation detectors, and Geiger counters described in Chapter 6; and other devices.

15.9.1 *Detection and Measurement.* A distinction is made between *detection* and *measurement* of radiation. A field of radiation is detected, its dimensions approximated, and its relative intensity roughly determined by means of a scanning survey with a sensitive G-M counter, proportional counter, scintillation counter, or ionization chamber. An instrument used for scanning or detection cannot be used for measurement of radiation

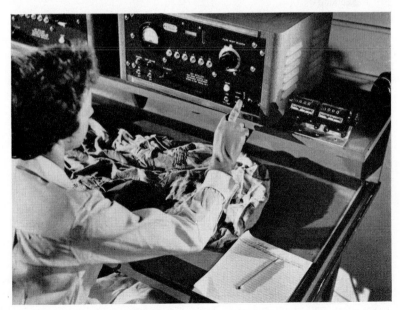

Fig. 10. Monitoring laundry (Oak Ridge, Tenn.)

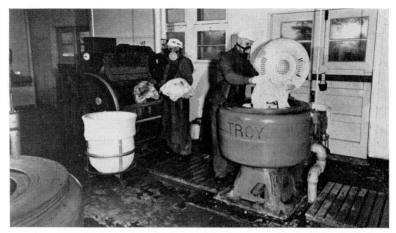

FIG. 11. Decontimation laundry (Los Alamos, N. Mex.)

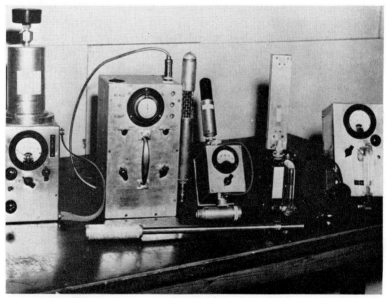

FIG. 12. Portable radiation instruments. Left to right: "neut" (fast neutron counter); G. M. scaler; $\beta\gamma$ meter; α detector; "Juno", general purpose meter (Hanford, Wash.).

unless it has been calibrated against a source of the approximate strength of the radiation under conditions similar to those which exist where the radiation is found. Detection of beta and gamma radiation may be accomplished with a suitable thin-walled Geiger counter. To distinguish between

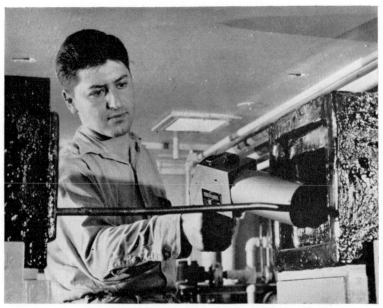

Fig. 13. Monitoring face of pile (Oak Ridge, Tenn.)

the beta and gamma components of a radiation field, the G-M tube should be equipped with a movable shield capable of stopping the β particles, but which will allow the gammas to penetrate to the tube. Since the walls of the Geiger tube are too thick to allow alpha particles to get through, these must be detected by means of an instrument such as the proportional counter, ionization chamber, or scintillation counter, whose sensitive elements can be made with windows of nylon or other thin materials. An equivalent thickness of 0.5 mg/cm² is needed for satisfactory alpha detection while a window of 3 mg/cm² or more is suitable for betas.

15.9.2 *Neutron Detection.* The detection of neutrons requires specially constructed instruments. For slow neutrons, a proportional counter lined with boron carbide or filled with boron trifluoride is probably best, since, this instrument discriminates against other radiations, but various other instruments can be used. For neutrons of intermediate or high energies, the counter may be surrounded by a suitable layer of paraffin, which moderates some of these fast particles to thermal energies, so that they may be detected by absorption in the boron. (Reaction: B^{10} (n, α) Li^7. The emitted α particle is what the counter detects.)

All detection instruments must be frequently checked against a known source.

15.9.3 *Area Monitoring and Radiation Surveys.* Quantitative measurement of radiation is accomplished by the collection of ions in an air-filled ionization chamber. In the case of gamma radiation, the chamber should have "air-equivalent" walls of such thickness as to prevent the escape of the secondary electrons, while for the measurement of alpha or beta radiation the chamber should have a window thin enough to permit the entry of these particles.

All radiations may be detected and measured by a properly calibrated Lauritsen electroscope. Even thermal neutrons may be measured by the use of an electroscope with a boron-coated chamber.

Beta and gamma radiations may be measured in units of rep or milli-rep per hour. Alpha particles are reported as counts or disintegrations per minute per cm^2. Neutrons are recorded in terms of flux, or number of neutrons per cm^2 per second.

Radiation monitoring is carried out in one or more of several ways. First one may list the method known as area monitoring, by which gamma and often beta-radiation levels in a work area are continuously measured and if desired recorded as a permanent record. For area monitoring, either portable or permanently mounted instruments of the Geiger-Müller counter or ionization chamber type are employed. Their output can be used to operate audible or visual warning signals when a given level of radiaton is exceeded. Then we have the method of surveying an area by means of portable detection and measurement instruments of the types described

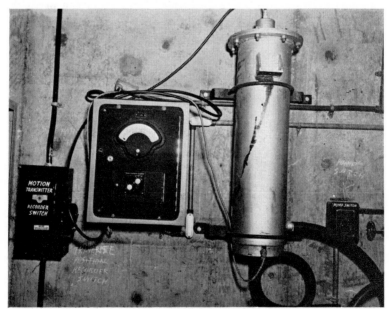

FIG. 14. Fixed ionization chambers for monitoring air (Hanford, Wash.)

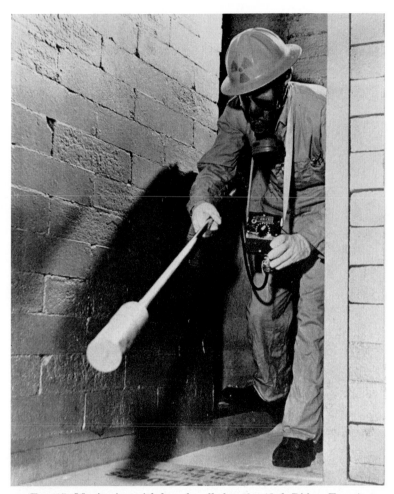

FIG. 15. Monitoring with long-handled probe (Oak Ridge, Tenn.)

above. Actually a radiation survey means more than the use of portable instruments to determine the location and intensity of sources of alpha, beta, gamma, and neutron radiation. A thorough survey should include a study of operating procedures, personnel work habits, radiation dosage rates, and other pertinent details, and should be completely presented as a written record, with recommendations for changes if indicated.

In conjunction with area monitoring and radiation survey techniques, it is often necessary to conduct tests to determine the concentrations of airborne radioactivity, which may be present in the form of radioactive gases or vapors, and also particulates. Properly designed ionization cham-

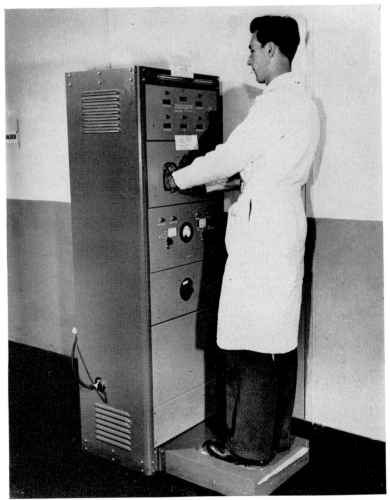

Fig. 16. Hand and foot counters (Brookhaven National Laboratory, Upton, N. Y.).

bers through which a measured flow of air is drawn can be installed for monitoring gaseous activity. Various filtration devices of either the continuous or intermittent type may be used to collect samples of radioactive particles, which may then be counted either automatically or as a separate laboratory procedure.

15.9.4 *Personnel Monitoring.* Finally, there is the practice of personnel monitoring, by which we attempt to arrive at an approximation as to the amount of radiation which the worker may receive in the performance of his tasks in the plant or laboratory. For this purpose, use is made of small

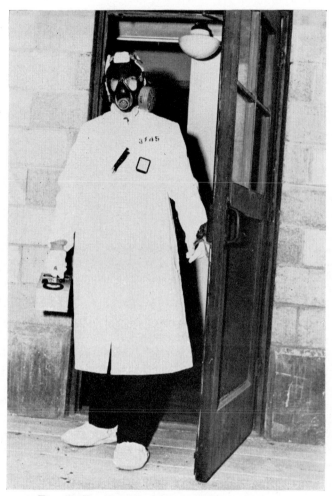

FIG. 17. Emergency monitoring (Hanford, Wash.)

fountain-pen-sized ionization chambers, * of either the non-indicating or self-indicating type. These instruments are received by the worker, fully charged, as he begins work for the day, and are read at the end of the day, or at any other appropriate time. Also, very wide use is made of dental-film-sized *"film badges"* or *"film badge meters"*. These film badges are available in a variety of emulsions, suitable for radiation intensities as shown in Table XI. They can be used to monitor an area or a process as well as the person of the worker and can be adapted for any type of radiation. The films have the advantages of economy, lightness, sensitivity, and

* Usual type of "Pocket Dosimeter."

TABLE XI
Approximate Useful Exposure Ranges of Some Radiation—Monitoring Films**

FILM TYPE	RANGE IN r UNITS	
	100–200 kv	Mv Region
Dupont types:		
Medical x-ray film, xtra fast, 508.........	0.002–1.8	0.05–6.
Medical x-ray film, par speed, 502.........	0.0025–2.2	0.1–10
Industrial x-ray film, very fine grain, 510...	0.03–5.	1–50
Microfilm, positive, 606................	0.5–140	15–700
Eastman Kodak types:		
Industrial x-ray film, type K............	0.0015–1.1	0.05–8.
Fine grain release positive, 5302.........	0.45–22	15–700
Dental x-ray film, periapical, extra-speed..	0.002–6	0.05–25
Spectroscopic film, 548–0, double-coated...	100–2400	1,000–15,000

* When developed in Kodak liquid x-ray developer for 5 min. at 20°C. Film sensitivity varies with a factor the order of 10 in 100–200 kv range. Data from N.B.S. Handbook 60, Dec., 1955.

of providing a permanent record. Their disadvantage is mainly in that they must be carefully calibrated, and processed and examined by special technics before the exposure can be determined.

In many installations workers are able to measure residual contamination of their hands, clothing and footgear by means of special instruments provided at places of exit from radioactive buildings and areas. By the use of such devices, the worker can avoid the possibility of spreading contamination and can be assured that he is himself properly decontaminated.

In some kinds of work, it may be possible for the individual to inhale or otherwise absorb small quantities of radioisotopes. For this reason, it is common practice for such workers to undergo periodic medical examinations, including the examination of body wastes for traces of radioactivity. Specimens of urine and feces, and sometimes breath samples, are processed by special methods and the samples counted by appropriate counting techniques.

Film badges and Pocket Dosimeters cover a wide range but there is need for more rugged devices unaffected by the elements, including submersion in water, and durable, to approximate the more heavy doses of emergency type. Of these, *silver-activated phosphate glass* presently appears most useful. This material becomes luminescent under ultra-violet light in proportion to the amount of dosage, the response being linear at least up to 1500 r. Special readers are required and available with a range of 10–600 r which could be extended to 20,000 r. Energy dependence is present but

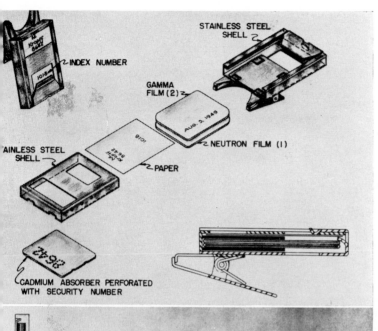

FIG. 18A
Film badge

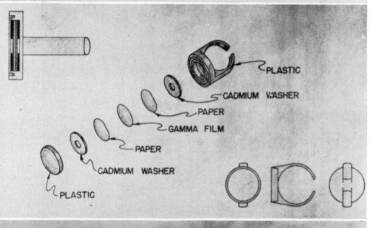

FIG. 18B
Film ring

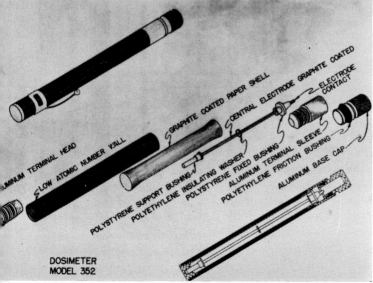

FIG. 18C
Dosimeter

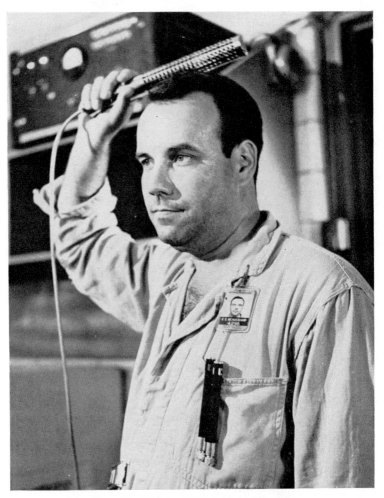

Fig. 19. "Frisker" (Oak Ridge, Tenn.).

reduced by placing the glass between lead shields. An opening of 0.107 inches improves response in the low energy range. Accuracy is ±20% between 80 Kev and 5 Mev. Shelf life is indefinite. Direction dependence is not appreciable above 1.25 Mev. Readers are fairly accurate, variations not exceeding 5% or 5 r. Size of glass $\frac{3}{4}$ x $\frac{3}{4}$ x $\frac{3}{16}$ in. Final readings can be made at 4 hours. Immediate readings are 10–20% low and 2 hours' readings 5% low.

15.9.5 *Laboratory counting technics* are of great importance in all phases of radiation work. Unfortunately even a brief description of the fundamentals of these techniques would be quite beyond the scope of this presen-

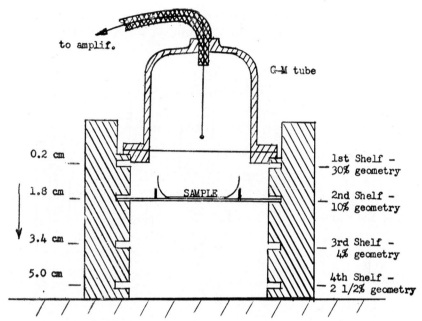

to amplif.

G-M tube

0.2 cm   1st Shelf –
                                         30% geometry

1.8 cm   SAMPLE   2nd Shelf –
                                         10% geometry

3.4 cm   3rd Shelf –
                                         4% geometry

5.0 cm   4th Shelf –
                                         2 1/2% geometry

FIG. 20. Arrangement for β counting with thin mica window GM tube (after ref. 2).

tation. However, it may be of some value to enumerate the various factors which must be considered in order to determine the validity of an individual count.

The radioactive sample is mounted or deposited upon a thin plate, or in a small dish, which is placed on a shelf in the tube-mount (see Fig. 22). The tube, usually a thin-end-window Geiger tube, but possibly a proportional counter or scintillation counter, is connected to a scaler via an amplifier. The tube mount may or may not be shielded depending upon the radioactivity of the sample and the level of laboratory background activity.

It is necessary to determine the total number of counts required or, stated otherwise, the length of time the sample must be counted at the rate of a given number of counts per unit time. Radioactive disintegration is a statistical process and the number of background counts in a given time as well as the number of disintegrations in the sample in the same length of time will follow statistical laws.

To determine the probable error, P, of a count a simplified formula has been used.

$$P = 0.675 \frac{\sqrt{\text{sum of counts}}}{\text{sum of counts}}$$ (15.25)

This expression is approximately correct when the total counting rate is over 5 times the background rate. For example, if the background rate is 40 counts/min and the total count (background + sample) is 200, the probable error is

$$\frac{0.675\sqrt{200}}{200} = .0477 \simeq 5\%$$

$$.05 \times 200 = 10 \text{ counts}$$

The precise count is therefore

$$200 \pm 10 \text{ ct/min.}$$

Now the probable error of a count is inversely proportional to the square root of the count, thus:

$$\frac{P_1}{P_2} = \frac{\sqrt{C_2}}{\sqrt{C_1}} \tag{15.26}$$

That is:

$$C_2 = \frac{P_1^2 C_1}{P_2^2} \tag{15.27}$$

Therefore, if we wished to reduce the probable error in the above example to $\pm 1\%$, the required number of counts would be:

$$C_2 = \frac{(.05)^2 (200)}{(.01)^2} = 5000$$

Since the counting rate of the sample is only 200 ± 10 ct/min the counting time would be approximately 25 minutes.

A count of the required accuracy having been obtained, it is then necessary to apply certain correction factors before the net count of the sample can be stated.

1. Geometrical efficiency. While it is theoretically possible to calculate the geometrical efficiency of an arrangement of tube and sample, in practice this would be very difficult. Tube and tube-mount geometries are therefore experimentally determined with respect to sample area and distance of sample from the window (Fig. 20).

2. Backscatter. A fraction of the particles will be directed away from the counting window and toward the container in which the sample is placed. Some of these particles will then be scattered upward, toward the window. The correction to be applied to a count because of this effect may also be determined by experiment with known sources, placing the source on a thin film and taking counts with and without the backing provided by the type of sample-holder used.

3. Absorption in window and in air. A number of the weak beta particles in a source will be absorbed by the mica window and by the layer of air between the sample and the window. Absorption curves may be plotted to be used in correcting for this effect.

4. Self-absorption. In a similar manner, curves may be prepared for use in correcting for the absorption of particles because of the thickness of the sample itself. This factor is of special importance in alpha counting.

5. Coincidence losses. These are losses in counts due to the arrival in the counter of another particle, while the counter is inoperative during its "dead time". The correction factor is determined experimentally by counting weak sources individually and together.

6. Variation in counter efficiency, which will occur from day to day, can be corrected by checking the counter against a long-lived standard reference source.

7. The background count must then be deducted.

Other corrections are necessary for special counting procedures, as, for example, the correction for the thoron content of air in sampling the air for long-lived alpha-emitters.

It is well to note that the precision of the final count will not exceed that of the counts made in determining the various correction factors mentioned above.

15.10 Disposal of Radioactive Wastes

One of the most troublesome problems encountered in working with radioactive materials is that of proper disposal of active waste materials. Not only do these wastes appear in countless forms, from ore tailings and lathe turnings to laundry wastes and body excreta, but sometimes it is not even possible to decide on permanent disposal—if indeed there actually is such a thing as permanent disposal. For example, accumulations of radioactive fission products of long or intermediate half-life, for which there is at present no profitable, or even feasible use, may one day become quite valuable if an industrial use for them should be developed. Presently expensive recovery processes may one day be simplified. Technical improvements may make it more profitable to use low grade feed materials in atomic energy plants. For such materials, controlled storage, rather than permanent disposal, is the preferred choice.

As a matter of fact, there are perhaps only one, or possibly two methods of permanent disposal. The surest method appears to be the one used by a West Coast laboratory where waste materials are mixed with concrete in steel drums and the drums are sunk in deep water in the Pacific Ocean. It is concluded that once the drums are buried in a number of feet of bottom ooze, there would be only the slowest diffusion of radioactivity throughout the ooze, even after the steel drums and the concrete should disintegrate. A second possibly permanent method of disposal is that of mixing the wastes with concrete and dumping into deep concrete vaults, constructed in a location of known geological formation, where no likelihood of eventual seepage through loose strata is foreseen. Such burial sites, of course, have to be guarded.

These and similar methods of disposal are suitable for solid or fairly concentrated liquid wastes, but in the case of dilute radioactive liquids other means must be devised for disposal. First of all, liquids containing short-lived isotopes may be stored in suitably guarded tanks or basins until the activity has decayed to safe levels. These liquids may then be discharged at a rate consistent with safety, into sewage systems. If it is not possible to dispose of all of the waste at such rates, or if the radioisotopes are of long half-lives, the liquid must be concentrated by evaporation, or the active material otherwise removed by chemical treatment or ion-exchange methods. The waste may then be disposed of as a solid.

Sometimes the discharge of radioactive wastes into sewage and drainage systems may be safely accomplished if the active isotope is diluted with stable isotopes of the same element. In this event the dilution should be such that no more than 4.15 ergs per gram of element per day are released as radiation. It is thought that in this dilution the radioisotope can no longer be reconcentrated by natural means.

Gaseous wastes, usually resulting from air-cooling of nuclear reactors, must be dealt with by still other methods. First, the solid particles must be filtered out of the air or gas which may then be discharged through tall stacks into the air, provided that meteorological conditions are satisfactory and the maximum permissible concentration of the isotope in the air is not exceeded. The solid filtrate must of course be handled like other radioactive solids.

It can be seen that the safe disposal of radioactive waste materials is not only bothersome, but also expensive. Research and development may bring about improvement in methods and in lower costs. Public safety, as well as conservation of wild-life and protection of domestic animals and crops, demands the most careful appraisal and solution of this problem.

At the Washington Conference on Waste Disposal, which was convened in September, 1948, methods of disposal of certain isotopes used in medicine were formulated. It was agreed that 10^{-5} microcuries of $C^{14}O_2$ per cc of air could be discharged provided that there was no particulate activity. It was also agreed that 5×10^{-4} $\mu c/cc$ of I^{131} could be discharged by an institution into the public sewer provided that the total activity was not more than 200 mc/wk. Similarly 10^{-4} $\mu c/cc$ of P^{32} could be so discharged with the provision that each millicurie was diluted with 10 grams of natural phosphorus as phosphate, the total not to exceed 200 mc/wk (10). These

TABLE XII*
Elimination of P^{32} and I^{131}

DOSE	MAX EXCR FIRST 24 H
mc	*mc*
P^{32}	
0.5	0.1
5.0	1.0
I^{131}	
5.0	4.5
60	54

* After A. E. C. Bulletin TID-388.

recommendations have been adopted by the National Bureau of Standards Advisory Committee which has prepared a special report on this subject (35). The radioactive discharge from the institution into the sewer should be less than 0.5 μc/liter for I^{131} and less than 0.1 μc/liter in the case of P^{32}. With the installation of a constant flow drip bottle to discharge the radioactive waste into the hospital drains, 100 *mc* may be disposed of in a 6-hour interval into a community sewage system with an average dry weather flow of 1 million gallons per day, with the discharge for other sewage flows proportional to these amounts.

Table XII will provide an indication of the rates of excretion of I^{131} and P^{32}.

Disposal of body excretions of these isotopes may be made by normal use of toilet facilities, or by dilution of urine to 1 gallon in a jug which may then be poured into a sink drain, provided that the sewage flow from the hospital is sufficient to reduce the concentration to the levels indicated above. Methods of calculation are given in NBS Handbook 49.

The disposal of other isotopes should be such as to result in concentrations no higher than those indicated for areas beyond control.

It may be well to point out that while the disposal of radioactive wastes is a serious matter, requiring expensive and time-consuming procedures which must be absorbed by any project in which they are used, the problem is not too greatly different from that of the disposal of other poisonous or potentially harmful waste materials. The prevention of stream pollution and air contamination from all causes is a problem which may ultimately call for a single solution.

15.11 Conclusion

Even as the disposal of radioactive wastes is a problem not greatly different from other forms of noxious waste disposal so the whole field of radiation protection is based upon principles which are similar to those governing the protection of individuals and communities against the hazards of industrial and technical origin. These problems are being met with constantly-improving methods of solution.

In the presentation of the material contained in this chapter no claim can be made for originality. The purpose has been to collect a variety of information which, it is hoped, will prove useful to those readers with an interest in the ever-expanding field of protection against atomic and nuclear radiations.

ADDENDUM

ILLUSTRATIVE EXAMPLE

15.12 NA²⁴ as Index to Exposure

A physicist, working on an unshielded nuclear assembly, was exposed to a large flux of external radiation when the assembly accidentally became over-critical. The total time of the radiation "flash" was considered to be very much less than one second. Estimate the dose of total body irradiation received by the victim if the NA²⁴ content of his blood serum, measured 6 hours after the accident, was 5.0 disintegrations per second per milligram of total sodium.

Calculations of this type are subject to many uncertainties. However, Hempelmann et al. have reported a series of nine similar cases (36) and conclude that the specific activity of the serum sodium offers a valid indication of the neutron flux received by the body. On this basis it was possible for Hempelmann and his co-workers to calculate the total body exposure from "prompt" neutrons and gamma rays, and their findings were presented as summarized in columns 1, 2, 3, and 4 of the tabulation in this section.

The methods of calculation are not indicated, but we may add the values

1	2	3	4	5
		WHOLE BODY		
CASE	SPECIFIC ACTIVITY OF SODIUM CORRECTED FOR DECAY (D/S PER MG NA)	80-KV X-RAY DOSE EQUIVALENT (ROENTGENS)	γ RAY DOSE (ROENTGENS)	COL. 3 PLUS COL. 4
1	18.0	480	110	590
2	1.1	31	0.14	31.14
3	73.6	1930	114	2044
4	13.3	390	26.4	416.4
6	7.1	186	10.7	196.7
7	3.8	140	8.7	148.7
8	2.03	55	4.37	59.37
9	1.54	42	2.72	44.72
10	1.22	33	2.41	35.41

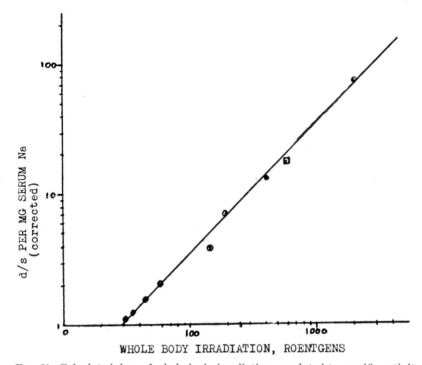

WHOLE BODY IRRADIATION, ROENTGENS

Fig. 21. Calculated dose of whole-body irradiation as related to specific activity of serum sodium (after Hemplemann et al, 1952).

in Column 3, which represent equivalent dosages due to neutrons, to those in Column 4, which are the prompt gamma dosages (except that in Case 1 the γ dose seems to include delayed gammas). Plotting these results, we obtain the curve shown in Fig. 21.

The relation appears to be linear, so that each disintegration per second per milligram of serum sodium represents approximately 30 r of neutron and gamma irradiation.

To correct the count of 50 d/s per mg Na to obtain the activity at $t = 0$ we use the expression

$$N_0 = \frac{N}{e^{-\lambda t}} \quad \text{where} \quad \lambda = \frac{.69}{\text{effective half-life}}$$

The effective half-life for Na[24] (Table XI) is 0.61 days. Then

$$N_0 = \frac{50}{e^{-\frac{.69}{.61} \times \frac{6}{24}}} = 6.7 \text{ d/s per mg Na}$$

Accordingly, the physicist in our example obtained a total body dose of

$$6.7 \times 30 = 201 \text{ r}$$

REFERENCES

Effects of Nuclear Weapons, Government Printing Office, Washington 25, D. C. 1957.

GLASSTONE, S.: *Sourcebook on Atomic Energy*. New York: Van Nostrand, 1950.

LAPP, R. E. AND ANDREWS, H. L.: *Nuclear Radiation Physics* (2nd ed.). New York: Prentice-Hall, 1954.

National Bureau of Standards Handbooks: Supr. of Documents, Govt. Printing Office, Washington 25, D. C.

7.B — Protection Against Neutron Radiation up to 30 Mev. 1957.

42 — Safe Handling of Radioactive Isotopes. 1949.

48 — Control and Removal of Radioactive Contamination in Laboratories. 1951.

49 — Recommendations for Waste Disposal of Phosphorus[32] and Iodine[131] for Medical Users, 1951.

51 — Radiological Monitoring Methods and Instruments. 1952.

52 — Maximum Permissable Amounts of Radioisotopes in the Human Body and Maximum Permissable Concentrations in Air and Water. 1953.

54 — Protection against Radiations from Radium, Cobalt[60] and Cesium[137], 1954.

56 — Safe Handling of Cadavers Containing Radioactive Isotopes. 1953.

58 — Radioactive Waste Disposal in the Ocean. 1954.

59 — Permissable Dose from External Sources of Ionizing Radiation. 1955. (Revision now about Ready—1958).

60 — X-Ray Protection. 1955.

Phosphate Glass Dosimetry: Federal Civil Defense Administration Technical Bulletin, TB-11-15, July 1954.

Note: In this Text, Chapters 6, 12, 13, 14 and 21 are especially pertinent to the subject.

16►

Survival Methods in Atomic Disaster

O. Schneider, M.D.

Revised by Charles F. Behrens, M.D. (Ed.)

16.1 Introduction*

This subject in all its ramifications would require volumes for complete coverage and also more time than all but a few people care to devote to it. It thus appears appropriate to provide this brief summary of the more important aspects.

16.2 General Considerations

Plans and programs of all types and on all scales have been made and abundantly discussed. A vast literature on the subjects now exists. The congressional report on "Civil Defense for National Survival" (2946 of 1956) gives a good picture of the situation. Much discussion now relates to the roles and possibilities of heavy shelter programs and evacuation.

16.2.1 *Shelters.* Increasing emphasis is being placed on the value of sturdy underground shelters because of the likelihood that warning intervals are apt to be greatly curtailed by resort to guided missiles with nuclear warheads. There are also notable and difficult complications to be anticipated from fallout radiation in the event of surface bursts with megaton weapons.

Shelters of sturdy type capable of withstanding virtually all stress save in the crater area itself, can be built and a detailed description and plan of such a shelter, developed by the F.C.D.A. is given in the "Effects of Nuclear Weapons." The specifications call for an underground structure with a covering of 5 feet of earth, built of reinforced concrete with walls 15 inches thick and roof 21 inches thick. The door is of structural steel and concrete, 8 inches thick. Ventilating ducts are equipped with filters and

* 16.1 and 16.2 by Editor.

antiblast closures to resist up to 100 psi. Capacity is 30 persons but dimensions could be increased to house more.

A great difficulty is the cost and diversion of materials associated with an extensive heavy shelter program and so strenuous opposition on such scores develops to further handicap efforts already impeded by familiar attitudes ranging between apathy, indifference, hopeless fatalism and finally the optimistic feeling that "it simply can't and won't happen." Accordingly ambitious shelter programs languish. Less expensive expedients have been mentioned such as roadside trenches 2 feet wide and 3 feet deep, concrete pipes 4 or more feet in diameter covered by 3 feet of earth, and light concrete structures reinforced by steel also covered by 3 feet of earth. These would be located along main roads. It has also been suggested that householders 15 miles from target areas construct backyard or basement shelters.

In general it is to be borne in mind that even light shelters and basement protection are bound to be of enormous value in the event of extensive fallout especially since an interval of several hours may elapse before heavy fallout begins. Attenuation effects are listed in the Effects of Nuclear Weapons (Table 9.37) as follows: Frame house factor of 2 for first floor and 10 for basement; multistory reinforced concrete buildings, factor of 10 on lower floors and 1000 or more in basements below ground level. The main peril as noted in other chapters is from γ rays.

16.2.2 *Evacuation.* Considerations mentioned above greatly diminish the prospective value of large scale evacuation as the sole or principle reliance in avoiding enormous casualties. However, regardless of shelter availability more or less evacuation may prove inevitable or advisable. It may be advisable, in the face of likely attack to evacuate all but essential workers from a given area. Again complete evacuation remains a valuable solution if sufficient warning is obtained. Following an attack it may be necessary to relocate large numbers of people rendered homeless.

16.2.3 *Dispersal and Construction.* Wide dispersal and blast resistant structures are of obvious value. The common and compelling objections relate to cost and, as regards dispersal, dislocation, loss of efficiency, transportation difficulties and housing availability. Prohibitive costs are envisioned, but it is worthy of note that the volume of new construction is such that valuable results are possible on a gradual basis if we will put our minds and hearts in the effort. We need to avoid the "all or nothing" outlook which conduces to doing nothing because we can't do what we would like, fast and without much trouble and expense.

16.3 Individual Survival

In the event of an atomic attack much will depend on the behavior of individual citizens. Each man, woman, or child who succeeds in escaping death or injury will not only help himself, but make available the services of a number of rescue, first aid, and other personnel, to help another who may not have been so fortunate. Thus the person who survives unhurt becomes an asset, while he who becomes a casualty only creates more work for all. The survival of the individual stands not merely as the goal of any system of civil defense, but as the first and most essential phase of such a system.

In the opinion of the writer each person must act upon the principles summarized below, in order to maximize his chances of survival during and after an atomic bomb attack. He must:

1. Learn the rules which have been adopted for his safety by his local civil defense organization.

2. Learn the fundamentals of first aid, fire-fighting, and rescue.

3. Learn the locations of designated shelters at his home and place of work, and to recognize warning signals.

4. Discipline himself to act calmly in an emergency, to proceed to his shelter or to his post of duty automatically and without saying or doing anything which might cause panic among others.

5. Know the hazards of the atomic bomb and observe all safety precautions regarding the effects of heat, the dangers of damaged buildings and the hazards of radiation.

6. Keep physically fit and develop the habit of mental alertness.

7. Keep in contact with his civil defense organization and, if required, do his part in this organization in accordance with his own talents and capabilities. He should be a regular donor of the blood procurement program.

8. Wear adequate clothing at all times. In summer, when out of doors, light-colored, loose-fitting garments should be worn which cover as much of the body as possible. A hat with a brim is recommended. In winter, ordinary street clothing is satisfactory.

9. Carry or wear some clearly legible personal identification, giving at least name and address, and the name and address of next-of-kin, or of the person to be notified in emergency. If a device for universal identification is adopted, one must carry it in accordance with instructions. The use of such a "dog tag" should not be regarded as an invasion of private rights. All military personnel are required to wear identification tags in battle, and many civilians have such tags made up for them at considerable expense. There should be no objection to wearing a tag issued by one's own civil defense authorities. In the event of disaster, the information provided upon it will save much time and effort for all concerned including the injured victim, his family, and the medical units who take care of him.

10. Practice taking cover. Given a few minutes warning, there is no reason why nearly everyone should not be able to find adequate shelter,

providing all act calmly and rationally. Most large downtown buildings
have designated shelter areas in basements and sub-basements. Many
cities have subway stations, tunnels or other protected locations. Suitable
shelters are also provided in many factories and other industrial buildings.
Most residential buildings and houses have basements which can be converted into good, or at least satisfactory shelters. Occupants of houses
without basements can rely upon a neighbor's shelter or can, without too
much difficulty, construct one of their own, following directions available
at their civil defense headquarters.

Even if there is only a few seconds' warning, persons indoors can dodge
beneath a desk, table, or bed, or behind a counter, safe, machine, or bench,
while those out in the open can crouch in a doorway or beside the wall of
a sturdy building, or in a ditch or gutter, or beneath a parked auto or
truck. Even if no warning has been given and no shelter whatever is at
hand, one can drop flat upon the ground at the flash of the bomb, face down,
covering the head with his coat-tails and cradling his face in his arms. Such
a position will prevent him from being thrown about by the blast and
should be maintained for half a minute or so, until the blast waves are over
and flying objects have ceased to fall.

It should be always borne in mind that the majority of atomic bomb injuries are likely to be due to mechanical violence. Lying prone upon the
ground will greatly reduce the chances of such injury. Keeping the head
and other exposed parts of the body covered will protect them against
flash burns and will keep foreign particles out of the eyes, nose and mouth.

It is true that if the victim happens to be within roughly a half mile
of the bomb his chances of survival are not good, but on the other hand,
if he is between one and two miles from the explosion his chances are, on
the average, very good. No one can predict just where an atomic bomb will
explode, and even after its intense flash has illuminated the entire area, it
will be very difficult to judge how far away from the burst one happens to
be. The best thing is to act intelligently, and without confusion, and take
cover instantly.

After a minute or two, when the air is clear of flying debris, the immediate
danger is past, and one may get up if unhurt and, using proper methods of
first aid, try to help others who may have been injured. If police, firemen, or
civil defense wardens are about, one should be guided by their instructions.
The individual must maintain his efforts to keep calm, must not shout or
rush aimlessly about, and must refrain from saying or doing anything which
might cause a panic.

People within ranges for serious, lethal or supralethal radiation dosage
are obviously candidates for radiation illness and death but the picture is
complicated by factors of shielding and other injuries. Many gradations of

exposure are likely along with various other injuries and burns. It is to be remembered that persons within lethal radiation ranges are not likely to survive other effects unless protected in substantial structures. Those potentially exposed to dangerous amounts require medical supervision even though not ill or only temporarily so. After a symptom free interval of perhaps several weeks many may become seriously ill from delayed effects. These people, too, are adversely affected by heavy exertions and exposure to extremes of temperature.

11. Finally, each householder should learn what steps to take to minimize damage to his property and injury to members of his household, and this he should do, not only for protection of his family, but to be able to save himself such worry and anxiety on their account as might lead him to behave rashly, with disastrous consequences to himself and others.

16.4 Atom Bomb Protection in the Home

16.4.1 *Subsurface Burst.* If an atomic bomb is detonated on or under the ground, or beneath the surface of a body of water, its blast effects will be radically reduced. The result will be fewer houses and buildings destroyed, and fewer fires started. Accordingly, fewer people will be killed or injured. But owing to the dispersal and surface deposit of radioactive fission products and debris, the radiation hazard will be much greater than in the case of high air burst. Many persons, caught in the open and subjected to a deluge of radioactive spray or rain, may receive a fatal dose of radiation before they can gain shelter where decontamination is possible. The initial intensity is enormous. Fortunately most fission products and other radioactive isotopes decay very rapidly, so that this form of atomic bomb hazard is necessarily of relatively short duration. In any case ordinary houses and buildings offer more or less protection against the fission product hazard, providing that doors and windows remain intact and closed, and that any ventilating systems are shut off or properly filtered. The roofs and outside surfaces of buildings will of course become contaminated—dangerously so for the first few hours;—due to gamma rays (0.7 mev average) even substantial structures will permit of serious exposures, in particular to those remaining near outer walls and roofs. This is an important shelter factor in areas subject to this type of danger. In general, however, where due regard can be and is paid to this hazard there will probably be, even in the most heavily contaminated areas, sufficient time "to seek shelter" before anyone receives a dangerous dose. It is chiefly a matter of keeping distance and barriers between oneself and the contamination. The civil defense authorities can be relied upon to issue the instructions as to where to go and what routes to follow. Until such instructions are received it is essential to remain indoors. The time spent in waiting may be occupied by preparations whenever possible; putting on overshoes or wrapping the shoes with several layers of rags, securing raincoats, gloves, and hats, packing a bag with cans of food and a first aid kit, and in other ways preparing for departure from the radioactive area. If there is a radio available one should listen constantly for instructions. It is expected that limited re-occupation of the contaminated area would commence within a few days.

Many people may be reluctant to leave valuable and cherished possessions unprotected. This should not be allowed to become a cause of delay, worry, or hysteria. The police and other authorities will keep an eye on their premises, so that these may well have as good, or better, protection than in normal times. Household pets should be placed on a leash and taken or carried along. Civil defense workers will have other things to do than to rescue or feed abandoned animals. The family car should if possible be parked off the street; however even if uncontaminated it should not be driven away unless permission has been broadcast to do so. Unauthorized usage of automobiles will have only one result—an impassable and dangerous traffic jam which might result in widespread panic and would certainly interfere with rescue and salvage work in the stricken area.

The safety of thousands of people—including members of one's own family—will depend upon orderly and prompt obedience to the instructions of proper authorities.

16.4.2 *Air Burst.* Against such a burst most ordinary buildings, aside from those of reinforced concrete construction, offer insufficient protection. It is therefore prudent for each householder to arrange a shelter area in his basement or cellar. This should be cleared of heavy, sharp, or fragile objects which might fall, shift or become missiles when the house is subjected to blast. If the floor above is not adequately supported, it should be reenforced by a strong beam and stanchion. Alternate means of exit should be provided, and the basement shelter should be equipped with emergency food, water and first aid supplies, flash lights, a radio and, if space is available, cots and blankets. If the supply of electricity is to be cut off, the radio of the family car might be left on if near enough to be heard. Portable battery-operated radios are helpful but it should be remembered that fresh batteries are likely to be scarce during wartime. In any case the wardens will pass along all needed information. An axe should be available in case it should be required to escape through a blocked exit, and a shovel and several buckets or boxes of sand are useful to fight fire. If no toilet facilities exist in the basement, a suitable covered vessel should be provided for use during an alert. Other emergency equipment and supplies, as recommended by civil defense authorities, may be stored in the shelter, including warm outer clothing, overshoes, gloves, hats, ready for use if the house must be evacuated.

The rest of the house should be cleared of all unneeded accumulations of paper, cleaning fluids, and other inflammables. On each floor and in the attic fire-fighting equipment should be provided.

At the sound of an air-raid warning signal, occupants of the house should immediately proceed to their shelter unless the house is afire. In this rare contingency, if the blaze cannot be rapidly extinguished, shelter must be found elsewhere. Whether or not the light switch should be opened or the gas shut off depends upon local regulations; usually water, gas, and electricity are all to be shut off. All open flames must be put out. In the basement, it is a good idea to fill the washing machine or laundry tub with clean water, immediately after the alert has sounded, for use in case of interruption of the water supply. A bathtub upstairs may be filled if this can be done without hazard or delay in seeking cover. The water supply should then be shut off.

Unless otherwise instructed, all persons should remain under cover until the all-clear is sounded. The urge periodically to leave the shelter to go outside and look up and down the block should be strongly resisted.

16.5 Group Shelter (See also 16.2.1)

Dwellers in apartment houses, hotels, auto courts, housing developments, or densely settled residential sections, inmates of hospitals, prisons and other institutions, theater patrons, and other gatherings or congregations will probably find that community shelter areas have been designated in their immediate vicinity. In many cities air-raid precautions have been adopted by the school systems and school children have been drilled for some time in procedures for taking shelter.

It is desirable to emphasize that regular drills and practice alerts will be most helpful in determining the most practical techniques to be adopted by a civil defense organization and by individual citizens alike, not only in the matter of shelter, but for other phases of protection as well.

The protection of workers and property in industrial plants, warehouses and large mercantile or other business establishments must necessarily constitute a large and crucial portion of any community disaster plan. Each plant will be found to have its own peculiar problems and the reader must be referred to the bibliography for a number of excellent references which are available on this subject. The principle of using the utmost foresight in preventing injury from blast, fire, and radiation is of course the keynote of industrial disaster preparedness as it is in any other type of plan. In the case of industrial and commercial establishments, the necessary preparations, drills, and rehearsals will be costlier than in residential buildings, but such preparedness is none-the-less necessary if maximum safety is to be provided. During World War II the workers of Great Britain were said to have stayed on the job in many war plants during enemy air raids but, then again, they had only ordinary high explosive bombs and fire-bombs to contend with. The chances of an industrial plant escaping serious damage from an atomic blast one or two miles away are almost nil. Without adequate bomb proofing or relocation of the plant, which in most cases is out of the question, there is no alternative but work stoppage to permit employees to seek shelter during an alert. This factor has been given deep consideration by industrial planners. Industrially, atomic defense may be regarded as an extension of existing arrangements for plant safety.

16.6 The Warden Service

If self-protection and household protection are the building-stones of the wall of civil defense, the warden service is the mortar which holds the structure firmly together. While it is entirely possible and even mandatory for individuals and families to adopt means successfully to survive an atomic attack, it is almost equally necessary that the community services and organizations also survive. Neither end could be achieved without a properly functioning warden service. Furthermore, the warden serves as the lifeline, the source of help if need be, between the individual and his civil defense organization.

It is not too much to say that the over-all effectiveness of a community diaster plan may be judged by the efficiency of its warden service and by the quality and training of its personnel. The World War II figure of the arm-banded, tin-hatted "air-raid warden" idly swinging his baton or flashlight during an "alert" or a "blackout" must be replaced with a person of far greater stature and authority in his job.

Indeed, the warden service is the feature of a civil defense organization which distinguishes it from the normally functioning protective services of a community. Fire protection, police protection, and health protection are always present to a degree. But the warden service exists only in civil defense, as a necessary bond to make the facilities of the community available to its citizens in time of great danger.

Block or building wardens must be selected with the greatest care and judgment on the part of the community civil defense authorities. It would probably be better to have no wardens at all than to appoint persons who are not well known or respected among their neighbors or co-workers. There is much that a warden must learn about rescue, fire fighting and first aid, and he must take time to learn all pertinent facts about the houses, buildings and people in his block. He must be able to extend his training to his neighbors and in many other ways secure their cooperation, and at the same time be able to offer all assistance to police, fire-fighters, rescue workers and others during a disaster. He must possess, in short, adequate qualities of leadership.

Principles governing the selection, organization, training and functioning of wardens may vary somewhat in different communities, but it is believed that best results will be obtained if wardens are granted sufficient authority to carry out their jobs. The public, also, must be made to understand that the safety of all may depend to a large extent upon the effectiveness of their cooperation with their wardens.

16.7 Community Problems (See also 16.8)

These are many and varied and in general fairly well recognized. It is proper to note here however that the perils of the day make it an urgent matter that all communities, and not merely the large ones, take stock of their individual circumstances and problems. If not prime targets themselves, they may well be in fallout areas. Again they may be called on for support and the housing of evacuees.

The problems relating to rescue and care of injured are naturally foremost in mind but it must not be overlooked that serious public health problems must also be met. These relate to such matters as food, water, housing, waste disposal, immunization, decontamination, radiological surveys and care of dead. Complex administrative problems will require solution especially where more than one city or state is concerned in a metropolitan area.

Cooperation of neighboring communities in limiting traffic to or from a threatened city is also important.

The lesson is clear. In order to be prepared for atomic attack, a community must possess a system of clearly audible sirens or other warning devices, and must have enough well-trained civil defense manpower to be able to control and to manage the situation promptly. Important as the medical or other portions of a disaster organization may be, there can be no substitute for avoidance of injury in the first place. The way to avoid injury is to take shelter.

16.8 Medical Plans and Problems

16.8.1 *Casualty Estimates**. It is recognized that these are bound to be high, but some approximation on a local basis is valuable for guidance in action. Lt. Col. Steer, U. S. A., describes a practical method based on early inspection by helicopter or light plane and assuming prior planning and knowledge of population density. The center of bomb damage, size of

---

* 16.8.1 contributed by editor.

crater and zone of complete destruction are reported along with visability. From these casualty probabilities are derivable and are based on zones. The zone of complete destruction results from overpressures of 15–35 psi or more plus 40–1000 or more cal/sq. cm. flash heat. This zone is likely to show 90 % killed and 10 % injured. A second zone with 10–15 psi and 10–40 cal/sq. cm. heat shows severe damage to all but heavily reinforced structures with 60 % killed, 30 % injured and 10 % uninjured. A third zone with 5–10 psi and 3–8 cal figures for 35 % killed, 50 % injured and 15 % uninjured. The fourth zone with 2–5 psi and 3–8 cal would show collapse of frame buildings with 10 % killed, 30 % injured and 60 % uninjured. Warning should reduce the number killed by 10–15 %.

The various zone areas are related to the zone of complete destruction as follows:

RAD. COMPLETE DESTRUCTION IN MILES	ZONE AREAS IN SQUARE MILES			
	I	II	III	IV
0.4	0.5	0.3	0.3	2.7
0.6	1.1	0.7	0.7	6.6
0.8	2.0	1.1	1.4	10.7
1.0	3.1	1.7	2.2	15.8
1.3	5.3	2.7	3.3	25.0

On a *national basis* figures from "Operation Alert" quoted in a congressional report suggest 12 million casualties surviving the first day after an all-out attack on the U. S. and its possessions, with about ⅓ eventual recoveries. Deaths were estimated at 3.9 million from fallout radiation out of a total of 16¼ million dead. This would indicate an approximate 25 % addition to the customary estimate of 15 % fatalities based on Japanese experience with radiation casualties.

As to severity, estimates indicate the probability of 40 % minimal cases returnable to duty at once, 20 % requiring immediate care to save life or limb, 20 % who can wait for delayed care, and 20 % so-called "expectant" cases requiring complicated and prolonged care.

In the face of such possibilities our C. D. stockpiles are now substantial but in need of considerable increase. Supplies for three weeks care of 4¼ million casualties were reported as available early in 1956 and have been increased since. It is also good to note that *emergency hospital units* have been designed and made available. Characteristics are as follows: Transportation, single motor trailer truck; storage space 2000 cu feet; assembly time 4 hours by professionals with auxiliary aid; minimum floor space 14,000 sq. feet; equipment for 3 operating rooms; generator; 500 gal. nylon tank.

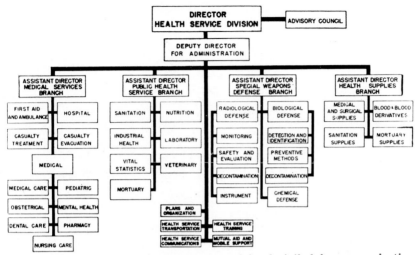

Fig. 1. Health service functions. State and local civil defense organizations (Through the courtesy of the Federal Civil Defense Administration.)

TABLE I

CITY	TOTAL STRUCTURES REPORTED	TYPES OF STRUCTURES BY EXTERIOR MATERIAL (UNITED STATES CITIES)			
		Wood	Brick	Stucco	Other Materials*
New York...............	591,319	236,879	229,482	41,661	13,297
Washington...............	156,359	48,971	95,939	5,764	5,685
Chicago..................	382,628	131,148	238,959	5,797	6,724
Detroit...................	267,677	165,488	94,333	1,923	5,933
San Francisco.............	105,180	61,172	2,334	40,902	722

Source: Sixteenth Census of the United States (1940), Vol. II.
* Includes blast-resistant buildings.
From: The United States Strategic Bombing Survey: The Effects of Atomic Bombs on Hiroshima and Nagasaki. Washington, D. C.: U. S. Government Printing Office, 30 June, 1946.

16.8.2 *Mutual support* is another aspect of planning which requires special effort. The persistent tendency for medical, dental, and allied professional people to collect themselves in several "professional" buildings of a city is still a characteristic of urban practice. This means that the services of most of these practitioners should not be depended upon in an atomic attack—only the blindest good fortune will prevent them from playing the roles of casualties. Instead, their places in the medical relief organization should be filled by personnel of mobile support teams from outlying communities. This is a most serious problem for every city.

Not only is a loss of medical personnel likely in the event of an atomic bombing, but a loss of facilities, vehicles, and supplies is probable. These deficiencies likewise will have to be made up by the equipment of mobile support teams.

Needless to add, all anticipated losses must be most carefully calculated in advance, to allow for adequate planning, organization, equipment and training of mobile teams. In addition, the requirements of all adjacent communities must be met by proper coordination on the part of the appropriate county, state, or interstate civil defense authorities. There is some indication of coordination in such matters as traffic control, fire-fighting and police aid, but similar efforts are needed for emergency medical services.

Almost every important community in the country has at the time of this writing been provided with some form of disaster plan, including

TABLE II

Population Densities

CITY	POPULATION DENSITIES, UNITED STATES AND JAPANESE CITIES		POPULATION DENSITY PER SQ. MILE
	Population	Area sq. mile	
New York.....................	7,492,000	322.8	23,200
Manhattan (day)...............	3,200,000	22.2	145,000
Manhattan (night).............	1,689,000	22.2	76,000
Bronx........................	1,493,700	41.4	34,000
Brooklyn.....................	2,792,600	80.9	34,200
Queens.......................	1,340,500	121.1	11,000
Staten Island.................	176,200	57.2	3,000
Washington...................	663,091	61.4	11,000
Chicago......................	3,396,808	206.7	16,500
Detroit......................	1,623,452	137.9	11,750
San Francisco................	634,536	44.6	14,250
Hiroshima....................	340,000*	26.5	12,750
Center of City...............	140,000†	4.0	35,000
Nagasaki.....................	250,000*	35.0	7,000
Built-up Area................	220,000†	3.4	65,000

* Prewar.

† As of 1 Aug. 1945.

Source: New York: Fortune, July 1939; other United States cities: Sixteenth Census of the United States (1940).

From: U. S. Strategic Bombing Survey: The Effects of Atomic Bombs on Hiroshima and Nagasaki. Washington, D. C.: U. S. Government Printing Office, 30 June, 1946.

TABLE III

Critical Target Areas of a Million or More Population (based on 1950 census)

Baltimore, Maryland	1,337,373
Boston, Massachusetts	2,369,986
Buffalo, New York	1,089,230
Chicago, Illinois and Indiana	5,495,364
Cleveland, Ohio	1,465,511
Detroit, Michigan	3,016,197
Los Angeles, California	4,367,911
Minneapolis-St. Paul, Minnesota	1,116,509
Philadelphia, Pennsylvania, New Jersey	3,671,048
Pittsburgh, Pennsylvania	2,213,236
New York and N.E. New Jersey	12,911,944
St. Louis, Missouri, Illinois	1,681,281
San Francisco-Oakland, California	2,240,767
Washington, D. C.-Maryland-Virginia	1,464,089

From F.C.D.A. list of Metropolitan target areas, July 1, 1953.

among its most important features a plan for medical care of the population. Space simply will not permit adequate critical discussion of such plans and, in any event, it must be accepted that a medical plan which suits one community will not necessarily be adequate or appropriate for another community. It is desired, however, to state as a matter of opinion that few of the plans which have been studied by the writer provide sufficiently for change of plan to meet changing needs. No preparations must be made which are so inflexible that they can not be altered to meet changing conditions. It is indeed well that a plan for medical care be as all inclusive and as anticipatory of details as practicable but the inclusion of all the innumerable requirements which must be met at the time of disaster must by no means be so rigorously observed as to prevent appropriate action to meet unforeseen eventualities. To take liberties with the poet, the really "best laid plans" do not "gang aglee." In order to insure that a plan will meet changing needs, constant review is necessary and arrangements which are thereby found to be inadequate or improbable of successful application must be properly changed at no matter what cost.

16.9 Minimum Requirements

It is hoped that the following paragraphs will be of service to acquaint the reader with minimum needs which must be met "when the chips are down" at the time of disaster.

16.9.1 *Rescue.* Authorities wisely consider that the rescue of trapped and injured people from burning or damaged structures is properly a task for specially trained and equipped personnel using, if necessary, cranes, shovels, and other heavy equipment. This is not to say that an uninjured person

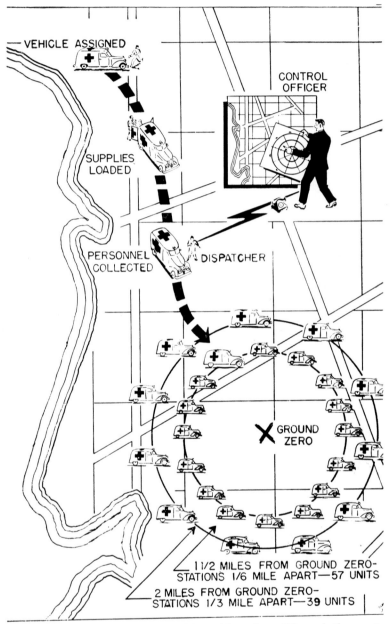

FIG. 2. Mobilization and location of first aid services. (Through the courtesy of the Federal Civil Defense Administration.)

must await the arrival of a rescue team before extricating an imprisoned victim if he can do so without injuring the latter or increasing the extent of his entrapment. In the event of an atomic bombing there will be many instances of rescue in which delay would have proved fatal. On the whole, however, it may properly be said that rescue operations are not a function of medical personnel.

16.9.2 *First Aid.* Most plans provide that first aid to an injured victim must be applied by the first person who reaches him whether it be his nearest uninjured neighbor, a member of a rescue team, a stretcher bearer, or any other. It is actually mandatory and not merely desirable that all persons receive some form of first aid training. Civil defense authorities urge that every one possible be given training in the American Red Cross first aid training program. The American Red Cross has had many long years of experience in the establishment of first aid training courses and in providing this most necessary instruction. At this time in our preparations for national civil defense there would be little profit in debating the merits of this or that system of rendering first aid treatment for hemorrhage, shock, burns, or any other injury or condition. The methods of the American Red Cross should be accepted as standard. Finally let us remember that elementary training on a broad basis must be supplemented by advanced and thorough training of a considerable group. These workers will be needed for supervision and instruction and also for aid in many capacities. Doctors and nurses will be overwhelmed and need lots of really able assistance— the type of assistance we find notably in the Services and in particular the Navy where the possibility of independent duty necessitates high level training of enlisted personnel of the hospital corps. Highly skilled personnel of this type should not however be detailed to rescue groups but utilized in the emergency stations and hospitals.

16.9.3 *Emergency Stations.* The chief activities here relate to: (1) sorting of casualties or triage, a most important matter; (2) prompt care of minor injuries and return of such cases to duty or effective status; (3) emergency treatment for shock and initial care of seriously injured. This may call for use of plasma, plasma expanders, serum albumin and possibly type O whole blood. This last procedure however may have to be reserved for hospitals. There will be great shortages initially. (4) Relief of pain; (5) immobilization of fractures; (6) tetanus and other prophylaxis; (7) antibiotics as indicated; (8) possibly decontamination; (9) sedation; (10) dispatch of cases to appropriate hospitals for definitive treatment; (11) ancillary matters such as records, registration, care of valuables, mortuary arrangements, communications, information.

A considerable staff is required for a large station and comprises 3 doctors, 2 dentists or veterinarians, 3 nurses, 8 nurses' aides, 20 first aid technicians, and 1 chaplain plus orderlies, clerks, an administrative assistant and a field force of 105 litter bearers, 27 first aid men, 16 ambulance drivers, along with orderlies and messengers.

16.9.4 *Definitive Treatment of Disaster Victims.* Definitive care of victims of an atomic disaster can only be provided at a temporary or permanent hospital. It is assumed that all communities which have formulated disaster plans have recognized that the existing permanent peace-time hospitals must be augmented by an adequate number of emergency hospitals appropriately dispersed throughout the area. The designation of such emergency hospitals, whether they be located in school buildings, warehouses, stadiums, auditoriums, or any other type of structure, must be followed up by the addition of a supply facility for the storage of beds and other needed hospital furniture and equipment. This furniture and equipment must be quickly available at the emergency hospital site or it is likely that there will be none at the time of disaster. Likewise, non-perishable food supplies and adequate quantities of medical and surgical stores to meet the needs of the first 4 to 24 hours of operation must be on hand. After the first few hours, of course, supplies may be replenished from central civil defense supply centers.

The emergency hospital must be able to provide all the services of a permanent hospital including all forms of emergency and after-care, perhaps in some instances convalescent care. Certainly, provision must also be made for care of the dead. Again the importance of a standardized system of record-keeping must be stressed and means must be available for the movement of recovered persons to their homes or other shelter.

While special wards or facilities for the care of radiation victims may not be necessary at once, it would be well to keep in mind that such cases will occur, and that materials and methods must be provided for this purpose. The heretofore accepted figure of only 15 % of fatalities from radiation will prove far too low in the event of heavy fallout and there will be huge numbers of non-fatal cases. Some persons may even be the victims of blast, burns, and radiation. In an atomic bombing, the factor of radiation injury will inevitably be one of great magnitude for the civil defense organization.

16.9.5 *Rehabilitation.* While the economic rehabilitation of bombing victims is not properly a medical matter, it is not difficult to foresee that the psychological and physiological aspects of rehabilitation will ultimately be a major concern of the medical services of a stricken community. For this and other reasons the closest cooperation is urged between the disaster medical organization and those of other services and agencies involved in the rehabilitation organization.

16.9.6 *Panic.* The occurrence of panic need not be considered as inevitable given a well organized and trained disaster organization and a well informed public. As in so many other aspects of civil defense the prevention and control of panic may be met by the execution of an appropriate program of training and preparation. This is a specialized problem requiring the participation of several services of the civil defense organization, including those of public information, medical service, police and warden service among others. It need not be feared that every disaster must be characterized by the same mass hysteria which led to the tragedy of the Cocoanut Grove fire in Boston. Psychiatrists and psychologists believe that panic is preventable.

16.9.7 *Routine Medical Care.* In every sizable community a certain proportion of the population is at all times under medical care, either ambulatory or as bed patients, in their homes or in hospitals. Of this number a smaller proportion is acutely, seriously, or critically ill. Means must be found to care for these people even during the height of any disaster. Those who are too gravely ill to be moved to a place of shelter must nevertheless be sheltered and protected from additional harm in every way possible. Shelter wards should be established without delay in all permanent hospitals. To these wards all bed patients capable of being moved may be transferred if there is sufficient time. Patients capable of helping themselves must be provided with assistance and guidance to places of shelter. Medical societies should establish a system of providing those who are sick at home with necessary medical and surgical care. This may prove to be one of the most difficult problems confronting the medical profession in time of disaster and has not been given sufficient consideration in civil defense planning.

In a similar manner, the routine requirements of public health and sanitation must be met even while extraordinary public health measures are being instituted.

16.9.8 *Other Special Weapons.** In keeping with the general orientation of this volume this chapter has dealt only with nuclear weapons. However, before closing it is appropriate to make brief reference to other special weapons.

Chemical or biological warfare could readily be used in an "all out" attack to complicate and aggravate the effects of atomic bombs. Mass casualties are possible from chemical warfare, particularly the nerve gases. Biological warfare has many possibilities for evil and lends itself readily to sabotage. These possibilities must be taken into serious account in connection with plans for atomic defense.

Nerve gases are really liquids which can form lethal vapors or aerosols and also be directly absorbed. They rapidly disorganize the functional mechanism of nerve endings. This mechanism produces a nice balance

* Par. 16.9.8 contributed by editor.

between production of acetylcholine as needed for stimulation and its destruction by the enzyme cholinesterinase to prevent excessive effects. The nerve gases irreversibly inactivate cholinesterinase and accordingly acetylcholine persists and accumulates, thereby causing gross over-stimulation.

The clinical picture that develops first features parasympathetic disturbances resulting in smooth muscle spasm and hypersecretion. The eyes show miosis and ciliary spasm. Breathing becomes difficult. There is watery nasal discharge. In severe cases symptoms progress toward cyanosis and asphyxia, nausea, diarrhea, muscular twitchings, convulsions, paralysis and death.

The sovereign remedy is atropine early and in liberal doses of $\frac{1}{30}$ gr repeated as the situation may call for.

Anticonvulsants will be needed; also many people familiar with resuscitation methods. The newer back pressure arm lift method (Holger Nielsen) adopted by the Armed Services, is preferable to the old Shaeffer method which is particularly ineffective when paralysis is present.*

Biological warefare possibilities demand chiefly alertness to any atypical epidemiological features of the various diseases of people, animals and plants and prompt reporting.

Laboratories of the cities, States and Public Health Service can be prepared to deal promptly with identification problems and provision, as appropriate of immunological materials.

16.10 Conculsion

The appalling possibilities for mass destruction which confront the world at the present time must not be met by hopeless resignation nor by the consoling idea that things will somehow turn out all right and that we need not "cross our bridges until we get to them." Such lines of thinking can lead only to the unnecessary magnification of the disaster when it occurs. True, there is no wrong in hoping that an atomic war will never materialize, but no plan should be based on over-optimism. Conceding that atomic bombing of crowded industrial and metropolitan centers constitutes the worst possible kind of disaster, plans for civil defense have wisely been based upon this premise. But since no plan is better than its capability of being put into action, it is not too much to say that our only guarantee of successful survival in a possible atomic war is in the will of people to contribute their best efforts toward the execution of the plan. This means participation by virtually everyone, before disaster strikes. Since the aim of civil defense is to assure survival of the people and their institutions against military or other catastrophe, the medical and allied

---

* Mouth to mouth methods either direct or via some simple device now being advocated.

professions bear a responsibility second to none—a responsibility which must ever demand the maximum efforts of all of their members.

REFERENCES

Civil Defense for National Survival. House Report No. 2946, 84th Congress, 2nd Session 1956, Supr. of Documents, Washington 25, D. C.

Effects of Nuclear Weapons, 1957, U. S. Department of Defense, Published by U.S.A. E.C., For Sale by Supr. of Documents, Washington 25, D. C.

F.C.D.A. Items, Procurable from Supr. of Documents, Washington 25, D. C.

Atomic Energy and Civil Defense Price List of Publications, 2nd Ed., April, 1957, PL 84.

Civil Defense Household First Aid Kit (revision) 1954, FCD 1.3: 11-12.

Emergency Medical Treatment 1953, FCD 1. 6/3: 11-8.

Evacuation Check List 1955, Technical Bulletin, FCD 1.3: 27-2.

Evacuation of Civilian Populations in Civil Defense Emergencies, 1955, FCD 1.3: 27-1.

Family Action Program, Home Protection Exercises, revised, 1956, 1957.

Interim Guide for Design of Buildings, Exposed to Atomic Blast, Revised 1956, FCD 1.6/3: 5-3.

National Plan for Civil Defense Against Enemy Attack, F.C.D.A.

Operational Planning, TM-8-2.

Operation Cue for Survival, 1956, FCD 1.2: Op2/2.

Role of Warden in H-Bomb Era, 1955, FCD 1.3: 27-3.

Role of Warden in Panic Prevention, Revised 1955, FCD 1.3: 7-1.

Target Areas for Civil Defense Purposes, Official List as of July 1, 1953.

What To Do Now About Emergency Sanitation at Home, Revised 1957, H-11-1.

What You Should Know About Radioactive Fallout, Revised 1956, FCD 1.17/2: 7.

HARTGERING, J. B.: Lt. Col. MC, U. S. Army, Sorting and Classification of Casualties. *Military Med. 118:* 4, 307–310, 1956.

NABATH, R. P.: Cdr. (MC) U. S. Navy: Some Rules of Thumb in Estimating Radiologic Hazards. *Armed Forces M. J. VI:* Aug. 1955.

Project East River—The Strategy of Civil Defense. *Bull. Atomic Scientists. IX:* No. 7, 1953.

SHILLING, C. W.: Twentieth Century Warfare. In: "The Human Machine". U. S. Naval Institute, Annapolis, Maryland 1955.

SMITH, R. L.: Emergency Medical Care. *Military Med. 118:* 4, 311–313, 1956.

STEER, A.: Casualty Estimates in Nuclear Warfare. *Military Med. 118:* 4, 300–304, 1956.

WHITNEY, J. M.: Initial Aid and Rescue. *Military Med. 118:* 4, 305–306, 1956.

17▸

Particle Accelerators

LAWRENCE H. LANZL, PH.D.

17.1 Introduction

During the last quarter century, the particle accelerator has been one of the primary tools of nuclear and radiation physics research. It is used to produce high-energy particles which are the projectiles for nuclear scattering and disintegration experiments, and which are used for the production of high-energy x-rays.

Some of the early types of accelerators are the cyclotron, Cockcroft-Walton generator, Van de Graaff generator, and betatron. Over the past decade, several new types have been developed, including the synchrotron and the traveling-wave linear accelerator. As the operational reliability of these machines has improved, due to advances in accelerator engineering, new uses for them have been emerging, among them applications to medicine.

This chapter starts with a resumé of some of the basic principles of physics governing the operation of accelerators. The middle portion consists of a description of some of the various types. The final section is a brief discussion of some of the medical and biological uses of accelerators including supervoltage therapy.

17.2 Physical Principles and Components Basic to All Particle Accelerators

Particle accelerators are needed for the production of high-energy particles or high-energy x-radiation. In the acceleration process, energy is imparted to electrically charged particles or ions by the force exerted upon them when they are placed in an electric field. Although the atoms of any of the elements can be electrically charged by the addition or subtraction of orbital electrons, and these in principle could be accelerated, the present-day accelerators have been designed primarily for the acceleration of the very lightest atoms and of electrons. One of the chief reasons for this is that nuclear disintegration is much more readily achieved by the use of light rather than heavy high-energy particles. In the collision of a heavy ion with a target nucleus, a large portion of the energy of the projectile ion is spent in setting the target nucleus in motion, leaving only a small fraction of the energy available for disintegration.

The light particles under discussion here include electrons, and the nuclei of the hydrogen atom (proton), of heavy hydrogen (deuteron), and helium (alpha particle), although some heavier ones, namely, oxygen, nitrogen, and carbon, are in present-day use. On the other hand, electrically neutral particles (neutrons, neutrinos, neutral mesons) and photons (x-rays, gamma rays) do not experience a force from an electric field and, therefore, do not undergo acceleration directly. They in turn are produced by high-energy charged particles. (The physical properties of some of the light particles are given in the table of par. 5.16.)

17.2.1 *Ion Sources.* A component common to all accelerators is the ion source. Its purpose is not only to provide a sufficient number of ions to be accelerated, but also to supply them to the accelerator at the proper location and at the proper time.

The ion source for electron accelerators is composed of a hot wire or filament with a directing grid. Oxide coated and pure tungsten filaments are among those which have been successful. The mechanism of electron release in the filament wire is identical to that in a vacuum tube, namely, by the process of "boiling off" of electrons due to an elevated temperature.

The ion source of a positive ion accelerator is somewhat more complex. A tank of hydrogen is needed for a proton source, and helium for an alpha source. A small continuous and controllable supply of gas must be fed into an air-free region. One of several methods, which is used for hydrogen, is to admit the gas by means of an electrically heated palladium tube. The amount of hydrogen which diffuses through palladium depends on the temperature. Since the temperature is easily controllable and also can be held constant fairly easily, such a palladium leak provides the necessary conditions for the gas supply.

There are several methods of ionizing the gas. One is by the use of radiofrequency, another by means of an electric arc. The hydrogen or helium arc is supported by a hot filament. The positive ions are extracted by means of a negative voltage placed on a probe, which attracts the positive ions and injects them into the accelerator proper.

17.2.2 *Vacuum Chamber.* Each accelerator has a vacuum chamber in which the ions undergo acceleration. Its form depends on the type of accelerator. The chamber is evacuated to provide an air-free region to prevent the ions from losing energy and from being scattered by collision with the constituent gas molecules of air. Scattering must be minimized because the ions must maintain a definite orbit for proper acceleration.

Accelerators operate in vacua of the order of 10^{-4} to 10^{-6} mm of mercury. The lower figure represents a pressure approximately equal to one-billionth of atmospheric pressure. Some of the electron accelerators have sealed-off accelerating tubes. However, heavy ion accelerators demand tubes which are continuously pumped since the ion source continually admits gas to the accelerator. Here the necessary low pressures are obtainable by means of a mechanical forepump operating in series with a diffusion pump. A rather recent development is the getter or evapor-ion pump, which sometimes requires only intermittent degassing of the accelerator tube.

17.2.3 *Electric Field—the Accelerating Agent.* The force on an ion is equal to the product of the electric field strength and the charge of the ion. The energy gain is the product of the distance through which the ion moves and the component of force in the direction of motion of the particle. The total energy of a particle is given by Einstein's well-known expression, mc^2, where m is the mass of the particle and c, the velocity of light. If we consider an example in which a particle is accelerated from rest, the energy gain is found by subtracting the rest energy from the total energy. The rest energy is equal to the rest mass times c^2. (The mass of particles quoted in tables of mass is the rest mass—see table, par. 5.16.)

The energy gain can thus be written as follows:

$$qEd = mc^2 - m_0c^2, \tag{1}$$

where q = the charge of the particle,
  m_0 = the rest mass of the particle,
  m = the mass of the particle after acceleration,
  c = the velocity of light in a vacuum,
  E = the magnitude of the electric field in the direction of motion,
  d = the distance traversed by the particle while being accelerated by the field E.

Example (1). This equation may be illustrated by an example. If an accelerator produces an electric field E in the direction of motion of, say, an alpha particle, of 2,000,000 volts per meter and the particle travels a distance d of 20 meters, and if the charge is equal to twice the charge of the electron, the energy gain will equal

$qEd = 2 \times$ electron charge $\times$ 2,000,000 [volts/meter] $\times$ 30 [meters]

  $= 120,000,000$ electron (charge) volts

  $= 120$ million electron volts [mev].

Since the rest energy of an alpha particle is 3,730 mev, the gain in energy of 120 mev represents a small fractional increase in total energy or mass.

Example (2). If an electron, on the other hand, were to be subjected to the same conditions, the energy gain would be

qEd = 1 × electron charge × 2,000,000 [volts/meter] × 30 [meters]

= 60 mev.

Since the rest energy of an electron is only 0.51 mev, an energy gain of 60 mev is a substantial one indeed and represents a mass increase of almost 12,000 %.

For these two examples, it is interesting to calculate the final velocity of the particle. This is done by means of another well-established physical law expressed by Einstein, namely,

$$m = m_0 \frac{1}{\sqrt{1 - \dfrac{v^2}{c^2}}}, \qquad (2)$$

where m, m_0, and c are defined as above and v is the velocity of the particle. Using the values of the above examples and the value $c = 3 \times 10^8$ meters/sec., one finds that the velocity of the alpha is 0.74×10^8 meters/sec. and that of the electron, 2.99×10^8 meters/sec. It is to be noted that the velocity of the alpha particle is small compared to the velocity of light, but that the velocity of the electron almost equals that of light.

17.2.4 *Electric Field, Magnetic Induction—the Steering Mechanism.* In the above section, the mechanism of the acceleration process was discussed. In this section, the concept of guiding or controlling the ions so that they may proceed in their proper path during acceleration will be considered. If it were possible to direct the ion initially and then have it proceed with no uncertainty of path, steering forces would not be so necessary in an accelerator. However, since this is not possible, due to such causes as initial direction, slight field irregularities, and residual air scattering, steering forces are needed except in special situations where the deviations from the ideal path are small compared with the distance through which the particle is accelerated.

Steering is achieved by means of a component of force transverse to the direction of the beam. This component is zero at the proper path of the particles but has some finite value away from it such that the direction of the force is to return the particle to its orbit.

Steering or focusing forces are either electric or magnetic or a combination of both. The force on a charge in an electric field was discussed in the above section and is pictorially represented in Fig. 1. If a particle of posi-

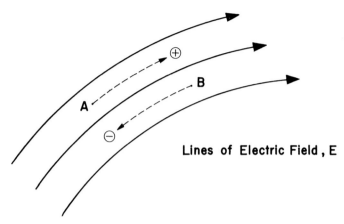

Lines of Electric Field, E

FIG. 1. *Particle movement in electric field.* A particle with a positive electric charge at position A, in an electric field E, will move (broken arrow) in the direction of the field lines (solid arrows). A particle at position B with negative charge will move in a parallel, but opposite direction.

tive electric charge is placed at position A, it will travel along the dotted line which is in the direction of the electric field, represented by solid arrows. On the other hand, a negatively charged particle at B will also travel along the electric field lines, as shown by the dotted line, but in the opposite direction.

The above representation assumes that the particles are initially at rest and are not scattered due to collisions with air. Both particles will gain energy as they move along in an electric field.

The force on a charge in an electric field is quite different from that in a magnetic field. The magnetic field is characterized by its induction B. If the induction is constant and the electric charge is not moving, for example, there is no force on the charge. If the particle is moving along the induction lines, there still is no force on it. However, if the particle is moving at some arbitrary direction to the magnetic induction, then there will be a force on it. For the case of a positive ion with velocity v in a field of induction B, the direction of the force is illustrated in Fig. 2. The direction is perpendicular to the plane formed by v and B. Since the force will change the direction of the particle, a circular orbit will be described for the case of a uniform magnetic field. Unlike the situation with an electric field, the force of magnetic induction does not add energy, nor does it take away energy from the particle since it is at right angles to the motion of the particle.

The sum of the electric and magnetic forces is combined in a single expression known as the Lorentz force,

$$\vec{f} = q(\vec{E} + \vec{v} \times \vec{B}), \tag{3}$$

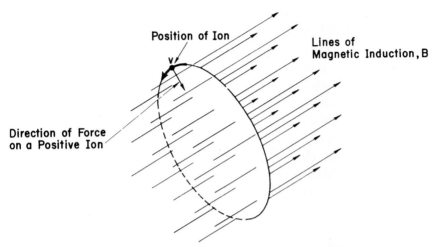

Position of Ion

Lines of
Magnetic Induction, B

Direction of Force
on a Positive Ion

FIG. 2. *Ion movement in magnetic field.* A positively charged ion moving in a magnetic field of induction B, at a velocity v, experiences a force perpendicular to both B and v, in the direction indicated.

where $\vec{E}$, $\vec{B}$, and $\vec{v}$ are vector quantities which have not only magnitude but also direction.

Besides the concept of steering or focusing which implies positional stability, another one, namely, time stability, is quite important in accelerator design. Time stability has meaning in the case of a periodic electric accelerating field. If an ion lags behind its proper phase angle in a periodic field and thereupon is subject to a greater field, it will advance in phase. If, on the other hand, the ion advances ahead of its proper phase angle and thereupon is subject to a smaller field, the reduced field will result in a lagging of the ion and its return to its proper phase angle. This condition is called phase stability.

Proper steering or focusing and phase stabilization are necessary for any accelerator. The conditions for these are not covered to any great degree in the description of the accelerators to follow. However, the references given discuss these points in some detail.

17.2.5 *Internal Target or Beam Extractor.* The accelerated electron or heavy particle emerges or is extracted from an accelerator and may be brought through a thin window, usually of metal and a few thousandths of an inch thick. The purpose of using a thin window rather than a thick one is to minimize both energy loss and scattering of the emergent particles.

In the use of internal target bombardment, the target material may be introduced into the vacuum chamber by means of a suitable air lock. In some cases, the internal target is used in electron accelerators merely for the production of x-rays and, therefore, need not be made removable.

17.3 Classification of Accelerators

A convenient way to classify accelerators is to divide them into two groups, namely, cyclic and linear. In the cyclic accelerator, the particles travel in circular orbits and undergo multiple transversals of the accelerating field. The cyclic accelerators include the cyclotron, synchrocyclotron, betatron, synchrotron, microtron, and fixed-field alternate-gradient accelerator. The group of accelerators in which acceleration occurs along a line are subdivided into electrostatic and linear. The electrostatic units include the Cockcroft-Walton, resonance transformer, and Van de Graaff. The linear accelerators include standing-wave and traveling-wave machines. The following sections will describe briefly the basic features of some of these types.

17.3.1 *Cyclotron.* The first successful cyclotron was constructed in 1931 by E. O. Lawrence and M. S. Livingston (1). At the present time, there are 26 in operation in the United States and 18 in other parts of the world (2). The energy range of these cyclotrons is from 1.8 mev to 200 mev, and they accelerate ions of hydrogen, deuterium, tritium, helium, nitrogen, carbon and oxygen.

A sketch of the cyclotron is shown in Fig. 3. The ion source is located in the geometrical center of the cyclotron. Within the vacuum tank, two hollow dee-shaped conducting electrodes are connected to a high-frequency voltage source. This voltage source supplies an alternating electric field, E, between the straight portions of the two "dees." A constant magnetic in-

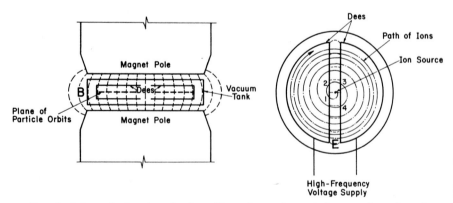

Fig. 3. *Schematic drawing showing side and top views of the central portion of a standard cyclotron.* The left-hand drawing is a side view of the magnet poles (the complete magnet is not shown) with the vacuum tank containing the dees. The magnetic induction B is indicated by the dashed lines between the poles. The right-hand drawing is a top view giving the position of the ion source and the path of the ions being accelerated. The high-frequency voltage supplies the accelerating field E shown by the dashed lines between the dees.

duction, B, is supplied at right angles to the dees by means of a magnet with poles above and below the vacuum tank. After positive ions leave the source, they are accelerated to position 1 shown in Fig. 3. Here they enter the dee, whose interior is free of electrical field but does contain a magnetic field. The ions, due to the magnetic induction, travel in a circular orbit to position 2. During this time, the high-frequency voltage supply has gone through one-half cycle, so that the direction of the electric field across the dees has now reversed. The ions undergo further acceleration in their path from position 2 to 3. From position 3 to 4 they are again acted upon solely by constant magnetic induction. By the time position 4 is reached, the electric field has again reversed and the field is yet again in a direction to cause further acceleration. This process is continued until the particles reach the outer edge of the dee, where they hit a target or are extracted from the cyclotron. The target or extraction device is located near the terminus of the ion path shown in the figure.

At any instant of time, when the ions are traveling in a circular orbit, the centrifugal force on the ions is balanced by the force due to the magnetic induction. This balance of radially directed forces is written in equation form,

$$\frac{mv^2}{r} = qvB, \tag{4}$$

where r is the radius of curvature of the path of the ion, m is the mass of the ion, and the other symbols are as defined above. This equation may be rewritten as follows:

$$r = \frac{mv}{Bq}. \tag{5}$$

Thus, for constant or nearly constant magnetic induction, constant mass, and, of course, charge, the radius of curvature increases as the ion velocity increases, as is indicated in Fig. 3. The angular velocity of the ion is equal to

$$\omega = \frac{v}{r} = \frac{Bq}{m}. \tag{6}$$

From this equation, one can see that the angular velocity is independent of the linear velocity, v, which means that an ion requires the same time to complete one revolution no matter whether it is traveling slowly near the center of the dees or fast close to the outer edge.

Figure 4 is a photograph of the cyclotron (3) of the Argonne National Laboratory which is located near Chicago. This unit is one of the largest conventional cyclotrons that it is practical to build. The hazy line in the

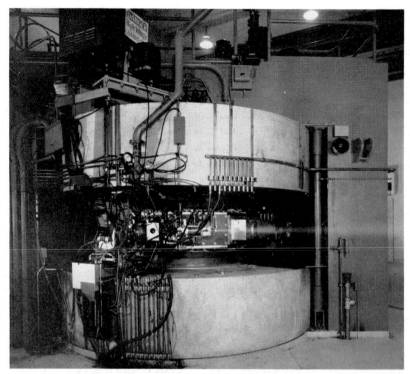

Fig. 4. *Overall view of the 158-cm-diameter cyclotron of the Argonne National Laboratory.* The exterior of the vacuum chamber is shown in the center of the picture, with the magnet poles immediately above and below it. The magnet energizing coils are housed in the large cylindrical boxes above and below the poles. The magnet yoke surrounds the entire unit, with the lower part below floor level. The ionization in air due to the emergent beam is visible toward the right. (Photograph through the courtesy of Argonne National Laboratory.)

center of the photograph is due to air ionization of the beam as it emerges from the vacuum tank. Directly above and below the vacuum tank are the magnet poles. The diameter of the poles is 1.58 meters. The rather large cylindrical-shaped boxes above the top pole and below the lower pole contain the magnet coils consisting of 1,099 turns of wire. The magnetic induction, B, between the poles has the value of 1.49 webers per square meter. Deuterons reach an energy of 21.6 mev with a beam current of 2×10^{-4} amperes with this machine. The high-frequency voltage supplies a potential of 240 kilovolts at a frequency of 11.2 megacycles per second.

17.3.2 *Synchrocyclotron.* As a consequence of equation (6), as mentioned above, when the magnetic induction B, the charge q, and the ion mass m remain constant, the time which it takes an ion to complete one revolution remains constant. However, as the energy of the particle increases, the mass also increases. For example, deuterons accelerated to 20 mev experience a mass increase of a little over 1 %. Thus, under actual conditions, the time to complete one revolution increases as the energy of the accelerating particle increases. Therefore, in a cyclotron whose high-frequency voltage is constant, the electric field across the dees will get out of synchronism with the ions crossing the dees. However, if the frequency of the voltage is reduced (modulated) and synchronized with the accelerating particles, they will continue to be accelerated and reach higher energies than with a fixed-frequency cyclotron. The concept of frequency modulation was suggested by Veksler (4) and independently by McMillan (5), and is used in the accelerator called the synchrocyclotron. In other respects, the synchrocyclotron operates like a standard cyclotron.

At this writing there are sixteen synchrocyclotrons throughout the world. The most energetic of these will accelerate protons to 680 mev.

17.3.3 *Betatron.* The cyclotron and synchrocyclotron are heavy ion accelerators, whereas the betatron is an electron accelerator. In principle, a betatron could be built to accelerate heavy ions, but it would require a magnet of enormous size and weight which would be uneconomical to build.

Like the cyclotron, the betatron is a cyclic accelerator. However, there are two fundamental differences between the two machines. These are: (1) The accelerating electric field is not produced by a high-frequency voltage source but by a time-varying magnetic flux, ϕ; and (2) the particles do not travel in ever increasing circular orbits but in an orbit of constant radius, R.

The first successful betatron was built by D. W. Kerst at the University of Illinois (6). Figure 5 is a sketch showing some of the major components as well as electron beam positions within the vacuum chamber which is called a "doughnut" because of its shape. The electron source within the vacuum chamber ejects electrons when the magnetic induction is very low. The electrons are magnetically focused and held in an equilibrium orbit during acceleration. The magnetic induction at the position of the equilibrium orbit increases proportionately with the magnetic flux within the orbit. Mathematically, this essential condition is written

$$\frac{\partial \phi}{\partial t} = 2\pi \, R^2 \, \frac{\partial B}{\partial t}, \qquad (7)$$

where $\partial\phi/\partial t$ is the time derivative of the flux, ϕ, enclosed by the equilibrium orbit of radius, R, and $\partial B/\partial t$ is the time derivative of the magnetic induction, B.

The magnetic induction undergoes rapid changes, producing eddy currents, which are prevented by the use of a laminated magnet as in the standard transformer. The space in the center of the vacuum doughnut is suffi-

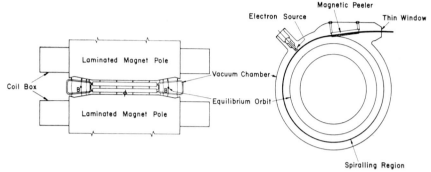

Fig. 5. *Schematic drawing of portions of a betatron.* The figure on the left is a cross sectional view of the vacuum chamber in position between the magnet poles and energizing coil boxes (the complete magnet is not shown). The direction of the magnetic induction B and flux ϕ is that of the arrows between the poles. The right-hand drawing is a sketch of the vacuum chamber showing the relative positions of the electron source, equilibrium orbit, spiraling region, magnetic peeler, and the window through which the electrons emerge. A doughnut for the production of x-rays alone would not contain a magnetic peeler, but instead a metal target.

ciently filled with magnetic material to satisfy the relationship given in equation (7).

After the electrons reach the desired energy, the conditions are changed to expand the orbit. The electrons on expansion reach a spiralling region where they either strike an internal target to produce an x-ray beam or are brought out of the machine. One means of beam extraction (7) employs a magnetic peeler which, placed in the spiralling region, provides a path free of magnetic induction through which the electrons pass, thus ceasing their cyclic motion and emerging as an external beam.

The electron energy of the various betatrons throughout the world ranges from 6 mev to 340 mev. Figures 6 and 7 are photographs of a 24-mev unit which is commercially available in the United States. The design of this machine closely resembles that of Kerst's second betatron. It has an equilibrium orbit with a radius of 0.2 meters and produces 180 electron pulses per second. The vacuum chamber has a cross section of 9 cm by 4 cm and is permanently sealed off.

17.3.4 *Synchrotron, Electron and Proton.* In both the electron and proton synchrotrons, acceleration is achieved by means of a radiofrequency electric field, while the particles are guided by a time-varying magnetic induction. Thus, the synchrotron utilizes the method of acceleration of the cyclotron and the guiding method of the betatron.

The electron synchrotron was proposed independently by three physicists in different parts of the world. These were V. J. Veksler (4) of Russia, E. M. McMillan (5) of the United States, and M. L. Oliphant (8) of Australia.

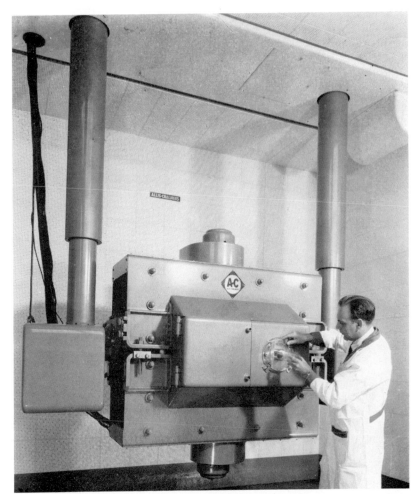

FIG. 6. *Photograph of a commercial 24-mev betatron.* The x-ray beam emerges from the opening indicated by the operator's hands. The protruding center section is a steel covered lead shield located in front of the vacuum doughnut. The magnet and its housing surround the doughnut. This betatron is mounted on a double telescoping suspension system and may be rotated about a horizontal axis. (Photograph through the courtesy of Allis-Chalmers Manufacturing Company.)

Electron and proton synchrotrons differ in regard to the radiofrequency electric field. In most of the electron synchrotrons now in existence, the frequency of the electric field is held constant. The electrons are first accelerated to about 3 mev by betatron action before the synchrotron action takes over further acceleration. Since the electron velocity at 3 mev is very close to the velocity of light, it remains almost constant as the energy in-

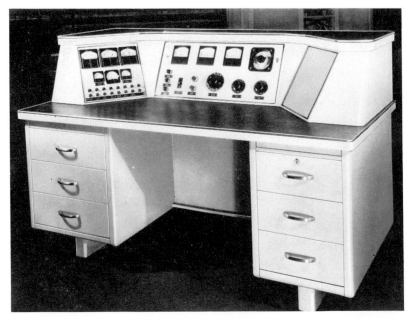

FIG. 7. *Betatron control console.* The console is located outside the shielded betatron room to protect the operator from stray radiation. (Photograph through the courtesy of Allis-Chalmers Manufacturing Company.)

creases. Now, since the electrons move in an equilibrium orbit with constant radius, the frequency of revolution is constant.

In the proton synchrotron, on the other hand, although the radius of the equilibrium orbit is constant, the proton velocity at which synchrotron acceleration takes over is only a small fraction of the velocity of light. Therefore, an electric field with variable frequency is needed for synchronism with the changing frequency of revolution of the protons. The reason for this was pointed out in the discussion on the synchrocyclotron.

The energies to which electrons are accelerated in the synchrotrons of today range from 13 mev to 500 mev. The radius of the equilibrium orbit of the 500-mev unit which is located at the California Institute of Technology is 3.5 meters.

The proton synchrotron is the most energetic of all the existing accelerators. At present there are three in operation, although seven others are in the advanced design stage or under construction. The largest unit in the United States is located at the University of California. It has an orbit with a radius of fifty feet and a maximum proton energy of 6,200 mev.

A rather recent development in the design of proton synchrotrons has been the guiding of the high-energy particles by means of a strong focusing technique using a series of magnets with alternate gradients. Several machines incorporating this technique are in the design stage. Several small scale models are in operation. They are called by the Midwest Universities Research Associates fixed-field alternate-gradient accelerators (9).

17.3.5 *Electrostatic Generators.* The group of accelerators known as electrostatic generators includes the Cockcroft-Walton (C-W), Van de Graaff, and various transformer types. The name "electrostatic" comes from the fact that this group of accelerators gains energy from an electrostatic field; that is, in these accelerators, the particles gain energy from an electric field which does not vary with time. Strictly speaking, a number of the widely used x-ray machines are of the electrostatic type, but this chapter deals only with units which accelerate charged particles to energies of 1 mev and above.

The *Cockcroft-Walton generator* (10) was developed almost thirty years ago, and it was with this machine that protons were first accelerated. The high electric field for this unit is developed by means of diode rectifiers and a transformer combined with a voltage multiplication circuit which employs condensers and additional rectifiers. The method employed by Cockcroft and Walton for voltage multiplication was first worked out by Greinacher. Of the nearly forty C-W generators in use today, only one is for electron acceleration, the rest being used for positive ions. These units are mostly in the one million-volt range, but several are designed to reach 1.4 mev.

Another type of accelerator which has proved to be quite satisfactory for electron acceleration in the region of one to two mev is the *resonant transformer*. This unit was developed in 1939 by E. E. Charlton (11) and is available commercially as an x-ray machine. The high voltage is produced on the secondary side of a transformer which is suitably tapped to give the correct voltages for both focusing and accelerating the electron beam. The vacuum tube is a multisectioned one which contains focusing electrodes not unlike the one pictured in the following section on the Van de Graaff generator. The simplicity of this unit makes it a highly reliable one with low maintenance requirements.

17.3.6 *Electrostatic Generator: Van de Graaff.* The Van de Graaff generator is a widely used type of accelerator. There are over 100 Van de Graaffs in physics laboratories alone, and of the order of 30 in hospital use, while numerous others are employed in industrial and biological research.

The Van de Graaff generator is named for Professor R. J. Van de Graaff, who built the first unit in 1931 (12). The first generators were placed in open air. In 1937, Herb (13) et al. enclosed a generator inside a pressurized

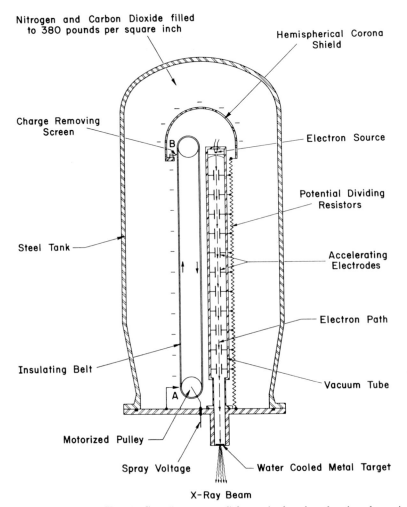

Nitrogen and Carbon Dioxide filled
to 380 pounds per square inch

Hemispherical Corona
Shield

Charge Removing
Screen

B

Electron Source

Potential Dividing
Resistors

Steel Tank

Accelerating
Electrodes

Electron Path

Insulating Belt

Vacuum Tube

A

Motorized Pulley

Spray Voltage

Water Cooled Metal Target

X-Ray Beam

FIG. 8. *Diagram of Van de Graaff generator*. Schematic drawing showing the major
components of a Van de Graaff electron accelerator. The functions of the various indicated parts are described in the text.

tank. This greatly reduced the space occupied by the unit since the distance
from the high-voltage terminal necessary to prevent unwanted sparking and
corona discharge decreases with increasing gas pressure.

Figure 8 is a schematic drawing showing the major components of the Van
de Graaff generator. This sketch illustrates the basic operation of an electron or negative ion unit, but the description of the operation is identical
for positive ions if proper voltage reversals are made. Between some pointed
conductors at point *A* and a conducting pulley wheel, there is a fast-moving

belt made of insulating material. By means of an external power supply of the order of 20,000 volts, a potential is placed on the metal pulley wheel. This potential produces an electric field sufficient to ionize the gas in the vicinity of the spray points. Electrons are attracted to the pulley, but are deposited on the belt which carries the charge to the high potential side of the accelerator shown at the top of the figure. At point B, a conducting screen is in rubbing contact with the moving belt. Due to their mutual repulsion, the electrons leave the belt and screen and gather on the hemispherical corona shield. The storing of charge on the corona shield results in the development of a high potential of the order of millions of volts between the shield and the steel tank. Within a vacuum tube and at the high potential terminal, an electron source (or proton source) is located. The electric field existing between the high potential source and a series of accelerating electrodes causes electrons to be accelerated in a focused beam toward the bottom or target end of the vacuum chamber. The electrons, upon striking a target which, incidentally, has to be water-cooled to prevent melting, produce x-rays. On the other hand, electrons may be extracted directly by replacing the target with a thin window. Not shown in the figure is a voltmeter which automatically controls the spray voltage in such a manner as to keep supplying the correct number of electrons to give an extremely constant high voltage.

The 380 pound per square inch pressure of nitrogen and carbon dioxide indicated in the figure is a nominal value of the High Voltage Engineering Corporation's 2-mev Van de Graaff. Figure 9 is a photograph showing one of their 2-mev units. The exit port, which is surrounded by a lead collimator, is shown in the lower central part of the picture. The pressurized tank extends upward and to the rear of the photograph. The apparatus attached to the left-hand side of the accelerator houses the vacuum system which is composed of a diffusion pump, a mechanical pump, and two cold traps. This particular unit is supported from the ceiling for ease of maneuverability.

Although the Van de Graaff generator produces a continuous, high intensity, monoenergetic beam, the maximum energy is several million electron volts due to present-day limitations of insulator technology. The highest energy Van de Graaff reported in the literature is the 6.5-mev unit at the Los Alamos Scientific Laboratory.

17.3.7 *Linear Accelerator.* The development of radar during World War II contributed considerably to the interest in developing the linear accelerator. This development was aided by advancements in techniques of producing high power radiofrequency pulses and greater understanding of electromagnetic field distributions within metal cavities. In the middle forties, a number of physicists at various universities and other institu-

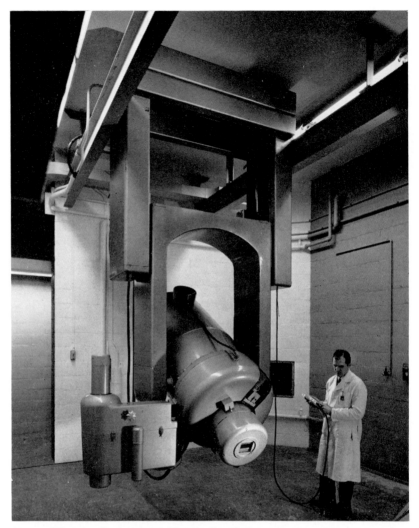

FIG. 9. *Photograph of a 2-mev Van de Graaff electron accelerator for medical use.* This unit may be employed for electron as well as x-ray therapy. (Photograph by Hedrich-Blessing.)

tions were actively engaged in electron linear accelerator development. Among these were F. F. Rieke at Purdue University, H. L. Schultz at Yale, G. R. Newbery at Hammersmith Hospital in England, D. W. Fry of the Atomic Energy Research Establishment in England, J. L. Lawson at General Electric Company, J. C. Slater at Massachusetts Institute of Technology, W. W. Hansen and E. L. Ginzton of Stanford University, and their associates. This section will describe briefly the features of the linear accelerator developed by the Stanford group (14), since it is one of the most outstanding.

The fundamental principle of operation of the Stanford type linear accelerator involves two important facts. First, an electromagnetic wave, produced when a radiofrequency pulse is directed into a hollow metal tube called a waveguide, can be made to travel through the inside of the tube parallel to its axis in such a way that its velocity is equal to that of electrons injected into the tube. Second, a sufficiently high fraction of electrons which are injected will remain in the hollow tube and will be accelerated to the desired energy.

Figure 10 is a schematic drawing of the linear accelerator of the Argonne Cancer Research Hospital (15), which is of the Stanford design. The figure indicates only some of the radiofrequency components. The vacuum, high voltage, metering, and other systems are not shown. The accelerator proper consists of two evacuated sections of waveguide, each 2.43 meters in length. Each section is supplied with radiofrequency power from a separate 20-megawatt klystron. These two klystrons act as power amplifiers and are both driven by a single magnetron oscillator at a frequency of 2,857 megacycles.

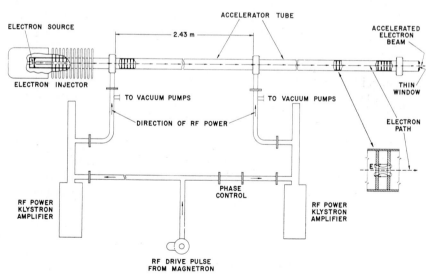

Fig. 10. *Schematic drawing of a 50-mev electron linear accelerator* including some of its essential radiofrequency (rf) components. Short rf pulses from the magnetron are guided to two klystron amplifiers, and from there to the accelerator tube. Electrons are injected into the tube simultaneously with these pulses. The inset to the right shows the shape of the traveling wave electric field E for one particular instant.

The klystrons are pulsed 60 times per second. Their output power is fed into the accelerating waveguide and proceeds to fill it with power until a maximum is reached. The electron source then injects electrons into the first section of the accelerator where their energy increases from the injection energy (usually around 80 kilovolts) to approximately 25 mev. Upon leaving the first section, they enter the second and are further accelerated to 50 mev. The force on the electrons is in the direction of the axis of the waveguide over its entire length. The inset of Figure 10 shows the general shape of the traveling wave electric field E for one particular instant. This field distribution travels toward the right within the accelerator tube. The linear path of the electrons is also indicated.

The figure also shows a series of disks whose function it is to "load" the waveguide in such a way that the phase velocity is reduced to the velocity of light in free space since this is the velocity with which electrons, after attaining a few mev, will travel. If the phase velocity were not equal to that of the electrons, the electrons would be acted upon by periodic forces which would be directed not only away from, but also toward the electron source. Of course, any force toward the injector would prevent the electrons from reaching full energy.

In some accelerator applications, it is desirable to have a variable electron energy. One way to achieve this is by means of a phase control. If, within the radiofrequency pulse, the phase relationship of the electric fields of the two accelerator sections is such that their peaks are not synchronized, the electrons when traveling through the second section will not receive the maximum possible energy. Thus, by controlling the relative phase, one can control the energy of the emergent beam.

Figure 11 is a photograph of the 50-mev electron linear accelerator. The accelerator proper is located within the long protective housing on the left-hand side of the picture. The three identical components in the right foreground are two operating and one spare klystron stations. The high-voltage protective cage, which is seen in the rear, contains a number of power supplies including the high-voltage, high-current supply which is necessary for the klystrons, and the high-voltage supply for the electron injector. The conventional waveguide, which carries the radiofrequency power from the magnetron to the klystrons, is shown affixed to the outside of the high-voltage cage. Also, a conventional waveguide can be seen between the klystron stations and the accelerator tube. The magnetron pulse driver is located to the right of the cage, and the accelerator vacuum system is visible behind the accelerator housing. In this unit, the phase control permits a variable electron energy from 5 to 50 mev.

Unlike cyclic accelerators, a linear accelerator may be made more energetic merely by adding successive sections. At the present time, Stanford

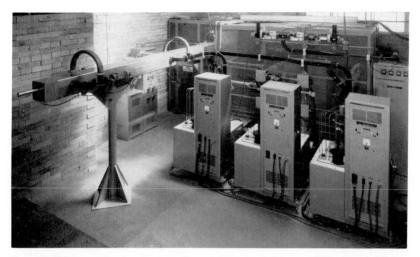

Fig. 11. *Photograph of a 50-mev electron linear accelerator.* This unit is located at the Argonne Cancer Research Hospital and is of the Stanford traveling wave type. (Photograph through the courtesy of the High Voltage Engineering Corporation.)

University has an accelerator whose energy exceeds 630 mev and which is being extended to 1000 mev.

Linear accelerators are not as widely used as other accelerators at the present time. The total number, both in the United States and Europe, is not greater than twenty. They range in energy from $\frac{3}{4}$ mev to 630 mev.

The discussion above has dealt with electron linear accelerators only. There has been success, also, in the development of a proton accelerator, notably by Alvarez (16). This accelerator operates with a standing rather than a traveling wave. To avoid decelerations, the protons travel alternately through regions containing an accelerating electric field and regions in which no forces act upon them. This is accomplished by the use of properly spaced small tubes called drift tubes, whose interior is free of electric field, located wherever the field would have a decelerating effect. At present, there are only two such units in the United States: one a 32-mev and the other a 68-mev machine. The highest energy unit being planned at present is a 1000-mev one at the Moscow Physical Institute in Russia (17).

17.3.8 *Cobalt-60 Therapy Unit.* By no stretch of the imagination could a radiation unit using radioactive cobalt-60 as a source be considered a particle accelerator. On the other hand, a short description of a cobalt-60 unit will be given to approach completeness for the discussion to follow on the various high-energy radiation sources used in biological research and medical therapy.

Space does not permit a full review of the development of all the cobalt units; however, the unit which was designed at the Argonne Cancer Research Hospital (18) will be discussed briefly.

Radioactive cobalt-60 is produced by the neutron capture of cobalt-59. The only supply of neutrons in sufficient abundance for this purpose is in a nuclear reactor. After a suitable fraction of the cobalt is transmuted to cobalt-60, the cobalt is removed from the reactor. In the decay of cobalt-60 to stable nickel-60, a beta particle and two gamma rays with energies of 1.17 and 1.34 mev are emitted. It is the gamma rays which are used for irradiations by cobalt units. Unlike an accelerator, which requires an elaborate and complicated apparatus to produce radiation, the source strength of cobalt-60 remains the same after its removal from the reactor except for its natural decay which has a half-life of 5.3 years. This decay amounts to a 1% decrease in activity per month.

During irradiation, a collimated beam of gamma rays emerges through an aperture in an absorbing shield which closely surrounds the source. To turn the beam off, an absorbing shutter is placed in the aperture.

Figure 12 is a photograph of the unit at the Argonne Cancer Research Hospital. This unit consists of a single shielded source which can revolve continuously in a vertical plane about a horizontal axis. The shield containing the source is visible in the upper left-hand portion of the unit. The shield and attached variable collimator are made of natural uranium metal to minimize bulk and weight. From the center of the shield, a collimated beam is directed to the center of the vertical circle or, by angulation of the shield, to any point on the axis of revolution. In therapy, the patient is placed on the cot shown in the center of the picture, in a recumbent position and on the axis of rotation of the source. Treatment does not necessarily need to be by full revolution, but may use an arbitrary sectorial field or conventional stationary fields.

The treatment cot can be positioned by one rotational motion about a vertical axis and three orthogonal linear motions. This movement permits the placing of any portion of a patient in a position within the gamma-ray beam.

Source rotation requires that the collimator should be at some distance from the patient. This necessitates that the source of radiation be made physically as small as possible, to avoid undesirable penumbra effects. To be consistent with present-day radiation therapy standards of intensity and penumbra, this unit was designed to contain a cylindrically shaped source, 0.75 cm in diameter and 3 cm long, and activated to a specific activity of the order of 150 curies per gram, or 1,750 curies total. The initial activity of this source is then equivalent to 1,750 grams of radium. Although the half-life of radium is over 300 times that of cobalt, the volume occupied by radium would be prohibitively large for this type of unit.

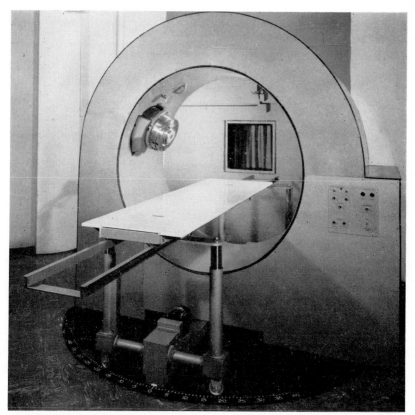

Fig. 12. *Photograph of the cobalt-60 therapy unit of the Argonne Cancer Research Hospital. In this view, the source shield, which revolves in a vertical circle, is shown on the left-hand side of the unit.*

A variety of other designs of cobalt-60 therapy units are in existence. References to some of these can be found in reference (18).

17.4 Medical and Biological Applications of Particle Accelerators

As was pointed out earlier, particle accelerators were developed primarily for nuclear physics research. However, applications have been found for some of these instruments both in biological research and in medical therapy. A few of the biological applications will be mentioned here, with a somewhat longer discussion of therapeutic uses, since probably the greatest single use of accelerators in either biology or medicine is for radiation therapy.

17.4.1 *Heavy Particle Accelerator Applications.* The application of heavy particle accelerators in medical therapy is still in preliminary stages of experimentation. However, applications are numerous in biological investigations. A few examples are given here.

A 2-mev proton Van de Graaff has been used extensively by Zirkle and Bloom (19) to bombard individual living cells with a very small beam of protons. The number of protons per cell involved in these irradiations has been from about 10 to tens of thousands. Using the most advanced machine shop and microscopic techniques, Zirkle and Bloom have been able to record on motion picture film the life cycle of normal and bombarded cells. From this work, new facts regarding such things as the function of the spindles in cell division have been discovered.

Pollard has used the Yale cyclotron for biophysical studies of large molecules. From these, methods for measuring shapes and cross sections of phage particles and enzymes have been developed.

Biological studies have been made by Warshaw and Oldfield (20) using protons from a synchrocyclotron. These studies included measurements of the relative biological effectiveness (RBE) of protons slowed down from 460 mev to a mean of 90 mev. They report an RBE of 1.75 ± .23 for a mouse spleen weight change, using 250 kev x-rays as the base of comparison.

C. A. Tobias and his associates have used 340-mev protons from a synchrocyclotron in a human therapeutic investigation (21) involving localized irradiation of the human pituitary gland. Localization was obtained by a combination of multi-port and rotational application of the proton beam. Definite evidence of depression in pituitary hormone output was achieved. The patients undergoing the treatment were advanced cases of metastatic carcinoma of the breast. Both 340-mev protons and 190-mev deuterons from the synchrocyclotron were used for radiation hypophysectomy of animals. Tobias has also been able to produce small brain lesions (of the order of one cubic millimeter) in animals by heavy-particle bombardment. He has pointed out that this can serve as a tool for studying the physiological functions of various loci of the central nervous system.

Figure 13 shows a central axis depth dose distribution for 180-mev deuterons with a 10-mev energy spread. This distribution was calculated by Warshaw and Oldfield (20) from measurements made by Tobias using a synchrocyclotron. The energy spread was introduced because a monoenergetic deuteron beam has a very narrow dose peak in the depth which would not be useful in therapy. When the energy is spread over several mev, this peak is broadened and the dose to the overlying region becomes relatively higher. The peak for the curve shown occurs at 11 cm. The surface dose is 65% of the maximum, and the radiation falls off rapidly beyond the peak.

Besides their use for direct irradiation of biological material, heavy-particle accelerators are employed for the production of certain medically ap-

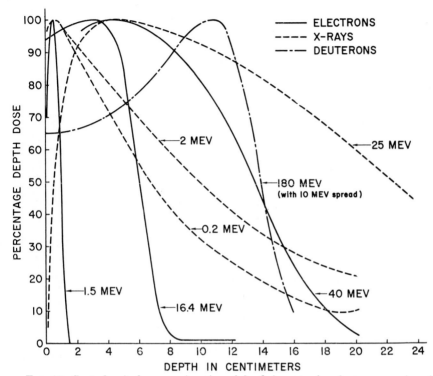

Fig..13. *Central axis dose as a function of depth in water* for electron energies of 1.5 mev (Van de Graaff), 16.4 mev (betatron), and 40 mev (synchrotron); peak x-ray energies of 0.2 mev (typical x-ray machine), 2 mev (Van de Graaff), and 25 mev (betatron); and a deuteron energy of 180 mev with a 10-mev spread (synchrocyclotron).

plied isotopes which cannot be made by neutron bombardment in nuclear reactors. For example, sodium-22, iron-55, iron-59, and iodine-130 are produced in a cyclotron. The cyclotron shown in Fig. 4 is designed specifically for isotope production.

17.4.2 *Electron Accelerator Applications.* In contrast to heavy-particle accelerators, electron accelerators are used extensively not only as biological research tools, but also as sources for radiation therapy with x-rays and electrons. The biological experiments will not be listed here, although they would make a formidable list indeed, but some of the characteristics of the radiations from electron accelerators which are relevant to therapy will be discussed.

Numerous accelerators throughout the world are devoted exclusively to biological and medical applications. Approximately ten 24-mev betatrons are currently in use. In a number of European countries, 15- and 31-mev betatrons are in operation. In the neighborhood of 30 Van de Graaff generators are in medical use. About a half dozen 4- to 15-mev linear accelerators are being employed in England for x-ray therapy; and in the United States, three in the 30- to 60-mev range for electron therapy as well as one 6-mev unit for x-ray therapy. There is one 70-mev synchrotron in this country and several others at lower energies are in clinical use abroad. Cobalt-60 therapy units are far more numerous, having come into widespread use in a great many countries.

Although there are several disadvantages in using high-energy accelerators in place of conventional low-energy x-ray equipment, such as high initial cost, maintenance, and developmental problems, these are offset from the physical point of view by a number of advantages. For high-energy compared to low-energy x-rays, these include, for example:

(1) As the energy of an x-ray beam increases, the peak dose does not remain at the surface but occurs at a progressively greater depth within the irradiated material (see Fig. 13). This effect, known as build-up, is of value in the treatment of deep-seated lesions by bringing about a reduction of skin reaction.

(2) The penetrating power of radiation is greater at high than at low energies. Thus, for equal dose to a deep-seated lesion, the dose to the overlying tissue becomes smaller for increasing energies.

(3) Also due to the greater penetrating power at high energies, the ratio of tumor dose to integral dose is higher.

(4) When using multiple beams or rotation at high energy (see Fig. 16), the beam can be directed toward the lesion rather than to a point deeper than the lesion, as the highest dose will always occur in the volume at which the beams are directed. This simplifies treatment planning.

(5) Lateral scatter is less for high than for low energy. This means that high-energy beams irradiate only a sharply defined region. This is also a contributing factor to (3).

(6) The absorption of radiation at high energies is more nearly independent of the atomic number of the absorbing material. Therefore, in the treatment of tissues other than bone, bone receives relatively less radiation at high energies.

(7) High-energy x-ray beams, properly compensated, produce dose distributions which are readily calculable since the isodose surfaces are flat.

High-energy electron beams have been used less extensively than high-energy x-ray beams in therapy. At low energies, i.e., 250 kev, the range of electrons in tissue is so small that electron beam therapy would be impractical. At high energies, however, the physical properties of electron beams have definite advantages.

For a given absorbing material, electrons have a definite range, which is a function of their energy. Beyond this range, the dose falls off very rapidly to a negligible amount. Therefore, by controlling the electron energy, one can control the depth of tissue to which the electron beam will penetrate, thus sparing the underlying tissue. At the present time, the linear accelerator most readily affords such control.

As in the case of high-energy x-rays, the isodose surfaces for electron beams are flat. Here, also, absorption does not depend strongly on the atomic number of the absorber. The physical determination of the absorbed dose is simpler for electrons than for high- or low-energy x-rays.

Figure 13 illustrates some of the above points. It shows the dose absorbed along the central axis of various beams directed into a container of water, as a function of depth within the water. (It is conventional in radiation therapy to make measurements in water, since, for certain types of radiation, water is similar to many body tissues as well as being a universally available material.) All curves are normalized to a peak dose of 100%.

The figure includes curves for electron beams of three different energies, namely, 1.5, 16.4 and 40 mev. As is shown, there is a rather sharp fall-off in the depth dose, although the effect of radiation straggling (electrons being removed from the beam through x-ray production) becomes evident in the 40-mev curve. The increase in penetration with increasing electron energy is clearly visible.

For a peak x-ray energy of 0.2 mev, which is in the range of conventional x-ray energies, the maximum dose occurs essentially on the surface. At a depth of about 7 cm, the dose has decreased to 50% of the maximum. For 2-mev x-rays, the peak dose is at about 0.5 cm, while the 50% dose is not reached until 10 cm. The 25-mev curve exhibits a very low surface dose, a peak of approximately 4 cm, and the 50% level at 22 cm.

The curves in this figure were procured from a variety of accelerators. The data for 1.5-mev electrons were obtained by Trump (22) from an electron Van de Graaff generator. Measurements of the 16.4-mev electron beam were made by Skaggs (23) using a 22-mev betatron. The 40-mev electron curve was obtained from a 70-mev electron synchrotron by Pollock (24) et al. The data for 0.2-mev x-rays are based on measurements by H. E. Johns (25) with a conventional x-ray therapy machine. Measurements for the 2-mev x-ray beam were made by Rozenfeld (26) using a Van de Graaff generator with an internal target. The 25-mev curve is from a betatron with an internal target.

Although not shown in this figure, the central axis depth dose for cobalt is very similar to the 2-mev peak x-ray distribution. This is to be expected, since the cobalt radiation consists of 1.17- and 1.34-mev gamma rays, whereas the 2-mev x-ray beam consists of an entire spectrum of energies whose maximum is the energy listed.

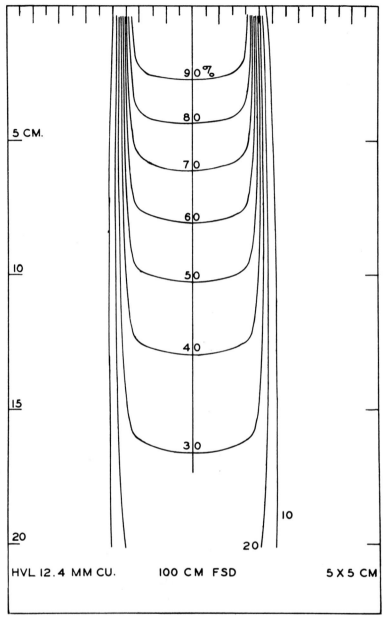

FIG. 14. *Experimental depth dose distribution for 2-mev peak x-rays* (half value layer 12.4 mm copper) from Van de Graaff. Distance from target to water surface: 100 cm. Field size at surface: 5 cm by 5 cm. Isodose lines in percent of maximum dose, which is located 0.5 cm beneath water surface.

Figure 14 is an example of a two-dimensional isodose plot, measured in water with a 2-mev x-ray beam from a Van de Graaff (26). This demonstrates the sharp lateral fall-off of absorbed dose at the edge of a beam at sufficiently high energy. The per cent isodose lines in this curve have been normalized to 100% at a peak which occurs on the central axis at 0.5 cm below the water surface. The target-to-surface distance was 100 cm, the cross section of the beam was a square of 5 by 5 cm, and, as indicated in the figure, the half value layer was 12.4 mm of copper. (The half value layer notation is a commonly used method of specifying the quality of x-ray beams.)

Figure 16 indicates the advantages of rotation therapy in being able to minimize the dose outside the region being irradiated and maximizing the dose within that region. Figure 15 shows a setup for the measurement of rotational depth dose distributions which was used with the cobalt unit of the Argonne Cancer Research Hospital (18). A section of the human body is simulated by an elliptically shaped Presdwood phantom placed on the treatment cot. A radiation detector is placed within the phantom material.

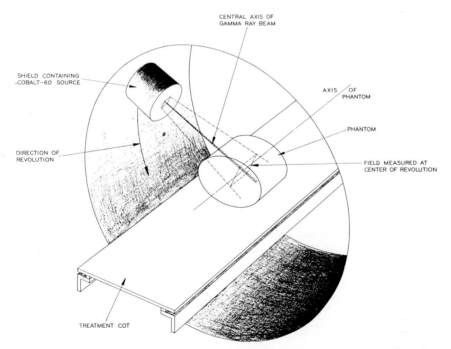

FIG. 15. *Diagram of cobalt-60 unit being used for measurement of depth dose* distributions with revolving source. The shape and location of Presdwood phantom simulate patient irradiation conditions.

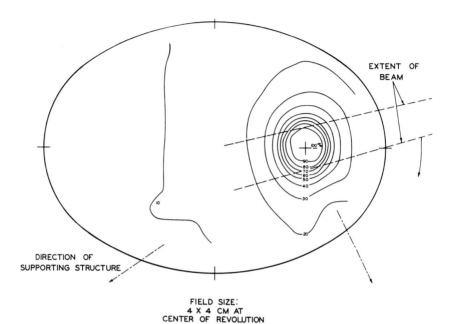

EXTENT OF
BEAM

DIRECTION OF
SUPPORTING STRUCTURE

FIELD SIZE:
4 X 4 CM AT
CENTER OF REVOLUTION

REVOLUTION SECTOR
360°

CENTER OF REVOLUTION
10 CM TO RIGHT OF
GEOMETRICAL CENTER ALONG
MAJOR AXIS OF ELLIPSE

Fig. 16. *Typical isodose plot obtained by the method of Fig. 15,* with elliptical phantom and 360° source revolution. It is to be noted that the radiation is limited to a rather sharply defined region.

Figure 16 shows dose measurements made by the author with the cobalt unit, using photographic film, of a field of 4 by 4 cm, with the phantom described above. The source was made to revolve completely around the phantom. The center of revolution is 10 cm to the right of the geometrical center, along the major axis of the ellipse. The extent of the beam is indicated by the dotted lines. (The direction of the supporting structure of the treatment cot disturbs the distribution slightly.) It should be noted that the peak dose of 100% is very near the center of revolution, and that the 80% iosdose line coincides closely with the geometrical edge of the beam. The dose received by the region outside the 4-cm circle, whose center is located at the center of revolution, falls off rapidly.

This is one example of the dose distributions which can be obtained with rotational therapy at high energies. Depending upon the location of a lesion and of the neighboring vital organs, a particular energy and type of radiation may be preferred.

17.5 Conclusion

This discussion is brief as far as the biological and medical use of accelerators is concerned. Nevertheless, it is hoped that the reader has gained some insight into the development of accelerators which exist today, and the applications being made. The development of the various accelerators to satisfy radiation therapy requirements continues to be an active endeavor for the radiation physicist. These new radiation instruments provide the physician with additional means of treating disease.

REFERENCES

1. LAWRENCE, ERNEST O. AND LIVINGSTON, M. STANLEY: A method for producing high speed hydrogen ions without the use of high voltages. *Phys. Rev. 37:* 707(A), 1931.
2. *American Institute of Physics Handbook.* New York: McGraw-Hill, 1957.
3. Specifications and photograph from the Argonne National Laboratory by personal communication from W. J. Ramler.
4. VEKSLER, V.: A new method of acceleration of relativistic particles, *J. Phys., U.S.S.R. 9:* 153, 1945.
5. MCMILLAN, EDWIN M.: The synchrotron—a proposed high energy particle accelerator. *Phys. Rev. 68:* 143, 1945.
6. KERST, D. W.: Acceleration of electrons by magnetic induction. *Phys. Rev. 58:* 841, 1940.
   An interesting history of the development of the betatron was published by Dr. Donald W. Kerst: Historical development of the betatron. *Nature, 157:* 90, 1946.
7. SKAGGS, L. S., ALMY, G. M., KERST, D. W. AND LANZL, L. H.: Removal of the electron beam from the betatron. *Phys. Rev. 70:* 95, 1946.
   SKAGGS, L. S., ALMY, G. M., KERST, D. W. AND LANZL, L. H.: Development of the betatron for electron therapy. *Radiology 50:* 167, 1948.
8. OLIPHANT, M. L., GOODEN, J. S. AND HIDE, G. S.: The acceleration of charged particles to very high energies. *The Proceedings of the Physical Society 59:* 666, 1947.
9. SYMON, K. R., KERST, D. W., JONES, L. W., LASLETT, L. J. AND TERWILLIGER, K. M.: Fixed-field alternating-gradient particle accelerators. *Phys. Rev. 103:* 1837, 1956.
10. COCKCROFT, J. D. AND WALTON, E. T. S.: Experiments with High Velocity Positive Ions. *Proc. Roy. Soc., London, s. A. 129:* 477, 1930.
11. CHARLTON, E. E., WESTENDORP, W. F., DEMPSTER, L. E. AND HOTALING, GEORGE: A new million-volt x-ray outfit. *J. Appl. Phys. 10:* 374, 1939.
12. VAN DE GRAAFF, ROBERT J.: A 1,500,000 volt electrostatic generator. *Phys. Rev. 38:* 1919, 1931.
13. HERB, R. G., PARKINSON, D. B. AND KERST, D. W.: Development and performance of an electrostatic generator operating under high air pressures. *Phys. Rev. 51:* 75, 1937.
14. CHODOROW, M., GINZTON, E. L., HANSEN, W. W., KYHL, R. L., NEAL, R. B., PANOFSKY, W. K. H. and the staff. Stanford high-energy linear electron accelerator (Mark III), *Rev. Scient. Instruments 26:* 134, 1955.
15. SKAGGS, LESTER S., NYGARD, JOHN C. AND LANZL, LAWRENCE H.: Design and initial operation of a 50-mev microwave linear accelerator for electron beam therapy. *Radiology 64:* 117, 1955.

16. ALVAREZ, LUIS W., BRADNER, H., GORDEN, H., PANOFSKY, WOLFGANG, K. H., RICHMAN, CHAIM AND WOODYARD, JOHN R.: Berkeley proton linear accelerator. University of California Radiation Laboratory (UCRL-236), U.S. Atomic Energy Commission Document, AECU-120 (November 30, 1948).

17. ROSENBAUM, E. P.: Physics in the U.S.S.R. *Scient. Am. 195:* 29, 1956.

18. LANZL, L. H., DAVISON, D. D. AND RAINE, W. J.: Kilocurie revolving cobalt-60 unit for radiation therapy. *Am. J. Roentgenol. 74:* 898, 1955.

19. ZIRKLE, RAYMOND E. AND BLOOM, WILLIAM: Irradiation of parts of individual cells. *Science 117:* 487, 1953.

20. WARSHAW, S. D. AND OLDFIELD, D. G.: Pretherapeutic studies with the Chicago synchrocyclotron. Semiannual Report to the U.S. Atomic Energy Comission, Argonne Cancer Research Hospital, ACRH no. 5, 54, (March, 1956).

21. TOBIAS, CORNELIUS A., ROBERTS, J. E., LAWRENCE, J. H., LOW-BEER, B. V. A., ANGER, H. O., BORN, J. L., McCOMBS, R. AND HUGGINS, CHARLES: Irradiation hypophysectomy and related studies using 340-mev protons and 190-mev deuterons. Proceedings of the International Conference on the Peaceful Uses of Atomic Energy, United Nations, Volume 10, 95 (August, 1955).

22. TRUMP, J. G., VAN DE GRAAFF, R. J. AND CLOUD, R. W.: Cathode rays for radiation therapy. *Am. J. Roentgenol. 43:* 728, 1940.

23. SKAGGS, L. S.: Depth dose of electrons from the betatron. *Radiology 53:* 868, 1949.

24. POLLOCK, H. C., HEBB, M. H. AND NOBLE, P. C.: The extraction of the electron beam from the 80-mev synchrotron. General Electric Research Laboratory, Report No. RL-546 (May 31, 1951).

25. JOHNS, HAROLD E.: *The Physics of Radiation Therapy.* Springfield, Ill.: Thomas, 1953, p. 231.

26. ROZENFELD, M. L.: 2-Mev isodose curves from a Van de Graaff x-ray generator. Semiannual Report to the U.S. Atomic Energy Commission, Argonne Cancer Research Hospital, ACRH No. 3, 34 (March, 1955).

18▶

Radioisotopes as Biologic Tracers

RICHARD PAUL SPENCER, LT. MC USNR

18.1 Introduction

A biologic tracer is any substance that can be used to follow ("trace") a metabolic pathway or compartment. A widely used tracer has been the dye Evans blue (T-1824). This compound principally binds itself to plasma proteins, and can be employed as an indicator of the magnitude of intra-vascular volume. Prior to the introduction of radioactive isotopes in medi-cine, the only tracers available (such as dyes) necessitated optical or chem-ical methods for their detection. Large sample quantities were required, and estimation of the amount present was time consuming. More serious however, the number of such tracers was distinctly limited.

Radioisotopes have completely altered this picture. Because they are de-tectable in minute quantities, radionuclides provide an elegant tool for following the metabolism of biologically interesting compounds, or estimat-ing the extent of various body compartments. The basic technics have been known for a number of years, but progress lagged until a variety of radio-isotopes were available in quantities sufficient for research. One of the first isotope biologic tracer studies was undertaken by Hevesy in 1923, when he made use of a naturally occurring isotope of lead to follow distribution of the metal in plants. During the late 1930 period, a group under Schoen-heimer initiated studies of biologic interactions, by means of deuterium. This isotope of hydrogen, although not radioactive, was the first nuclide to be systematically employed in research in the life sciences.

The discovery of artificially induced radioactivity (Joliot and Curie, 1934), indicated that isotopes other than those occurring in nature could be produced. Lawrence's development of the cyclotron, and the construc-tion of the first uranium pile by Fermi and co-workers (1942), provided the means for obtaining radioisotopes in a variety and abundance suitable for biologic studies.

Intensive research has resulted in the accumulation of hundreds of reports on the role of radioactive materials as biologic tracers. Books on the subject have been written by Hevesy, Kamen, Sacks and Siri; numerous symposia have been held, to deal with specific phases of radioisotope tracer technics. Each year reviews and abstracts appear (such as Nuclear Science Abstracts and the Annual Review of Nuclear Science) to help in keeping readers abreast of the latest developments. Recently technical journals have appeared, which are entirely devoted to biologic applications of radioisotopes. This chapter is intended to serve as a guide for those who are not familiar with such tracer technics, and as an introduction to the extensive and detailed literature.

18.2 Isotopes

Precise measurement of the molecular weight of various elements revealed values that were not always integers. One of the reasons for this was explained when Aston, using a mass spectrometer, showed various elements to exist in more than a single form. These forms of an element differed from one another only in their weight. That is, they could not be distinguished by chemical differences, but only by the physical property of having a variant weight.

Forms of an element which differ from one another in their weight, are called isotopes. This fact, simple as it may seem, has profound implications, and is the basis for the use of isotopes as tracers. All of the isotopes of an element have an identical number of protons in their atomic nuclei. In the orbits around the nucleus are electrons similar in number to the nuclear protons. Since it is the orbital electrons which largely determine chemical properties, and these are identical in number in all the isotopes of an element, all isotopes of a given element react in precisely the same chemical manner. The weight difference between isotopes of an element is accounted for by one or more neutrons in the nucleus. Neutrons may be viewed as having no electric charge, and hence contribute only to the mass of the atom, not to its chemical properties. Certain combinations of nuclear protons and neutrons are unstable. As the nucleus rearranges to a more stable configuration, emissions (energy or particles) are given off. Isotopes having this property are called radioactive.

18.2.1 *Radioactive and Stable Isotopes.* As a convenient shorthand, the atomic number of an element is written as a subscript, and its atomic weight as a superscript. Thus, magnesium, the 12th element in the periodic table, having an atomic weight of 24, may be designated $_{12}Mg^{24}$. An isotope of magnesium with a weight of 25 mass units is also known to occur ($_{12}Mg^{25}$ or simply Mg^{25}). Atoms of Mg^{25} are one mass unit heavier than those of Mg^{24}, but are chemically indistinguishable from the former. Mg^{25} is also a stable isotope, and does not undergo spontaneous disintegration. There is an isotope of magnesium (Mg^{27}) which is radioactive (half-life 9.5 min.). Each element is known to have at least one radioactive isotope, and certain elements only exist in radioactive forms.

Stable Isotopes. Stable nuclides occur in nature. For example, Mg^{24}, Mg^{25} and Mg^{26}, all stable, can be found in native magnesium. The relative quantity of each is referred to as the "fractional abundance". For magnesium

78.8 per cent occurs as Mg^{24}; fractional abundance is 0.788.

10.1 per cent occurs as Mg^{25}; fractional abundance is 0.101.

11.1 per cent occurs as Mg^{26}; fractional abundance is 0.111.

Total fractional abundance is 1.000.

A number of elements exist in only one form in nature, such as Na^{23}, P^{31}, I^{127}; this single type is of course "100 per cent abundant." Stable isotopes can sometimes be produced by bombardment of a precursor material with subatomic particles. Thus, Mg^{25} may be formed by the action of neutrons on Mg^{24}: $_{12}Mg^{24} + {_0}n^1 \rightarrow {_{12}}Mg^{25} +$ gamma ray. However, all stable isotopes which can be produced by artificial means, already exist in nature.

Radioactive Isotopes. A limited number of elements having one or more stable forms, also possess naturally occurring radioactive isotopes (such as C^{14}, K^{40}, Nd^{144}). In addition, all ements above atomic number 83 exist only in radioactive forms. Despite this, the total of naturally occurring radioisotopes is small (about 55), when compared with the total number (over 1000) which are produced by means of the cyclotron and nuclear reactor. This availability of multiple artificially produced isotopes has opened the door to biologic research.

18.2.2 *Decay of Radioisotopes.* Isotopes possessing an unstable combination of nuclear particles undergo spontaneous rearrangement (isomerization) or breakdown (disintegration) to more stable forms. The rate of disintegration can be described statistically:

$$Q = Q_o e^{-\lambda t}$$

Q represents the quantity remaining after a given time t, if an original quantity, Q_0 was present. The number e (2.718...) is the base of the natural logarithms. The decay constant, λ, is related to the half-life of the isotope by the following expression:

$$\text{half-life} = \frac{0.693}{\lambda}$$

By half-life of a radioisotope is meant the period of time required for half of any given number of atoms to disintegrate. The half-life is expressed in units of time, and λ has the units of reciprocal time (1/time). Each radio-isotope has an invariant half-life which may be used in its characterization. The mechanics of nuclear disintegration have been treated elsewhere in this book. The majority of radioisotopes of biologic importance decay by emission of one or more of the following rays or particles.

Gamma ray: an energy emission, no weight.

Beta particle: electron, possessing negative charge and slight weight, depending upon velocity.

Positron: a positively charged electron. Unstable, combines with an electron, causing an "annihilation" with emission of 2 gamma rays.

Alpha particles: nucleus of helium atom, carrying a double positive charge.

Each emission has a particular energy, which is usually expressed in terms of million electron volts (mev). By means of the half-life, type of emissions, and energy of the emissions, a radioisotope may be accurately identified. As will be pointed out, the various emissions have the ability to traverse distance and penetrate matter. Hence, they can be detected with suitable equipment. Such terms as "tagged", "labeled" and "radioactive indicator" are used to indicate their detectability.

18.2.3 *Choice of Isotope.* Stable isotopes can be used as tracers, but usually not as conveniently as radioactive nuclides. A number of elements have both stable isotopes and radioactive forms, and the investigator therefore has a choice. Stable nuclides are advantageous in that they emit no ionizing radiations which may disturb a sensitive system. On the debit side though, they are difficult to obtain, need cumbersome spectrometric equipment for their estimation, and can only be detected by actually sampling a biologic preparation under study. Isotopes which emit gamma rays, on the other hand, can be detected externally to the source, and have been employed during *in vivo* studies.

TABLE I

Principal Isotopes of Carbon, Hydrogen, and Sulfur, Used in Research

ELEMENT	ISOTOPE	STABILITY	TYPE EMISSION	mev ENERGY	HALF-LIFE
Hydrogen	H^2	Stable			
	H^3	Radioactive	Beta	0.018	12.26 years
Carbon	C^{13}	Stable			
	C^{14}	Radioactive	Beta	0.158	5600 years
	C^{11}	Radioactive	Positron	0.51*	20.5 min.
Sulfur	S^{36}	Stable			
	S^{35}	Radioactive	Beta	0.167	87 days

* Energy from annihilation gamma rays.

Some elements have no convenient radioactive isotopes. By "convenient" is meant readily available, and with a half-life from one-half day to 100 days. Oxygen and nitrogen fall into this group. In such instances, a rare stable isotope may have to be relied upon. It is unfortunate that hydrogen, carbon and sulfur, all of great interest, do not have many isotopes well suited to studies in the biologic sciences (Table I).

In certain cases, more than one radioactive isotope is available for an element under study. Iodine, with only one stable isotope, has 20 radioactive isotopes; of these, 4 have been used in studies of thyroid function.

IODINE ISOTOPE	HALF-LIFE	EMISSIONS
I^{128}	25.0 min.	beta, gamma
I^{130}	12.6 hr.	beta, gamma
I^{131}	8.0 days	beta, gamma
I^{132}	2.3 hr.	beta, gamma

When such a choice is present, a number of ancillary factors must be considered, including availability. Since I^{131} is produced in a nuclear reactor, it is the easiest of the above isotopes to obtain. Half-life is important, and I^{128} is impractical for a laboratory at a distance from the production site (the radionuclide would be dissipated before reaching the area of utilization). There are also limits to the upper value for the half-life; if the isotope is to be used for human research, the physical half-life should preferably be under 100 days in order not to subject the host to prolonged radiation (thus Na^{24} with a half-life of 15.0 hours, is preferred to Na^{22} with a $T_{1/2}$ of 2.6 years).

When performing *in vivo* studies, most laboratories prefer to use gamma ray emitting isotopes, since they can be detected externally to the source. Other considerations in the choice of an isotope include the available chemical form of the material and its specific activity (the ratio of the number of radioactive atoms to the number of stable atoms). With most isotopes now available for biologic studies, the latter presents no problem as the specific activity is high (that is, most of the material is in the radioactive form, with little nonradioactive "carrier").

18.2.4 *Assumptions in Isotope Tracer Procedures.* There are a number of basic assumptions involved in tracer work with radioisotopes. Transgressions beyond the limit of an assumption often lead to erroneous results, and hence these concepts will be briefly presented.

(1) *Nondiscrimination against the isotope.* By "nondiscrimination" is meant that the biologic system fails to distinguish between the radioisotope and the element as it occurs in nature. If there were even slight discrimination, the radionuclide would be handled in a manner which differs from that

of the native element. In most biologic situations, there is probably equal facility for working with any isotope of an element. Notable exceptions occur, particularly the inability of lower forms to utilize deuterium-water in a manner similar to natural water.

(2) *No excess irradiation to local area or whole body.* Early in the development of tracer technics, the observation was made that a number of systems that had received radioisotopes, reacted in a different chemical manner than untreated systems. Subsequent studies revealed that in such instances, the radioisotope had delivered a large does of radiation to the area under study, with alteration of the chemical composition. An essential requisite of tracer work is that the tracer does not adversely affect the site under scrutiny. If this is violated, spurious results may occur. With sensitive radiation detection devices, minimal quantities of radioactivity are employed, and the possibility of organ damage is reduced.

(3) *High specific activity.* Specific activity has been mentioned as the ratio of radioactive atoms to nonradioactive atoms in a sample. The ratio is generally expressed as millicuries per gram (mc/gm). A specimen containing only "hot" atoms, and no carrier, is called "carrier-free". A number of isotopes of biologic interest (such as I^{131}) can be obtained in carrier-free form. Such preparations have the advantage of bringing only a minute quantity of the chemical under consideration into the body. This precaution is necessary when only traces of the element are normally present in the body. As an example of how a biologic system may be overburdened, consider a study in which radiocopper (Cu^{64}) was used to follow the uptake of copper by brain tissue. The Cu^{64} had a specific activity of 500 mc/gm. In terms of stable copper, since each animal received 5 mc, 5 mc/500 mc $\times$ 1 gm or 0.01 gm of stable copper was administered per animal. A 300-gram rat contains about 0.003 grams of copper, and hence the "tracer dose" contained sufficient carrier to overload the copper handling mechanism. Results from such a study may not correlate with the true situation *in vivo*. Whenever possible, carrier-free isotopes should be employed. When not carrier-free, the highest specific activity available can be used, if calculations indicate excess stable material is not being introduced.

(4) *Sufficient time for equilibration.* No matter how rapidly biologic reactions proceed, a finite period is required. Depending upon the system investigated, a greater or lesser period will be necessary for equilibration. If the system is sampled too soon after administration of an isotope, equilibration may not have occurred, and an erroneous impression can be obtained as to the kinetics of the event. To avoid this pitfall, samples may be drawn at repeated intervals, and radioactivity present plotted as a function of time.

(5) *Equilibration is physiologically possible.* Closely associated with the

concept of allowing sufficient time for equilibration is the idea that an equilibrium must be attained under physiologic conditions. For instance, during short term experiments, all of the sodium in the body does not come into equilibrium with administered radiosodium (Na^{24}). Admixture of body stores with radiosodium is uneven, and a large portion of body sodium (perhaps 30 per cent) is in bone and relatively inaccessible to the isotope. Hence, there is no justification in speaking of the "sodium space" by isotope dilution. All that is measured by use of radiosodium is a fraction of body sodium; this is designated "exchangeable sodium."

18.2.5 *Precautions in Tracer Work.* The use of radioisotopes can not be entered into carelessly. It should be reserved for individuals with sufficient understanding of the procedures involved so that no hazard arises to either the investigator or the test subject. Principles of radiation safety, similar to those enunciated elsewhere in this book, must be strictly followed.

Mention has been made that very short half-life isotopes (under 12 hours) can not be readily used in laboratories far from the site of manufacture, because of rapid decay. There is also a limit to the upper range of half-life, when an isotope is to be used for human study. Generally it is not desirable to employ an isotope with a half-life longer than 100 days. This is because longer lived nuclides subject the experimental host to irradiation for a prolonged period. For sensitive work, in addition to the physical half-life, an investigator must consider the distribution of the isotope, its effective period in the body, the energy of the radioemissions, and their range in tissue.

In all cases, administered radiation must be low, and constant surveillance is the keyword. Low level counting methods for isotopic tracers have been described, and should be employed so that the administered dose may be kept at a minimum.

18.3 Physical, Effective and Biological Half-Life in Relation to Use

If radioiodine is injected into an animal, and counts taken over the thyroid gland after maximum accumulation has occurred, a progressive decline in activity will be observed. Part of this decrease is of course due to radioactive decay of the iodine isotope. In addition, secretion of iodine occurs from the thyroid gland. If secretion did not occur, the activity in the gland would correspond to the amount originally present minus the quantity lost through radioactive decay.

The amount of radioactivity in the thyroid can be plotted as a function of time. At some point, activity will be reduced to one-half of the quantity originally present. This is referred to as the "effective half-life," and represents the dual factors of radioactive decay and biologic excretion. The term "biologic half-life" is often used in the literature. This is a quantity which can not be precalculated, but may be determined once the effective half-life is known, by use of the relationship:

$$\frac{1}{\text{Biologic half-life}} = \frac{1}{\text{Effective half-life}} - \frac{1}{\text{Physical half-life}}$$

Iodine[131] has a physical half-life of 8 days, and an average effective half-life of 6 days (the effective half-life may be equal to the physical half-life, but it can never be greater). For iodine under these conditions:

$$\frac{1}{\text{Biologic half-life}} = \frac{1}{6} - \frac{1}{8}$$

Biologic half-life = 24 days. The interpretation of this is that if I[131] did not undergo decay, its activity would still be reduced to one-half (by excretion), and this would require 24 days. Certain isotopes (such as radiogold in the peritoneal cavity), do not leave the body once introduced. Hence, their effective half-life and biologic half-life have no meaning, and the stay of the material within the body is determined solely by the physical half-life.

The concept of effective half-life is important in tracer studies for two reasons. First, it allows calculation of the biologic half-life, which is an indication of biologic handling of the element. Second, if counting of a system is to be done some time after a dose has been given, sufficient activity must be administered initially so that a significant counting rate remains after decay and secretion have occurred. By knowing the effective half-life, the magnitude of the required initial dose can be calculated.

18.3.1 *Commonly Employed Biologic Tracers.* Listed in Table II are the isotopes most commonly used in biologic tracer studies. It can be seen that only five of these have a physical half-life greater than 100 days (H[3], C[14], Co[60], Ca[45], Zn[65]). However, only in the case of Ca[45] and possibly C[14] is the effective half-life greater than 100 days.

The listed isotopes emit either beta particles alone (H[3], C[14], P[32], S[35]), or various combinations of beta and gamma rays. Arsenic[74] and Cu[64] emit positrons, which are quickly annihilated with the emission of two gamma rays. None of the listed nuclides emit alpha particles. Because of the tendency of isotopes which emit alpha particles to have a prolonged residence in bone, and the damage which can result from such particles, these nuclides are not routinely used in human tracer studies (but they have found applications in experimental work with animals). The worker handling such radionuclides must exert utmost caution, since even slight contamination might create a serious health hazard.

18.3.2 *Preparation of Radioisotopes.* After production in either the nuclear pile or the cyclotron, radioisotopes are separated by various combinations of physical and chemical procedures. The manifold problems of production,

TABLE II

Radioisotopes Commonly Employed as Biologic Tracers

ISOTOPE	PHYSICAL HALF-LIFE	APPROXIMATE EFFECTIVE HALF-LIFE	USE
Pure Beta Emitters			
H^3	12.3 years	19 days	Body water estimation
C^{14}	5.6×10^3 years	35 days (fat)	Labeling compounds
		180 days (bone)	Labeling organic compounds
P^{32}	14.5 days	14 days	Incorporation into tissues; labeling
S^{35}	87 days	18 days	Extracellular fluid; compound labeling
Sr⁹⁰	*28 yrs.*	*15 days*	
Ca^{45}	160 days	151 days	Calcium metabolism
Isotopes Which Emit Gamma Rays (with or without beta particles)			
I^{131}	8.1 days	7 days	Thyroid function, protein tagging, tumor localization
Cr^{51}	27 days	22 days	Red cell tagging
Fe^{59}	45 days	40 days*	Iron absorption; erythrokinetics
K^{42}	12.5 hr.	0.5 days	Potassium exchange; membrane transport
Na^{24}	15.0 hr.	0.6 hr.	Exchangeable sodium, transport.
Cu^{64} (p)	12.8 hr.	0.5 days	Brain tumor localization; transport
As^{74} (p)	17 days	5 days	Brain tumor localization
Co^{60}	5.2 years	8 days	Vitamin B_{12}-Co^{60}
Ca^{47}	4.7 days	4.5 days	Calcium metabolism
Zn^{65}	245 days	21 days	Zinc metabolism
Ga^{72}	14.1 hr.	0.5 days	Incorporation into bone, osseous tumors
Au^{198}	2.7 days	2.5 days	Phagocytosis, uptake into lymphatics
Rb^{86}	18.6 days	15 days	Parallels potassium
Cl^{38}	37.3 min.	0.5 hr.	Chlorine transport
Br^{82}	35.9 hr.	30 hr.	Bromine transport

(p) = positron emission.
* Iron may not leave body, except via bleeding or interchange with ingested iron molecules.

isolation, refinement and synthesis into compounds, had in the past been handled by a limited number of radiochemists and physicists. Because of the increased use of isotopes in biologic fields, within the past few years leading pharmaceutical concerns have begun processing radionuclides, so that they can be obtained in a variety of forms with a high degree of chemical purity; such preparations are "radioactive pharmaceuticals."

For a number of isotopes, once preparation in the pile or cyclotron has been accomplished, their processing is complete (aside from sterilization if parenteral use is contemplated). Certain nuclides are of use in biology only after incorporation into complex molecules. For instance, C^{14} is often of interest only following its synthesis into an organic compound. Three techniques for accomplishing such syntheses are available: (1) hot atom chemistry; (2) exchange reactions; (3) biosynthesis.

"Hot atom chemistry" has been in existence since the days of the Manhattan Project. Its technics, brought to bear on biologically important materials, has yielded handsome results. The first problem of the radiochemist is to separate the radioisotope from the many other materials present. Use of the type reaction described by Szilard and Chalmers (and designated by their names) has been employed in obtaining carrier free isotopes. The Szilard-Chalmers reaction depends upon the bombardment of a compound containing the element under study. By use of the proper compound, when the element becomes radioactive, it splits off from parent molecule, and hence is carrier-free. The second task is to incorporate the isotope into the final compound. The chemical technics used for this purpose are ingenious and often complex.

Exchange reactions for the preparation of labeled compounds have come into use only recently. As an example, Wilzbach observed that molecules containing hydrogen, after being in contact with gaseous tritium, became "tagged." Apparently hydrogen in the molecule had exchanged with tritium. This technic provides a potentially valuable method for labeling complex substances which otherwise would resist synthesis de novo from a radioisotope.

Biosynthesis is the third method for producing tagged molecules. The term biosynthesis implies that the manufacture has been carried out by a viable organism (higher palnts, bacteria, animals, and so on), or their enzyme systems. From simple radioactive precursors, highly complicated tagged molecules can often be obtained from biologic systems. For example, Anfinsen was able to obtain a C^{14}-tagged enzyme, ribonuclease. Biosynthesis has been of particular value when the substance desired is too complex to permit chemical synthesis (as with enzymes), or when the standard synthetic methods are too involved to be rapidly feasible (as in the preparation of certain vitamins, hormones, and medicinals).

The greatest bulk of biologically important compounds contain carbon, and C^{14} has been a favored starting point for biosynthesis. The carbon may be burned in oxygen, producing radioactive carbon dioxide. Upon growing in an atmosphere which contains $C^{14}O_2$, plants incorporate some of the radiocarbon into their molecules. Radioactive digitoxin and nicotine have been obtained in this manner. In each instance, the final product must be isolated and purified according to rigid radiochemical criteria. By employing different biosynthetic systems, it is possible to obtain two or more forms of a compound, each labeled at different sites. Thus, Villee and Hastings incubated $C^{14}O_2$ with liver slices and produced radioglucose labeled in the 3 and 4 carbon positions, from glycogen. These investigators obtained a distinct form of radioglucose labeled in all positions by growing leaves in $C^{14}O_2$.

18.3.3 *Correction for Radioactive Decay.* During the course of an experiment, radioactive decay is dissipating the number of detectable events from a radioisotope. The relationship governing this statistical breakdown has been discussed elsewhere. To correct for such decay, four courses are open.

(1) If the isotope has a very long half-life, no correction is necessary for decay during a short interval. Carbon[14] has a half-life of 5600 years, and a negligible quantity is dissipated in 1 day.

(2) Samples drawn at various intervals may be saved, and counted at the same time. Hence, no correction is necessary for breakdown, since all specimens have decayed to the same extent. Values obtained in this manner are usually expressed in terms of a percent of the initial dose.

(3) A standard may be prepared, which is identical with the administered dose. Samples can be counted as they are withdrawn, and compared with the standard. Since the result is expressed as a fraction of standard activity, no further correction is necessary.

(4) Absolute standards are sometimes employed. They may be of value if precise information as to the administered dose is desired. The quantity of an isotope present may be calculated at each interval that a sample is withdrawn. Carefully calibrated sources are available from the National Bureau of Standards. In addition, a number of calibrated isotopes are obtainable through commercial sources. In tracer work, the microcurie (3.7×10^4 disintegrations per second) is the standard most commonly used.

Radioactive decay becomes a particular problem when short half-life isotopes are used. For example, C^{11} has a half-life of 20.5 minutes. Separation from its production site, synthesis into desired materials, and administration, must be performed within a few hours. Prior to the availability of C^{14}, the C^{11} isotope was the only one available for radiocarbon tracer investigations. By use of rapid handling, C^{11} was made to serve in the study of intermediary metabolism in animals, and the investigation of photosynthesis in plants. Because of its emission of positrons, which are annihilated to produce gamma rays, C^{11} may be detected at a distance from the biologic sample in which it resides; the C^{14} isotope emits only a weak beta particle, and its counting poses a problem. Thus in certain instances a short half-life isotope may possess definite advantages. Provided an investigator has the proper facilities, short lived isotopes may be as useful as longer lived species.

In addition, their activity is rapidly dissipated, and creates less of a problem from the viewpoint of health physics.

18.4 In Vivo and In Vitro Counting

True *in vivo* studies can be performed only by use of gamma emitting isotopes, which permit their recognition at a distance from the specimen. Counting of isotopes which emit only beta particles necessitates sampling the system, and placing the material in a sensitive low background instrument.

The efficiency of detecting gamma rays has been greatly improved by the use of scintillation crystals (such as sodium iodide, activated by thallium). With such devices, small amounts of gamma emitting isotopes may be used to obtain a significant counting rate. Gamma rays are photons traveling with the speed of light. They have a great range in air and tissue, and are absorbed in exponential fashion. Because of this ability to traverse tissue, gamma rays may be detected outside of an organ, whereas beta particles are usually absorbed in the tissue. This principle underlies the use of I^{131} for *in vivo* thyroid studies. Beta particles of the isotope are dissipated in the thyroid, while the majority of gamma rays pass through and can be detected.

Alpha particles, heavy, densely ionizing and limited in range, require special devices for their detection, and are of little practical importance in most biologic tracer studies.

Beta particles however, are of great significance in tracer work. These electrons, of nuclear origin, are emitted with various energies, and may have a range in air up to many centimeters. When passing through an absorber, the range of a beta particle depends upon its energy, and is inversely proportional to the denisty of the absorber. Range is expressed in terms of weight per unit area of absorber. When stated in such a manner, thickness of absorber in centimeters can be calculated from: $\dfrac{\mathrm{gm/cm}^2}{\mathrm{density}}$ = thickness in cm. This assumes that beta particles from an isotope have the same energy. Actually, a spectrum of energies exists, from a maximum value down almost to zero. The average energy of the beta particles emitted by an isotope is about one-third the maximum energy. For energetic beta particles, the range is appreciable. The 1.7 mev beta emission of P^{32} travles about 760 mg/cm². In Figure 1 is plotted the absorption curve for P^{32}, as a function of the thickness of absorber. The line is not straight, but can be approximated by a straightedge. The beta particle of C^{14}, with an energy of 0.155 mev, has a range of only 35 mg/cm². Since the average particle possesses an energy only one-third of this, it is imperative to bring the isotope close to the counting device, with little interposed absorbing material. "Thin

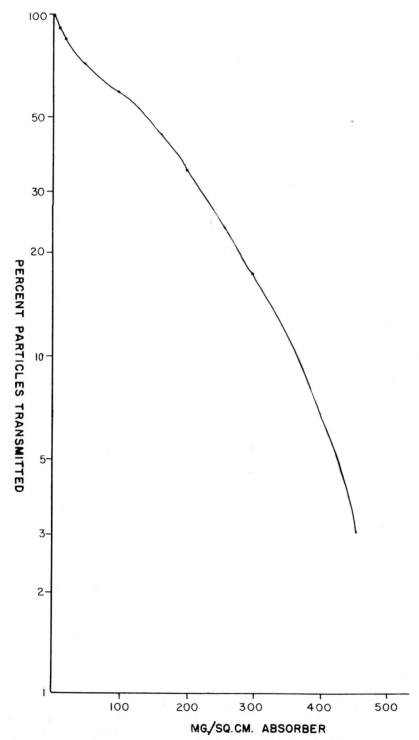

Fig. 1. *Gamma ray spectrum* of a mixed sample of Fe[59] and Cr[51]. Because of a contribution from radio-iron at the radiochromium peak, a correction is necessary when counting in this area.

window" Geiger tubes are available, which absorb but few of the low energy particles. The isotope, tritium (H^3), emits a beta particle with maximum energy of only 0.011 mev. This is absorbed in 0.25 mg/cm^2 (less than 1 mm in tissue). For tritium counting, very sensitive devices are necessary, and special technics are used.

(1) If tritum is part of a molecule in the solid state, the compound can be placed in a liquid beta scintillation counter. This is a medium which scintillates each time it is struck by a beta particle; surrounding the liquid is a sensitive crystal for detecting the light flashes. (2) Gaseous tritium may be introduced directly into the sensitive area of a counting device, such as a Geiger tube. As a further aid to *in vivo* counting, collimated scintillation crystals are employed to detect gamma rays from specific regions of the body. The collimator is a device in a heavy metal (usually lead) so arranged that it shields out "stray" gamma emissions and allows counting only of rays from the area under study. Total number of counts per minute at various times after the isotope has been administered, may be recorded. Thus, uptake and disappearance can be followed (but counts must be corrected for decay). The technic is often not quantitative in that the exact amount of isotope beneath the probe is uncertain. If the geometry of the area is known, a standard can be produced and counted, and the "uptake" of standard and unknown compared.

All other technics depend upon taking a sample of tissue, fluid or excreta, and introducing it to the detection apparatus (a photographic emulsion, or electronic counting devices). For quantitation, gamma emitting isotopes do not have to be in thin sections, as is necessary for beta emitters. This is more fully discussed in a later section.

18.4.1 *Multiple Labeling.* There is no theoretical limit to the number of radioactive tags, that may be introduced into a compound. We have already mentioned glucose in which all of the carbon atoms have been C^{14}. In a sense, this is multiple labeling. The term however is generally reserved for cases in which two or more different isotopes are incorporated into a molecule.

Several situations exist in which multiple labeling is of importance. (1) Two or more parts of a compound are to be studied metabolically (such as the phenyl rings and the iodine, of thyroxin). (2) Information is to be gathered concerning the handling of a substance in the presence of previous loading of the material (such as the absorption of iron, following a high iron diet—in this case two iron isotopes are readily available—Fe^{55} and Fe^{59}).

Following the successful labeling of a molecule with more than one radioisotope, the basic problem is to distinguish between the nuclides. Three technics to accomplish this are in use. (1) If there is a marked difference between the half-life of the isotopes, they may be counted together and the more rapidly dissipated one allowed to decay. After this, the second nuclide can be estimated. This is especially useful when the longer lived isotope is a beta emitter, which would have been masked by a shorter lived gamma emitting nuclide. (2) Differences in the types or energies of the emissions may be utilized by means of different absorbers. Numerous examples are found in the literature. Thus, a compound labeled with both S^{35} and I^{131} was counted by comparing the activity before and after an aluminum absorber was placed over the detection device. The aluminum filter stopped nearly all of the beta particles from the S^{35} while allowing over half of the I^{131} counts to pass. The isotope of Fe^{55} has been estimated in the presence of Fe^{59} by the different sensitivity of various window thicknesses to the various emissions. (3) The availability of gamma ray and beta ray spectrometers has permitted distinction to be made between two or more isotopes present in a specimen, as long as the energy of their emissions is sufficiently different.

A gamma ray spectrometer is essentially a scintillation crystal which, by varying the applied voltage, can be made more or less sensitive to different energy gamma rays. One of the commonest medical uses of the spectrometer has been distinguishing between Fe^{59} and Cr^{51} in blood during erythrokinetic studies. To elucidate the life history of red blood cells, Fe^{59} is used to "tag" plasma while Cr^{51} is employed as a red cell "label".

Prior to the availability of gamma ray spectrometers, Fe^{59} studies could not be performed while the isotope Cr^{51} was present in the specimen. The two radionuclides have almost identical gamma emissions. Figure 2 shows the gamma ray spectrum of Fe^{59} and Cr^{51} mixed together. Gamma ray spectroscopy can also be used to distinguish between isotopes in tissue. Spencer and Mitchell followed the uptake of K^{42} and Cu^{64} in brain tissue, by distinguishing between their gamma emissions, and this paper may be consulted for the technic and sample calculations.

Beta ray spectrometers work on the same principle. The intensity of the

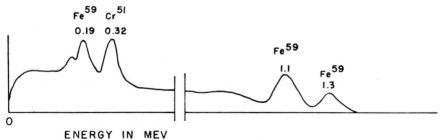

FIG. 2. *Absorption curve for beta particles from* P^{32}. Observe that the plot does not give a straight line.

scintillation produced in a liquid medium is proportional to the energy of the beta particle. This is picked up by a crystal, magnified, and recorded. The device can be set up to count only pulses due to particles of a particular energy.

18.4.2 *Beta Counting.* Carbon[14] is one of the most widely employed isotopes in tracer studies. Since C^{14} emits only a weak beta particle the investigator must be prepared to do beta counting.

Absolute beta counting, that is determining the total number of emissions, is a tedious task, and of little practical importance to the biologist. What is used in its place is relative counting. In relative counting, having all factors constant, the activity in a sample is compared with a standard, or with an aliquot of the administered dose.

$$\left(\frac{\text{Activity in sample}}{\text{Total activity administered}} \times 100 = \text{per cent activity in sample} \right).$$

Factors influencing beta counting are numerous, and are usually controlled by using an identical set up from one trial to the next. Among the factors, which may vary if care is not taken, are:

(1) *Geometry.* Particles from a radioactive source travel in all directions, forming a "sphere" of emissions. If the source is at the center of a spherical detector, then potentially all particles may be detected. In most devices, the detector is in the form of a hemisphere around the source, and hence its sensitive volume does not detect particles leaving the "bottom." Spherical detectors are referred to as having 4 π geometry (since the area of a sphere is $4\pi r^2$), and the hemispherical detectors are termed 2 π. For relative counting, 2 π counters are sufficient, as long as the geometry is not altered from sample to sample.

(2) *Scattering.* In standard 2 π counters, a number of emissions which are directed downward and theoretically not detectable, strike the rear surface, and "scatter" back into the sensitive volume of the apparatus; detectable counts will be higher than the number expected. By using the same apparatus, and keeping sample sizes identical, scattering may be kept approximately constant. Back scatter increases with increased atomic weight of the sample holder. Materials with a low atomic weight (aluminum, Lucite) are thus used to hold the sample and reduce scattering factor.

(3) *Ionization.* To be detected, an emission must produce an "ionization" (either a true ionization in a gas, or a "collision" and scintillation in a scintillating medium). The probability of such an event is low for a gamma ray, but very great (close to unity) for a beta particle. By keeping the medium invariant for a given isotope, the ionization factor may also be reduced to an invariant.

(4) *Absorption.* This factor has been discussed in a previous section. Ex-

cept in cases when the radioisotope is introduced directly into the sensitive volume of a detector, the emissions must pass through a "window" in order to gain access. The window itself, air, and other intervening materials, will absorb emissions and reduce the total count. A simple technic has been employed in order to correct for this absorption. Thin filters are successively introduced in front of the radioisotope, reducing the counts. After several points have been plotted (per cent transmission against mg/cm² absorber), the curve may be extrapolated back to "zero" absorber (Figure 1). When counting weak beta particles, thickness of the window should be less than 2.5 mg/cm².

(5) *Self-absorption.* Weak energy beta particles are absorbed in small quantities of matter, including the thickness of the sample itself. A layer only one atom thick would have no "self-absorption." As additional layers are added, some of the beta particles from the deeper strata are absorbed, and fail to gain the surface. With the continuing addition of layers, more self-absorption occurs until a certain point (called "infinite thickness") is reached, beyond which all particles from deep layers are completely absorbed. It is of the utmost importance to keep samples thin, and to maintain the same thickness from sample to sample.

18.4.3 *Preparation of Samples.* To obtain significant and reproducible counts from a weak beta emitter, samples must be prepared so that, (1) there is minimal extraneous foreign material (which can act as an absorber) (2) there is uniform distribution of the radioisotope over a small area. Preparation of the sample is aimed at eliminating inert materials. Methods employed depend upon the isotope present, its chemical form, and the suspending medium.

(1) *Drying.* An isotope, if diluted in a liquid, may be prepared simply by drying on a planchette. Should the nuclide tend to evaporate during the procedure, a "stabilizer" may be added, or drying may be attempted under conditions of reduced pressure (to lower the temperature required).

(2) *Ashing.* Extraneous organic material can often be gotten rid of by ashing the biologic specimen (the method is not useful if the isotope itself volatilizes). "Wet ashing" consists of treating the sample with a strong acid or other reagents to oxidize organic material. "Dry ashing" is nothing more than incineration at high temperatures. Ashed specimens may be further treated to concentrate the isotope.

(3) *Precipitation.* Technics are available for precipitating a number of radioisotopes. Most of these require the isotope to be in a distinct chemical form, and hence pretreatment is necessary (Table III tabulates some of these methods).

Such procedures are of course most necessary in the case of isotopes which emit beta particles. For a number of gamma emitting nuclides, pre-

TABLE III
Methods of Preparing Some β-Emitting Isotopes from Specimens

BETA EMITTING ISOTOPE	PRETREATMENT	PRECIPITATION METHOD
P^{32}	Add inactive sodium phosphate in quantities to produce uniform weight of samples after precipitation (this keeps self-absorption at a constant value).	Precipitate as magnesium ammonium phosphate.
S^{35}	Oxidize tissue organic sulfur to sulfates.	Precipitate as benzidine sulfate.
C^{14}	Oxidize tissue to yield $C^{14}O_2$.	Precipitate as insoluble barium carbonate (or count $C^{14}O_2$ directly in sensitive volume of detector).

cipitation methods are also available, and may be used for accurate work with small quantities.

(4) *Other methods.* For handling specific problems, a number of ingenious technics are available. *a. Ion exchange.* By use of a suitable ion exchange resin, a desired anion or cation can be selectively taken from a specimen, and held to the resin "column." The material may then be eluted by suitable acid or alkali, concentrated, and counted. Resins are made by a number of commercial concerns who furnish descriptive literature. Trace elements have been particularly concentrated by this method. *b. Chromatography.* When a mixture of compounds is poured into a column containing an absorbing substance (such as alumina), and a suitable solvent is added the compounds migrate downward at different rates, depending upon their affinity for the column. This difference in rate of mobility may be utilized to separate a compound or element from interfering substances. "Column" chromatography, "paper" chromatography (see a later section for a more complete description) and "electrochromatography" are all variants of their basic procedure. *c. Additional physical techniques.* A number of additional physical methods have been used for concentrating isotopes. Iron and certain metals may be electroplated from a solution onto a planchette; this leaves the majority of impurities behind. Differences in solubility and diffusion, have also been applied to the concentration of isotopes.

18.5 Autoradiography

By autoradiography is meant the exposure of a suitable photographic emulsion by a radio-active material. Becquerel produced the first autoradiograph in 1896 when uranium ore placed on top of a photographic film resulted in "fogging" of the emulsion. Hence, autoradiography dates to the time of the discovery of radioactivity. The term "autoradiography" appeared as early as 1904, and hence has a certain historical sanction. It is to be preferred to "radioautography" which furthur suffers from having four vowels in a row.

Autoradiography is the ultimate method, so far, for localizing radioactive deposits on the microscopic level. Boyd has provided a valuable book on the method, which may be consulted for additional details and references.

The principal technic of autoradiography consists of placing a specimen (gross or microscopic) in contact with a photographic emulsion for a period sufficient to allow exposure of the silver halide grains. The emulsion is developed, and the tissue section is stained. Superimposition of the developed autoradiograph and the tissue section, allows determination of the areas responsible for darkening of the film.

An autoradiographic "emulsion" is really a gelatin suspension of a silver halide, such as AgBr. Occasionally dyes are added to render it less sensitive to visible light.

Emissions striking a grain of silver halide cause a change to occur which allows the grain to be "developed" by suitable chemicals. A developer is a material which changes the silver ions on the activated grain to metallic silver, producing a visible image. Thus a "picture" is produced, which may be compared with the standard histologic section.

Alpha particles, heavy and producing much ionization, result in straight paths of exposed silver grains. Beta particles, faster moving, have a lesser probability of meeting a grain. Beta autoradiographs are thus of necessity performed on film that has a larger grain size. Emulsions for beta work have a thickness of 5 to 10 microns. Silver grains themselves are 0.1 to 1.0 microns in diameter, and resolution of a nuclear event is ultimately limited by this factor. Gamma rays have little probability of striking a silver grain (low ionization and great range). Films designed for beta autoradiography are of slight use for isotopes which emit only gamma rays. A thicker emulsion, and larger grains, may prove successful in detecting gamma events.

To obtain a significant number of interactions between radioemissions and silver grains, long periods of time (often many days) may be required. Throughout this period, the tissue must be held in close approximation to the emulsion. Any space between the two will result in a loss of counts, and poor resolution. Initially, tissue containing radioactivity was placed on a slide and pressed against film. However, the two had to be separated in order to develop the emulsion and stain the tissue. Realigning tissue and its autoradiograph was difficult and inexact. Three technic have been developed for keeping tissue and emulsion in precise alignment.

(1) Melted emulsion may be poured over the tissue (Belanger and Leblond). Emulsion thickness can then be varied as desired. There is little difficulty in subsequently developing the emulsion or staining the tissue.

(2) Tissue can be mounted directly on the photographic emulsion (Endicott an Yagoda). Alpha emitting isotopes (such as polonium), beta emitting nuclides (as C^{14}), and mixed beta-gamma emitters (as I^{131}) have been successfully studied using this technic. Staining and fogging of the emulsion during histologic processing of the autoradiograph has been common in this method as well as with the melted emulsion technic. Because of this, the "stripping film" was introduced

(3) Stripping film is composed of three layers.

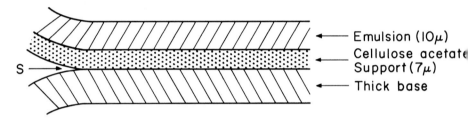

Emulsion (10μ)
Cellulose acetate
Support (7μ)
Thick base

DIAGRAM OF STRIPPING FILM

The emulsion and support can be stripped away from the thick base at the point marked S in the diagram. In practice, a histologic section is mounted on a slide and paraffin removed with xylol and absolute alcohol. A section of film is "stripped" and turned upside down, so that the emulsion is facing the water. The film gradually spreads out without wrinkles. The slide is placed under water and brought up so that the emulsion covers the histologic section. Exposure and development of the film is allowed to proceed. Sections may often be studied by phase contrast microscopy, without staining. If staining is necessary, depending upon the technique, it may be stained directly, or the section can be turned over and stained.

Numerous tissue samples, including the formed elements of blood, have been studied by autoradiography. While valuable information is obtained as to the distribution of radioactive materials, there are also three serious limitations.

(1) *Autochemography.* The finding of silver grains capable of being developed is not in itself sufficient evidence that radioactivity is present in a sample. It can be demonstrated that a number of nonradioactive compounds will "expose" silver grains in an emulsion. Among these substances are terpene hydroxides and reagents containing sulfhydryl groups. Exposure of a photographic emulsion by chemicals in a tissue is termed "autochemog-

raphy." To avoid this pitfall, a section of nonradioactive tissue should be used as a control.

(2) *Physical development.* During chemical development of an emulsion, silver grains are swept away from nonexposed areas, and may be deposited (as artifacts) in the tissue being studied. This "physical development" depends on such factors as pH changes, and can be a source of misinterpretation.

(3) *Latent image changes.* Autoradiography depends upon development of the latent images engendered on silver halogen grains by a source of energy. Any sufficient threshold of energy, irregardless of type, can potentially induce latent images. Among these sources, static electricity and mechanical pressure, may cause changes in the grains. This induction of artifacts is furthur added to by stray cosmic rays which strike the emulsion. Furthur complicating the picture, is the fact that latent images are not permanent, but fade over a period of time. Fading is accentuated in a moist atmosphere, and hence use of a desiccant is advisable.

18.6 Studies of Transport and Metabolism by Tracers

When a radioisotope is added to a biologic system, it is diluted into the pool of the stable element or compound. Even though the specific activity may be reduced several fold by this dilution, the radioisotope is usually still readily detectable. For example, if only one microcurie was used (3700 disintegrations per minute), activity could easily be detected after a 1 to 1,000 dilution. The atoms in 1 microcurie of a biologic tracer generally weigh less than one billionth of a gram. Radioactive isotopes may be detected by their emissions in quantities too small to assay by weight or chemical reaction. Again, it must be emphasized that carrier-free isotopes should be employed whenever possible, to avoid burdening the system with stable carrier.

Upon administration to an animal, a sample of a C^{14}-amino acid may have a specific activity of 3×10^5 counts per milligram. A definite time interval after injection, the liver may contain 1×10^2 counts per milligram. Hence one milligram of liver contained $\dfrac{1 \times 10^2}{3 \times 10^5}$ or 0.033 per cent of the administered dose. The specific activity of the compound has been altered. It may be possible to fractionate the liver still furthur (proteins, polypeptides, amino acids), and express the specific activity of each fraction (counts/mg) as a function of time. Such comparisons provide valuable information as to the quantitative distribution of compounds, and the nature of their precursors. This extremely important application of isotopes will be further discussed in the section on intermediary metabolism.

18.6.1 *Exchange.* Radioisotopes which are present in ionic combination within a compound, may dissociate in solution, and "exchange" with stable ions of the element. The compound $Na^{24}Cl$ dissociates into sodium and chlorine ions, and the metabolic fate of one ion may be quite different from that of the other. Exchange has been used to obtain information as to the reaction rates in varied chemical kinetic studies. For this purpose they are a unique tool.

Bonds other than simple ionic may not necessarily undergo exchange. The ester linkage between glycerol and phosphoric acid is stable, and the phosphate may not readily exchange. However, esterase enzymes split off phosphate, which is then free to exchange. In fact, liberation of P^{32}-phosphate from an ester can be employed as a means of quantitatively estimating esterase activity. Hydrogen atoms in water and in amines undergo exchange, while hydrogen linked directly to carbon is less active. In some cases, the interrelations are complex, and only part of a reaction may involve exchange. Thus, each system must be studied individually.

18.6.2 *Concept of Turnover.* Although the external appearance of the body may be static, there is evidence that tissue components are in a state of dynamic change. Starting with the early investigations of Schoenheimer, many experiments using isotopes have shown that there is a continuing and rapid interchange of chemicals within cells and extracellular components. Metabolic pools are drawn upon and replaced in a precise fashion which usually leaves their net extent unchanged. No longer can structures such as bone and cartilage be viewed as "inert." They are in metabolic activity at all times, with materials entering and leaving.

Of the various technics available for calculating the rate of exchange, perhaps the simplest, when applicable, is determination of the "half-time." This is based on the assumption that the total concentration of the material is not changing, and that as labeled molecules are removed, they are replaced by an equal number of unlabeled molecules. An example will be used to illustrate this point. Stable iron, and radioactive iron (Fe^{59}), are bound to a globulin found in plasma proteins. Plasma can be withdrawn, incubated in vitro with Fe^{59} and reinjected. If samples of blood are taken at 10-minute intervals after this, and the plasma separated, it will be found that the radioactivity (counts/ml plasma) is declining. Plotting the results on semilogarithmic paper, with time as the abscissa and counts/ml as the ordinate (Fig. 3), a straight line results (at least during the first few hours, after this the curve is more complex). Considering initial counts/ml plasma to be 100 per cent, then a point on the curve can be found which represents 50 per cent of the initial activity. The time corresponding to this 50 per cent point is called the "half-time," since it represents the interval required for activity to fall to one half of its original value.

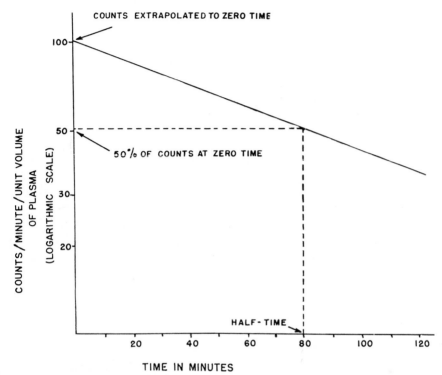

Fig. 3. Diagrammatic representation of the method involved in calculating "disappearance half-time."

The average half-time for Fe^{59} disappearance from plasma is 60 to 120 minutes. Taking as an example a half-time ($T_{1/2}$) of 80 minutes, we can determine a "decay constant" corresponding to this value. It will be recalled that the decay constant of a radioactive material was defined as:

$$\lambda = \frac{0.693}{T_{1/2}}$$

Where $T_{1/2}$ represents the half-life expressed in any convenient time unit. Since radioiron is disappearing from plasma in exponential fashion, as though it were "decaying," a constant (K) may be defined so that

$$K = \frac{0.693}{T_{1/2}}$$

In the case of a half-time of 80 minutes:

$$K = \frac{0.693}{80.} = 0.00866/\text{min.}$$

The reciprocal of this value is the "turnover time" (T_t):

$$T_t = \frac{1}{K} \qquad T_t = \frac{1}{0.00866/\text{min.}} = 115 \text{ min.}$$

This figure is used in calculating the number of turnovers (N_t) per day. Remembering that the time unit being used is the minute, and that there are 1440 minutes per day:

$$N_t = \frac{1440}{T_t}$$

$$N_t = \frac{1440 \text{ min.}}{115 \text{ min.}} = 12.5$$

The interpretation of this is that Fe^{59}, if it truly represented serum iron turnover, would be fully exchanged 12.5 times per day.

Still another important quantity, the actual amount of iron passing through plasma, may be evaluated by means of these figures.

$$\left[\begin{array}{l}\text{Amount of iron passing} \\ \text{through plasma per day}\end{array}\right] = \frac{(N_t) \text{ (plasma volume) (plasma iron concen-}}{\text{tration)}}$$

In the above case: Amount = (12.5) $(4,000 \text{ ml})$ $(1 \mu g/\text{ml}) = 50,000 \mu g/\text{day}$. This technique of determining turnover has also been employed in following the disappearance of phospholipids-P^{32} from plasma, and the disappearance of iodine.

A biologic system can, for purposes of evaluation, be subdivided into spaces called pools or compartments. These divisions, which refer to physiologic and biochemical subdivisions, do not always conform to anatomic units. The blood volume approximates the space within the vascular tree, but the sodium pool is just as definite, although not so precisely defined in anatomic terms.

Most pools are not in free connection, one with another. Rather, there are constraints on the passage of materials, and therefore the flow of substances follows a distinct path and definite regulation. Models of biologic systems have been devised using either catenary (series) or mamillary (parallel) circuits. These models have been useful in calculating the rate of exchange of substances. For example, consider a simple model.

$$A \underset{K_2}{\overset{K_1}{\rightleftarrows}} B \underset{K_4}{\overset{K_3}{\rightleftarrows}} C$$

Three distinct compartments are represented by A, B and C. During the "steady state" the rates of transfer of the material under study are constant. In the diagram, the "rate constants" are represented by K and a subscript. A rate constant signifies some quantity per unit of time (as grams per hour, milliequivalents per minute). During "nonsteady states", the rates of transfer vary, and the values of the K's change.

By the use of radioisotopes, the transfer of materials from one compartment to another may be followed and quantitated. Often, there is a complex interplay of multiple compartments, and the data obtained falls on a curve not readily expressed by a simple mathematical expression. In such instances, a model may be set up, as above, and various rates tried by trial and error, until the resulting data matches that of the original experiment. Electric analogue computers are devices which are suited to this "curve matching," and have been increasingly employed in biologic studies. If a curve is obtained which corresponds to the experimental values, it indicates that a useful model has been obtained. It does not necessarily signify that an exact one to one correlation has been defined.

18.6.3 *Turnover of organic compounds.* Almost all compounds of biologic interest contain carbon, and hence C^{14} has been a commonly employed tracer. Radiosulfur and radiophosphorus also enjoy wide use. Basic facts of body chemistry have yielded to tracer techniques, and it has become clear that a number of previously held concepts are not correct. For example, carbon dioxide rather than being an inert end product, has been demonstrated to be used in the synthesis of all major classes of nutrients.

In the homeostatic individual, most chemical reactions are at equilibrium; that is, the majority of systems are undergoing anabolism to the same extent that they are being broken down or transported away. Turnover rates can be determined in such equilibrium reactions. If a labeled precursor is added to a system, the end product will also bear the radioactive tag, and an estimate of the reaction can be obtained by plotting specific activity of the end product against time.

If the above procedure were performed by injecting a single dose of P^{32} labeled phosphate, the specific activity of tissue organic phosphate would be observed to increase and then decrease. This has been shown to be due to the fact that specific activity of inorganic phosphate in plasma is not constant, but decreases with time. If a constant infusion of P^{32} is used, tissue organic phosphate specific activity approaches that of the inorganic component. By the use of such a method, Hahn and Hevesy found that the rate of phospholipid turnover was greatest in the liver and small intestine.

Inaccuracies of the technique of constant infusion have been pointed out (Zilversmit et al.). Mathematical relationships are available for determining if one compound is the precursor of another on the basis of the rate of change of specific activity following a single injection. Bollman and coworkers studied phospholipid turnover (in rat liver) by means of both the single injection and constant infusion techniques. They defined a proportional turnover rate as:

$$\text{Rate} = \frac{\text{change in specific activity of phospholipid/hour}}{\text{mean sp. act. inorganic P-mean sp. act. phospholipid P}}$$

the values of R as calculated by the two different technics (single injection and constant infusion), agreed closely.

18.6.4 *Determination of site and nature of turnover.* The permeability of cells is not a passively determined factor, but depends upon the functioning of an intact biologic membrane. If the permeability for a compound under consideration (as inorganic phosphate) were low, concentration of the material in interstitial fluid would be higher than that within cellular fluid. Hence, gross counting of "tissue" (which includes both cells and interstitial fluid) might give erroneous results. Inorganic phosphate does not readily enter skeletal muscle. To compensate for this, Kalckar and associates perfused muscle with phosphate-free cold Ringer's solution (one might question if this upset membrane equilibrium), in order to wash out phosphate of interstitial fluid. Under such conditions, comparison of the specific activity of inorganic tissue phosphate with organic phosphate, indicated a large turnover of muscle organic phosphate.

To obtain significant results in any study involving the transfer of a tagged material, it is essential to demonstrate that the reaction is a metabolic one, and not simply "exchange" by collision between labeled and unlabeled materials. In a number of cases, the true metabolic nature was shown by inactivating the enzymes responsible, and demonstrating that no significant exchange occurred. By such techniques, the incorporation of phosphate by the liver, the production of proteins by hepatic slices from amino acids, and the uptake of iodine by thyroid sections, have been shown to be enzyme mediated reactions.

18.6.5 *Water and Electrolyte Movement.* Electrolytes in plasma may or may not enter tissues. If transfer does occur then it happens in both directions across cell membranes, and at equilibrium the rates of entrance and removal are balanced. Tissues contain some sodium, which exchanges with injected Na^{24}. Activity in the blood stream rapidly falls, and then reaches a level that is fairly constant, as the specific activity of tissue sodium approaches that of sodium in the blood. From the blood value of Na^{24} it is possible to calculate the "space" within which the isotope was diluted. By no means is this "sodium space" the total extent of body sodium. There are sodium stores (particularly in bone) which do not readily equilibrate with administered Na^{24}.

Dilution of heavy water (or electrolyte) given intravenously, occurs in a complex fashion. The plot of activity versus time results in a curve. Such a curve can be expressed by an exponential function (see Flexner et al.), and it is possible to calculate the extent of water and electrolyte transfer. The subject can also be approached by removing tissue sections after administration of an isotope, and following the increase in radioactivity. Techniques are available for estimating the extent of "exchangeable" electrolytes by comparing urine radioactivity with that of the blood.

The curve (activity versus time) can have more than two components, if the material enters multiple distinct compartments. The problem of evaluating the extent of these compartments is difficult, and recourse must be made to such techniques as trying to match the curve with similar curves produced by an analogue computer.

Other applications of tagged electrolytes in transfer studies have included their use in determining the entrance of materials into cerebrospinal fluid, the degree of uptake from the gut, and the quantity of passage through partially occluded vessels.

One of the basic approaches to the determination of body composition, has been the estimation of total body water by means of tritiated water (THO). Labeled water is administered, and an interval allowed for equilibration to occur. If account is made of any tagged water lost in urine or feces, then the amount of radioactivity in a unit of blood can be used as an indication of the extent of body water by the dilution formula:

$$A_1 V_1 = A_2 V_2$$

Where A_1 is the counts/minute/ml of tritium injected, V_1 is the volume of injection, A_2 is the counts/minute/ml of plasma after equilibration, and V_2 is the unknown volume of water within the body. By the use of such technics, about two-thirds of the human body has been shown to be composed of water. Discussions of this method and the use of isotopes in the determination of body composition have been presented by Siri and by Moore.

The dilution formula has also been employed in determining the blood volume of an individual. Red blood cells are tagged with Cr^{51} and 20 minutes after reinjection, an aliquot of blood is withdrawn and its radioactivity determined.

18.6.6 *Tracers in the Study of Intermediary Metabolism.* Ingested nutrients are degraded by enzyme systems to simpler compounds, which then become available to body tissues. Investigation of these metabolic pathways, biologic intermediates, and end products of metabolism, has been one of the brightest areas in the use of radioisotopes as a research tool.

A substrate of known composition, containing a radioactive tag, can be administered to the system under study. Care must be taken that the substrate is of high specific activity, and conditions are kept as physiologic as possible. Following a suitable time interval, excreta and tissues are analyzed and various fractions separated. Isolation of a pure compound which contains the radioactive tag, means that at least part of the initial labeled compound was converted to this substance. Simply finding the tag in a new material tells little of its manner of formation. For instance, if radioactive C^{14} were found in a 3 carbon chain, it could be present in any one or more of seven combinations:

$$
\begin{array}{ccccccc}
*\text{C—A} & \text{C—A} & \text{C—A} & *\text{C—A} & *\text{C—A} & \text{C—A} & *\text{C—A} \\
| & | & | & | & | & | & | \\
\text{C—B} & *\text{C—B} & \text{C—B} & *\text{C—B} & \text{C—B} & *\text{C—B} & *\text{C—B} \\
| & | & | & | & | & | & | \\
\text{C—D} & \text{C—D} & *\text{C—D} & \text{C—D} & *\text{C—D} & *\text{C—D} & *\text{C—D}
\end{array}
$$

Where the asterisk indicates the radioactive carbon atoms. Because of this multiplicity of forms, precise chemical degradation is necessary to determine the location of the radiolabel.

When a tagged carbon compound is placed in a metabolic pool (tissue slices or an intact organism), both dilution and degradation take place. Any intermediates will of necessity have a specific activity less than that of the original substrate. In practical terms, this means that a small quantity of low specific activity material is sought in the presence of a "hotter" substrate. It is obvious that great care must be taken, so that the biologic intermediate is obtained free of contaminants. Two technics have been particularly employed to gain radiochemical purity.

(1) Repeated precipitation, crystallization, or solvent extraction, may rid a material of radiocontaminants. Preferably, more than one procedure is used, so that contaminants which survive the first step will be disposed of in subsequent stages. When a compound shows a constant concentration of radioisotope per unit weight (constant specific activity), it is assumed to be in a pure state. Closely related compounds have been known to precipitate together, and care must be taken in interpreting studies which use only a single operation in purifying materials.

(2) By the use of an excess of a nonradioactive material similar in chemical makeup to a known radiocontaminant, the carrier may "wash out" the radioactive impurity. This technic has gained wide application in both organic and inorganic tracer studies. As an example, it has been reported that after the incorporation of C^{14}-alanine by hepatic slices, an excess of the unlabeled amino acid was added to "wash out" unbound alanine. Chromatography, a third technic used to insure radiochemical purity, will be discussed in a later section.

Employment of labeled molecules has elucidated the nature of a number of intermediate compounds, and has led to the use of carriers in isolating minute quantities of these materials. For example, it has been reported that C^{14} in the methyl group of methionine can be detected in epinephrine, after the former compound was administered to rats. By adding carrier epinephrine and recrystallizing it was possible to obtain a constant specific activity.

18.6.7 *Special Technics: Isotope Dilution.* Mention has been made of the addition of a stable carrier to facilitate the isolation of labeled materials. A variant of this procedure has also been used, and has been called "isotope dilution."

A tagged compound is added to the system under study, allowed to equilibrate, and then isolated along with the stable material present. During chemical isolation and purification of a compound, variable losses occur, and difficulty is encountered in estimating the quantity originally present. With the tagged material present as a "marker," the desired compound may be isolated and purified until constant specific activity occurs. The initial quantity of unlabeled compound in the system can then be calculated.

$$Q_{orig} = \left(\frac{Sc}{Ss} - 1\right) Q_{label}$$

where Q_{orig} is the quantity of unlabeled material originally present, Q_{label} is the quantity of labeled carrier added, Sc is the specific activity of the carrier, and Ss is the specific activity of the isolated substance.

The value and versatility of the procedure depends on the fact that no correction has to be applied for loss of the compound, as long as enough remains to be accurately weighed and assayed for radioactivity. An extension of the technique has been proposed by Bloch and Anker, so that the quantity and specific activity of intermediate compounds can be determined. Different, but known amounts of an unlabeled carrier are added to aliquots of the system. Intermediates are then separated. The isotope dilution formula is applied to the two or more concentrations that were employed. Two unknowns are involved (specific activity and quantity), but at least two equations are available, and these can be solved simultaneously. Further applications can be obtained from the literature.

18.6.8 *Special Technics: Chromatography.* Even minute amounts of radioimpurities would interfere with the estimation of a specific tagged molecule. Intensive efforts have therefore been made to assure complete separation and accurate identification of materials; two technics used were previously discussed. One of the ultimate methods thus far devised for delineating a series of related compounds is chromatography.

Chromatography is a term loosely applied to a number of analytic procedures which differ in their basic principles. Four methods are in greatest use (adsorption chromatography, partition chromatography, ion exchange

chromatography and electrochromatography). Generally, chromatography
is any process which permits the resolution of mixtures by separating part
or all of their components in areas or phases different from those in which
they originally were found.

Adsorption chromatography is performed by pouring the mixture to be
separated into an adsorption column (such as alumina, fuller's earth and
so on, depending upon the nature of the compounds). Substances in the
original mixture may show different degrees of affinity for the absorbent,
and hence become separated as the mixture moves down the column.
Separated components may be obtained in pure form by cutting apart the
zones of the column, or by adding a liquid solvent to "elute" the materials
(wash them from the adsorbent). Adsorption chromatography has been
employed for both qualitative and quantitative separation of organic and
inorganic compounds.

In partition chromatography, the technics resemble those used in the
adsorptive technic, but the principle is quite different. Partition chromatography results in the separation of materials because of differences in partition coefficients between two solvents. The most widely used application
of this is in paper chromatography. Cellulose fibers of filter paper serve as
a supporting structure for water. An organic solvent (developer) migrates
through, carrying materials of the mixture.

In one dimensional chromatography, a drop of the mixture to be assayed
is placed on a corner of filter paper. The bottom edge of the paper is placed
in a trough containing the organic solvent, which migrates upward; the
solvent may also be started at the top of the paper, and allowed to run
downward. Solvent migration is slow, about 1 cm per hour. Since the average paper strip is 20 to 30 cm in length, about 1 day must be allowed for
most chromatographic separations. Paper and solvent are usually placed
in a covered jar, to prevent evaporation. At the conclusion of the migration
period, the paper strip is dried, and then processed to make the compounds
visible.

Often unidimensional chromatography is insufficient to separate closely
related compounds. To handle this situation, two-dimensional chromatography was evolved. The mixture is run as with one dimensional chromatography, the paper is dried, rotated 90 degrees, dipped in a second solvent,
and chromatographed again. Since the flow of materials may be different
in the second solvent, greater separation is possible (Fig. 4). The usefulness
of the two-dimensional technic was shown by Gross and Pitt-Rivers, when
they showed that crude "thyroxin" contained traces of triiodothyronine.
The importance of the choice of adsorbent and solvent can not be over-
estimated, and the success or failure of a chromatographic run will be determined by these choices.

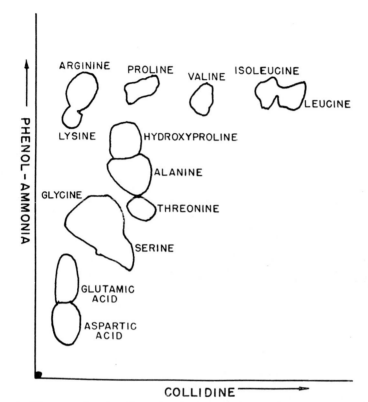

FIG. 4. *Diagram of a two-dimensional chromatogram,* using an hydrolysate of gelatin. The paper was sprayed with ninhydrin to make the amino acids visible. The acid most likely to have made the spot is marked.

For positive identification of materials on a chromatogram, several procedures have been tried.

(1) If sufficient pure compound is present in the chromatographic system, it may be eluted, and subsequently analyzed chemically.

(2) A standard can be prepared, and run simultaneously with the "unknown". If the two spots are at corresponding points, identity is presumably proven. However, difficulty arises if the solvent system employed was not sufficient to separate two closely related compounds.

(3) Spots on the paper can be sprayed with various reagents, and the nature of the material surmised from such "spot tests."

(4) Reliance has often been placed on calculation of the Rf value of the compound. By Rf is meant the "rate of flow," which is the ratio:

$$Rf = \frac{\text{distance of given compound from origin}}{\text{distance of solvent front from origin}}$$

Values of Rf vary with different solvents and must be interpreted accordingly.

Ion exchange chromatography, and electrochromatography, are special applications of the methodology, and multiple examples are present in the literature. The first depends upon different affinities of materials for an ion column, while the second procedure relies upon the different rate of flow of substances in an electrical field.

Chromatographic techniques have been applied to problems of separating tagged metabolites, with handsome results.

(1) Taurog, Tong, and Chaikoff administered I^{131} to rats and performed one-dimensional chromatography on thyroid hydrolysates, 24 hours later. The amount of radioactivity was plotted against the distance of each spot from the starting point of the chromatogram. Radioactive diiodotyrosine, tyroxine and inorganic iodide were demonstrated.

(2) Borsook and associates prepared a paper chromatogram from guinea pig liver homogenates incubated with lysine-C^{14}. A radioactive spot was noted which did not correspond to any then known lysine metabolites. Studies indicated the material to be alpha-amino adipic acid, an intermediate in lysine degradation.

Separation of radioactive metabolites prepared by biosynthesis, and the testing of radiochemical manufactured by other techniques, have been entrusted to chromatography. The growing literature on the subject testifies as to its many applications.

18.7 Neutron Activation Analysis

The technic of neutron activation analysis is a special application of isotope procedures, useful in determining the electrolyte composition of samples (biologic or otherwise). A substances placed in a neutron flux has its component nuclei react with bombarding neutrons. Of the isotopes so produced, some are are unstable and give off emissions. Detection and quantitation of these emissions permits identification of the isotope and estimation of its elemental precursor. The advantages of the method include:

(1) The sample does not have to be separated into its components.

(2) Since the procedure is nondestructive, the sample may be reassayed or kept for other studies.

(3) Minute quantities of anions and cations are detectable, and the neutron activation technique is one of the most accurate analytic methods known.

Low flux intensities (2.5×10^8 neutrons/cm²/sec.) can be used for the analysis of a number of electrolytes. This flux level is obtainable from small nuclear reactors, van de Graaff-beryllium sources, and radium-beryllium mixtures. Hence the method should be available to an increasing number of laboratories. Spencer, Mitchell, and King have presented data on the neutron activation analysis of blood and tissues, and this paper may be consulted for details.

18.8 Summary

Radioactive isotopes have multiple applications as biologic tracers. These "tags" have been employed to estimate the extent of body compartments and to elucidate the compounds involved in intermediary metabolism. Employed cautiously, with their limitations in mind, radioisotopes are an invaluable analytic tool.

SELECTED REFERENCES

General:

HEVESY, G.: *Radioactive Indicators.* New York: Interscience, 1948.
KAMEN, M. D.: *Isotopic Tracers In Biology* (3rd ed.). New York: Acad. Press, 1957.
SACKS, J.: *Isotopic tracers in Biochemistry and Physiology.* New York: McGraw-Hill, 1953.
SIRI, W. E., editor: *Isotopic Tracers and Nuclear Radiations with Applications to Biology and Medicine.* New York: McGraw-Hill, 1949.

Preparation Labeled Compounds:

ANFINSEN, C. B.: Radioactive crystalline ribonuclease. *J. Biol. Chem. 187:* 827, 1950.
GEILING, E. M. K., ET AL.: Biosynthesis of radioactive drugs using carbon 14. *Science, 108:* 558, 1948.
WILZBACH, K. E.: Tritium labeling by exposure of organic compounds to tritium gas. *J. Am. Chem. Soc. 79:* 1013, 1957.
WOODRUFF, N. H. AND FOWLER, E. E.: Biological synthesis of radioisotope labeled compounds. *Nucleonics, 7(2):* 26, 1950.
VILLEE, C. A. AND HASTINGS, A. B.: The metabolism of C^{14} labeled glucose by the rat diaphragm in vitro. *J. Biol. Chem. 179:* 673, 1949.

Multiple Labeling:

BURR, W. W. AND WIGGANS, D. S.: Direct determination of C^{14} and S^{35} in blood. *J. Lab. & Clin. Med. 48:* 907, 1956.
GIBSON, J. G., II, ET AL.: The measurement of post-transfusion survival of preserved stored human erythrocytes by means of two isotopes of radioactive iron. *J. Clin. Invest. 26:* 704, 1947.
LeROY, G. V., GOULD, R. G., BERGENSTAL, D. M., WERBIN, H. AND KABARA, J. J.: Studies on extrahepatic cholesterol synthesis and equilibration in man with a double labeling technique. *J. Lab. & Clin. Med. 49:* 858, 1957.
MITCHELL, T. G., SPENCER, R. P. AND KING, E. R.: Use of radioisotopes in diagnostic hematological procedures. III. Simultaneous Fe^{59} and Cr^{51} studies. *Am. J. Clin. Path. 28:* 461, 1958.
SPENCER, R. P. AND MITCHELL, T. G.: Simultaneous uptake of radiocopper and radiopotassium by rat brain. *J. Neuropath. & Exper. Neurol. 17:* 479, 1958.

Low Level Methods and Beta Counting:

DAVIDSON, J. D. AND FEIGELSON, P.: Practical aspects of internal-sample liquid-scintillation counting. *Int. J. Applied Radiation & Isotopes, 2:* 1, 1957.

FULLER, R. C.: Modified end-window counting tube for paper chromatograms. *Science, 124:* 1253, 1956.

FUNT, B. L. AND HETHERINGTON, A.: Suspension counting of carbon-14 in scintillating gels. *Science, 125:* 986, 1957.

JOHNSTON, W. H.: Low-level counting methods for isotopic tracers. *Science, 124:* 801, 1956.

SOFTKY, S. D. AND NATHER, R. E.: Low-background counter for solid β-emitting isotopes. *Nucleonics, 15:* 90, 1957.

Autoradiography:

BELANGER, L. F. AND LEBLOND, C. P.: Method for locating radioactive elements in tissues by covering histological sections with a photographic emulsion. *Endocrinology 39:* 8, 1946.

BOYD, G.: *Autoradiography in Biology and Medicine.* New York: Acad. Press, 1955.

ENDICOTT, K. M. AND YAGODA, H.: Microscopic historadiographic technic for locating and quantitating radioactive elements in tissues. *Proc. Soc. Exper. Biol. & Med. 64:* 170, 1947.

Other Tracer Applications:

BLOCH, K. AND ANKER, H. S.: An extension of the isotope dilution method. *Science, 107:* 228, 1948.

SCHOENHEIMER, R.: *The Dynamic State of Body Constituents.* Cambridge, Mass.: Harvard Univ. Press, 1942.

Turnover and Its Analogues:

MACDONALD, J. R., PERRY, E. G., MADISON, L. L. AND SELDIN, D. W.: An electrical analogue for analysis of tracer distribution kinetics in biological systems. *Radiation Res. 6:* 585, 1957.

ROBERTSON, J. S.: Theory and use of tracers in determining transfer rates in biological systems. *Physiol. Rev. 37:* 133, 1957.

STANBURY, J. B. AND BROWNELL, G. L.: Multi-compartmented biologic models. *J. Clin. Endocrinol. 14:* 1079, 1954.

ZILVERSMIT, D. B. ET AL.: The turnover rate of phospholipids in the plasma of the dog as measured with radioactive phosphorus. *J. Gen. Physiol. 26:* 333, 1943.

Neutron Activation Analysis:

SPENCER, R. P., MITCHELL, T. G. AND KING, E. R.: Medical Applications of neutron activation analysis. *Int. J. Applied Radiation & Isotopes 3:* 104, 1958.

SPENCER, R. P., MITCHELL, T. G. AND KING, E. R.: Neutron activation analysis of sodium in blood serum. *J. Lab. & Clin. Med. 50:* 646, 1957.

19▲

Radiophosphorus and Radioiodine

Charles F. Geschickter, M.D. and Murray M. Copeland, M.D., D.Sc.

19.1 Radiophosphorus

19.1.1 *The Nature of P^{32}*. The nucleus of stable phosphorus (P^{31}) contains 15 protons and 16 neutrons. When bombarded with neutrons moving at high speed the neutron goes into the nucleus to give P^{32} with 15 protons and 17 neutrons. This unstable element undergoes nuclear transformation with the emission of an electron given off as a beta ray and becomes stable sulfur (S^{32}). This transformation makes the element P^{32} radioactive. The element has a half life of 14.5 days.

When the usual form of administering ionizing irradiations is used (roentgen therapy) the biologic effects partly depend on the liberation of secondary electrons when the primary roentgen rays penetrate the tissues. Radioactive phosphorus is a beta-emitter and produces high speed electrons with identical biologic effects. The difference is in the distribution of the ionizing irradiations of the isotope which penetrate only a few millimeters and therefore are confined largely to the skeletal tissues which concentrate P^{32}. In addition to these two attributes (the form of irradiation used and its distribution), there is a third factor which contributes to the effects observed. This is the radiosensitivity of the biologic structures. (When P^{32} is used, the most radiosensitive tissue, because of its proximity and biologic properties, is the marrow, whether normal or having malignant changes.

Radioactive phosphorus was the first artificial isotope to find widespread application to the cancer problem. It has been applied as a tool for elucidating the nature of the disease as well as a therapeutic instrument in curtailing its progress.

19.1.2 *P^{32} Metabolism*. The use of P^{32} as a tracer has emphasized the rate of turnover of cellular materials or metabolites in normal tissues. Thus, although the brain and liver as organs contain equal amounts of phosphorus in organic combination, the liver takes up about six times as much P^{32} per unit of time as does the brain. This correlates with the higher metabolic turnover of food stuffs in the liver and with the fact that hepatic epithelium undergoes continual replacement, whereas the ganglion cells of the brain do not. The use of P^{32} as a tracer has confirmed also the histologic observation that cancer renews itself more rapidly than the corresponding normal tissue. This replacement of tissue is roughly proportional to the number of mitoses per thousand cells in a stained section. The mitotic count is increased in malignancy. This increased rate of cellular reproduction is reflected in the P^{32} take-up. The lymph nodes and spleen of leukemic mice take up roughly three times as much radioactive phosphorus as the corresponding organs of normal mice. This is further evidence that the cycle of tissue regeneration is foreshortened in malignancy. Thus, the normal cycle for renewal of the polymorphonuclear leukocyte is 15 days; in leukemia the cycle is roughly five days or less, according to whether the leukemia is chronic, subacute or acute. Moreover, the rate of metabolic turnover as indicated by P^{32} uptake is shifted to the nuclear protein as against the lipid fraction. This indicates that in cancer the major energy expenditure is for nuclear growth and reduplication as against cytoplasmic differentiation.

19.1.3 *Use of Radiophosphorus in Metabolic Studies.* In addition to the usefulness of P^{32} in the study of benign and malignant cellular growth, it has been applied extensively as a biologic indicator in metabolic research.

In the mineral metabolism of bone and of growing teeth, approximately 75 per cent of body phosphate is stored in these organs. Eighty per cent of this phosphate is deposited as a stable portion of the teeth and bones and 20 per cent as a superficial labile portion which is in dynamic equilibrium with the phosphates of the blood plasma. This exchange takes place by surface absorption and comes to equilibrium in about two hours after intravenous injection as shown by the use of P^{32} (Neuman and Riley). In rachitic rats it has been found that vitamin D favors the deposition of absorbed phosphate in the bones as against the soft tissues, and partially inhibits the re-excretion of phosphate in the intestine. A single dose of vitamin D exerts its maximum effect on P^{32} uptake in rachitic bone in 54 to 72 hours.

In animal experimentation with radioactive phosphorus, the growing epiphyses of bones have been found to turn over phosphorus in a ratio of four to one, as compared with the shafts of the bones. In phosphorus deficiency, there is a shift of phosphorus concentration from bone to the soft part tissues. At the same time there is a decrease in urinary phosphorus excretion and a corresponding calciuria. Where calcium deficiency obtains, less phosphorus is deposited in the bone but a larger amount is excreted in the urine.

Osgood points out that in the human adult only about 8 per cent of the phosphorus in the body is in equilibrium. Very little of the P^{32} from the labeled pool of phosphorus is in the skeleton, in contradistinction to studies made in young animals, where the majority of the radioactive phosphorus is found in bone. He points out the common mistake of transferring tracer studies from one species to another, or one age group to another in the same species.

Tracer studies with radiophosphorus have confirmed the important role that phosphorus plays in carbohydrate metabolism. As a result of such studies, Sachs concludes that the absorption of glucose by cells (such as muscle cells, probably the mucosa of the small intestine and renal epithelium) takes place by the formation of the glucose-6-phosphate derivative on the cell membrane, with the glucose portion directed toward the cell interior and the phosphate portion directed away from the cell. The hydrolysis of the compound then results in the entry of the glucose molecule, while the phosphate molecule remains outside the cell. On the other hand, the phosphate molecule enters the cell by the formation on the membrane of other organic phosphate compounds with a reversal of spatial arrangements. Once in the interior of the cell, the phosphorus metabolic exchange in the cytoplasm is five to 100 times more active than the exchange of phosphorus across the cell membrane. This is true of the interactions of the PO_4 ion with such molecules as phosphocreatine (PC), adenosine triphosphate (ATP) and hexose monophosphate (HMP).

It has been found that insulin accelerates the transfer of P^{32} as PC and ATP across the cell membrane of muscle; but not in traumatic shock. Thyroid hormone also accelerates this transfer while hypothyroid states diminish it.

In regard to lipoid metabolism, Flock and Bollman showed that glycerophosphate in the liver acquires administered P^{32} first, but later the phosphorus is transferred to the liver phospholipids. The magnitude of phospholipid formation in the organs is highest in liver, kidney and small intestine in descending order. The phospholipids of the blood plasma are supplied and removed by the liver. The rate of removal of phospholipids from the plasma (10 per cent per hour) rapidly declines when the liver is excluded from the circulation. These and similar studies indicate that phosphorylating reactions are involved in fat transport and in fat metabolism, but that phosphorylation is not an obligate stage in fat transport. Thus, hepatic phospholipids account for only 3 per cent of the fat undergoing transportation. The phospholipids in the thoracic duct come mainly from the intestine; a smaller portion from the liver.

Bollman and Flock in a study of phospholipid turnover in the liver of the rat, found that the rate of P^{32} phospholipid turnover per hour per 100 gm. of body weight was remarkably constant and uninfluenced by changes in the composition of the diet, which influenced instead the total hepatic lipid content. Partial hepatectomy increased the turnover per gram of liver, while CCl₄ poisoning decreased it though the livers were larger, but neither affected the rate in relation to body weight. The administration of choline increased the turnover rate in the fatty livers of rats placed on a previous choline-free diet, but not in rats with normal livers.

Work with P^{32} in lipoid metabolism has been handicapped because phosphoric esters upon injection undergo rapid hydrolysis. Labeled plasma phospholipids may be injected intravenously but phospholipids found in the tissues when reinjected act as foreign bodies and are concentrated in the macrophages of the spleen and lungs. The phospholipids of muscle are acquired by transport, not by synthesis.

Adrenalectomized rats have normal rates of phospholipid formation in the intestine. Roosters treated with estrogen showed an increased rate of phospholipid formation in the liver and a higher rate of transfer to the plasma.

The turnover rate of lecithin is higher than cephalin in normal and neoplastic tissues.

Radiophosphorus has been used in the study of muscle protein metabolism. The ribosenucleic acids of the cytoplasm are found to undergo metabolic turnover. Desoxyribosenucleic acids in the nuclei are increased and take up P^{32} during tissue growth. This uptake of P^{32} parallels mitotic activity in regenerating liver following partial hepatectomy and in experimental hepatoma (Brues, Tracy and Cohn).

The uptake of radiophosphorus is greatest in normal tissues that form new cells throughout life such as bone marrow, intestinal epithelium, etc. (Andreasen and Ottesen).

The teeth utilize and exchange a relatively low amount of phosphorus under normal conditions, and this occurs through the pulp and dentine. Very little phosphorus is picked up through the intact enamel unless there are areas of tooth decay.

Brachet emphasizes the striking parallelism between the intensity of the alkaline phosphatase reaction and the turnover rate of desoxyribosenucleic acid phosphorus in various organs. This strongly suggests that the nuclear alkaline phosphatase may be responsible for the replacement of phosphorus in the desoxyribosenucleic acid molecule.

Tweedy et al. studied the role of parathyroid hormone in excretion of phosphorus by the kidneys in rats. Parathyroidectomized rats were given P^{32} and were found to excrete no radioactive phosphorus in the urine. Following the administration of parathyroid hormone, the rats were found to excrete P^{32} in the urine. When the parathyroidectomized rats were subjected to bilateral nephrectomy they showed no fecal excretion of P^{32}. The administration of parathyroid hormone and P^{32} failed to bring about any change in fecal excretion in these nephrectomized animals. Conclusion drawn was that while the role of parathyroid hormone in phosphorus excretion is important, it is not controlling.

Irradiation with x-rays decreases the uptake of P^{32} in nuclear desoxyribosenucleic acid in normal tissue, but following irradiation the rate rapidly returns to normal.

19.1.4 *Dosage, Absorption and Distribution of* P^{32}. Kenney, Marinelli and Woodward in studying the uptake of phosphorus (P^{32}) by breast carcinoma, osteogenic sarcoma and lymphosarcoma found that osteogenic sarcoma concentrated P^{32} more effectively than did normal bone, but that the amount which was concentrated did not deliver sufficient radiation to destroy the tumor. They also found that primary breast cancer concentrated P^{32} to a lesser extent than did the metastatic nodes or even normal nodes in the same patient. Lymph nodes involved by lymphosarcoma showed a selective concentration of phosphorus.

It would appear that the uptake and retention of phosphorus is definitely related to the phosphorus present in the tissues, and to the relative rate of metabolism of phosphorus within the tissues. It, therefore, holds that neoplastic tissues with a high rate of mitotic division will utilize increased amounts of phosphorus, which is readily observed by studies with radioactive phosphorus (P^{32}).

Erf, et al., Lawrence, et al., Tuttle, et al., and Low-Beer, et al., report tracer studies with radioactive phosphorus which indicate that the element is rapidly utilized by red blood cells and lymphocytes in normal individuals, and in patients with leukemia and polycythemia rubra vera. In the first 48 hours following tracer P^{32} absorption, the erythrocytes contain more phosphorus than the leukocytes. After 48 hours, there is a decline in the amount of radioactive phosphorus contained in the red blood cells of both normal individuals and in patients with leukemia or polycythemia rubra vera. In leukemia patients, however, more P^{32} is found in the whole blood than in normal subjects or patients suffering with polycythemia rubra vera. Leukemia patients show an increasing uptake of P^{32} absorption by leukocytes. Ultimately, these patients reveal a concentration of P^{32} in the leukocytes five times greater than in the erythrocytes present. The plasma concentration of P^{32} is similar in normal subjects and in patients with leukemia and polycythemia. Under the same circumstances of time and administration, the bone marrow shows a higher concentration of phosphorus (P^{32}) than does the peripheral blood. Myelocytes and lymphocytes differ in their proclivities for the uptake of P^{32}. The nuclei of myelocytes concentrate larger amounts of P^{32} than the cytoplasm, while in lymphocytes the uptake seems to be the same in both the nucleus and cytoplasm. The permeation of red blood cells by inorganic phosphorus appears to be a link in the dynamics of cell metabolism, rather than simple diffusion. Body temperature, hemolysis and certain drugs affect the transfer rate of phosphorus from plasma to red blood cells and reflect changes in cell membrane permeability.

Radioactive phosphorus has been used extensively in metabolic studies, other than those previously mentioned. *Those of diagnostic importance include* the use of P^{32} in the localization of brain tumors. Selverstone, Solomon and Sweet found that it was necessary to devise a miniature Geiger-Müller counter that could be inserted directly into the brain tissue, because of the short effective range of the beta radiation emitted by radioactive phosphorus (P^{32}). Good differentials were obtained between normal and pathological areas, and the method holds promise as a part of the neurosurgeon's diagnostic armamentarium.

Locksley et al., in a comparative clinical and laboratory study in localization and treatment of brain tumors, demonstrated that with P^{32}, K^{42} and sodium borate, there was a close agreement in the concentration ratios observed between tumor and brain.

Bakay has utilized P^{32} to determine whether or not a blood-brain barrier exists at birth. Rabbits were used as experimental animals, 50 of which were pregnant and four used as controls. He concluded from this investigation that the existence of a blood-brain barrier is dependent upon capillary development and metabolic requirements. The cerebral level of P^{32} is high for the first few post-natal weeks and then drops to adult level. There is a higher and more generalized uptake by the foetal embryonic tissues.

Bauer, Moss and Richardson suggested, as the basis for a technic to distinguish between benign and malignant origin of an effusion, the P^{32} activity of the pleural fluid. The method depends on the increased uptake of P^{32} by nucleoprotein in rapidly growing neoplastic, acute inflammatory or actively regenerating normal tissue. A "P^{32} index" is arrived at which, the authors claim, will distinguish between increased metabolic activity due to benign and malignant causes.

Wilson, in an uptake radioactive phosphorus study, by the knee-joint and tibia of 6-week old mice, and the effect of x-rays upon the uptake, has provided base-line data for the quantitative assessment of radiation damage to bone. These data can be used to evaluate various dosage levels, time-dose relationship and other radiation variables. For instance, it was noted that there was a depression of phosphorus uptake produced by 2000 roentgens of 200-kv x-rays administered as a single dose. Subsequent recovery was slow and incomplete at 22 weeks. The reasons for this chain of events are postulated.

Wilkinson and Leblonde, in a study of deposition of radiophosphorus in fractured bones in rats, showed by the use of radioautographs that the trabeculae of new bone fix radiophosphorus most actively. This would indicate that the trabeculae calcify rapidly, playing an early role in strengthening the fractured bone. They further deduce from this study that dissolution and reprecipitation of crystalline material occurs not only in the fractured bone, but also in normal bones far from the seat of injury.

Clinical studies on the uptake of tracer doses of radioactive phosphorus (P^{32}) on tumors of the breast have yielded some interesting observations. McCorkle, Low-Beer and their associates have found that malignant tumors of the breast and related metastatic deposits show an increased absorption of radioactive phosphorus (P^{32}). Inflammations of the breast also show an increase in the absorption of phosphorus. This is of some diagnostic significance if the cancer or inflammation is not situated deeper than 0.5 cm. from the surface.

Radioactive phosphorus (P^{32}) has also been effectively used in the study of peripheral vascular disease. Friedell, Schaffner and their associates studied 100 patients in the Cook County Hospital. They found that P^{32} was concentrated more rapidly in the tissues of extremities of persons with arteriosclerosis than in tissues of subjects with apparently normal circulation. From this they postulated that the radioactive ion diffused more rapidly into the tissues of older patients and in those individuals with abnormal circulation. The authors feel that they have established the presence of vasodilation in the capillary bed, associated with arteriosclerosis, and in all persons in whom arterio-elasticity has diminished.

Arden and Veall have utilized P^{32} for investigating the blood supply of the femoral head. One to two cc. of P^{32} is given intravenously one hour before the nail operation utilized in treating fractures of the neck of the femur. At operation, a sample of bone is removed from the trochanteric region (for control), and from the head of the femur. These samples are analyzed for radioactive content. More recently, a needle Geiger counter has been utilized to take direct readings at the time of operation. By this means the investigators feel that it is possible to decide, at the time of operation, the status of the femoral head, blood supply.

Corrigan and Hayden consider tracer technique an exceptionally valuable means of diagnosis, when used carefully in cooperation with other methods. They point out the use of I^{131} for identifying toxic retrosternal thyroids. When the I^{131} test is negative, on a mediastinal mass, it is their standard procedure to administer 100 microcuries of radioactive phosphorus. The radioactive iodine will clear from the bloodstream within 48 hours and, thereafter, if the mediastinal shadow is due to an actively growing tumor, a good concentration of P^{32} can be found. These authors discuss factors which lead to error and give suggestions for arriving at accurate diagnosis in complicated cases.

Krohmer, et al., consider P^{32} uptake studies as valuable adjuncts to careful clinical evaluation of suspected eye tumors, but not as a conclusive diagnostic test. Five-hundred microcuries of P^{32}, in sterile isotonic saline is injected intravenously. Immediately following injection, a counting tube is placed directly in contact with the eye, at the closest point to the suspected tumor. The authors conclude that a selective uptake ratio of 1:4 or higher in the anterior segment of the eye is suggestive of tumors, while a ratio of less than 1:2 indicates a non-neoplastic process. The uptake ratio for posterior tumors of the eye was less reliable.

Woodward and Kenney have studied the relationship of phosphatase activity in bone tumors to the deposition of radioactive phosphorus. Some bone tumors were found to contain little or no alkaline phosphatase and apparently lacked the capacity to lay down calcium phosphate. The majority of osteogenic sarcomas, however, contained large amounts of alkaline phosphatase. It appeared that the more rapid the growth and the greater the osteoplastic tendency, the higher the alkaline phosphatase activity present. Many of the metastases from such tumors contained large amounts of phosphatase. The presence of great phosphatase activity suggested that larger amounts of P^{32} would be picked up by both the primary lesion and the metastases. Such proved to be the case. In some osteogenic sarcomas, however, with high phosphatase activity, unknown factors present prevented the deposition of calcium phosphate. It was pointed out that this fact connoted a poor prognosis. It was also noted that this peculiar lack of calcium phosphate deposition would prevent the possible use of radiophosphorus in the treatment of such bone tumors.

Radioactive phosphorus has not proven successful, alone, in the treatment of primary bone tumors, though its supplementary use with other forms of irradiation has been suggested.

Radioactive phosphorus is usually administered intravenously as the isotonic aqueous solution of disodium acid phosphate. It can also be administered orally. About 1 out of 500,000 molecules is radioactive. The beta ray emitted has a maximum energy of 1.8 million electron-volts with a maximum range of tissue penetration of approximately 0.7 cm.

As stated above, when P^{32} enters the body the rate and amount of its uptake are dependent on (1) the exchangeable P content of the tissues, (2) the rate of turnover of exchangeable P, and (3) the rate of reproduction of tissues. They also depend on (1) the dose and form in which P^{32} is given and (2) the mode of administration.

By intravenous administration there is fairly constant relationship between retention and excretion. Approximately 25 per cent is excreted the first three days after intravenous administration. The amount retained at the end of the third day is called the retention dose. Between the fourth and 14th days about 5 per cent of the retention dose is lost daily so that 50 per cent is left on the 14th day; 33 per cent on the 21st day and 19 per cent on the 30th.

Besides this factor of elimination, there is the one of decay. At the end of two weeks half of the retained dose, or 37.15 per cent, is present. But it has only one-half of its former radioactivity. Thus, only 18.5 per cent of the initial dose remains.

By 6 weeks the patient will receive negligible radiation from any previous dose, barring gene mutations from unpredictable threshold exposure.

In the use of radioisotopes for tracer studies and clinical application certain precautions should be taken which include knowledge of radiation dosage and its safety limits, the avoidance of contamination as a factor in unreliable experimental data, and the avoidance of contamination as a health hazard.

In present-day usage most radioisotopes are administered orally or parenterally in soluble form. Marinelli and his co-workers, while emphasizing the difficulty involved, feel that, in some cases at least, a satisfactory estimate of tissue dosage can be made when the factors of half-life, radiation energy and the physiologic factors of uptake and secretion are known.

Radioisotopes, which are beta-ray emitters only, such as P^{32}, render dosage which is essentially confined to the regions or tissues actually containing the material. When a substance is a gamma-ray-emitter the rays released in a unit of tissue expend most of their energy elsewhere along their paths, and present problems closely akin to interstitial radium gamma ray dosage.

A safe tracer concentration is considered the number of microcuries per kilogram of tissue which will result in a whole tissue dose of 0.1 r the first day (due to the beta rays alone).

Physiologic information on the distribution of the radiation in tissue depends on the amount of isotope administered, the type of animal, the mode of administration, the chemical form of the radioactive element, the state of the metabolism of the organism and metabolic elimination.

The differential absorption ratio of various tissues is most important in calculating the safe dose of tracers. The safe dose is assumed to be 0.3 r per week for the entire body. If one of the tissues absorbed 10 times as much as another, this could well lead to dosage in the tissue absorbing the greater amount much beyond the factor of safety. This might be desirable in considering therapy. Many complications enter such calculations, for which the reader is referred to appended literature on this subject.

Marinelli and his co-workers indicate that the actual amounts of the safe concentrations of many radioisotopes in tissue may not vary greatly but that the intervals at which they can be repeated do. A reasonable interval between full radio-tracer doses of any particular element would be four or five effective half lives, unless the material is excreted completely in a much shorter period. Phosphorus (P^{32}), for instance, could be repeated in 2 months. It also must be understood that the individual is receiving no radiation from any other source.

The rate of elimination of a radioisotope by a given tissue obviously will affect the dosage, since a portion of the radioisotope in the tissue will not disintegrate there, but will be eliminated. The rate of concentration, as affected by both elimination and decay, must be obtained by actual measurements. The decrease is exponential but is more rapid than if there were no excretion of radioactive material. Such measurements of radioactivity in vivo represent the effective disintegration rate of the isotope and determine the effective half life of the radioisotope to be less than the physical half life.

Inorganic and colloidal suspension forms of P^{32} have been used. Phospholipids, pentonucleotides, glycerophosphates, etc., have not been tried in therapy. Their absorption and distribution require investigation.

19.1.5 *Therapeutic Applications of Radioactive Phosphorus.* Treatment of Polycythemia: Without going into detail in regard to the experimental evidence, it is generally agreed that the distribution of radioactive phosphorus in the tissues is dependent, as stated above, on the following factors: (1) the exchangeable phosphorus content of the normal differentiated structure (in this regard bone has the highest chemical concentration, containing roughly 75 per cent of the total body phosphorus); (2) the rate of turnover of metabolized phosphorus utilized for ordinary caloric requirements, such as the combustion of carbohydrates; (3) the rate of cellular reproduction in the tissues or the amount of phosphorus used for nuclear and cytoplasmic reconstruction.

Although radioactive phosphorus was introduced in the treatment of leukemia by Lawrence and his co-workers over ten years ago, practically no attempt has been made to influence the physiologic processes which control the uptake and distribution of this highly potent therapeutic agent in the human body. As a result, although malignant tissue utilizes more than its normal proportion because of its increased rate of cellular reproduction, the chemical composition of the bone outweighs this pathologic factor. Moreover, the cells in the marrow normally multiply rapidly. Hence, the danger of bone marrow suppression following the administration of P^{32} imposes a severe handicap to its usefulness as a therapeutic agent.

To date the therapeutic application of radiophosphorus has been largely limited, in the larger clinics, to polycythemia vera and chronic leukemia.

A smaller number of cases of multiple myeloma, Hodgkin's disease and lymphomas have been treated. The number of cases of polycythemia vera treated and reported run into several hundred. Reports include those from the Crocker Radiation Laboratory of California; from the Mayo Clinic; from the Mallinckrodt Institute of St. Louis, from Mt. Sinai Hospital in New York, from University of Oregon Medical School in Portland and many other papers have been reviewed summarizing the therapy of polycythemia vera with radiophosphorus.

Treatment with radiophosphorus varies as to details but, in general, a single initial dose is given intravenously or by mouth followed, subsequently, by repeated dosages as necessary for the control of the disease.

The disease having been carefully verified, an initial dose based on 100 microcuries per kilogram of body weight is a satisfactory approach to dosage. This may be increased 25 % if given by mouth. Fractionation into three daily portions when given by mouth has been utilized in maintaining a better biological half life for the dosage. The average dose by this method varies between 4–10 millicuries. A larger single dose than 10 mc is not recommended, and from 2 to 3 months are allowed to elapse before a second or successive dose is given.

Osgood and Associates use the following plan for dosage of P^{32} given intravenously: for patients weighing 125 to 175 pounds, the dose of radioactive phosphorus is 4 mc; for patients weighing over that, 5 mc are given; for patients weighing less than that, 3 mc are given. The patient may be treated again in 4 weeks and at 8 weeks, if necessary for control, if symptoms and findings indicate.

Retreatment, after satisfactory control, is rarely necessary, before 1 to 3 years. Osgood retreats with the same scale of dosage and, in a few cases, has had to use larger doses at more frequent intervals. In the greater percentage of cases not only did the red count fall from an average high of 7.25 million to between 4 and 5 million, but a corresponding relief was noted in the symptoms of fatigue, headache, dizziness, bone and splenic pain, pruritus, visual disturbance and paresthesia.

In general, these patients have been followed between five and thirteen years. The symptomatic relief and control of the blood count (both red and white cells) have been striking. From the studies of Lawrence, Berlin and Huff, and also of Stroebel, it is apparent that, with any of the methods currently in use for treating polycythemia rubra vera with radioactive phosphorus, a life expectancy of nearly normal duration may be expected. The best method to use is still to be evaluated with the use of comparative data not yet available.

The treatment of polycythemia with radiophosphorus is not without its complications. A large proportion of the cases at some time during treatment developed leukopenia, thrombocytopenia or anemia because of the suppressive action on the bone marrow. Such complications occur in about 20 per cent of the individuals treated. Deaths after therapy were attributed to leukemia, hypoplastic anemia, pneumonia, and to cancer of the stomach, pancreas and kidney. Tuberculosis, peritonitis and various forms of hemorrhage also accounted for some of the deaths. The incidence of leukemia following radiophosphorus therapy (3 per cent) is probably higher than in cases treated by other methods.

The increased longevity of patients treated by this method, however, renders the complications less formidable and makes the method acceptable until some better therapeutic approach is demonstrated.

Palliation of the symptoms of chronic leukemia may be obtained by therapy with various substances. It is felt by some that, in chronic myelocytic or monocytic leukemias of the Naegeli type, roentgen irradiation, radiophosphorus and several chemotherapeutic agents are useful. In chronic lymphocytic leukemia and in chronic monocytic leukemia of the Schilling type, chemotherapy and external roentgen therapy are preferred. Watkins doubts that any known treatment prolongs the life of a chronic leukemia patient. Except for Osgood's reported results from titrated, regularly spaced P^{32} therapy, patients with chronic leukemia, irradiated by ordinary means, live about 3.5 years. The average duration of fatal cases treated by P^{32} is 3.6 years.

Osgood treats both chronic myeloid and lymphocytic leukemia by means of titrated, regularly spaced P^{32} dosage, intravenously. The initial dose of P^{32} is not an average dose but a small one, arrived at by experience, as not being too much for patients with more radiosensitive cells. The average first dose is 20 microcuries per kilogram in lymphocytic leukemia cases, and 40 microcuries per kilogram in treating chronic granulocytic leukemia. The interval between treatments is rarely shorter than a week. At each subsequent visit, essential information is obtained concerning the patient's condition, after which the next interval and dosage are decided upon. The object is to maintain the patient at his usual occupation and recreation, keeping his ideal weight, with leucocyte count between 10,000 and 20,000, and not over 1(+) enlargement of nodes, very little enlargement of spleen and liver, and patient free of and bleeding tendency. Once a steady improvement is established, the dose and interval are determined which maintain the patient in a uniform status.

Osgood, in discussing results of therapy in selected groups of cases under his care, indicated that of 100 previously "untreated" patients who received total body x-ray treatment, or were treated with P^{32}, 39 were living with a mean survival period of 58.4 months. Osgood further states there is now evidence that the chronic lymphocytic leukemia cases will show a somewhat longer median and mean survival time than those with granulocytic leukemia, with the range of survival periods for both types almost completely overlapping. He feels there is no evidence for the statement that P^{32} is not the best therapy available for the treatment of lymphocytic leukemias.

Certainly, the titrated, regularly spaced whole body irradiation is an interesting and promising proposal for refinement of radiation therapy of chronic leukemia. Advances in the chemotherapy of this condition are also encouraging. As yet, neither is out of the research stage, nor is there total agreement on the best methods of treatment for the chronic leukemias.

19.1.5.2. P^{32} in Other Diseases: In the treatment of acute and subacute leukemia, P^{32} is not considered satisfactory by most investigators. Osgood, however, reports that, when combined with continuous cortisone therapy, P^{32} has given better results, in his experience, than any other method he has investigated.

There have been only indifferent results in treating multiple myeloma, Hodgkins disease, and lymphosarcoma.

Rusche and Jaffe have treated 80 patients having inoperable prostatic carcinoma with the interstitial injection of radioactive colloidal chromic phosphate. These patients have been observed over a 3-year period. Two patients have excellent results with no clinical evidence of residual disease. Thirty-seven patients have had marked clinical improvement. The usual dosage was 0.3 to 0.5 millicuries of chromic phosphate per gram of prostatic tissue. The average amount of isotope injected was 25 millicuries. These same authors report irradiation of seven bladder carcinomas with interstitial colloidal chromic phosphate. Two patients are living and free of clinical disease for 18 and 30 months.

Intracavity use of colloidal chromic phosphate has been employed in the treatment of serous effusions of the pleural and peritoneal cavities, as a substitute for radioactive gold suspensions. Preliminary clinical studies indicate a significant degree of dissociation of the labeled phosphorus behaving like inorganic phosphate with a similar distribution. Only a small amount is present in the blood at any one time. A considerable amount of the chromic phosphate migrates to dependent portions of the cavity treated. Clinical results have been reported as favorable, but the use of chromic phosphate is still in the experimental phase. Jaffe feels that the results with radiochromic phosphate compare favorably with the reported results of palliative treatment with radiogold and that it is more convenient to use.

19.1.5.3 *Complications of P^{32} therapy.* Potential hazards are to be encountered in the use of any form of ionizing radiation which entails generalized distribution of the irradiation or its toxic products. Radiation sickness is perhaps the most common complication. Other more serious complications include: Hypoplasia of the bone marrow, with suppression of the erythrocytic, granulocytic and/or thrombocytic series of cells. Combinations of suppression in these groups are often noted. Stroebel, at the Mayo Clinic, reports 8 cases of leukemia in treating polycythemia vera by radioactive phosphorus, among 251 patients. Osgood reports two such cases among 100 cases of polycythemia vera. At times, thrombocytic or granulocytic or granulocytic hypoplasia in which the leukocyte count has dropped below 4000, or the thrombocytic count below a critical level that leads to purpura, has been observed and requires remedial therapy before any further irradiation is indicated. Ultimate irreversible depletion of bone marrow must be recognized promptly, for further ionizing radiations are contraindicated.

19.2 Radioiodine

19.2.1 *Physical Properties and Distribution.* The principle radioisotope of iodine, commonly used, is iodine (I^{131}) with a physical half-life of 8 days. The other radioisotopes of possible medical use are iodine (I^{124}) with half-life of 4.5 days (Cyclotron); iodine (I^{126}) with half-life of 13 days (Cyclotron or pile); iodine (I^{130}) with half-life of 12.6 hours (Cyclotron); iodine (I^{132}) with half-life of 2.3 hours (pile); iodine (I^{133}) with half-life of 21 hours (pile); and iodine (I^{135}) with half-life of 6.7 hours (pile). Iodine (I^{131}) is a product of fission of uranium. It emits negative beta rays with a maximum energy of 0.6 mev and gamma rays of 0.080 to 0.73 (cascade of 6 gamma) mev. The isotope has proven satisfactory for autographic identification and is easily traced with measuring instruments such as the Geiger counter.

The unusually high concentration of iodine in the thyroid gland, with its distribution in the other organs at a much lower level, makes radioiodine ideal for radioisotopic experimental and clinical use. Iodine is not abundant in nature and is found in quite minute amounts in foodstuffs and in the water supply used for human consumption. Likewise, the body requires little of this element, but when the intake of iodine is below the normal threshold, thyroid dysfunctions appear with either simple or complex physical changes in the gland.

The physiologic utilization of iodine by the thyroid gland and its fate in the human body have been the subject of extensive experimentation. A review of the literature gives evidence that the iodide entering the thyroid in physiologic amounts is rapidly fixed to protein molecules containing tyrosine groups and that the resulting diiodotyrosine groups are chemically combined to yield thyroxine. A catalytic agent of the enzyme system governs these reactions. When large doses of iodine are administered to individuals the thyroid gland becomes saturated rapidly and does not accept more iodine. As little as 0.5 per cent of the dose may enter the gland.

The iodine absorbed by the gland is stored as iodide. Any excess of iodide retained inhibits thyroxine synthesis and thus causes a depression of the basal metabolism.

19.2.2 *Iodine Metabolism*. The use of radioactive iodine, beginning with the work of Hertz and Roberts, Evans and also Means (1938–1948), has revealed many of the intricacies of iodine metabolism. Hertz and his co-workers repeated many of the classic studies made by Marine (1915–1916). They observed the avidity of the thyroid for iodine; they observed that thyroids which were made hyperplastic by the administration of thyroid-stimulating hormone concentrated a greater percentage of administered iodine than did the thyroids of similar controlled animals. Leucutia (1946) emphasized the findings of Hertz that both the normal and hyperplastic thyroid took up a larger portion of a small dose than of a large dose of iodine. The amount of radioiodine found in the thyroid at any given time was smaller than the total amount going through the gland. Experiments by Hertz and his associates revealed that in Graves' disease, which takes up large amounts of iodine, the gland did not tend to become saturated with iodine by the summation of small amounts, but tended to take up iodine and then secrete it.

Leblond and Sue (1940) observed that thyroids treated with thyrotropic hormone had an increased affinity for iodine which was decreased following hypophysectomy. The thyrotropic hormone represents the principal mediating hormone through which most factors involving the thyroid gland act. There are, however, a group of drugs, commonly known as antithyroid drugs, which affect or act directly upon the thyroid tissue. Thiourea, sulfonamides and other related substances, when given in sufficient amounts, produce functional thyroidectomy and lower the basal metabolic rate. Radioiodine studies of the thyroid gland in such cases indicate that the transformation of iodine into thyroxine is suppressed through the inhibition of the oxidative system responsible for the chemical change.

Studies by Keating, Rawson, Peacock and Evans (1945) indicated that the first changes to occur in the thyroid as the result of treatment by thyroid-stimulating hormone were hypertrophy of the thyroid cells and loss of thyroid iodine. Leblond suggested that in the loss of thyroid iodine the thyroglobulin present in the colloid of thyroid follicles was hydrolyzed by a proteolytic enzyme system and thus was transformed into small molecules (thyroxine and diiodotyrosine) which diffused through the thyroid cells and reached the blood stream. Keating and his co-workers further demonstrated that the thyroid weight increased slightly during the early phase of administration of thyrotropic hormone, and that only after 72 hours did one note a precipitous increase in the weight of the gland. The increased avidity of the gland for iodine was not apparent until 24 hours had elapsed, and was maximum only 48 hours after the maximum loss of iodine was noted. This, of course, raises the question as to whether the increased absorption of iodine by the gland is dependent on a previous exodus of the thyroid's normal iodine, rather than upon any function of the thyroid-stimulating hormone. It would seem that a balance is established between thyroxine released by the thyroid gland and thyrotropic hormone released by the hypophysis: a rather stable equilibrium, easily adjustable to physiologic changes.

The thyroxine which enters the circulation is rapidly deposited in the gastro-intestinal tract and liver. The stomach and duodenum excrete large amounts which pass down the gastro-intestinal tract. However, only small amounts of radioiodine are found in the feces, indicating the great absorptive capacity of the lower gastro-intestinal tract for iodine. Hertz and his co-workers found that the uptake of iodine by the thyroid reached a maximum in 10 to 15 minutes, and further observation for as long as an hour and a half did not show great increase in the amount absorbed. They further estimated that, in the rabbit, the normal thyroid gland collected up to 80 times the quantity of iodine found in other tissues. Moreover, the thyroid seems equipped, physiologically, to prevent the addition of more than 10 to 20 mg. per cent of iodine over and above its pre-existing supply. When such a condition prevails, the gland is said to be "saturated." The fate of a pharmacologic dose of radioiodine is interesting and experiments have shown that there is a free interchange of iodine ions from the blood to the extracellular fluids and back again. However, the thyroid and the excretory organs actually absorb the iodine into the cells of the respective organs. The excretory organs concerned include the liver, stomach, intestines and kidneys. Large quantities of iodine are excreted by the kidney after the administration of iodine, and close to 100 per cent of a large dose may be found in the urine over a period of several days. Most of the elimination in the urine takes place within the first few days following administration and probably represents the rapid fall of radioiodine in the blood and in the extracellular spaces of the body. Hamilton and Soley in 1940 observed that a physiologic dose of radioiodine was excreted in the urine at the rate of 12 per cent after 12 hours and 37 per cent after 18 hours. The feces showed less than 1 per cent excretion of iodine after four hours, but 17 per cent had appeared in the feces after 18 hours. As a general rule, the amount of radioiodine found in the urine may be used as an index of the activity of the thyroid, that is, the more iodine absorbed by the gland, the less will be found in the blood and urine. The radioiodine in the urine is used as a check, in many clinical institutions, to determine the thyroid activity.

Hamilton and Soley compared the uptake of radioiodine in normal human controls with patients suffering from various thyroid diseases. The laboratory technics included Geiger counter determinations of radioiodine activity in the thyroid. The urine and feces also were studied for radioactive iodine over a period of five days. The iodine was given orally and was found to be absorbed rapidly from the gastro-intestinal tract. Radioactivity was noted in the thyroid gland within 20 minutes after ingestion. Over a five-day period, normal individuals had a urinary excretion of 80 per cent of the administered dose. In the first 24 hours, 60 per cent of the radioiodine was excreted. Myxedematous patients studied during the five-day period of observation showed a urinary excretion of 89 per cent to 91 per cent of the iodine administered. They excreted only 45 per cent to 50 per cent of the labeled iodine during the first 24-hour period. Other observers have noted that hypothyroid children without goiters collected very little iodine, while patients with hyperthyroidism or Graves' disease showed large resorption of iodine and relatively low excretion. Keating and his co-workers observed that normal subjects excreted an average of 65 per cent of the dose in the urine and that the rate of excretion leveled off between 25 and 36 hours after the administration of the iodine. Myxedematous subjects were found to excrete between 85 per cent and 90 per cent of the iodine, but at a much slower rate of excretion. Hyperthyroid states showed the rate of excretion to be much less than in normal individuals, with the rate leveling off much more quickly.

Quimby and McCune studied 54 subjects, including infants and children, ranging in age from one to 14 years. Radioactive iodine (I^{131}) in the form of a weak solution of sodium iodide was administered to these patients. It was found that the concentration and retention of iodine (I^{131}) in the thyroid gland varied from 12 per cent in those patients without evident thyroid disorders to several times this value in those with hyperthyroid states. Hypothyroid cases had less than 1 per cent concentration and retention of iodine (I^{131}). Some normal thyroid patients also gave low values. This variability limited the interpretation of iodine (I^{131}) levels, but the investigators felt that more specific results could be obtained by a more rigid standardization with respect to the patient's state of health and previous iodine intake.

G. E. Moore, in 1947, described a compound, diiodo^{131} fluorescein, made from the dye, fluorescein, and iodine (I^{131}), which is now being used as an aid in the diagnosis and localization of brain tumors. This dye localizes to a great extent in brain tumor tissue and is excreted by the gastro-intestinal tract. Marvin and Moore (1948) have reported on the experimental evaluation of the physical limitations of this substance. An aqueous solution of diiodo^{131} fluorescein, containing 1 mc. of radioactivity per 10 cc. of 2.0 per cent solution, was used for injection. Five hundred to 600 μc. of radioactivity were injected intravenously. It was found that the dye definitely localized in the tumor tissue, often in a concentration as high as 17 times that in the normal brain. Technical difficulty was encountered in the matter of accurate calculation of the radioactive dye concentration. This was overcome to a considerable extent by modifying a Geiger counter to fit the conditions encountered. Brain tumors which retained increased amounts of radioactive iodide compound could be detected with the Geiger counter, provided that the tumor volume exceeded 20 cc. and approached 40 cc.

Davis, Martin and their co-workers have utilized radioactive diiodofluorescein in the study of 200 patients with the diagnosis of a space-occupying lesion of the central nervous system. The results reveal a 95.5 per cent accuracy in diagnosis in lesions verified by surgical intervention or corroborated by pneumography or angiography. This study included a positive radio-dye test in 5 of 6 verified tumors of the spinal cord. The investigators used approximately 1.1 millicuries of radioactive diiodofluorescein intravenously, made up in an 8 to 10 per cent sterile solution. They noted that, within a minute or two after the injection of the dye, the radioactivity at the surface of the head was at a maximum and then slowly declined. The most significant counting rates occurred within one-half to two hours after the administration of the radio-dye. At the end of two to four hours, the readings were only confirmatory, for the differential concentrations were no longer striking.

Peyton, Moore and Associates (1951), reported their results from the beginning of the development of the localization of intracranial lesions by diiodofluorescein and then, later, using radioactive iodinated human serum albumen and the scintillation counter. The accuracy was greatly improved by the latter method, and increased from 62 to 75 per cent on the cases done in mid-1951. They pointed out that, if the clinical data were used in conjunction with the counts, the accuracy rose to 94 per cent.

Chou, Moore and Marvin recently (1952) have employed the oral administration of about 300 microcuries of NaI in patients suspected of having brain tumors and who have been "lugolized" to block the thyroid. They have demonstrated that I^{131} as NaI may be used orally in place of radioactive diiodofluorescein and that it gives very satisfactory results. The head survey is started one hour after administration of the drug. After "lugolization", the thyroid uptake of I^{131} by the end of twenty-four hours is less than 1 % of the administered dose. The NaI is excreted rapidly through the urine (30–70 % in first 24 hours). These authors have determined that diiodofluorescein and radioactive iodated human serum albumen are not specific for cerebral tumor tissue and that localization obtained is merely indicative of an area in the brain in which the blood barrier has been disrupted allowing extravascular diffusion of anions which are bound to abnormal protein radicals in the tumor tissue. It would appear that the NaI per se supplies more available I^{131} and accounts for the high difference of uptake over the previous iodine preparations. The advantages of its use are enumerated to include (1) economy (2) adequate localization and (3) ease of oral administration.

Many other investigators since have studied radioactive iodine, perfecting the methodology and determining the metabolism of the drug, evaluating its usefulness as a diagnostic and tracer agent.

Using tracer doses of from 25 to 100 microcuries of radioactive iodine, hyperthyroid individuals have been found to concentrate over 50 per cent of the radioactive material in 24 hours, as contrasted with 10 to 20 per cent in normal individuals. Studies are available on the metabolism of I^{131} and its conversion to protein bound thyroxine. It has been found that hypothyroid individuals have a six to ten per cent conversion, whereas hyperthyroid persons have a conversion of from 50 per cent and up to 90 per cent in severe thyrotoxic states.

Kriss studied the uptake of radioactive iodine after intravenous administration. Forty to 100 microcuries of radioactive iodine in 5 or 10 c.c. of isotonic sodium chloride solution were administered to hyperthyroid individuals as well as to controls. The thyroid uptake one hour after the tracer doses correlated satisfactorily with the activity of the thyroid gland and with clinical toxicity, permitting differentiation between euthyroid and hyperthyroid states. The method apparently offers advantages over the 24 hour oral method by the rapidity of the test and its diagnostic accuracy. It reduces the overlap in values between normal and hyperthyroid persons.

Tracer uses of radioactive iodine include the work of Chapman, Corner, Robinson, David and Evans, who have studied the transfer of radioiodine from the mother to the human fetus. They observed that during the first 12 weeks of pregnancy, the fetus does not compete with the maternal available iodine supply, and concluded that a woman, during this phase of pregnancy, may be treated safely with radioactive iodine therapy.

Rugh and Booth have conducted experiments to determine if thiouracil, methimazole or thyrotropic hormone treatment will protect offspring in utero from expected thyroid damage when radioiodine is injected into the mother. Pregnant mice were used. The protecting drugs were used prior to radioiodine injection and it was found that they did modify the radiation damage to both maternal and foetal thyroids. The protection was brief and transient. Thiouracil, on histological gland studies, seemed to offer more protection against radioiodine induced necrosis.

Corrigan and Hayden and also Hummon and Magalotti have shown that, when functioning thyroid tissue is present in the superior mediastinum, the tracer readings show a different pattern of diminishing Geiger tube readings in the area surrounding the usual anatomical location of the thyroid gland. By establishing normal "fall-off" values, or a normal pattern of tracer values within which normal thyroids fall, the presence of a functioning substernal thyroid gland is more easily evaluated.

Grispell, Porter and Nieset in 1950 reported a very close correlation of the blood volume values, determined simultaneously, using Evans Blue and radioactive iodinated serum albumen. Sklaroff, in a study (1956) of the normal aged, using the radioactive iodinated serum albumen test, was able to show that the blood volume values are generally below the average quoted for advancing age. Such facts are of importance in the management of the elderly during surgical procedures.

Yuhl and Stirrett, in a clinical evaluation of hepatic radioactivity, utilized 287 patients. The method employed the intravenous injection of a tracer amount of I^{131} human serum albumen and the subsequent detection of areas of increased activity in the liver. Successive counts over coordinated areas of thorax and abdomen were compared with normal values determined in persons without disease. Areas of increased radioactivity were considered to represent sites of neoplastic disease. The overall diagnostic accuracy was 96% in 187 patients where no lesion was found. In 53 patients with known liver metastases, an increase in radioactivity was found in 93%, as compared with 43% accuracy of diagnosis when conventional liver tests were used.

Katz, in a re-evaluation of Legg-Calvé-Perthes' disease, to determine the relation of thyroid hypofunction or toxic adenoma to the disease, used protein-bound radioactive iodine as tracer in the study. Previous investigators had reported that many children with the Legg-Perthes' disease had shown either thyroid hypofunction or toxic adenoma. The authors were unable to verify any connection with thyroid disease in a study of 32 patients with Legg-Perthes' disease.

Wainwright and Associates confirmed the findings of *in vitro* I^{131} penetration studies in teeth by *in vivo* studies on patients who had tooth extractions following large doses of I^{131} from 5 to 15 days previously. The I^{131} was given by oral administration. The authors showed that, in human subjects, I^{131} will rapidly and diffusely penetrate intact normal enamel, dentin and cementum, as well as enamel lamellae and damaged portions of the tooth. No differences in the amount of localization could be detected in teeth extracted 5 hours or 19 days after the administration of I^{131}. No turnover of I^{131} was noted in the teeth for at least the first two weeks.

Thode and Associates describe a method for measuring the uptake of I^{131} by the salivary glands. They have noted that the uptake of iodine is related inversely to that of the thyroid. The authors expect that this test will be valuable in the diagnosis of hypothyroidism, inasmuch as it augments the 24-hour uptake measurements over the thyroid gland and the conversion ratio studies currently used.

Bauer and Associates, (1953), reported a method for studying some of the morphological characteristics of the frontal profile of the human thyroid gland in its normal and abnormal states. The method he uses is iodine (I^{131}) and a directional scintillation counter. The outline of the thyroid gland obtaind is called a "scintigram." A dose of carrier-free I^{131}, ranging from 100 to 300 microcuries is given by oral administration. The scanning procedure is carried out 24 to 48 hours later. The tracing resulting from the scanning is a record of the activity of the tissue examined. This procedure is advocated as a routine clinical procedure in hyperthyroidism, simple goiter, solitary or multiple nodules, carcinoma of the thyroid gland and aberrant thyroid tissue.

Goodwin and Associates utilized a scintiscanner to estimate the weight of the thyroid gland, which is considered a more accurate method than previous approaches to the problem. A scintigram is obtained after the oral administration of some 250 microcuries of I^{131}. An actual size scintigram of the gland is obtained. An estimate of the thyroid gland weight is then determined by applying a formula: i.e., the weight of the gland in grams is equal to $0.32 \times$ the area of the scintigram in square centimeters $\times$ the maximum length of the lobe in centimeters.

In addition to the ever-increasing utilization of radioiodine for tracer studies, considerable therapeutic trial and experience have been recorded in the use of radioiodine in the treatment of hyperthyroid states and tumors of the thyroid gland.

19.2.2.1 *Radioiodine in thyroid diagnostic tests.* Most diagnostic procedures employing tracer doses of radioiodine, (between 1 and 40 microcuries), are designed to estimate the secretory activity of the thyroid from the uptake of I^{131} by the gland, or from I^{131} uptake at some fixed interval following administration. Frequent dissociation between iodine accumulation and hormone release, in the healthy as well as in the diseased thyroid, have stimulated investigators to develop clinically useful procedures to measure the secretory rate in the thyroid directly. These methods determine, at some fixed interval after administration of radioiodine, the rate at which the radioiodine appears in the organic fraction of plasma or the concentration of protein-bound radioiodine.

The determination of I^{131} collection by the thyroid, utilizing direct measurement over the gland at 24 hours after administration of the isotope, is probably the simplest and most expeditious method for the appraisal of thyroid function by radioiodine. In 80 to 85 per cent of the patients tested, the procedure reflects the true status of the thyroid function. In those individuals where the test does not establish the diagnosis, or which is at variance with the clinical appraisal, the protein-bound iodine tests can be run without additional dosage of I^{131}. A minimum of 15 microcuries oral dose is necessary where the combined uptake-PBI studies are to be made. The PBI test measures with considerable accuracy the concentration of thyroxin in the circulating blood and, at the present time, represents the best available measure of thyroid activity. It is also applicable to children, psychotic and unconscious patients. The great difficulty of utilizing the test is that it requires considerable proficiency on the part of the technical personnel, which is not always available in the average laboratory. In the interpretation of PBI results, great care must be used to rule out disorders originating outside of the thyroid gland. The 72-hour PBI determination offers about 90% correct diagnosis when compared with the final clinical evaluation.

The ratio between the total amount of radioiodine in the plasma and that amount fixed in the plasma protein 24 hours after the isotope has been given by mouth has proven useful in differentiating hyperthyroidism and euthyroidism. It does not separate euthyroidism from hypothyroidism. This appears to be due to the fact that euthyroid individuals may have a distinctly low conversion ratio. The results are expressed as the ratio of radioactivity in the protein fraction in counts per second to the total plasma radioactivity in counts per second.

The identification of discrete nodules in the thyroid by the uptake of radioiodine, as compared with the uptake of radioiodine in the remainder of the gland, is of value in clinically assessing the nature of the underlying pathologic condition. One may detect a hypofunctioning nodule; a relatively non-functioning nodule, which may be carcinoma; and hyperthyroidism with a nodular goiter, where it is difficult to distinguish, clinically, between Graves' disease and a non-functioning nodule, or hyperthyroidism due to a hyperfunctioning nodule.

Such localization techniques are assessed by directional counting over three sites: (1) over the nodule; (2) over other areas of uninvolved tissue; and (3) over tissues at a distance from the gland. Scintigrams are extremely satisfactory for recording and interpreting the uptake of I^{131}.

19.2.2.3 *Radioiodine Therapy in Hyperthyroidism.* Chapman, Skanse and Evans, between 1943 and 1947, used available iodine (I^{130}) with a half life of 12 hours, to treat 65 patients with hyperthyroid states. They observed that it had been used effectively, alone, in a single retaining dose averaging 0.45 mc. per estimated gram of thyroid. Ninety per cent of the radiation dose was delivered in the first 36 hours. They report no relapse or recurrence of hyperthyroidism, although the authors continue to keep the patients under observation. The toxic effects of the short-lived form of radioactivity were found to be nausea, slight fever, swelling and tenderness of the thyroid for a few days. Myxedema was produced in some cases. Histologic changes which were observed subsequently in some of their patients showed fibrosis and regenerative hyperplasia. Chapman and his co-workers further stated that effective doses of radioiodine (I^{130}) given in the fourth or fifth month of pregnancy had not produced any recognizable changes in the children, who still appear healthy. However, they advised against the use of the isotopes in pregnancy after the third month.

19.2.3 *Radioiodine Therapy.* Miller, Dailey and McCorkle, (1952), reported the results of the treatment of 100 consecutive cases of hyperthyroidism, using I^{131} therapy. The dosage calculation of I^{131} was based on maximum uptake of a tracer over the thyroid gland, biological half-life and estimated weight of the gland. After experience, the dose of radioactive iodine was increased so that the authors gave 120 microcuries of I^{131} as the initial dose per estimated gram of thyroid tissue. The majority of patients received between 2 and 10 millicuries, by mouth. The response in this group was satisfactory with from one to three doses; 18% required four or more doses.

Clark and Rule have established the following criteria for the use of radioiodine in the treatment of hyperthyroidism: recurrent or persistent hyperthyroidism following thyroidectomy; hyperthyroidism, complicated by other concurrent diseases; uncomplicated hyperthyroidism in patients over 40 years of age; refusal to accept surgical therapy; severe exophthalmos; and patients with idiosyncrasies to anti-thyroid drugs. The authors emphasize the following contraindications: hyperthyroidism in children; large, toxic, nodular goiter; hyperthyroid state complicated by pregnancy and lactation; hyperthyroidism associated with a clinical solitary nodule; and non-toxic, diffuse or simple goiter.

It is not practicable to measure radioiodine dosages delivered to the thyroid tissue, but considerable information is available by which practical dosage formulas may be evolved. Certain factors must be taken into account in establishing these formulas which include the lack of uniformity of distribution of the isotope throughout the thyroid gland, and the fact that the isotope does not remain fixed in the gland to decay according to the physical half-life of 8 days. This introduces, therefore, the factor of the biologic half-life, which is the number of days required for half of the isotope to disappear from the gland, corrected for physical decay. Quimby has developed the following formula:

$$\text{Average Dose} = \frac{\mu c.\ \text{administered}}{\text{Gm. gland}} \times \%\ \text{retained} \times \text{effective half life} \times 20,$$

in reps.

When toxic goiter is treated with 3 to 4 millicuries of I^{131}, taken by mouth, two-thirds of the patients become clinically quiescent in about 4 months time. Occasionally, a patient will become hypothyroid. Werner points out that 85 % of patients show remission or become hypothyroid after a second dose of 3 to 4 millicuries. It is usually safe to repeat treatment 2 months after the first dose, providing a test for the uptake of I^{131} reveals abnormally high absorption of iodine. If the patient is mildly hypothyroid, it is usually better to wait 4 months before considering retreatment. About half of the remissions are achieved with radiation dosages between 7500 and 10,000 reps. Hypothyroidism, however, has resulted in as little as 2500 reps. Because of the biological variability in resistance to radiation effect, and in order to limit the radiation dose to the thyroid, Werner uses a narrow range of doses of I^{131}. Between 1 and 8 millicuries are given initially, with 4 millicuries as an average dose. A patient with mild hypothyroidism and a small gland receives the least, and the patient with a large nodular gland, and severely toxic, receives the most. If remission is not induced by the first dose, it is repeated according to the same criteria, 2 months later. If the gland has diminished in size, a smaller dose may be sufficient the second time. Uptake must be tested as a preliminary step to retreatment. Occasionally, three or more doses are indicated. If the hyperthyroidism is refractory, a larger dose is then given (between 3 and 25 millicuries). There is less chance of developing hypothyroidism at this stage because of the inherent resistance of the gland. The larger dose is indicated in order to prevent extreme resistance which may follow repeated inadequate radiation dosage.

Werner and his co-workers determined the status of patients with thyroid disease by means of tracer studies of radioiodine (I^{131}). Normal uptake is 15 per cent to 30 per cent of the administered tracer dose of 1 to 40 μc. Anything with an absorption rate of more than 40 per cent is regarded as definitely indicating hyperthyroidism; anything less than 10 per cent is regarded as hypothyroidism. There appears to be no definite relationship between the basal metabolic rate and the percentage uptake in the gland at the end of 24 hours.

The cause of failure to control the disease in this group of cases appeared to be related to inadequate dosage and an unusually high basal metabolic rate. The inadequacy of the dosage frequently was due to the large size of the gland for the total dose given.

19.2.3.1 *Complications.* Complications following radioiodine therapy for thyroid conditions include: (1) Hypothyroidism, the symptoms of which usually put in their appearance in the third to fourth month after the ingestion of iodine; when the condition is transient it usually clears up within the space of a month; in several instances, however, persistent myxedema has been produced. (2) Tender gland. (3) Sore throat, with tracheal irritation; these symptoms appear 10 days to two weeks after treatment and subside in from one month to six weeks later. (4) Exacerbation of toxicity; this phenomenon has usually indicated that the patient will need a second course of therapy.

19.2.3.2 *Radioiodine therapy in cardiac disease.* Blumgart, Freedberg and Kurland, (1955), reported on the treatment of 1070 patients with angina pectoris or congestive heart failure. These authors previously (1948) proposed the use of large doses of radioiodine to produce a hypothyroid state as a palliative procedure for the treatment of angina pectoris and congestive heart failure which did not respond to routine therapeutic measures. Doses of from 10 to 20 millicuries of I^{131} were established as the dosage to be given at weekly intervals of 3 weeks, followed by repeated doses at intervals of 1 to 2 months until a definite hypothyroid state was achieved. The larger doses of I^{131} are to be discouraged because of the possibility of temporary hyperthyroidism occurring 2 or 3 weeks after the dose, due to the sudden release of hormone. In angina pectoris, about 40 % of the patients showed a marked improvement, and a significant response was noted in another 35 %. In congestive heart failure a good response was noted in about 38 % of the patients treated, with marked improvement in about 20 % of patients.

The myxedema developing from treatment with I^{131} is controlled by giving oral thyroid medication in carefully controlled doses.

The I^{131} treatment does not alter the basic pathology involved but, by decreasing the thyroid function, brings about lessened circulatory requirements, which are adequately served by a diminished cardiac reserve.

Jaffe, Rosenfeld and Associates, (1955), reported 231 new thyroid cardiac patients treated with I^{131}. These authors favor the use of small weekly doses of I^{131}, as contrasted to the higher dosages, for the following reasons: to avoid sudden release of thyroxin from destroyed gland; to avoid the possibility of bone marrow destruction; to avoid radiation thyroiditis; and to minimize the necessity for hospitalization in treatment of the patient. The patients received a thyroid uptake examination, having been given 5 microcuries of I^{131} orally. Following this, the patients received 500 microcuries of I^{131} orally, and 24 hours later a scintigram was made to estimate the size and activity of the gland. The patients then received, orally, 6 millicuries of I^{131} weekly, until a total of 30 millicuries were given. One month after conclusion of the first course, a scintigram was again made. If the gland still showed normal function, a similar second and even third course were given. The best results were in angina pectoris, with 56 % of patients revealing excellent results and 37 % good results. In the patients with conges-

tive heart failure, 53 % showed excellent results; 28 % good results. Patients
with combined disease had about a 50–50 chance of showing excellent results; and 30 % good results.

The mechanisms by which thyroidectomy increases the exercise tolerance
in cardiac disease appears obscure. The resting cardiac output is reduced,
partly by increased efficiency of oxygen utilization and, partly, by diminished oxygen demands of the tissues. These factors do not explain why an
angina patient, after treatment, can increase his cardiac output by several
times the resting rate and have no pain.

19.2.3.3 *Radioiodine in Carcinoma of the Thyroid.* Frantz, Ball, Keston
and Palmer (1944) reported the first cases of metastatic thyroid carcinoma
to take up radioactive iodine, demonstrated by Geiger counter and radio-
autograph. Seidlin, Marinelli and Oshry (1946) reported a case of metasta-
sizing hyperfunctioning cancer of the thyroid gland which was treated by
radioiodine with subjective and objective improvement. Rawson and Skanse
(1948) made a study of 21 cases of thyroid cancer and found that there was a
measurable pick-up of iodine in only 10 out of the 21 cases. The iodine
absorption by those tumors in which it was measurable was extremely low
when compared to the pick-up of iodine by normal thyroid tissue.

Marinelli, Foote, Hill and Hocker (1947) have shown that certain types
of thyroid cancer possess the ability to accumulate radioactive iodine,
while others do not. Autoradiographic studies were used to demonstrate
the relationship of the structural qualities of the gland to radioiodine
concentration. Thyroid glands with more or less normal or orderly cell
arrangement, having follicle formation and the presence of colloid-like material, showed the highest percentage of radioiodine uptake. Tumors with a
more cellular growth or with absence of normal gland arrangement revealed
either smaller amounts or the absence of radioactive iodine deposited in
the gland. Such observations do not warrant overoptimism by those interested in treating cancer of the thyroid with radioactive iodine.

Frantz, Quimby and Evans (1948) reviewed the previous experience of
the Columbia-Presbyterian Medical Center in using postoperative irradiation for thyroid carcinoma, and made a preliminary report up to May
first, 1948, on their studies of iodine (I^{131}) as used in nontoxic thyroid
lesions, benign and malignant. Thirty-two patients with thyroid lesions,
out of 68 cases suspected of having cancer, were proved to have thyroid
carcinoma. The relatively undifferentiated tumors, i.e., graded II and III
by the pathologist, showed no uptake of radioiodine. No pure papillary
carcinoma nor Hurthle-cell tumor, benign or malignant, has shown uptake
of radioiodine to date. The malignant adenoma group of thyroid tumors
was quite variable in the absorption of radioiodine. This fact caused

Quimby and her co-workers to hold, *sub judice*, the hypothesis that the greater the degree of differentiation, the higher the functional activity. Mixed papillary and adenomatous tumors showed some iodine uptake but were apparently a less favorable group than the adenomas for therapy with iodine (I^{131}).

Rawson, Skanse, Marinelli and Fluharty (1949) studied the differentiation of function in benign and malignant tumors and in both primary malignant thyroid cancers and their metastatic deposits. Patients on whom thyroidectomy was to be performed were given from 100 to 2000 microcuries of iodine (I^{131}) one to seven days prior to operation. Surface measurements indicated that the capacity to collect iodine is characteristic of thyroid tissue, and that the function of concentration parallels the degree of differentiation of the tumor. The metastases from the thyroid cancer develop function, frequently, after the surgical removal of the primary tumor and thyroid gland. This has been interpreted as an activation of function in the metastases which had been non-functioning prior to the time of thyroidectomy.

Meckstroth and Curtis, in a consecutive study of 47 cases of thyroid carcinoma, (1953), noted only 7 % of lesions with sufficient uptake of I^{131} to cause reduction in size of the tumor. The authors concluded that there are three indications for extensive therapy with I^{131}, i.e.: (1) functioning metastases; (2) non-functioning metastases, the treatment being directed at destruction of normal functioning thyroid tissue, thus bringing into play the mechanisms which encourage metastatic deposits to take up and retain iodine; and (3) for studying uptake in surgical or autopsy specimens.

Wollman states forthrightly that most metastatic thyroid tumors do not accumulate enough I^{131} to be destroyed. A calculation was made of required I^{131} per gram of thyroid tissue, assuming that it is desirable to completely destroy the tumor with a single dose. Few tumors of the thyroid gland in man have been reported as having received the estimated required dose. Wollman concludes, "it appears that complete destruction of functional metastatic thyroid tumors may be a rare event." This, however, is not the determining factor as to whether therapy should be undertaken.

Trunnell, Marinelli and associates studied 25 cases with proved metastases from carcinoma of the thyroid gland (pulmonary and skeletal). They found it was necessary to remove the thyroid gland in all but one case, in order that the metastases would concentrate sufficient I^{131}. Thyrotropic hormone was given in 30 mgm. doses daily, for five or more days, to six patients. This resulted in an increased avidity for radioactive iodine in the metastases of three of the six patients. Thiouracil and propylthiouracil were given over a period of months in ten thyroidectomized patients with metastases. These patients had metastatic lesions which had already developed increased avidity for I^{131}. The thiouracil drugs, however, resulted in a further pronounced increase in radioactive iodine uptake.

Of especial interest in furthering the treatment of thyroid carcinoma by iodine (I^{131}) have been the two following groups of thyroid tumors:

1. Lateral aberrant thyroid neoplasms, i.e., mixed papillary and adenomatous carcinomas, with multiple foci in the lateral neck and with or without obvious involvement of the gland itself.

2. Malignant functional adenomas with distant metastases, chiefly to bone.

The mortality of patients with lateral aberrant thyroid carcinoma is high, except for one group. There is a striking incidence of lateral aberrant thyroid carcinomas in the young, with long survival rates of these patients after various forms of therapy. Frantz, Quimby and Evans list 10 such patients with ages varying from four to 23 years. One of these patients was living 14 years after the onset of disease. Evidence has accumulated that, in both the mixed papillary and adenomatous carcinomas and the malignant adenomas, ablation of the primary focus by an elective total thyroidectomy will enhance the function or physiologic demand of local or distant tumor foci, improving the uptake of radioactive iodine. This may be further stimulated by administration of thyrotropic hormone. Frantz and her co-workers have used dosages of from 50 to 100 mc. of iodine (I^{131}) in patients with bone metastases. In those patients with only local disease in the neck radically removed at operation, but with possible small foci remaining, much smaller doses (5 to 10 mc. of iodine [I^{131}]) were used.

It is obvious that specification of dosage and technics cannot be laid down as yet because of the problems which must be overcome in determining distribution of radioiodine within all the tumors; whole body radiosensitivity; delivering therapeutically effective dosage without producing irreparable damage to normal body structure; determining the tumor dose by reasonably accurate estimates of tumor volume and means of decreasing isotope concentration in the sputum, gastric juice and urine without lowering the concentration in the tumors. Marinelli and others have been carrying out investigations in connection with iodine (I^{131}) therapy, keeping these factors in mind. The Department of Clinical Investigation at Memorial Hospital has performed tests which show radiation damage to marrow, kidneys, gonads and liver. There is transient impairment of salivation; dryness of the oral mucous membranes and occasional symptoms of cystitis. Rall, Foster, et al., in a study of hematopoietic damage from radioactive iodine, concluded that the lymphocyte count has been found to be the most sensitive and reliable index of the degree of radiation damage. The blood count is correlated with the integrated blood concentration of I^{131}, plus an empirical factor derived from the integrated amount of isotopes retained in the body. The lymphocyte fall is not well correlated with the millicuries of the isotope administered. Doses as high as 186 mc. of iodine (I^{131}) have been given within a period of one week. In one case, 550 mc. of iodine (I^{131}) was given in a period of 10 months. Several patients have received single doses of approximately 200 mc. of iodine (I^{131}). There is a possible causal relationship between radioiodine therapy for hyperthyroid states and subsequent proved cancer. Quimby, in a recent personal communication, indicated that the group at the Columbia-Presbyterian Medical Center sent out questionnaires to some 120 specialists in an attempt to discover whether the possibility of late radiation damage leading to malignant change had ever been observed following x-ray therapy to either a normal or hyperfunctioning thyroid gland. Over 100 replies were received of which an analysis revealed 8 cancers of the thyroid, 4 of which might possibly have been related to the administration of previous x-ray therapy. It must be remembered, however, that the concentration of iodine (I^{131}) in the thyroid may offer greater concentration of radiation dosage to the gland and increase the hazards of developing carcinoma. It was also pointed out that a definite percentage of thyroid adenomas which showed malignant change have had no exposure to radioactivity.

19.2.3.4 *Radioiodine in other malignant tumors.* Kriss and Associates have treated nine cases of multiple myeloma with I^{131}. Two forms of therapy were used: (1) massive dosages of isotope in patients pretreated with stable iodide, and (2) radioactive iodinated serum albumen. The total dose per patient ranged from 150 millicuries, given as a single does, to 510 millicuries given in five doses. Four of the nine patients gained strength and were relieved of pain. Seven patients were given a total of 12 doses of radioactive iodinated serum albumen intravenously. The dosage ranged from 14 millicuries, given in one dose, to 42 millicuries given in four doses. Three of the patients obtained definite relief of pain. RISA proved much easier to handle from the standpoint of personnel protection and patient management. Relapse in 3 to 4 months was the rule, but retreatment was usually effective. Mild radiation sickness occurred in about one-third of the cases; recalcification of bone did not occur; and no lasting change was noted in the serum protein pattern. Anemia was not improved.

The investigators feel that I^{131} or RISA may be given in multiple myeloma (1) if the lesions are diffuse and pain generalized; (2) if skin tolerance does not permit further x-ray treatment; or (3) if patient is not ambulatory and cannot be moved for x-ray therapy.

Kory and Associates report that radioactive iodine, given orally, to eight patients with malignant metastatic melanoma, in doses of 50 to 65 millicuries, revealed no visible alteration in the course of the disease.

19.2.4 *Radiologic Hazards of Radioiodine.* Careful studies on radiation hazards from the use of radioactive iodine in treating patients indicate that reasonable care in handling the administration of the drug is the chief concern. Measurements taken on patients in whom the present dosages of the drug have been assimilated reveal that the patient, individually, is not a radiation hazard to surrounding personnel. It would seem wise, however, not to concentrate large numbers of such patients in the same area. Individual patients under such treatment may be placed in the ward with other patients without producing undue radiation hazard. Their excretion collections, likewise, offer little hazard when placed in a laboratory reasonably well separated from personnel until disposed of. Remember that the radiation hazard to surrounding personnel is much greater during the treatment of patients with radium emanation or radium element applications of any kind.

The evidence at hand certainly seems to justify iodine (I^{131}) therapy in the treatment of metastatic thyroid cancer in selected cases and indicates that dosage calculations are still in the experimental state.

REFERENCES

Phosphorus:

ABELS, J. C., ET AL.: Postirradiation Changes in Levels of Organic Phosphorus in Blood of Patients with Leukemia. *Cancer Research, 1:* 771, 1941.

ALLEN, H., HEMPELMANN, L. H., JR., AND WOMACK, N. A.: The Effect of Insoluble Radiophosphorus (Chromium Phosphate) When Applied Interstitially in the Treatment of Adenocarcinoma of the Mamma in Mice. *Cancer Research, 5:* 239, 1945.

ANDREASEN, E., AND OTTESEN, J.: Studies on the Lymphocyte Production. Investigations on the Nucleic Acid Turnover in the Lymphoid Organs. *Acta Physiol. Scandinav., 10:* 258, 1945.

ANDREWS, G. A.: *Treatment of Pleural Effusion with Radioactive Colloids. Therapeutic Use of Artificial Radioisotopes.* New York: Wiley, 1956, p. 295.

ARDEN, G. P. AND VEALL, N.: The use of radioactive phosphorus in early detection of avascular necrosis in the femoral head in fractured neck of femur. *Proc. Roy. Soc. Med. 46:* 344, 1953.

BAKAY, L.: Studies on blood brain barrier with radioactive phosphorus. III. Embryonic development of the barrier. *A.M.A. Arch. Neurol. & Psychiat. 70:* 30, 1953.

BAUER, R. E., MOSS, I. H. AND RICHARDSON, A. D.: A study of radioactive phosphorus activities in pleural effusions. *Cancer 7:* 852, 1954.

BRANSON, H. AND BANKS, L. O.: The Turnover Time of Phosphorus in Normal Sickle Cell Trait, and Sickle Cell Anemia. Blood *in Vitro* as Measured with P^{32}. *Science, 115:* 89, 1952.

BRUES, A. M., TRACY, M. M., AND COHN, W. E.: Nucleic Acids of Rat Liver and Hepatoma; Their Metabolic Turnover in Relation to Growth. *J. Biol. Chem., 155:* 619, 1944.

BOLLMAN, J. L., AND FLOCK, E. V.: Phospholipids of Liver and Blood Studied with Radioactive Phosphorus. *J. Lab. & Clin. Med., 31:* 478, 1946.

BURSTONE, M. S.: The Effect of Radioactive Phosphorus Upon the Development of the Teeth and Mandibular Joint of the Mouse. *J. Am. Dent. Assoc., 41:* 1, 1950.

COHN, W. E., AND GREENBERG, D. M.: Studies in Mineral Metabolism with the Aid of Artificial Radioactive Isotopes. I. Absorption, Distribution, and Excretion of Phosphorus. *J. Biol. Chem., 123:* 185, 1938.

COPELAND, M. M.: Evaluation of radio-active isotopes as an adjunct to surgical diagnosis and therapy. *J. Bone & Joint Surg. 33-A:* 1021, 1951.

COPELAND, M. M.: The palliative care of inoperable and incurable recrudescent neoplasms. *J. Chronic Dis. 4:* 186, 1956.

COPP, D. H., AND GREENBERG, D. M.: Studies on Bone Fracture Healing. I. Effects of Vitamins A and D. *J. Nutrition, 29:* 261–267, 1945.

CORRIGAN, K. E. AND HAYDEN, H. S.: Failures, flops and false localizations in tracer technique. *Radiology 60:* 870, 1953.

CRAVER, L. F.: Treatment of Leukemia by Radioactive Phosphorus. *Bull. New York Acad. Med., 18:* 254, 1942.

DALS, M. J. L., ET AL.: Studies on Phosphorus Metabolism in Normal and Rachitic Rats with Radioactive Phosphorus Isotope. *Koninklijke Akad. Wettenschaff. Amsterdam, Proc., 50:* No. 6, 1937.

DIAMOND, H. D., CRAVER, L. F. AND PARKS, G.: Radioactive Phosphorus. I. In the Treatment of Lymphatic Leukemia. *Cancer 3:* 779, 1950.

DOAN, C. A., WISEMAN, B. K., WRIGHT, CLAUDE-STARR, GEYER, J. H., MYERS, WILLIAMS AND MEYERS, J. W.: Radioactive Phosphorus[32]. A Six-Year Clinical Evaluation of Internal Radiation Therapy. *J. Lab. and Clin Med., 32:* 943–969, 1947.

ERF, L. A.: Clinical Studies with the Aid of Radiophosphorus. II. The Retention of Radiophosphorus by Tissue of Patients Dead of Leukemia. *Am. J. M. Sc., 203:* 529, 1942.

ERF, L. A.: Primary Polycythemia: Remission Induced by Therapy with Radiophosphorus. *Blood, 1:* 202–208, 1946.

ERF, L. A., AND FRIEDLANDER, G.: Phosphorus Exchange in Tissues of Patients with Lymphoid Leukemia. *Proc. Soc. Exper. Biol. and Med., 47:* 134–136, 1941.

EEF, L. A., AND LAWRENCE, J. H.: Clinical Studies with the Aid of Radioactive Phosphorus. I. The Absorption and Distribution of Radiophosphorus in the Blood and Its Excretion by Normal Individuals and Patients with Leukemia. *J. Clin. Investigation, 20:* 567, 1941.

ERF, L. A., AND LAWRENCE, J. H.: Clinical Studies with the Aid of Radiophosphorus. III. The Absorption and Distribution of Radiophosphorus in the Blood of, Its Excretion by, and Its Therapeutic Effect on, Patients with Polycythemia. *Ann. Int. Med., 15:* 276, 1941.

ERF, L. A., TUTTLE, L. W., AND LAWRENCE, J. H.: Clinical Studies with the Aid of Radiophosphorus. IV. The Retention in Blood, the Excretion, and the Therapeutic Effect of Radiophosphorus on Patients with Leukemia. *Ann. Int. Med., 15:* 478, 1941.

ERF, L. A., TUTTLE, L. W., AND SCOTT, K. G.: Retention of Orally Administered Radiophosphorus by Mice. *Proc. Soc. Exper. Biol. & Med., 45:* 652, 1940.

FLOCK, E. V., AND BOLLMAN, J. L.: Phospholipid Turnover Following Administration of Diethylstilbestrol to Cocks. *J. Biol. Chem., 156:* 151, 1944.

FRIEDELL, M. T., SCHAFFNER, FENTON, PICKETT, W. J., AND HUMMON, I. W., JR.: Radioactive Isotopes in the Study of Peripheral Vascular Disease. I. Derivation of a Circulatory Index. *Arch. Int. Med.*, *83:* 608–619, 1949.

FRIES, B. A., AND CHAIKOFF, I. L.: Factors Influencing Recovery of Injected Labeled Phosphorus in Various Organs of the Rat. *J. Biol. Chem.*, *141:* 469, 1941.

GOLDECK, H., GROTH, H. AND HORST, W.: Radiation therapy with radiophosphorus in polycythemia rubra vera. *Klin. Wchnschr. 30:* 28, 1952.

HADEN, R. L.: Hematology (Recent Advances in Treatment of Cancer). *J.A.M.A.*, *136:* 308, 1948.

HAHN, P. F.: Selective Radiation Obtained by the Intravenous Administration of Colloidal Radioactive Isotopes in Diseases of the Lymphoid System. *South. M. J.*, *39:* 558, 1946.

HALL, B. E.: Therapeutic Use of Radiophosphorus in Polycythemia Vera, Leukemia and Allied Diseases. In the Use of Isotopes in Biology and Medicine, A Symposium, p. 353. Madison, University of Wisconsin Press, 1948.

HALL, B. E., AND WATKINS, C. H.: Radiophosphorus in the Treatment of Blood Dyscrasias. *Med. Clin. North America, 31:* 810–840, 1947.

HALL, B. E., WATKINS, C. H., HARGRAVES, M. M. AND GIFFIN, H. Z.: Radioactive Phosphorus in the Treatment of Polycythemia Vera. Results and Hematologic Complications. *Am. J. Med. Sciences, 209:* 712–717, 1945.

HOSTER, H. A., AND DOAN, C. A.: Studies in Hodgkin's Syndrome. IV. Therapeutic Use of Radioactive Phosphorus. *J. Lab. and Clin. Med.*, *30:* 678–683, 1945.

JACOBSON, L. O., SPARR, C. L., SMITH, T. R., AND DICK, G. F.: Radioactive Phosphorus (P32) and Alkylamines (Nitrogen Mustards) in the Treatment of Neoplastic and Allied Diseases of the Hemopoietic System. *Med. Clin. North America, 31:* 3–18, 1947.

JAFFE, H. L.: Treatment of malignant serous effusions with radioactive colloidal chromic phosphate. *Am. J. Roentgenol. 74:* 657, 1955.

JONES, H. B., WROBEL, C. J., AND LYONS, W. R.: A Method of Distributing Beta Radiation to the Reticulo-endothelial System and Adjacent Tissues. *J. Clin. Investigation, 23:* 783, 1944.

KENNEY, J. M.: Radioactive Phosphorus as a Therapeutic Agent in Malignant Neoplastic Disease. *Cancer Research 2:* 130–142, 1942.

KENNEY, J. M., AND CRAVER, L. F.: Further Experiences in the Treatment of Lymphosarcoma with Radioactive Phosphorus. *Radiology, 39:* 598, 1942.

KENNEY, J. M., MARINELLI, L. D., AND CRAVER, L. F.: Treatment of Lymphosarcoma with Radioactive Phosphorus: A Preliminary Report. *Am. J. Roentgenol.*, *47:* 217–226, 1942.

KENNEY, J. M., MARINELLI, L. D., AND WOODWARD, H. Q.: Tracer Studies with Radioactive Phosphorus in Malignant Neoplastic Disease. *Radiology, 37:* 683–690, 1941.

KIEHN, C. L., FRIEDELL, HYMER, BENSON, JERREL, BERG, MARVIN, AND GLOVER, D. M.: A Study of the Viability of Autogenous Frozen Bone Grafts by Means of Radioactive Phosphorus. *Ann. Surg., 132:* 427, 1950.

KROHMER, J. S., THOMAS, C. I., STORAASLI, J. P. AND FRIEDELL, H. L.: Detection of intraocular tumors with the use of radioactive phosphorus. *Radiology 61:* 916, 1953.

LAWRENCE, E. O., AND COOKSEY, D.: On the Apparatus for Multiple Acceleration of Light Ions to High Speeds. *Phys. Rev., 50:* 1131, 1936.

LAWRENCE, E. O., *et al.:* Initial Performance of the 60-inch Cyclotron of the William

H. Crocker Radiation Laboratory, University of California. *Phys. Rev., 56:* 124, 1939.

LAWRENCE, J. H.: Observations on the Nature and Treatment of Leukemia and Allied Diseases. *Proc. Inst. Med., Chicago, 14:* 30, 1942.

LAWRENCE, J. H., ET AL.: Studies on Neoplasms with the Aid of Radioactive Phosphorus. I. The Total Phosphorus Metabolism of Normal and Leukemic Mice. *J. Clin. Investigation, 199:* 267, 1940.

LAWRENCE, J. H., BERLIN, N. I. AND HUFF, R. L.: Nature and treatment of polycythemia; studies on 263 patients. *Medicine 32:* 323, 1953.

LAWRENCE, J. H., AND SCOTT, K. G.: Comparative Metabolism of Phosphorus in Normal and Lymphomatous Animals. *Proc. Soc. Exper. Biol. and Med., 40:* 694–696, 1938.

LAWRENCE, J. H., SCOTT, K. G., AND TUTTLE, L. W.: Studies on Leukemia with the Aid of Radioactive Phosphorus. *Internat. Clin., 3:* 33, 1939.

LAWRENCE, J. H., AND WASSERMAN, L. R.: Multiple Myeloma: A Study of 24 Patients Treated with Radioactive Isotopes (P^{32} and Sr^{89}). *Ann. Int. Med., 33:* 41, 1950.

LOCKSLEY, H. B., SWEET, W. H., POSOSNER, H. J. AND DOW, E.: Suitability of tumor bearing mice for predicting relative usefulness of isotopes in brain tumors; comparative clinical and laboratory study in localization and treatment of brain tumors with P^{32}, Na^{24}, K^{42}, and sodium borate. *A.M.A. Arch. Neurol & Psychiat. 71:* 684, 1954.

LOW-BEER, B. V. A., LAWRENCE, J. H., AND STONE, R. S.: The Therapeutic Use of Artificially Produced Radioactive Substances. *Radiology, 39:* 573, 1942.

LOW-BEER, B. V. A.: Surface Measurements of Radioactive Phosphorus in Breast Tumors as a Possible Diagnostic Method. *Science, 104:* 399, 1946.

LOW-BEER, B. V. A.: *The Clinical Use of Radioactive Isotopes,* pp. 54, 128, 212, Springfield, Illinois, Charles C Thomas, 1950.

LOW-BEER, B. V. A., BELL, H. G., McCORKLE, H. J., AND STONE, R. S., with the assistance of STEINBACH, H. L., and HILL, W. B.: Measurement of Radioactive Phosphorus in Breast Tumors in Situ; a Possible Diagnostic Procedure. Preliminary Report. *Radiology, 47:* 492–493, 1946.

LOW-BEER, B. V. A., LAWRENCE, J. H., AND STONE, R. S.: The Therapeutic Use of Artificially Produced Radioactive Substances. *Radiol., 39:* 573, 1942.

LOW-BEER, B. V. A., AND TREADWELL, A. DE G.: Clinical Studies with the Aid of Radio-Phosphorus. V. Early Effects of Small Amounts of Radio-Phosphorus on Blood Cell Levels, Uptake, and Excretion. *J. Lab. and Clin. Med., 27:* 1294–1305, 1942.

MARSHAK, A.: Uptake of Radioactive Phosphorus by Nuclei of Liver and Tumors. *Science, 92:* 460, 1940.

MARSHAK, ALFRED, AND BYRON, R. L.: A Method for Studying Healing of Bone. *J. Bone and Joint Surgery, 27:* 95–104, Jan. 1945.

MASOUREDIS, S. P., LOW-BEER, B. V. A., BIERMAN, H. R., CHERNEY, L. S., AND SHIMKIN, M. B.: The Partition of Radiophosphorus in Blood, Urine, and Tumor Tissue in Patients with Hodgkin's Disease and Lymphosarcoma Before and After Treatment with Nitrogen Mustard. *Journal of the Nat. Cancer Inst., 11:* 289, 1950.

McCORKLE, H. J., LOW-BEER, B. V. A., BELL, H. G., AND STONE, R. S.: Clinical and Laboratory Studies on the Uptake of Radioactive Phosphorus by Lesions of the Breast. *Surgery, 24:* 409–415, 1948.

MINOT, G. R., BUCKMAN, T. E., AND ISAACS, R.: Chronic Myelogenous Leukemia;

Age Incidence, Duration, and Benefit Derived from Irradiation. *J.A.M.A.*, *82:* 1489, 1924.

NEUMAN, W. F., AND RILEY, R. F.: The Uptake of Radioactive Phosphorus by the Calcified Tissues of Normal and Choline-deficient Rats. *J. Biol. Chem.*, *168:* 545, 1947.

OSGOOD, E. E.: Titrated, Regularly Spaced Radioactive Phosphorus or Spray Roentgen Therapy of Leukemias. *Arch. Int. Med.*, *87:* 329, 1951.

OSGOOD, E. E.: *Treatment of the Leukemias and Polycythemia Vera with Radioactive Phosphorus. Therapeutic Use of Artificial Radioisotopes.* New York: Wiley, 1956, ch. 7, p. 102.

OSGOOD, E. E., LI, J. G., TIVEY, H., DUERST, M. L., AND SEAMAN, A. J.: Growth of Human Leukemic Leukocytes *in Vitro* and *in Vivo* as Measured by Uptake of P^{32} in Desoxyribose Nucleic Acid. *Science*, *114:* 95, 1951.

OSGOOD, E. E. AND SEAMAN, A. J.: Treatment of chronic leukemias; results of therapy by titrated regularly spaced total body radioactive phosphorus or roentgen irradiation. *J.A.M.A.* *150:* 1372, 1952.

OSGOOD, E. E., SEAMAN, A. J. AND KOLER, R. D.: Natural History and Course of Leukemia. Third National Cancer Conference Proceedings, p. 366, published by J. B. Lippincott & Co., 1957.

OSGOOD, E. E., SEAMAN, A. J. AND TIVEY, H.: Comparative survival times of x-ray treated versus P^{32} treated patients with chronic leukemias under the program of titrated regularly spaced total body irradiation. *Radiology 64:* 373, 1955.

OSGOOD, E. E., AND TIVEY, H.: The Biological Half-life of Radioactive Phosphorus in the Blood of Patients with Leukemia. II. Plasma—With Deviations of Observations from Predicted Values, etc. *Cancer, 3:* 1003, 1950.

OSGOOD, E. E., AND TIVEY, H.: The Biological Half-life of Radioactive Phosphorus in the Blood of Patients with Leukemia. IV. Leukocytes—Radioactive Phosphorus Content and the Relation to Plasma P^{32} Levels. *Cancer, 3:* 1014, 1950.

REINHARD, E. H.: Artificially Prepared Radioactive Isotopes as a Means of Administering Radiation Therapy. *Am. J. Roentgen.*, *58:* 757, 1947.

REINHARD, E. H., ET AL.: Radioactive Phosphorus as a Therapeutic Agent. A Review of the Literature and Analysis of the Results of Treatment of 155 Patients with Various Blood Dyscrasias, Lymphomas and other Malignant Neoplastic Diseases. *J. Lab. & Clin. Med.*, *31:* 107, 1946.

RHOADS, C. P.: The Medical Uses of Atomic Energy. *Bull. Atomic Scientists, 2:* 22, 1946.

ROOT, S. W., TYOR, M. P., ANDREWS, G. A. AND KNISELEY, R. M.: Distribution of colloidal radioactive chromic phosphate after intracavity administration. *Radiology 63:* 251, 1954.

RUSCHE, C. AND JAFFE, H. L.: Palliative treatment of prostatic cancer with radioactive colloidal chromic phosphate: three years experience and results. *J. Urol. 74:* 393, 1955.

RUSCHE, C. AND JAFFE, H. L.: Treatment of prostatic carcinoma with radioactive colloidal chromic phosphate (P^{32}): a preliminary report. *J. Urol. 72:* 466, 1954.

SCHAFFNER, FENTON, FRIEDELL, M. T., PICKETT, W. J., AND HUMMON, I. W., JR.: Radioactive Isotopes in the Study of Peripheral Vascular Disease. II. Method of Evaluation of Various Forms of Treatment. *Arch. Int. Med.*, *83:* 620–631, 1949.

SCHWARTZ, H. G.: A Scintillation Counter for the Diagnosis and Localization of Intracranial Neoplasms. *Am. J. of Roentgenol.*, *67:* 351, 1952.

SELVERSTONE, B., SOLOMON, A. K., AND SWEET, W. H.: Location of Brain Tumors by Means of Radioactive Phosphorus. *J. Am. Med. Assn.*, *140:* 277–278, 1949.

SIMON, N.: Suppression of Gastric Acidity with Beta Particles of P^{32}. *Science, 109:* 563, 1949.

STROEBEL, C. F.: Current status of radiophosphorus therapy. *Proc. Staff Meet. Mayo Clinic, 29:* 1, 1954.

STROEBEL, C. F., HALL, B. E., AND PEASE, G. L.: Evaluation of Radiophosphorus Therapy in Primary Polycythemia. *J.A.M.A., 146:* 1301, 1951.

STURGIS, C. C.: Some aspects of the leukemia problem. *J.A.M.A. 150:* 1551, 1952.

TAYLOR, F. H. L., LEVENSON, S. M., AND ADAMS, M. A.: Studies of Phosphorus Metabolism in Man. II. A Study of the Permeability of the Human Erythrocyte to Inorganic Phosphate in Vitro by the Use of Radioactive Phosphate (P^{32}). *Blood, 3:* 1472–1477, 1948.

THEIS, J., AND BAGG, B.: Effect of Intravenous Injections of Active Deposit of Radium on Metabolism. *J. Biol. Chem., 41:* 515, 1920.

TIVEY, H.: The prognosis for survival in chronic granulocytic and lymphocytic leukemia. *Am. J. Roentgenol. 72:* 68, 1954.

TIVEY, HAROLD, AND OSGOOD, E. E.: The Biological Half-life of Radioactive Phosphorus in the Blood of Patients with Leukemia. I. Whole Blood—With Deviations from Predicted Values and an Estimate of Total-Phosphorus Turnover Rate. *Cancer, 3:* 992–1002, 1950.

TIVEY, H., AND OSGOOD, E. E.: The Biological Half-life of Radioactive Phosphorus in the Blood of Patients with Leukemia. III. Erythrocytes—With Deviations of Observations from Predicted Values. *Cancer, 3:* 1010, 1950.

TUTTLE, L. W., ERF, L. A., AND LAWRENCE, J. H.: Studies on Neoplasms with the Aid of Radioactive Phosphorus. Phosphorus Metabolism of the Phospholipid, Acid-soluble and Nucleoprotein Fractions of Various Tissues of Normal and Leukemic Mice Following the Administration of "Tracer" and "Therapeutic" Doses of Radiophosphorus. *J. Clin. Investigation, 20:* 577, 1941.

TUTTLE, L. W., SCOTT, K. G., AND LAWRENCE, J. H.: Phosphorus Metabolism in Leukemic Blood. *Proc. Soc. Exper. Biol. & Med., 41:* 20, 1939.

WATKINS, C. H.: Treatment of chronic leukemia. *M. Clin. North America, 40:* 1117, 1956.

WHITE, H. E.: *Classical and Modern Physics.* New York: D. Van Nostrand Co., Inc., 1940.

WILKINSON, G. W. AND LEBLOND, C. P.: The deposition of radiophosphorus in fractured bones in rats. *Surg. Gynec. & Obst. 97:* 143, 1953.

WILSON, C. W.: The uptake of phosphorus by the knee joint and tibia in six week old mice and the effect of x-rays upon it—variations of uptake with time after a dose of 2000 r of 200 k.v. x-rays. *Brit. J. Radiol. 29:* 86, 1956.

WOODWARD, H. Q., AND KENNEY, J. M.: The Relation of Phosphatase Activity in Bone Tumors to the Deposition of Radioactive Phosphorus. *Am. J. Roentgenol., 47:* 227–242, 1942.

Iodine:

ASTWOOD, E. B., AND BISSELL, A.: Effect of Thiouracil on the Iodine Content of the Thyroid Gland. *Endocrinology 34:* 282, 1944.

BARRETT, T. F., PECK, H., BAUER, F. K., LIBBY, R. L. AND JARRETT, S. R.: Evaluation of a thyroid panel; practical application of scintillation counter in diagnosis of diseases of the thyroid. *J.A.M.A. 152:* 1414, 1953.

BAUER, F. K., GOODWIN, W. E., LIBBY, R. L. AND CASSEW, B.: The diagnosis of morphologic abnormalities of the human thyroid gland by means of I^{131}. *Radiology 61:* 935, 1953.

BLOCH, H. S., AND RAY, F. E.: Organic Radioiodo Compounds for Cancer Research. *J. Natl. Cancer Inst.*, *7:* 61, 1946.

BLUMGART, H. L., FREEDBERG, A. S. AND KURLAND, G. S.: Treatment of incapacitated enthyroid cardiac patients with radioactive iodine; summary of results in treatment of 1070 patients with angina pectoris or congestive failure. *J.A.M.A.* *157:* 1, 1955.

BOYD, G. A.: The Physical Principles and Techniques of Autoradiographs. *Jour. Biol. Phot. Assn.*, *16:* 65, 1947.

CHAPMAN, E. M., CORNER, C. W., JR., ROBINSON, DAVID, AND EVANS, R. D.: The Collection of Radioiodine by the Human Fetal Thyroid. *J. Clin. Endocrinol.*, *8:* 717–720, 1948.

CHAPMAN, E. M.: Treatment of Graves' Disease with I[131]. *West. J. Surg.*, *56:* 1, 1948.

CHAPMAN, E. M., AND EVANS, R. D.: The Treatment of Graves' Disease with I[131]. *J.A.M.A.*, *131:* 86, 1946.

CHAPMAN, E. M., SKANSE, B. N., AND EVANS, R. D.: Treatment of Hyperthyroidism with Radioactive Iodine. *Radiology, 51:* 558, 1948.

CHOU, S. N., MOORE, G. E., AND MARVIN, J. F.: Localization of Brain Tumors with Radioiodine. *Science, 115:* 119, 1952.

CLARK, D. E. AND RULE, J. H.: Radioactive iodine or surgery in treatment of hyperthyroidism. *J.A.M.A. 159:* 995, 1955.

CLARK, D. E., TRIPPEL, O. H., AND SHELINE, G. E.: Diagnostic and Therapeutic Use of Radioactive Iodine. *Arch. Int. Med.*, *87:* 87, 1951.

COPHER, G. H., WALLINGSFORD, V. H., SCOTT, W. G., ZEDLER, G. G., HAYWARD, B., AND MOORE, S.: Direct Irradiation of Carcinoma of the Liver and Biliary Tract by the Use of Radioactive Iodine (I[131]) in Tetraiodophenolphthalein (An experimental and clinical study). *Am. J. Roentgenol.*, *67:* 964, 1952.

CRILE, G., JR.: Papillary Carcinoma of the Thyroid and Lateral Cervical Region. So-called "Lateral Aberrant Thyroid." *Surg., Gynec. & Obstet.*, *85:* 757, 1947.

CURTIS, G. M. AND SWENSON, R. E.: The significance of the protein bound blood iodine in patients with hyperthyroidism. *Ann. Surg. 128:* 443, 1948.

DAVIS, LOYAL, MARTIN, JOHN, ASHKENAZY, MOSES, LEROY, G. V., AND FIELDS, THEODORE: Radioactive Diiodofluorescein in Diagnosis and Localization of Central Nervous System Tumors. *J. Am. Med. Assn.*, *144:* 1424–1432, 1950.

EVANS, T. C.: Preparation of Radioautographs of Thyroid Tumors for Study at High Magnification. *Radiology, 49:* 206, 1949.

EVANS, T. C.: Selection of Radioautographic Technique for Problems in Biology. *Nucleonics, 2:* 52, 1948.

FINDLAY, D., AND LEBLOND, C. P.: Partial Destruction of Rat Thyroid by Large Doses of Radioiodine. *Am. J. Roentgenol.*, *59:* 387, 1948.

FRANKLIN, A. L., AND CHAIKOFF, I. L.: The Effect of Sulfonamides on the Conversion *in vitro* of Inorganic Iodine to Thyroxine and Diiodotyrosine by Thyroid Tissue with Radioactive Iodine as Indicator. *J. Biol. Chem.*, *152:* 295, 1944.

FRANKLIN, A. L., CHAIKOFF, I. L., AND LERNER, S. R.: The Influence of Goitrogenic Substances on the Conversion *in vitro* of Inorganic Iodine to Thyroxine and Diiodotyrosine by Thyroid Tissue with Radioactive Iodine as Indicator. *J. Biol. Chem.*, *153:* 151, 1944.

FRANTZ, V. K., ET AL.: Thyroid Carcinoma with Metastases, Studied with Radioactive Iodine. *Ann. Surg.*, *119:* 668, 1944.

FRANTZ, V. K., QUIMBY, E. H., AND EVANS, T. C.: Radioactive Iodine Studies of Functional Thyroid Carcinoma. *Radiology, 51:* 532, 1948.

FREEDBERG, A. S., CHAMOVITZ, D. L., URELES, A. L., AND VAN DILLA, M. A.: The Direct Measurement of I¹³¹ Uptake in the Thyroid Gland; Further Observations. *J. Clin. Endocrinology, 10:* 910, 1950.

FREEDBERG, A. S., URELES, A. L., LESSES, M. F., AND GARGILL, S. L.: Pulmonary Metastatic Lesion Successfully Treated with Radioactive Iodine. *J.A.M.A., 144:* 16, 1950.

GOODWIN, W. E., CASSEN, B. AND BAUER, F. K.: Thyroid gland weight determination from thyroid scintigrams with post mortem verification. *Radiology 61:* 88, 1953.

GORBMAN, A.: Effects of Radiotoxic Dosages of I¹³¹ Upon Thyroid and Contiguous Tissues in Mice. *Proc. Soc. Exp. Biol. and Med., 66:* 212–213, 1947.

GORDON, E. S., AND ALBRIGHT, E. C.: Treatment of Thyrotoxicosis with Radioactive Iodine. *J.A.M.A., 143:* 1129, 1950.

GROSS, J., AND LEBLOND, C. P.: Distribution of a Large Dose of Thyroxine Labeled with Radioiodine in the Organs and Tissues of the Rat. *J. Biol. Chem., 171:* 309, 1947.

HAIGH, C. P., AND REISS, M.: Diagnostic and Therapeutic Uses of Radioisotopes. II. Some Applications of I¹³¹ and Na²⁴ to Clinical Diagnosis. *Brit. J. Radiol., 23:* 534, 1950.

HALL, B. E., AND WATKINS, C. H.: The Medical Use of Radioactive Isotope I¹³¹; Radioactive Isotopes in Hematological Disturbances and Neoplasms. *Am. J. M. S., 213:* 621, 1947.

HAMILTON, J. G., AND SOLEY, M. H.: Studies in Iodine Metabolism *in situ* by the Use of Radioiodine in Normal Subjects and in Patients with Various Types of Goiter. *Am. J. Physiol., 131:* 135, 1940.

HAMILTON, J. G., SOLEY, M. H., AND EICHORN, K. B.: Deposition of Radioactive Iodine in Human Thyroid Rissue. *Univ. Calif. Publ. Pharmacol., 1:* 339, 1940.

HAMILTON, J. G., ET AL.: Radioactive Iodine Studies in Childhood Hypothyroidism. *Am. J. Dis. Child., 66:* 495, 1943.

HAMILTON, J. G., AND SOLEY, M. H.: Studies in Iodine Metabolism by the Use of a New Radioactive Isotope of Iodine. *Am. J. Physiol., 127:* 557, 1939.

HAMILTON, J. G., AND SOLEY, M. H.: Unpublished data, referred to by Hamilton, J. G.: Radioactive Tracers in Biology and Medicine. *Radiology, 39:* 541, 1942.

HARINGTON, C. R.: Thyroxine: its Biosynthesis and its Immunochemistry. *Proc. Roy. Soc. London, 132:* 223, 1944.

HERTZ, S., AND ROBERTS, A.: Radioactive Iodine as an Indicator in Thyroid Physiology. III. Iodine Collection as a Criterion of Thyroid Function in Rabbits Injected with Thyrotropic Hormone. *Endocrinology, 29:* 82–88, 1941.

HERTZ, S., AND ROBERTS, A.: Radioactive Iodine as an Indicator in Thyroid Physiology. V. The Use of Radioactive Iodine in the Differential Diagnosis of Two Types of Graves' Disease. *J. Clin. Investigation, 21:* 31–32, 1942.

HERTZ, S., AND ROBERTS, A.: Radioactive Iodine in the Study of Thyroid Physiology. VII. The Use of Radioactive Iodine in Hyperthyroidism. *Jour. Amer. Med. Assn., 131:* 81, 1946.

HERTZ, S., AND ROBERTS, A.: Radioactive Iodine in the Study of Thyroid Physiology. VII. The Use of Radioactive Iodine Therapy in Graves' Disease. *West. J. of Surg., 54:* 474, 1946.

HERTZ, S., ROBERTS, A., AND EVANS, R. D.: Radioactive Iodine as an Indicator in the Study of Thyroid Physiology. *Proc. Soc. Exper. Biol. & Med., 38:* 510, 1938.

HERTZ, S., ROBERTS, A., AND SALTER, W. T.: Radioactive Iodine as an Indicator in

Thyroid Physiology. IV. The Metabolism of Iodine in Graves' Disease. *J. Clin. Investigation, 21:* 25–29, 1942.

HERTZ, S., ET AL.: Radioactive Iodine as an Indicator in Thyroid Physiology. II. Iodine Collection by Normal aad Hyperplastic Thyroids in Rabbits. *Am. J. Physiol., 128:* 565, 1940.

HUMMON, I. F. AND MAGALOTTI, M. F.: Substernal thyroid identified by a simple radioiodine (I^{131}) procedure. *Am. J. Roentgenol. 75:* 1144, 1956.

JAFFE, H. L., ROSENFELD, M. H., POBIRS, F. W. AND STUPPY, L. J.: Radioiodine treatment of euthyroid cardiac disease; four years of experience with two hundred thirty-one patients. *J.A.M.A. 159:* 434, 1955.

JOHNSON, T. B., AND TEWKESBURY, L. B., JR.: The Oxidation of 3,5-Diiodotyrosine to Thyroxine. *Proc. Natl. Acad. Sc., 28:* 73, 1942.

KATZ, J. F.: Protein-bound iodine in Legg Calve-Perthes disease. *J. Bone & Joint Surg. 37-A:* 842, 1955.

KEATING, F. R.: The Medical Use of Radioisotopes; Radioiodine and the Thyroid. *Am. J. M. Sc., 213:* 626, 1947.

KEATING, F. R., POWER, M. H., BERKSON, J., AND HINES, S. F.: The Urinary Excretion of Radioiodine in Various Thyroid States. *Jour. of Clinical Investigation, 26:* 1138, 1947.

KEATING, F. R., JR., ET AL.: Collection and Loss of Radioactive Iodine Compared with Anatomic Changes Induced in Thyroid of Chick by Injection of Thyrotropic Hormone. *Endocrinology, 36:* 137, 1945.

KELLAWAY, P. E., HOFF, H. E., AND LEBLOND, C. P.: Response to Thyroxine after Subtotal Hepatectomy. *Endocrinology, 36:* 272, 1945.

KORY, R. C., TUCKER, R. G. AND MENEELY, G. R.: Radioactive iodine in malignant melanoma. *Am. J. Roentgenol. 72:* 119, 1954.

KRISS, J. P.: Uptake of Radioactive Iodine After Intravenous Administration of Tracer Doses. *J. Clin. Endocr., 11:* 289, 1951.

KRISS, J. P., BIERMAN, H. R., THOMAS, S. F. AND NEWELL, R. R.: Treatment of multiple myeloma with radioactive iodine and radioactive iodonated serum albumen. *Radiology 65:* 241, 1955.

LEBLOND, C. P.: *Iodine Metabolism, in Advances in Biological and Medical Physics.* New York: Academic Press, Inc., 1948, vol. 1, p. 353.

LEBLOND, C. P., FORTMAN, M. B., PUPPEL, I. D., AND CURTIS, G. M.: Radioiodine Autography in Studies of Human Goitrous Thyroid Glands. *Arch. Path., 41:* 510, 1946.

LEBLOND, C. P., PERCIVAL, W. L., AND GROSS, J.: Autographic Localization of Radioiodine in Stained Section of Thyroid Gland by Coating with Photographic Emulsion. *Proc. Soc. Exp. Biol. and Med., 67:* 74, 1948.

LEBLOND, C. P., PUPPEL, I. D., RILEY, E., RADIKE, M., AND CURTIS, G. M.: Radioiodine and Iodine Fractionation Studies of Human Goitrous Thyroids. *J. Biol. Chem., 162:* 275, 1946.

LEBLOND, C. P., AND SÜE, P.: Passage de l'iodide radioactif (I^{128}) dans la thyröide stimulée par l'hormone thyréotrope de l'hypophyse. *Compt. rend. Soc. de biol., 133:* 543, 1940.

LEITER, L., ET AL.: Adenocarcinoma of the Thyroid, with Hyperthyroidism and Functional Metastases. *J. Clin. Endocrinol., 6:* 247, 1943.

LEUCUTIA, T.: The Medical Use of Radioactive Iodine. *Am. J. Roentgenol., 56:* 90, 1946.

LIVINGOOD, J. J., AND SEABORG, G. T.: Radioactive Isotopes of Iodine. *Physical Review, 54:* 775, 1938.

LOW-BEER, B. V. A.: *The Clinical Use of Radioactive Isotopes.* Springfield, Ill., Chas. C. Thomas, pp. 54, 128: 1950.

MACINTYRE, W. J., STORAASLI, J. P., KRIEGER, H., PRITCHARD, W. AND FRIEDELL, H. L.: I¹³¹ labeled serum albumen: its use in the study of cardiac output and peripheral vascular flow. *Radiology 59:* 849, 1952.

MANN, W., LEBLOND, C. P., AND WARREN, S. L.: Iodine Metabolism of Thyroid Gland. *J. Biol. Chem., 142:* 905, 1942.

MARINE, D.: Quantitative Studies on the *in vivo* Absorption of Iodine by Dogs' Thyroid Glands. *J. Biol. Chem., 22:* 547, 1915.

MARINE, D., AND ROGOFF, J. M.: Absorption of Potassium Iodide by the Thyroid Gland *in vivo* Following Its Intravenous Injection in Constant Amounts. *J. Pharmacol. & Exper. Therap., 8:* 439, 1916.

MARINE, D., AND ROGOFF, J. M.: How Rapidly Does the Intact Thyroid Gland Elaborate Its Specific Iodine-containing Hormone? *J. Pharmacol. & Exper. Therap., 9:* 1, 1916.

MARINELLI, L. D.: Dosage Determinations with Radioactive Isotopes. *Am. J. Roentgenol., 47:* 210, 1942.

MARINELLI, L. D., ET AL.: Retention of Radioactive Iodine in Thyroid Carcinomas. *Am. J. Roentgenol., 58:* 17, 1947.

MARINELLI, L. D., AND HILL, R. F.: Radiation Dosimetry in the Treatment of Functional Thyroid Carcinoma with I¹³¹. *Radiol., 55:* 494, 1950.

MARINELLI, L. D., AND HILL, R. F.: Radioautography; Some Physical and Radiobiological Aspects of the Technic as Applied to Thin Specimens. *Am. J. Roentgenol., 59:* 396, 1948.

MARINELLI, L. D., QUIMBY, E. H., AND HINE, G. J.: Dosage Determination with Radioactive Isotopes. II. Practical Considerations in Therapy and Protection. *Am. J. Roentgenol., 59:* 260, 1948.

MARINELLI, L. D., ET AL.: Factors Involved in the Experimental Therapy of Metastic Cancer with Iodine (I¹³¹). *Radiology, 51:* 553, 1948.

MARVIN, J. F., AND MOORE, G. E.: Localization of Brain Tumors with Radiodyes. *Nucleonics, 3:* 63, 1948.

MCARTHUR, J. W., ET AL.: The Urinary Excretion of I¹³¹ as an Aid in the Diagnosis of Hyperthyroidism. *Ann. Int. Med., 29:* 229, 1948.

MCCULLAH, E. P., GOLD, A., AND MCKENDRY, J. B. R.: Radioactive Iodine Uptake in the Hypermetabolism of Acromegaly. *J. Clin. Endocrinol., 10:* 687, 1950.

MCCULLAH, E. P., AND RICHARDS, C. E.: Radioactive Iodine in the Treatment of Hyperthyroidism. *Arch. Int. Med., 87:* 4, 1951.

MEANS, J. H.: The Use of Radioactive Iodine in the Diagnosis and Treatment of Thyroid Diseases. *Bull. New York Acad. Med., 24:* 273, 1948.

MECKSTROTH, C. V. AND CURTIS, G. M.: Criteria for therapy of malignant thyroid lesions with I¹³¹. *A.M.A. Arch. Surg. 67:* 187, 1953.

MILLER, E. R., DAILY, M. E. AND MCCORKLE, H. J.: Evaluation of treatment of hyperthyroidism with radioiodine. *A.M.A. Arch. Surg. 65:* 12, 1952.

MILLER, E. R., SOLEY, M. H., AND DAILEY, M. E.: Preliminary Report on the Clinical Use of Radioactive I¹³¹. *Amer. Jour. of Roentgenology and Radium Therapy, 60:* 45, 1948.

MOE, R. H., ADAMS, E. E., RULE, J. H., ET AL.: Evaluation of Radioactive Iodine in Treatment of Hyperthyroidism. *J. Clin. Endocrinol., 10:* 1022, 1950.

MOORE, G. E.: Fluorescein as an Agent in the Differentiation of Normal and Malignant Tissues. *Science, 106:* 30, 1947.

MOORE, G. E.: Use of Radioactive Diiodofluorescein in the Diagnosis and Localization of Brain Tumors. *Science, 107:* 569, 1948.

MOORE, G. E., CAUDILL, C. M., MARVIN, J. F., AUST, J. B., CHOU, S. N., AND SMITH, G. A.: Clinical and Experimental Studies of Intracranial Tumors with Fluorescein Dyes, with Additional Note Concerning the Possible Use of K^{42} and I^{131} Tagged Human Albumen. *Am. J. Roentgenol. 66:* 1, 1951.

MORTON, M. E., CHAIKOFF, J. L., AND ROSENFELD, S.: Inhibiting Effect of Inorganic Iodine on the Formation *in Vitro* of Thyroxine and Diiodotyrosine by Surviving Thyroid Tissue. *Jour. Biological Chemistry, 154:* 381, 1944.

MORTON, M. E., ET AL.: Radioactive Iodine as Indicator of Metabolism of Iodine. Effects of Hypophysectomy on Distribution of Labeled Thyroxine and Diiodotyrosine in Thyroid Gland and Plasma. *Endocrinology, 30:* 495, 1942.

MULLER, J. H. AND BRUNNER, C.: Normal birth of a healthy girl after successful treatment of metastasis of a struma maligna of the mother with radioactive iodine (I^{131}). *Schweiz. Med. Wchnschr. 83:* 54, 1953.

NICKSON, J. L.: Dosimetric and Protective Consideration for I^{131}. *J. Clin. Endocrinol., 8:* 721, 1948.

PATTERSON, R.: Diagnostic and Therapeutic Uses of Radioisotopes. V. The Treatment of Thyroid Carcinoma by Radioiodine. *Brit. J. Radiol., 23:* 553, 1950.

PERLMAN, I., CHAIKOFF, I. L., AND MORTON, M. E.: Radioactive Iodine as an Indicator of the Metabolism of Iodine; the Turnover of Iodine in the Tissues of the Normal Animal, with Particular Reference to the Thyroid. *J. Biol. Chem., 139:* 433, 1941.

PERLMAN, I., MORTON, M. E., AND CHAIKOFF, I. L.: Radioactive Iodine as an Indicator of the Metabolism of Iodine; the Rates of Formation of Thyroxine and Diiodotyrosine by the Intact Normal Thyroid Gland. *J. Biol. Chem., 139:* 449, 1941.

PEYTON, W. T., MOORE, G. E., FRENCH, L. A. AND CHOU, S. N.: Localization of intracranial lesions by radioactive isotopes. *J. Neurosurg. 9:* 432, 1952.

POCHIN, E. E., CUNNINGHAM, R. M. AND HILTON, G.: Quantitative measurements of radioiodine retention in thyroid carcinoma. *J. Clin. Endocrinol. 14:* 1300, 1954.

PORTMANN, U. V., HAYS, R. A., McCULLAH, E. P., AND RICHARDS, C. E.: Experience in the Treatment of Diseases of the Thyroid Gland with Radioactive Iodine. *Am. J. of Roentgenol., 66:* 179, 1951.

QUIMBY, E. H.: Physical aspects of radioiodine use. In: *Thyroid* (Sidney C. Werner, ed.). New York: Hoeber, 1955, ch. xv.

QUIMBY, E. H., AND McCUNE, D.: Uptake of Radioactive Iodine by the Normal and Disordered Thyroid Gland of Children. *Radiology, 49:* 201, 1947.

RALL, J. E., FOSTER, C. G., ROBBINS, J., LAZERSON, R., FARR, L. E., AND RAWSON, R. W.: Dosimetric considerations in determining hematopoietic damage from radioactive iodine. *Am. J. Roentgenol. 70:* 274, 1953.

RALL, J. E., SONENBERG, M. S., ROBBINS, J., LAZERSON, R., AND RAWSON, R. W.: The blood level as a guide to therapy with radioiodine. *J. Clin. Endocrinol. 13:* 1369, 1953.

RAWSON, R. W., MARINELLI, L. D., SKANSE, B. N., TRUNNELL, J., AND FLUHARTY, R. G.: The Effects of Total Thyroidectomy on the Function of Metastatic Thyroid Cancer. *J. Clin. Endocrinol., 8:* 826–841, 1948.

RAWSON, R. W., AND MCARTHUR, J. W.: Radioiodine: Its Use as a Tool in the Study of Thyroid Physiology. *Jour. of Clinical Endocrinology, 7:* 235, 1947.

RAWSON, R. W., AND SKANSE, B. N.: Radioactive Iodine: Its Use as a Tool in Studying Thyroid Physiology. *Radiology, 51:* 525, 1948.

RAWSON, R. W., SKANSE, B. N., MARINELLI, L. D., AND FLUHARTY, R. G.: Radioactive Iodine. Its Use in Studying Certain Functions of Normal and Neoplastic Thyroid Tissues. *Cancer, 2:* 279–292, 1949.

REINEKE, E. P., AND TUNER, C. W.: Effect of Certain Experimental Conditions on Formation of Thyroxine from Diiodotyrosine. *J. Biol. Chem., 162:* 369, 1946.

RICHARDS, C. E., CRILE, G., JR., AND MCCULLAH, E. P.: Radioactive Iodine in Treatment of Hyperthyroidism of Nodular Goiter. *J. Clin. Endocrinol., 10:* 1077, 1950.

RUGH, R. AND BOOTH, E.: Modification of maternal and foetal effects of radioiodine by pretreatment of the mother. *J. Pediat. 44:* 516, 1954.

SCHIFF, L., ET AL.: Gastric and Salivary Excretion of I^{131} in Man (Preliminary Report). *J. Natl. Cancer Inst., 7:* 349, 1947.

SCHULTZE, A. B., AND TURNER, C. W.: The Determination of the Rate of Thyroxin Secretion by Certain Domestic Animals. *Missouri Agricultural Experiment Station Research Bulletin,* 392, 1945.

SCOTT, K. G., AND STONE, R. S.: Tumor Host Studies. II. Increased Concentration of Tagged Iodotyrosins in the Gastrointestinal Tract of Rats Bearing Tumors. *Cancer, 3:* 722, 1950.

SCOTT, W. G., SEAMAN, W. B., MACBRYDE, C., GOTTLIEB, L., DAUGHADAY, W. H., AND SWEENEY, B. J.: Observations and Results in the Treatment of Hyperthyroidism with Radioactive Iodine (I^{131}). *Am. J. of Roent., 66:* 171, 1951.

SEED, L. AND JAFFE, B.: Results of treatment of toxic goiter with radioactive iodine. *J. Clin. Endocrinol. 13:* 107, 1953.

SEIDLIN, S. M., MARINELLI, L. D., AND OSHRY, E.: Radioactive Iodine Therapy. Effect on Functioning Metastases of Adenocarcinoma of the Thyroid. *J.A.M.A., 132:* 838, 1946.

SEIDLIN, S. M., OSHRY, E., AND YALOW, A. A.: Spontaneous and Experimentally Induced Uptake of Radioactive Iodine in Metastases from Thyroid Carcinoma; A Preliminary Report. *Jour. of Clinical Endocrinology, 8:* 423, 1948.

SHELINE, G. E., MOORE, M. C., KOPPAS, A., AND CLARK, D. E.: A Correlation Between the Serum Protein Bound Iodine and the Radioiodine Conversion Ratio in Various Thyroid States. *J. Clin. Endocrinol., 11:* 91, 1951.

SKANSE, B. N.: The Biological Effect of Irradiation by Radioactive Iodine. *J. Clin. Endocrinol., 8:* 707, 1948.

SKLAROFF, D. M.: Isotopic determination of blood volume in the normal aged. *Am. J. Roentgenol. 75:* 1082, 1956.

SMITH, P. E.: Hypophysectomy and Replacement Therapy in Rat. *Am. J. Anat., 45:* 205, 1930.

SOLEY, M. H., AND MILLER, E. R.: Treatment of Graves' Disease with Radioactive Iodine. *Medical Clinics of North America, 1–15,* January, 1948.

STANLEY, M. M., AND ASTWOOD, E. B.: Determination of the Relative Activities of Anti-Thyroid Compounds in Man Using Radioactive Iodine. *Endocrinology, 41:* 66, 1947.

STENSTROM, K., AND MARVIN, J. F.: Urinary Excretion of Radioactive Iodine in a Case of Severe Hyperthyroidism. *Proc. Soc. Exper. & Biol. Med., 66:* 47, 1947.

SWEENEY, B. J., DAUGHADAY, W. H., GOTTLIEB, L., SCOTT, W. G., AND MACBRYDE

C. M.: Radioactive Iodine Therapy of Hyperthyroidism. Determination of Optimum Dosage. *Southern Med. Journal, 44:* 648, 1951.

TAUROG, A., CHAIKOFF, I., AND FELLER, D.: The Mechanism of Iodine Concentration by the Thyroid Gland: Its Nonorganic Iodine-binding Capacity in the Normal and Propylthiouracil-treated Rat. *J. Biol. Chem., 171:* 189, 1947.

THODE, H. G., JAIMET, C. H. AND KIRKWOOD, S.: Studies and diagnostic tests of salivary gland and thyroid gland function with radioiodine. *New England J. Med. 251:* 129, 1954.

TRUNNELL, J. B., MARINELLI, L. D., DUFFY, B. J., JR., HILL, RUTH, PECOCK, WENDELL, AND RAWSON, R. W.: The Treatment of Metastastic Thyroid Cancer with Radioactive Iodine: Credits and Debits. *J. Clin. Endocrinology, 9:* 1138–1152, 1949.

WAINWRIGHT, W. W., BUTT, B. G., HAUPTFUEHRER, J. D. AND DUTE, H. L.: Deposition of radioactive iodine in teeth of persons treated for disease of the thyroid gland. *J. Am. Dent. A. 47:* 649, 1953.

WARREN, S.: Tumors of the Thyroid, *Bull. New York Acad. Med., 23:* 5, 1947.

WERNER, S. C.: Results in the treatment of hyperthyroidism with radioiodine (I[131]). *M. Clin. North America 36:* 623, 1952.

WERNER, S. C.: Treatment of Hyperthyroidism in: *The Thyroid* (Sidney C. Werner, ed.). New York: Hoeber, 1955, ch. 28.

WERNER, S. C., HAMILTON, H. B., LEIFER, E., AND GOODWIN, L. D.: An Appraisal of the Radioiodine Tracer Technic as a Clinical Procedure in the Diagnosis of Thyroid Disorders; Uptake Measurement Directly over the Gland and a Note on the Use of Thyrotropin. *J. Clin. Endocrinol., 10:* 1054, 1950.

WERNER, S. C., QUIMBY, E. H., AND SCHMIDT, C.: Clinical Experience in Diagnosis and Treatment of Thyroid Disorders with Radioactive Iodine (8-day Half-life). *Radiology, 51:* 564, 1948.

WINKLER, A. W., RIGGS, D. S. AND MAN, E. B.: Serum iodine in hypothyroidism before and during thyroid therapy. *J. Clin. Invest. 24:* 732, 1945.

WOLFF, J., AND CHAIKOFF, I.: The Inhibitory Action of Iodine upon Organic Binding of Iodine by the Normal Thyroid Gland. *J. Biol. Chem., 172:* 855, 1948.

WOLFF, J., AND CHAIKOFF, I. L.: Plasma Inorganic Iodide as a Homeostatic Regulator of Thyroid Functions. *J. Biol. Chem., 174:* 555, 1948.

WOLLMAN, S. H.: Analysis of radioiodine therapy of metastatic tumors of the thyroid gland in man. *J. Nat. Cancer Institute, 13:* 815, 1953.

YUHL, E. T. AND STIRRETT, LLOYD H.: Clinical evaluation of the hepatic radioactivity survey. *Ann. Surg. 138:* 857, 1953.

20▸

Radioisotopes of Medical Interest, Other than Radiophosphorus and Radioiodine

CHARLES F. GESCHICKTER, M.D. AND MURRAY M. COPELAND, M.D., D.Sc.

This chapter is concerned with the trace metals, alkali metals, alkaline earth tracers and other radioisotopes of medical interest.

20.1 Manganese

There are seven radioisotopes of Manganese: Mn^{50-54} and Mn^{56-57}. Manganese (Mn^{56}) has a half life of but 2.58 hours and is the only available manganese isotope produced by the chain reactor pile. The other isotopes are produced only by a charged particle accelerator. Manganese (Mn^{52}) appears in two isomeric states with half lives of 21 minutes and 5.7 days. Manganese (Mn^{54}) has a half life of 300 days. These are the radioactive isotopes of manganese best available for tracer studies and therapeutic trial. The 6.0 day Mn^{52} decays by positron beta ray (0.6 mev). Each positron is accompanied by a cascade of 3 gamma rays with energies of 1.4, 0.7 and 0.9 mev. Mn^{54}, with its 300 day half life, is a gamma ray emitter (0.84 mev). Because of the convenient half life of Mn^{52} it is best suited for treating diseases which involve the reticuloendothelial system. Either isotope may be used in tracer studies.

Manganese has been studied for its specific role in biologic processes and its essentiality for animal health has been established. Von Oettingen (1935), Maynard and Loosli (1943), McCance and Widdowson (1944), Maynard and Smith (1947) and Comar (1948) have reviewed the literature and detailed the role which manganese plays in metabolism, while indicating the possibilities of further study. Greenberg and Campbell (1940) used radioactive manganese in biologic tracer work. They found that in a normal diet the rat excreted 90 per cent of the manganese in the feces within 75

485

hours when given orally or intraperitoneally. Very little manganese was excreted in the urine.

Greenberg, Copp and Cuthbertson (1943), from bile fistula studies in rats, determined that about 75 per cent of injected manganese appearing in the feces is carried by the bile and that intravenous injections of manganese reached the liver and intestines in the same proportions as when the element was given intraperitoneally.

Greenberg and Campbell found that muscle and skin apparently are important sites for the storage of manganese that is absorbed. Bone and liver also seem to be important in the storage of manganese.

Burnett and his co-workers have confirmed that radiomanganese injected intravenously as $MnCl_2$ is localized in the pancreatic tissues of the rat, mouse and dog. The uptake of manganese by the pancreas is as rapid as the uptake by the liver at the end of one hour and continues to be at a high level over five hours; whereas liver begins to excrete its manganese after one hour. Therefore, manganese is excreted over a period of 72 hours in the pancreatic juice. The peak of excretion coincides with feeding time. They estimated that 11 per cent of injected manganese passes through the pancreas of the dog per day. The manganese was apparently secreted by the pancreas in the protein fraction of the pancreatic juice. It can be separated from the protein fraction by dialysis. These authors suggest that manganese activates pancreatic enzyme systems, although confirmatory evidence was not obtained.

Other studies indicate that manganese aids lactation and prevents atrophy of the testicles in rats, serves as an activator of enzymes and prevents "perosis," a nutritional disease in chickens. Hahn and Sheppard and also Motley have reported the clinical use of colloidal sols containing radioactive manganese in selective internal radiation therapy of diseases of the lymphoid system, with effective remissions in some of the lymphomatous diseases.

Radioactive manganese in colloidal form is found in higher concentrations in the liver, spleen and bone marrow than in other viscera and is excreted almost entirely in the feces. The isotope has been given in a highly dispersed colloidal suspension by intravenous injection. Motley reports the treatment of 14 cases of Hodgkin's disease, 9 cases of lymphoid leukemia and 3 cases of lymphosarcoma with Mn^{52}. The most favorable therapeutic results were obtained in Hodgkin's disease, particularly the febrile and abdominal types, with varying degrees of palliation. In cases of lymphoid leukemia treated with radioactive manganese the results were not superior to x-ray therapy. Two cases of lymphosarcoma showed little or no improvement after therapy. The range of dosage used by Motley averaged

12 mc. of Mn^{52} intravenously. Hodgkin's disease was treated at intervals of three to four months, when necessary.

Cyclotron Mn^{52} colloids were used about one year (1945–46) in the treatment of the leukemias and Hodgkins disease. While showing good clinical response, it was not practicable to produce it economically and in sufficient amount. Other satisfactory colloidal isotopes, such as $Gold^{198}$ have proven acceptable.

20.2 Iron

Radioisotopes of iron (6) include: Fe^{53}, Fe^{55} and Fe^{59}. The two heavier isotopes, Fe^{55} and Fe^{59}, are available for tracer work.

Iron (Fe^{55}) has a half life of 2.9 years and disintegrates solely by K capture, giving rise to Mn K x-ray. Iron (Fe^{59}) has a half life of 45 days, giving off both complex negative beta ray patterns, with maximum energies 0.27 to 1.56 mev, and also gamma rays with intensities of 1.3, 0.19 and 1.1 mev. Fe^{59} may be produced either by the cyclotron or pile reaction. When iron is bombarded by neutrons, both Fe^{55} and Fe^{59} are produced which is a disadvantage in some problems of metabolic research. Most studies carried out during the past eight years have been with iron (Fe^{59}).

18.2.1 *Metabolism of Iron.* Iron absorption is a function of the gastro-intestinal mucosa. Hahn and his associates found that the normal non-anemic dog absorbs little iron as compared with the dog which has chronic anemia and low iron reserve. The saturation of the mucosa by iron in the normal dog is rapid and blocks an absorption of a subsequent dose of labeled iron given a few hours later. Labeled iron incorporated in hemoglobin of normal dogs was discovered to be liberated by erythrocyte destruction and was immediately reutilized to form hemoglobin for new cells, rather than using iron from body stores which were ample. Children are found to utilize more iron during the growth period than are adults. Between the ages of seven and 10 years, calculations revealed requirements of 2 to 4 mg. of absorbable iron per day. Iron also has been found more efficiently utilized during the last half of gestation. In general, the normal body is efficient in utilizing iron and excretion is at a minimal level.

Austoni and Greenberg, in studying iron metabolism in rats, found that a single dose of iron passed from the stomach and small intestine in about 12 hours. In 10 days normal animals retained 30 per cent of the iron but anemic animals retained 50 per cent. After 0.7 mg. of iron (Fe^{55}) was administered parenterally to rats, excretion was found small. The urine contained 1.6 per cent, the feces 0.2 per cent and the bile 0.7 per cent. No adequate information on the distribution of iron has been made to date. Fair approximations have been achieved by Hahn and Whipple (1936) and by Austoni, Rabinovitch and Greenberg (1940) in the perfused tissues of the dog. Of total body iron, 64 per cent is distributed as blood hemoglobin iron, 16 per cent is found in muscle and other tissues, 15 per cent is located in the liver, spleen and marrow, which Hahn speaks of as available visceral storage, and 5 per cent is estimated available iron from other tissues.

Granick, Ball and Michaelis have recently established the nature of the reservoir iron in mucosa and other tissues as "ferritin." Ferritin consists of a protein fraction which is found to contain 23 per cent by weight of iron. It has been isolated from bone marrow, liver, spleen and gastrointestinal mucosa. Labeled iron has demonstrated the conversion of heme iron of the red blood cells into iron which could be identified as a constituent of crystalline ferritin.

As a result of these findings, Granick has hypothesized on the mode of iron absorption, transport and storage. The hypothesis includes: entry of ferric iron into the gastro-intestinal tract; the presence of reducing agents in the food to convert the iron to the ferrous state, absorption occurring mainly by the mucosal cells of the duodenum and jejunum; a compound, apoferritin, capable of combining reversibly with iron is present in the intestinal mucosa; the presence of iron in the body brings about an increase in apoferritin, a protein moiety which combines with iron to produce ferritin in the mucosa; and, finally, the ferritin is transported by the blood stream to be stored as reserve iron.

Labeled isotopes of iron have made it possible to acquire information as to the paths taken by iron in the body in both pathologic and normal states. Radioiron metabolism studies in pathologic states include polycythemia, pernicious anemia, hemolytic anemia, secondary anemia from infection and secondary anemia due to parasites and hemorrhagic iron deficiency anemias.

With labeled iron the life of the red blood cell is found to be 120 to 130 days (Shemin and Rittenberg). The protoporphyrin of hemoglobin prior to the incorporation of iron utilizes glycine in its synthesis. With labeled glycine it has been found that the red cell matures with maximum absorption of glycine for 20 days, remains constant as an adult red blood cell for 50 to 70 days, and then its life span drops with an S-shaped curve. From this data the average life span of a red blood cell in the human male is 120 days, and that in a woman 109 days.

In polycythemia vera, in spite of the increased number of red blood cells, the survival curve is normal with an average life span of 131 days, and the shape of the death curve is normal. Hence, there must be an increased rate of synthesis in cell formation. It was found according to glycine synthesis that the red cells are made and mature at $2\frac{1}{2}$ times that of normal. This is accompanied by hyperplasia of the bone marrow. In sickle-cell anemia there is increased rate of destruction, with an average life of red blood cells of 42 days. Both the rate of formation and the rate of destruction is 2.8 times normal. The rate of destruction is random. When whole blood from sickle-cell anemia patients is incubated with N^{15} labeled glycine, the heme was synthesized from glycine *in vitro*.

In pernicious anemia there was disclosed an abnormal pattern of red cell destruction with a low survival time. The rate of formation of circulating heme was 80 per cent of normal, and the rate of formation of circulating cells 50 per cent of normal. In other words, in pernicious anemia the cells are manufactured at one-half the normal rate, or stated better—are matured at one-half the normal rate.

Hahn et al. found that in polycythemia vera the total red cell mass greatly exceeded the predicted value, if the latter were based on hematocrit and body weight determinations, using radioactive iron, Fe^{59} to label the red cells. They found that the estimated red cell mass was 3400 cc in one patient and the actual determination 6200 cc. In the other patient, the estimated red cell mass was 2560 and the actual determination 3960. These are more accurate determinations of the size of the red cell mass resulting in the disease since in both these patients the red cell count per cu. mm. was misleading. In one the red cell count was 10.8 million per cu. mm., and in the other it was 7.

Inflammation and infection interfere with the body mechanisms for handling iron, limiting the effects of such therapy. Iron therapy in malaria is not effective because the anemia is due to a hemolytic process. The end products of hemoglobin disintegration are retained by the body and utilized in hemoglobin for new red blood cells without calling on body stores. In uncomplicated pernicious anemia and hemolytic anemia there is no iron deficiency involved, for the same reason. Increased iron uptake indicates some coincidental reason for iron deficiency, such as bleeding, which is basic in producing microcytic or hemorrhagic iron-deficiency anemia.

Horst and Schafer, by means of paper electrophoresis and radioautography, found that iron in the form of Fe^{59} and Fe^{55} is bound selectively by beta globulin in the serum of humans, rats and mice. If an excess of radioiron is applied to the human serum, some of it is carried with other globulins. The carrier protein is always found in the beta globulin, independent of the method of application. The selective binding of iron by the beta globulin is also found in the urine of patients with kidney diseases, in serous pleural exudates, ascites and in the cerebrospinal fluid of healthy humans. In these latter instances, the beta globulin, in general, is lower than in the serum. In both human and cow milk, the iron migrates with the total complex of immune globulins and not with beta lactoglobulin. Quimby points out that, since the iron in the plasma becomes bound to a globulin fraction, a direct intravenous injection of globulin labeled with Fe^{59} has appeared to be a more straightforward method for studying iron utilization. The iron leaves the plasma at a very slow rate in the blood dyscrasias where the production of red cells is grossly impaired. In polycythemia, however, the presence of greater than usual numbers of maturing red cells is accompanied by rapid iron clearance. Thus it would appear that the rate of plasma turnover of iron is an index of the degree of erythropoiesis. The complete story on iron storage and utilization is not yet available and awaits further investigation.

20.3 Cobalt

Cobalt has a number of radioactive isotopes with variable half lives and a variety of emission energies. Most of the isotopes of cobalt are both gamma and beta emitters. Co^{60} has a half life of 5.2 years. Its gamma emission has an energy of 1.17 and 1.33 mev and its negative beta ray of 0.31 mev. Because of its long half life and easy production by the atomic pile it has been suggested as a substitute for radium element in the treatment of neoplastic diseases. Co^{58}, which has a half life of 71 days, is available from the cyclotron only and is suitable for tracer work in cobalt studies. It exhibits K capture and is also both a gamma and positive beta emitter: Gamma 0.81 and 1.64 mev; positron 0.48 mev. Radiocobalt[60] disintegrates at a rate of 1.09 per cent of the original activity per month. It is a weak beta radiator and emits essentially monochromatic gamma rays with a mean energy of 1.2 mev. The beta radiation emitted is approximately 4 per cent of the emission in gamma radiation. One millicurie of cobalt[60] unfiltered delivers 13 gamma roentgens per hour at one centimeter distance. It has been estimated in terms of roentgens that the quantity of ionization produced by one millicurie of cobalt per hour is equivalent to that produced by approximately 1.4 milligrams of radium element.

In handling cobalt[60] the same precautions are used as in handling radium, including the storage containers and other matters of protection.

The metabolic role of cobalt is not well understood, though its absence is known to cause disease in cattle and other animals. It is stored in the hematopoietic tissues and also in the adrenals and kidney. Small amounts of cobalt after administration are largely stored and very little is excreted in the bowel and the feces; however, large amounts given intravenously are readily excreted by the urine (62 per cent) and represent the main path of excretion of internally metabolized cobalt (Sheline et al.). Schultz (1940) has reviewed the data which indicate that cobalt is essential to blood formation. Comar, Davis and Taylor (1946) have studied the distribution of cobalt in cattle following the administration of the radioactive element cobalt[60] (Co^{60}). Table I gives the distribution of labeled cobalt in cattle 10 days after administration.

Radioactive properties of cobalt make it a suitable isotope for external and interstitial radiation therapy. Its only disadvantage as compared with radium is the shorter half life of the radioactive cobalt. The advantages in using radiocobalt include the low energy beta radiation which can be screened easily; the gamma radiation of radiocobalt is almost homogeneous; there are no contaminating gaseous daughter products to be considered because cobalt[60] decays into a stable solid element; it is rapidly eliminated from the body; it is readily produced in the nuclear reactor in any desired quantity; it can be prepared in any shape or form; it can be electro-plated on any material, subsequently being activated for clinical use; it is readily soluble, therefore may be placed in thin wall containers or other applicators for interstitial or intra-cavity use; irregular volumes can be more easily implanted because of flexible nylon applicators that can be used; the cost of cobalt is less than that of radium; and behind a magnetic metal it can be handled with an electro-magnet.

As with other radioactive isotopes, radioactive cobalt is open to new applications in tracer techniques for the biologist and physiologist. In tracer quantities it is of interest in the studies of vitamin B_{12} in relation to hemoglobin and red blood cell formation. It has also been utilized in conjunction with radioactive sodium chloride and radioactive phosphorus[32] in determining the intermediate metabolism of these isotopes in both normal and abnormal individuals.

Parr, O'Neill and Krebs have studied the x-irradiation protection afforded by cobalt. Four hundred female Swiss albino mice were used. The animals which were kept on cobalt diet before irradiation showed a significant increase in their resistance against irradiation in comparison to the irradiated groups on Purina chow, only. Those surviving with cobalt diet had the appearance of the animals in the non-irradiated control group.

Hale and Stone have shown that whole body Co^{60} gamma irradiation, in sublethal doses, effectively destroyed the immunity to pneumococcus infection in mice, even with abundant specific antibody present. The authors believe the destruction in immunity was due to a drop in leucocytes.

Callender, Turnbull, et al., used Co^{60}-labeled Vitamin B^{12} in a study of the absorption of Vitamin B^{12} in the feces to make an estimate of the status of the intrinsic factor of Castle in healthy people and in pernicious anemia patients. An oral test dose of 0.5 micrograms was given. In 10 normal individuals, 31 % of the test dose was recovered from the feces. In patients with pernicious anemia, 88.7 % was recovered. This latter rate of recovery was reduced considerably by giving the patient sources of intrinsic factor.

Myers in 1948 first used radiocobalt as a source of interstitial radiation.

TABLE I

Cobalt in Mg./100 gm. of Fresh Weight of Tissue

TISSUE	HEIFER NO. 3 (2400 GAMMA INJECTED INTO JUGULAR VEIN)
Adrenals	3.1
Liver	2.2
Kidney	1.4
Lung	0.93
Red bone marrow (ribs)	0.78
Lymph nodes	0.76
Thyroid	0.64
Esophagus	0.64
Spleen	0.54
Heart	0.34
Reproductive organs	0.38
Bile	0.02
Gall bladder	0.57
Small intestine	0.49
Large intestine	0.21
Feces	0.15

Cobalt[60] alloy wire was cut to desired lengths, enclosed in gold needles which filtered out the beta radiation, and was used in the same manner as radium needles.

Morrison and Low-Beer devised beads consisting of 98.9 per cent metallic cobalt and 1.1 per cent contaminants (iron, nickel and sulphur), from 3 to 5 millimeters in diameter, and had them activated in the Oak Ridge nuclear reactor. These beads varied in strength from 0.6 to 6 millicuries in the smaller sizes and from 10 to 20 millicuries in the larger sizes. The beads were silver plated to a thickness of from 80 milligrams to 130 milligrams per square centimeter, or the equivalent of from 0.08 millimeters to 0.16 millimeters in thickness. Blais and Low-Beer estimated that under experimental conditions used by them the energy of one millicurie of cobalt[60] is equivalent to 1.4 milligrams of radium filtered with 0.5 millimeters of platinum. Beads were prepared in preference to needles and tubes so that they might approach more accurately "point sources" of radiation. It was felt to be advantageous in intra-cavity radiation. Results of the use of the radiocobalt beads are yet to be completely evaluated.

James, Williams and Morton since 1948 have been developing methods for the interstitial use of radioactive cobalt in cancer tissue. They point out the use of an applicator made of flexible nylon tubing. The external diameter of the tubing is 1.27 millimeters, which makes an applicator

slightly larger than No. 4 silk tension suture material. This flexible applicator can be implanted in irregular volumes of tissue around major blood
vessels. Beta particles are completely filtered out by the nylon applicator.
They felt that good dosage control could be had through accurate implantation and careful loading of the applicators. The nylon applicators are
sterilized by boiling. After heating, it is possible to stretch the ends of the
applicators thin enough so that they can be threaded through the eye of
appropriate needles. This stretching of the nylon is impossible after it
becomes cold. Guide needles are first implanted throughout the field to be
treated. They are either in the form of long Keith needles or curved tension
needles, depending upon the contour of the tumor volume to be implanted.
When all of the guide needles have been inserted, the ends of the nylon
applicators are threaded through the eyes of the guide needles. As the
needles are pulled through, the cobalt is pulled into proper position in the
tumor tissue. It is pointed out by the authors that it is possible to load the
applicators with cobalt so that by spacing them at one centimeter intervals
the various parts of the tumor will receive a total of 1000 roentgens per
day. The cobalt[60] is left in place for an average of 7 to 10 days, depending
upon the amount of radiation desired. At the end of that time the applicators can be easily withdrawn without the use of anesthesia. The nylon
applicators should be used within four weeks after preparation since the
beta radiation absorbed makes them brittle after this time. The authors
report that in 1950 forty cases of head and neck cancer were implanted with
radioactive cobalt. In each instance the cases had received previous treatment, in the form either of surgery or other types of radiation. The authors
point out that malignant tumors in the head and neck regions are best
treated primarily by surgical excision, and that post-operative radiation is
reserved for those cases in which there has been incomplete resection of the
tumor. They suggest that radioactive cobalt in flexible nylon applicators
should have a greater use in the treatment of head and neck tumors when
radiation is indicated, because very often the tumor mass presents itself in
an irregular form at or near major blood vessels. The longest interval that
patients have been followed after treatment was reported as eight months
with no evidence of residual carcinoma. One of the main limiting factors
in the method apparently is damage to the regional major blood vessels.
Experimental work is going on in their laboratory at this time to determine
the maximum amount of gamma radiation from cobalt[60] which the normal
vessels can tolerate.

Morton, Callandine and Myers also have pointed out Co[60] in nylon
tubing as a source of gamma ray energy to supplant radium needles. They
suggest the addition of aluminum spacers to increase the intensity of the
irradiation if desired. They point out that during surgery the radioactive

source may be placed anywhere that is deemed necessary. In internal cancers the long stretched inactive ends of the nylon tubing may be brought out through a puncture wound in the manner of a drain, allowing for the removal of the radiocobalt without further surgery. In placing circular implants they advocate the diameter of the circle must exceed 4 centimeters to prevent locking.

Becker and Scheer have developed a cohesive but non-adhesive plastic mass which can be molded at body temperatures and yet retain its shape in the absence of undue pressure. Powdered cobalt is dispersed in this mass and then the whole is worked on with wet wooden surfaces. A 5 millimeter layer of the cobalt[60] plastic mass has been encased in cellophane and taped to the area to be treated. Intra-cavity applicators have been shaped as required and then encased in sterilized beef gut and tied at each end like a sausage. Many other methods for the use of the cobalt[60] plastic mass are depicted. They expect to render a subsequent publication pointing out dosage distribution detail.

Bladder tumors are treated by Co[60] sources which can be placed at the geometric center of the bladder so that homogeneous irradiation covers the mucosa of the surface. Hinman, Schulte and Low-Beer reported, (1955), 34 patients treated by this method. Ten patients had lesions confined to the mucosa of the bladder or infiltrating less than half the thickness of the bladder muscle. Twenty-two patients had more extensive disease. Treatment with Co[60] was given in two sittings. The average dose per sitting was approximately 2500 gamma r. to 3000 gamma r. as measured at the mucosal surface. Nine patients with non-infiltrating tumors had adequate irradiation. Four of these patients are without evidence of disease up to four years from the time of initial treatment. In the infiltrating group of bladder cancers treated, 14 received what was considered adequate irradiation therapy. Ten are dead, and three have arrested disease at the time of the report. The infiltrating lesions cannot be treated by intracavity cobalt alone, but may be treated by this method plus external roentgen therapy, in some cases. The average dose of external irradiation, i.e. roentgen rays, averaged about 3500 r., fractionated over a period of 35 to 40 days. This therapy had qualities of 0.95 mm. of copper HVL, or 2.5 mm. of copper HVL. Most infiltrating bladder lesions are only temporarily arrested, even by the combined intracavity and external irradiation therapy.

Vermooten reports the use of radioactive cobalt nylon threads in bladder carcinoma, and, in a case of secondary carcinoma of the bladder from a primary lesion in the prostate, noted good immediate palliation.

Mayor reports the use of a solution of Co[60] chloride in a balloon within the bladder for malignant papillomatosis and other superficial tumors. Sixty cc. of "solution" were left in the bladder for 8 to 10 days and gave an estimated dose of from 9,000 to 12,000 gamma r. Sixty patients were treated, most of whom had advanced disease, but 22 patients had no cysto-scopic evidence of disease following three years of observation after treatment. The author emphasizes the necessity for accurate technical data to be employed in order to reproduce his treatment and results.

Cobalt[60] offers an interesting possibility in terms of external beam therapy. Grimmett points out the advantages of radioactive cobalt over radium therapy in general. He indicates that for reasons both physical and bio-physical there are advantages in the use of high energy radiation of the cobalt[60] type, which include simplicity and safety in loading the cobalt[60] into the machine; adequate protection for operators so that it will be possible to adjust patients for treatment without exposure; a simple ar-rangement for turning the gamma ray beam on and off; flexibility of the machine; provision for fitting the usual clinical accessories, such as duration indicators, range finders, etc. The Oak Ridge Institute of Nuclear Studies and the M. D. Anderson Hospital for Cancer Research have cooperated in building a 1000-Curie cobalt[60] irradiator for experimental radiobiology and for the treatment of human cancer.

Other investigators in both this country and in Canada are working along similar lines. Progress is being made in perfecting cobalt radiators for use in external radiation therapy. The fundamental design of the units is simple, consisting of a heavy metal cylinder, (lead tungsten alloy or uranium), of sufficient thickness to protect against giving more than a per-missible tolerance dose in the treatment room when the beam is in the "off" position; a mechanism for rotating the source wheel within the cylinder; a collimating device to keep the penumbra of the beam at a mini-mum; a stand of adequate dimensions to hold the cylinder and to permit rotation of the beam of therapy as much as possible; either movable shut-ters with a light localizer, or a set of cones which are interchangeable can be used. At least 15 cm. distance should separate the skin from the lead or tungsten parts of the portal, so that the thickness of air will absorb the secondary electrons originating from the metal.

Co[60] teletherapy units are used like 250-kv x-ray machines with either stationary fields or rotational type of therapy.* The clinical approach, how-ever, is different. Skin reaction is not a factor—(up to 5000 r., given in fractionated amounts over three weeks, does not give a sharp erythema). All treatments have to be planned on the basis of volume distribution. End dosage points are higher, but careful evaluation is still in progress as to how much more can be safely given. Fletcher feels that Co[60] therapy should be used to improve on the results obtained by 250-kv therapy and outlines, from his experience, the lesions best suited for such treatment:

* See also par. 17.3.8

(I) *In the head and neck:* differentiated squamous cell carcinoma of paranasal sinuses, nasopharynx, tonsil, base of tongue, oro- and hypopharynx, and some extensive carcinomas of the oral cavity and laryngopharynx; (2) *In the thorax:* squamous carcinoma of oesophagus, inoperable bronchiogenic carcinomas and metastatic mediastinal lymph nodes; (3) *In the abdominal cavity:* testicular tumor, metastases to retroperitoneal lymph nodes; (4) *In the pelvis:* advanced carcinoma of the cervix, body of the uterus and bladder.

There are many reports on the characteristics and use of cobalt-60 beam therapy. Johns, and also Watson report on an 1100-Curie unit in Saskatoon. Smith reports on a 1300-Curie unit in London, Ontario. He makes some interesting observations as follows: Co^{60} will not replace conventional methods of irradiation; it will expand the effectiveness of irradiation; it requires a radiation physicist; it places added emphasis on centralization of radiation therapy; it will place us closer to"State Medicine"; it or its equivalent will be a "must" for any department handling 500 new therapy cases a year.

Fedoruk, et al., reporting on isodose curves and depth dose data from an 1100-Curie Co^{60} unit, indicates that the unit produces a beam equivalent to about 3 mev, and delivers 33 r. per minute at 80 cm. distance. Due to the size of the cobalt source, a moderate penumbra results about each field. This, however, is no handicap and the isodose curves compare favorably with those of 2 to 3 mev roentgen rays.

Percentage doses of a Co^{60} beam are greater for the same size portals and source skin distance than x-ray therapy of one to three mm. copper HVL quality. For instance, at 80 cm., using a 20 cm. square field, the Co^{60} unit depth dose, at 10 cm., is 50 % of the dose 6 mm. below the skin surface, whereas, with 200 KV therapy, using the beam quality of 1 mm. copper HVL quality, at 80 cm. distance, and using a 20 cm. square field, the depth dose is only 23 % of the skin dose.

20.4 Copper

The importance of copper for the formation of blood has recently been stressed (Elvehjem, 1935). Like iron, copper is widely distributed in the tissues of the human body. It is normally stored in the liver, adrenal, kidney, spleen, red marrow and lymph nodes. It is interesting to note that copper is normally present in the lymph nodes, whereas iron is accumulated there only under pathologic conditions. Normally there are between 5 and 6 mg. of copper in the blood of an adult and, according to most observers, the major part of this copper is in the corpuscle fraction rather than in the plasma. Copper is largely excreted in the bile and feces after administration and practically none appears in the urine. In spite of its relatively

TABLE II

Mg. Copper per kg. of Dry Normal Tissue

Liver	24.9
Pancreas	4.3
Adrenal	18.0
Brain	17.5
Spleen	5.2
Kidney	17.5
Red marrow	4.4
Lymph nodes	10.8
Hair	15.1

Modes of Highest Excretion

Cat bile	22.7 mg./kg.
Dog bile	71.0 mg./kg.
Digestive tract	9.0 mg./kg.

high concentration in the skin, there is no evidence that it is excreted by this tissue. The following table on the distribution of copper in the human body is combined from Elvehjem's (1935) review and the work of Cunningham (1931).

Schultze (1940) has shown that the administratiod of copper increases the cytochrome oxidase activity of the bone marrow of rats, and Cunningham (1931) believes that copper is essential for the conversion of dihydroxyphenylalanine to melanin. The enzyme catalyzing this reaction is tyrosinase. Tyrosinase, prepared from domestic mushrooms, contains 0.13 per cent copper per dry weight. Cunningham (1931) found as much as 8 mg. of copper per kilogram of dry weight in a melanotic tumor.

In hematopoiesis, copper is concerned with the transformation of ingested iron into hemoglobin but does not aid in the absorption of iron.

Experiments with radioactive copper are handicapped by the brief half life of radiocopper (Cu^{64}), 12.8 hours. When radiocopper is given to normal anemic dogs it is concentrated in the blood plasma within five hours and then in the red blood cells during the next 48 hours. Only about 5 per cent of the copper fed is retained, the greatest retention being in the liver, kidney and bone marrow. Radiocopper (Cu^{64}) decays in three modes: by negative beta particle emission with a maximum energy of 0.57 mev, by K capture and positron emission with a maximum energy of 0.66 mev. Gamma rays of 1.34 mev energy are also reported.

Wrenn et al. in 1951 devised a scintillation counter, which enabled them to detect radioactive copper 64, which has a half-life of 12.8 hours. They were able to synthesize this into copper phthalocyanine, and found that it would penetrate only those areas of the brain in which there was altered tissue structure through injury. From the animal studies they believed this would be a good method of localizing brain tumors preoperatively from outside the intact skull. Wren and Good reported further progress on this project in 1952.

Brownell and Sweet (1953) discussed the theoretical aspects of the problem, described their equipment and gave an example of the successful use of Cu^{64} in detecting and localizing a recurrence of a meningiomatous tumor. The authors also used As^{74}, another positron emitter. Two scintillation counters were applied, one on each side of the head and pointing at each other. The recording equipment responded only when pulses were received simultaneously from both counters. Interpretation of recordings from such a coincidence counting technique is not fully evaluated but, theoretically, there appear to be advantages over the single pulse counting technics.

20.5 Zinc

Radioactive isotopes of zinc (8 + 2 isomers) include: Zn^{63}, Zn^{65} and Zn^{69}. The only tracer easily utilized is Zn^{65}, with a half life of 245 days, but Zn^{63} with a half life of 38 minutes has been used in experimental animal and clinical studies. Zn^{65} is produced by either the cyclotron or neutron bombardment of zinc and decays by positron emission, with a maximum energy of 0.33 mev (in addition to annihilation radiation) and K capture. The positron emission is accompanied by gamma rays with 1.12 mev energy.

Sheline et al. (1943) have studied the distribution and excretion of labeled zinc following the intravenous injection of 1 to 12 micrograms of zinc chloride into dogs. Similar work was carried out on rats. Most of the radiozinc was excreted by way of the gastro-intestinal tract. About 25 per cent was found in the feces in 12 to 15 dogs. Relatively little zinc appeared in the urine. Per gram of tissue, the pancreas took up the greater amount of zinc from the plasma, followed by the liver and kidneys. These latter organs lost the zinc concentration rapidly. In the case of the liver, the loss was not accounted for in the bile but indicated that the zinc was removed for uptake by other tissues. Such movements of zinc have not yet been fully explained.

Evidence has been presented by Montgomery et al. (1943) that the acinar portion of the pancreas is concerned with the metabolism of zinc. Radiozinc chloride was injected into the hind leg vein of several dogs, which had been prepared with biliary, pancreatic and duodenal fistulas in various combinations. About 11 per cent was excreted in the pancreatic juice within 14 days, while in the bile only 0.4 per cent was excreted in eight days. Vallee and Fluharty (1947) in studying zinc metabolism have found by external application of the Geiger counter that radiozinc injected into normal dogs is widely distributed throughout the body. Samples of blood, white cells and tissue from these dogs were dry-ashed and the zinc extracted with dithizone for photometric determination. The authors found no selective accumulation of the element in the heart, great vessels, muscle, cortical bone, marrow, spleen, lymph nodes, endocrines, respiratory organs, digestive organs, genito-urinary tract, plasma and whole blood. Following intravenous injection radioactive zinc was found sufficiently concentrated in circulating white blood cells for radioassay. The white blood cells necessary for bioassay were collected as leukocytic masses from at least 15 cc. of whole blood.

Muller reports the use of subcutaneous and intramuscular injections of radiozinc suspended in pectin solution. These suspensions are not followed by diffusion of radioactive substance outside the injected areas as checked by radioautographs and by counting the radioactivity of blood specimens.

The author found that zinc[63] infused intraperitoneally into mice did not diffuse beyond the peritoneum for a period of 2.5 hours when given as a sol. A homogeneous diffusion of the isotope was noted within the peritoneal cavity in a whole body radioautographic study. There was also observed a limited radiation effect on the peritoneum. Some histological changes were seen in the liver and kidneys. Later experimental studies in rabbits revealed no hematological changes over a period of months. The author was prompted by these studies to use zinc[63] in a few late cases of ovarian carcinoma with peritoneal involvement. Some general improvement was noted in the condition of the patient following treatment with radiozinc, with a decrease in the amount of ascites. A study of the tumor cells in the ascitic fluid revealed marked degeneration. The author suggested that the method might afford a useful purpose in irradiating tissues not accessible to treatment by the use of radium needles or implants. The complicating factors in the use of the method include the danger of over-irradiation of focal spots and total body effects from gamma irradiation.

Various authors have reported that some cancer tissues differ from normal tissues in zinc content. It has also been suggested that a marked difference exists between cancer patients and normal individuals with regard to the effect of zinc salts on the serum alkaline phosphomonesterase. In view of these suggested differences Banks, Tupper and Wormall investigated the distribution of Zn^{65} (245 day half-life) following the intravenous injection of various zinc compounds.

A method for the determination of Zn^{65} in animal tissues was described as used by Banks et al.

In a study made of the distribution of radioactive zinc[65] in the tissues of rabbits they found that approximately half of the zinc carbonate or phosphate used was concentrated in the lungs in 45 minutes. Small amounts only were found in the liver and kidney. No attempt was made to reduce the size of the Zn particles so that they approached colloidal size. In this way the distribution of relatively large inorganic particles injected in the blood stream could be followed.

An organic compound of Zn was felt more likely to localize in certain tissues. About 80 % of an injected organic compound zinc dithizone complex was present in the lungs after 24 hours and over 50 % remained there 10 days after the injection. The liver contained small amounts only (1.4–5.3 %) of the injected zinc.

Heath and Liquier-Milward in studies of the distribution of radioactive Zn[65] in the tissues of tumor bearing mice following its injection subcutaneously found an increased concentration in tumor tissues. In the sarcoma group of mice the age of the tumor influenced the uptake of Zn[65]/unit weight of tumor tissue. The nuclear desoxyribose nucleoproteins of both carcinomas and sarcomas contained appreciable quantities of zinc. A large part of the injected zinc remained localized at the site of injection; about 20 % being lost in 18 hours. The authors do not feel that Zn[65] can be used for tumor therapy from the absorbed isotope because the liver, pancreas, spleen, intestine and kidneys would receive much higher irradiation than does the tumor. The zinc preparation used in the experiments was Zn[65] as a chloride neutralized with NaOH and made up to a known volume with doubly distilled water. About 20 microcuries were used per 20 gram mouse.

Muller and Rossier also reported on a new method for the treatment of cancer of the lungs by using zinc[63] and gold[198]. They showed selective fixation of the artificial radioactive materials within the lungs. The procedure was carried out in six patients. Zinc[63] was used in two patients, and gold (Au[198]) in four. One was a case of pulmonary metastasis from hypernephroma; one patient had a pulmonary lymphogranuloma; and four patients had inoperable bronchial carcinomas. While the localization of the two isotopes within the lung tissue was similar, gold[198] was preferred because of its longer half-life. It was suggested that radioactivity could be localized to a certain part of the lung by injecting the radioactive solution into a catheter previously inserted through the heart into a selected pulmonary artery. They stated that up to 150 mc. had been injected in this way. The ultimate benefit of such a procedure is yet to be proved.

Müller, (1956), reports his previous experience with zinc[63]. He indicated that the use of the radioisotope involved a great deal of work and exposure on his part because it was necessary to perform the radiochemical separations and preparations in his own hospital. With the advent of radioactive gold, this use of cyclotron-produced zinc[63] has not been a factor in treatment of cases.

20.6 Arsenic

Little is known about the metabolism of arsenic or the role it plays in human physiology, although it is always found in minute amounts in human tissues.

DuPont, Ariel and Warren injected subtoxic amounts of labeled arsenic, intravenously, into rabbits. There was a rapid excretion in the urine, with maximum concentration in the liver and kidneys. The brain showed very low concentrations. At the dosage level of two mgs. little or no arsenic was retained after one week. Because of the variation in the time for distribution in the tissues from animal to animal, no conclusions were drawn as to the time pattern for distribution.

Studies on distribution of labeled potassium arsenite in animals and man have revealed some interesting findings. In the rat, 95 % of the arsenic in whole blood was localized in the red blood cells which seemed to be bound to a large molecule. The globin and heme fractions retained the arsenic. Radioarsenic disappears rapidly from the blood of all animals except rats. In the latter instance there is noted a long retention of arsenic in the blood. In the human, leukocytes average ten times the amount of arsenic found in erythrocytes. No appreciable accummulation appears to occur in rapidly growing tissues and the bulk of the arsenic is found in the protein fraction of tissues metabolizing it. The view that arsenic may replace phosphorus in proteins has not been supported. The excretion of arsenic in humans is almost entirely through the kidneys, less than ten per cent being found in the feces.

Ducoff, Neal and associates investigated the excretion of radioarsenic in two patients with Hodgkin's disease and leukemia, respectively. They also studied the excretion of radioarsenic in rats and rabbits, as well as the distribution of radioarsenic in the tissues of these animals and in one of the patients who came to autopsy. They found a highly selective concentration of the arsenic in the liver, kidneys, spleen and lungs. The uptake by tumor tissue was relatively low. The distribution pattern, however, was altered by the presence of transplanted tumors in some of the animals (mice).

Walinder suggests the introduction of colloidal $As_2^{76}S_3$ into the urinary bladder for the treatment of papillomatosis. The compound is a beta ray emitter and its use would entail less risk of fibrosis of the bladder wall than would be expected with more penetrating rays.

As^{74} like Cu^{64} is a positron emitter and produces annihilation radiation. It has been used for the localization of brain tumors. Because of its longer half-life—(17 days)—it is more satisfactory for some studies than is Cu^{64} with a half-life of 12.8 hours. As^{76} differs from As^{74} in that it does not emit positive beta particles.

Benda, David and Constans (1953) reported on the localization of brain tumors by As^{76} in the form of ammonium arsenate. A dose of 1 to 2 millicuries of As^{76} was used. Localization was possible after 3 hours, with external counting before operation, and differential counts between tumor and normal structure during operation with the use of a probe counter. In the opinion of these authors, As^{76} compares favorably with P^{32} for the detection of brain tumors.

The use of radioarsenic has shown that certain parasites concentrate the element and, therefore, that the parasite is affected by the element, per se.

Griffon and Barbaud report that in toxicology studies it is possible to detect arsenic in the hair of individuals by exposing a sample of hair to bombardment, producing radioactive arsenic in situ.

Arsenic is a simple element with one stable isotope (As^{75}). Numerous radioactive isotopes exist, but As^{76}, As^{71} and As^{74} are best suited for tracer investigation. The isotope (As^{71}) has a half life of 62 hours, with a maximum positron emission energy of 0.81 mev, K capture and 0.17 γ. Arsenic^{74} has a half life of 17 days, emitting positrons with a maximum energy of 1.53 mev., and negative beta particles with a maximum energy of 1.36 mev. There is also a gamma ray component, with energies of 0.6 and 0.64 mev. The radioisotope (As^{76}) is produced in the pile by neutron irradiation of some organic arsenical. It has a half life of 26.7 hours. The negative beta particles have maximum energies of 2.96 and 2.41 mev. There are five gamma radiations reported with energies from 0.55 to 2.1 mev.

20.7 Antimony

Because of the proved value of antimony compounds in the treatment of parasitic infections, the blood level and distributions of these compounds after administration have been investigated by several experiments with radioantimony. Antimony (Sb^{124}), with a half life of 60 days, and antimony (Sb^{122}), with a half life of 2.8 days, have both been used ($Sb^{124}\beta,\gamma$; $Sb^{122}\beta\gamma$, β^{+} and K)

Cowie and his co-workers injected organic antimonials intravenously into dogs in the amount of 0.8 mg. of antimony per kilogram of body weight, administering the compound daily, except Sundays. The tissue levels obtained by repeated injections were higher than those by a single injection. They found the concentration of antimony in the dog highest in the thyroid, liver and parathyroid, and next highest in the parasites (Dirofilaria). The spleen, lymph nodes, jejunum and kidney followed in degree of concentration. There was a continuous accumulation of the antimony compounds in the blood with daily injections, which supports the hypothesis that a certain threshold has to be reached in order to achieve therapeutic resulps. The concentration in parasites explains the usefulness of antimony ccmtounds in chemotherapy. Cowie et al. found that antimony concentration in the blood of the rat differed from that in dog and man.

20.8 Gold

Of the various gold radioisotopes, gold (Au^{198}) is of the most value. The distribution of gold in perfused rabbits was studied by Tobias et al., as quoted by Hevesy. The kidneys, spleen, adrenals, marrow, liver and synovial membrane were found to take up an appreciable amount of gold. A further study by Bertrand and Tobias, as reported by Dougherty and Lawrence, demonstrated that the uptake of radiogold sodium thiosulfate in the synovia and synovial fluid of a patient suffering from rheumatoid arthritis was marked, while in control animals it was less.

Because radioactive manganese was difficult to obtain, Hahn and Sheppard selected gold with similar properties of concentration in the reticulo-endothelial system for study. The half life of gold (Au^{198}) is 2.7 days and it emits both negative beta rays, with a maximum energy of 1.37 mev, and gamma rays, with energies of 0.42, 0.68 and 1.1 mev. The gamma radiation is of particular value in enabling the investigator to measure the localization and relative degree of concentration of the radioactive material. It was further felt that the half life of gold was ideal in therapy, since the patient received three-fourths of the radiation from a given dose in about 5.5 days.

The chemical behavior of gold in preparations of colloidal suspension sols is well known. They are stable and will withstand repeated autoclaving at 120° centigrade. They can be concentrated by boiling and a reasonable amount of dissolved salts does not appear to affect the stability. Hahn and his co-workers found that this was not true with sols of manganese oxide which must be dispensed under sterile conditions since they do not withstand subsequent sterilization.

Sheppard, Goodell and Hahn found that in the human being, particles of intravenously administered colloidal metallic gold are phagocytized by reticulo-endothelial cells with a higher concentration than is obtained with manganese. Under the conditions of using the sol, the toxic effects of ionic gold present no problem. Due to the insolubility of metallic gold, blood levels are low following its deposition in the body. If the dosage is limited to 4 milligrams or less of gold per dose an additional safety factor is achieved.

Sheppard, Goodell and Hahn point out that the chemical procedure in preparing radiogold sols is relatively simple. Metallic gold is converted to a solution of gold chloride and reduced to metallic gold in alkaline solution by adding ascorbic acid. The presence of gelatin, although not essential, increases the reliability of the procedure.

Intravenous administration of the sols is facilitated by the use of a saline infusion. The saline solution is run into the cubital vein in the usual manner and after satisfactory flow is established, the sol is poured into the solution by the use of tongs. This technique permits the maintenance of a safe distance by the worker at all times. The authors determined the radioactivity of each dose by measuring the gamma ray intensity at a distance of one meter, using a Lauritsen electroscope.

Sheppard, Wells and associates have reported a study of distribution of radioactive gold in tissues of patients in the terminal stages of acute and chronic leukemia, and other neoplastic diseases. Radioactive gold was administered intravenously in the form of highly dispersed colloidal sols shortly before death. In one patient it was found that the disappearance of the gold sol from the blood was complete 30 minutes after the injection. The uptake was found relatively high in the spleen and liver, intermediate in the kidney, and low in all other organs including the pancreas. It would appear that gold is distributed in the reticulo-endothelial system much as would be expected of any foreign material, and resembles in its distribution that of the iron colloids. Hahn and Carothers found in an attempt to treat a case of leukemia that the lymphadenopathy in the cervical region did not respond satisfactorily but that a leukemia cutis which existed in the skin showed a relatively good response to intravenous therapy. An attempt was then made to infiltrate directly the lymph nodes which could be reached with the radioactive gold sol. Successful diminution in their size was noted.

Since gold does not migrate about the body as do a number of other materials which are dissolved following phagocytosis, it was felt that direct infiltration of tumor tissue might be successful and a number of direct infiltrations were attempted. Many tumors, especially the cauliflower-like lesions of the female cervix, did not retain the solution injected. In metastatic hypernephroma and certain lesions of lymphosarcoma the areas were so vascular that the gold promptly gained access to the blood stream and ultimately appeared in the liver and spleen. It was found, however, that any well encapsulated or discrete mass offered fertile ground for the use of the isotope as a means of ionizing radiation therapy. Tissue tolerance in the use of radioactive gold has posed one of the chief problems in its use. Hahn and Carothers cite an example indicating a method that they have used in calculating dosage.

Hahn, Skipper, Carothers and Bernard in working with AK-4 leukemia in mice found that radioactive colloidal metallic gold of the order of 0.1 to 0.75 millicuries consistently increased the life span of the mice by a significant but small increment. They point out that in clinical trials with the isotope, one remission of one year and another of nine months have been obtained in a series of 13 patients with acute leukemia, but that in the overall picture it was an unsatisfactory method of treating the disease.

Hahn, Carothers, Hilliard and Bernard, (1956), reviewed 9 years experience in treating patients with leukemia by radioactive colloidal gold.

There were 78 patients with chronic myelogenous or lymphogenous leu-kemia. No selection of cases was used. In some instances the patients were moribund. An occasional case responded to as little as 10 millicuries of gold in one treatment. In other instances, experience prompted them to recom-mend an initial dose of 40 to 50 millicuries of colloidal radioactive gold in the average size individual with a white count in excess of 200,000 cells per cu.cm. Empirically, one should tentatively administer from 0.8 to 1.2 millicuries kilogram of body weight. Remissions averaged 6 months du-ration. No increase over the average 3.5 year life span was claimed for the agent. The investigators feel that Au[198] colloids constitute as convenient and satisfactory a method of treating chronic leukemia as any of the available agents at the present time.

Hahn and Carothers, in an extensive study of the problem of treating bronchiogenic carcinoma, have pointed out that Meneely, Quarles and Curtis demonstrated that when water soluble materials, tagged with radioactive iso-topes, are administered by the tracheal route, the water is rapidly absorbed by the alveoli of the lungs. When radioactive metallic colloidal gold solu-tions were administered under similar circumstances it was found that the fluid vehicle was absorbed and the gold remained for many days in the lung parenchyma. It did not gain access to the blood stream. These latter experiments, aimed at showing not only the distribution of the gold colloid but also in determining the tolerance of the animal to the radiation in selected portions of the lung. The experiments were carried out by using large doses of radioactive gold administered at therapeutic levels. It was found that the gold colloidal sol was drained very slowly by the regional lymphatics, taking from 10 days to 2 weeks to concentrate sufficiently to permit adequate radiation in the lymphoid tissues. The gold isotopes (Au[198] and Au[199]) having half lives of 2.7 and 3.15 days respectively, therefore were considered unsuitable for therapeutic trial in treating bronchiogenic carcinoma with regional lymph gland metastases, at least when used alone. Hahn and Carothers therefore considered other possible isotopes for ex-perimental use and among them was silver (Ag[111]) with a half life of 7.5 days. On trial it was found that the colloids of metallic silver were rapidly transported to the regional lymphatics of the lung following intrapulmonary administration. Unfortunately, the isotope of silver was difficult to produce in the pile by reaction of thermal neutrons on palladium since the cross section is none too good, and the parent palladium isotope is not highly abundant. The authors then decided to attempt to produce non-active silver-coated radioactive gold colloids, hoping the body would show a tendency to distribute the latter material according to the chemical and physiological activity of silver.

Silver-coated gold colloid was prepared by adding a fraction of a milliliter of metallic colloid gold[198] to a solution containing 50 milligrams of silver in the form of the nitrate and which already contained an excess of ascorbic acid. This resulted in the immediate dispersal of some of the silver. An additional three drops of 40 per cent sodium hydroxide and one milliliter of six per cent gelatin were added, followed by the addition of a solution of civatemic acid containing 250 milligrams of the latter reducing agent. Water was added to make up the total amount of fluid desired.

Dogs were used in the experiment to determinea distribution of the radio active colloid after its administration by the intrpulmonary route through a bronchoscope. It was found that it was rapidly removed from the lung parenchyma and a considerable proportion appeared in the lymph nodes draining the lung region.

Hahn suggests that, on the basis of the experimental evidence to date, he would outline a course of procedure in the use of the silver-coated gold colloids as adjuvant treatment to surgery in the management of primary lung tumor in the following terms:

He would instill the colloid about 14 days prior to the time of planned pneumonectomy which would permit lymphatic drainage and the irradiation of microscopic implants in the lymph nodes and prevent undue exposure to the surgeon during the period of the pneumonectomy. At the time of operation, blocks of tissue should be obtained from the lung and from the regional chains of lymph nodes for both the histological examination and determination of radioactivity content on a basis of activity per gram of fresh tissue. In the event that an individual is found to be nonresectable no harm has been done, for there is a strong likelihood that palliation and increase in life span may be effected. The chief advantages in the resectable cases would appear to be (1) that the extremely intense irradiation of the lymphatics can be accomplished without general irradiation of the whole lung area, and (2) no pleural adhesions or other undesirable sequellae may be anticipated.

Williams, Stanton, Jamison and Williams studied the distribution of radioactive gold colloid in rats, mice and transplanted mouse tumors. Injections of 200 to 500 microcuries of the active colloid into mouse sarcoma 180 and sarcoma 37 resulted in a satisfactory group of regressions. Occasionally poor distribution within the tumor resulted in a regression of the larger portion of the primary but a recurrence at one margin indicated that a small area of cells had escaped irradiation. Twenty-one complete regressions were obtained by gold[198] in 31 treated mouse tumors. Controlled transplants of the tumor done at the same time showed 6 regressions in 22 animals.

They also found that when the gold colloid was administered by the intravenous or intrasplenic route in mice and rats it is deposited largely in the liver and spleen, being retained by the Kupffer and reticulo-endothelial cells. Distribution of the radioactive material was uniform in all lobes of normal liver in mice and rats. When injected locally into tumors of mice under favorable conditions, the greatest portion remains in the tumor (88 to 100 per cent). In tumors of considerable vascularity or in the presence of necrosis, varying amounts of the gold sol leak into the general circulation. Uniform distribution in the solid tumors was difficult to obtain by needle infiltration. Tumor regressions in mice were obtained by a combination of nitrogen mustard and radioactive gold sol infiltration. It was pointed out that the particulate structure of the gold sols varies considerably and must be taken into account. The large particles go to the liver, the small ones are often found about the lungs. It was found, however, that with different doses of gold sols the authors obtained no difference in the distribution to the liver. As a speculation it was pointed out that the liver reticulo-endothelial system might be taking up the same portion of large and small particles of gold sol.

Sherman, Bonebrake and Allen have conducted animal experiments employing radioactive colloidal gold in pectin solution to find whether transplanted squamous cell carcinoma of the cervix in mice could be cured safely and completely by interstitial injection of the radioactive gold. This was proved in the affirmative. Their experiments showed that when the gold was injected into the paracervical tissues of rabbits, it entered the lymphatic system and reached the regional lymph nodes. They also studied tolerance levels by this form of therapy. Because of these findings they were encouraged to continue the experiments at a clinical level. Thirteen cases were selected; 10 cases of carcinoma of the cervix, one of carcinoma of the vulva and two of inguinal lymph node metastases.

During the preliminary experiments Sherman, Bonebrake and Allen found that at autopsy 50 to 60 cc. of colloid gold could easily be injected into each parametrium through the vagina. The technique of injection, simulating that of the insertion of radium needles into the parametrium, was developed and employed in all cases presented where gold was injected into the parametrium. The technique gave a rather uniform dispersion of the gold throughout the area to be treated. The patients were carefully observed following injections and showed no untoward reactions. The highest concentration found in the general circulation in any of the patients treated was 63 microcuries, which represents 0.12 per cent of the total injection. Many of the patients developed a peculiar purpuric urticarial rash of the erythema multiforme type which, although generalized, was chiefly confined to the lower extremities. Most of the patients were able to return to their work the following day. Dosages used in the parametria varied between 7.5 millicuries of radioactive gold to 16 millicuries of radioactive gold. In one instance 54 millicuries of radioactive gold was injected into the right parametrium and about 20 milliliters of inactive gold was injected into the left side. In this case the patient was subjected to a complete abdominal hysterectomy and pelvic lymphadenectomy 17 days later. At operation gold was seen infiltrating the entire parametrium on both sides and extended laterally to the pelvic walls and into the obturator fossae. It also extended up over the sacrum to the promontory of the pelvis. No areas of irradiation necrosis were identified, although definite radiation effects were noted throughout the right side of the pelvis. The results of the experiments qualified the use of radioactive colloidal gold as a supplementary treatment for carcinoma of the cervix and vulva and suggested the use of this material as an adjunct to present methods of radiation therapy in these diseases.

Allen, Sherman and Arneson, (1954), applied the method to humans in carcinoma of the cervix, mostly clinical stages I and II. The addition of diodrast to the radioactive material showed, on subsequent films, that volumes of solution of from 30 to 40 cc., injected in each parametrial zone, diffusely infiltrated the entire parametrial area and node bearing regions. Scintoscanner techniques indicated that the radioactive material remained localized in the areas. In 24 cases where the Wertheim hysterectomy and pelvic lymphadenectomy followed injections of 50 millicuries of Au^{198} the intensity of the radiation from the beta source was measured in the various groups of lymph nodes in the pelvis. The gamma contribution was determined to be about 1200 gamma roentgens to the cervix, bladder and rectum and 2200 gamma r. to the mid-parametrium. The beta source was measured in the obturator lymph nodes in the amount of 8400 rep to 99,000 rep. The smallest doses noted were received by the upper iliac lymph nodes and reported as bearing from 4400 rep to 15,000 rep. The authors believe that on the basis of the results obtained to date the Wertheim hysterectomy and lymphadenectomy, plus parametrial injection of radiogold give better results especially in stage II cases as compared with patients receiving radium and roentgen therapy alone.

Wish, Furth, Sheppard and Storey made a study of the disappearance rate of tagged substances from the circulation of roentgen-irradiated animals. Exaggerated phagocytic activity and increased permeability of the capillary wall are among basic changes noted in man and animals exposed to massive irradiation.

The disappearance rate of labeled homologous and heterologous plasma, homologous and heterologous erythrocytes, Evans blue and radiogold were studied in rabbits and mice. It was found that one day after irradiation all of these substances disappeared faster from the circulation of roentgen-irradiated animals than from the circulation of normal animals. This indicated a heightened capillary permeability caused by irradiation. The colloidal gold labeled with gold[198] was injected into normal and roentgen-irradiated rabbits 1, 3, 5 and 8 days after irradiation. These sols similarly prepared gave disappearance curves with a half value time of 1.5 to 2.5 minutes. Their results indicated that the ratio of permeability values of normal to roentgen irradiated animals ranges from 1.1 to 2 at 5 minutes, and from 3.2 to 8.7 at 20 minutes.

King, Spicer, Dowda, Bender and Noel studied the use of radioactive colloidal gold (Au[198]) in pleural effusions and ascites associated with malignancy. They have reported 16 cases treated with this material. Twenty-five per cent of the patients experienced marked relief, both from the standpoint of the reduction of fluid accumulation and relief of pain. Twenty-five per cent of the patients experienced moderate relief from the symptoms, and results in the remaining 50 per cent varied. Colloidal particles used by them were stated to be 0.003 microns in diameter. In determining the dosage of radioactive gold, three factors were considered: the amount of stable gold injected; the radioactivity in millicuries injected; and the approximate radiation dose to the tissues. For every 100 millicuries of radio gold there were approximately 20 milligrams of stable gold. Patients received from 46 to 107 millicuries of radioactive gold per injection. In some of the patients more than one injection of gold was given. One patient received a total of 157 millicuries to the right pleural space and a total of 138 millicuries to the left pleural space. One case received three injections totalling 242 millicuries. The authors point out that the calculation of the tissue dose of radiation was difficult. They felt that calculation of the tissue dose in terms of millicuries injected per 1000 square centimeters of serosal surface was the better approach and used Chamberlain's method noted in the Abbott brochure. They noted that excretion studies revealed practically no radiogold. Immediately after the injection of the material the patients were positioned on the left side for 15 minutes and on the right side for 15 minutes with the head of the bed elevated for 15 minutes and with the foot of the bed elevated for 15 minutes. This cycle was repeated for about 4 hours to insure distribution of the colloidal material over as much of the pleural or peritoneal surface as possible. About one-half the cases treated demonstrated a reaction ranging from mild nausea to nausea, vomiting, malaise and headaches. This usually occurred on the second or third post injection day and lasted about one day. Hemograms following the injection were difficult to evaluate as the patients were usually severely ill and anemic from their disease. It was noted, however, that a transitory leukopenia developed four to six weeks after therapy. Patients treated presented no special nursing problem.

The results of this study suggest that the intra-cavity use of radioactive colloidal gold should be accepted as a valid palliative radiotherapeutic procedure. No conclusions were drawn as to the prolongation of life or actual destruction of malignant tissue resulting from the use of radiogold in the series.

Remold, Siegert and Stamm, (1954), report 11 patients with peritoneal and pleural carcinomatosis from ovarian carcinoma, treated by intraperitoneal or intrapleural injections of radioactive gold. Excessive fluid was first aspirated and then doses of from 31 to 168 millicuries were administered in from one to three injections. Regression of the ascites occurred in only one patient. Tumor growth remained uninfluenced in all patients and the general condition of the patients deteriorated.

Müller reports 114 cases of ovarian carcinoma treated with colloidal gold, up to the end of 1954. The majority of these patients were treated first by surgery and then supplementary intraperitoneal colloidal radiogold, together with post-operative therapy consisting of a total depth dose of about 3000 to 4000 r. within the pelvic cavity and of 1000 to 2000 r. in the upper part of the abdomen. Most of these patients further received a vaginal radium application of from 1000 to 1800 mg.lhrs. Müller divided his patients into four stages for recording results: *Stage 1:* Patients in which a radical removal of the tumor was possible. Nineteen patients are well and free of disease from $3\frac{1}{2}$ to 5 years later. *Stage 2:* Patients in whom unilateral or bilateral ovarian cancer were removed with pelvic peritoneal tumor deposits remaining, but in which removal of implants was seemingly successful on occasion. Twelve of sixteen patients remain free of disease from one to $5\frac{1}{2}$ years. *Stage 3:* Includes patients with carcinoma of one or both ovaries, the disease having extended to the omentum and to the peritoneum beyond the pelvic area. Only partial resection could be carried out on this group. Fifteen patients, out of 36 cases treated, remain free of disease from six months to $5\frac{1}{2}$ years. *Stage 4 and 5:* Include cases of ovarian carcinoma with inoperable primary lesions and extended deposits in the whole abdomen. Out of a total of 41 patients, three lived for three years after the isotope treatment was started; one patient lived $2\frac{2}{3}$ years; two patients lived $1\frac{3}{4}$ years; three patients lived from 1 to $1\frac{1}{2}$ years. In Stage 1, from 50 to 225 millicuries of Au^{198} were given intraperitoneally per patient. In Stage 2, the average dosage of the radiogold was about 300 millicuries, divided into two doses. In Stage 3, 300 millicuries of radiogold were used, divided into two or three applications. In Stage 4, total doses of from 90 up to 560 millicuries of Au^{198} were administered intraperitoneally, and from 40 to 50 millicuries were administered intrapleurally.

The treatment of carcinoma of the prostate by interstitial injection of Au^{198} is limited to those patients with inoperable carcinoma, without distant metastases; patients who refuse radical prostatectomy; and patients who have some other contraindication to radical prostectomy for locally operable lesions. Flocks, Elkins and Culp report 389 patients who have been treated by radioactive gold. The majority of the patients had a local lesion which weighed less than 80 mg., and were treated with 80 millicuries of radioactive gold. The objective of the therapy was not only to destroy the local lesion but also to destroy the neoplasm in the surrounding fascia, in the regional lymph nodes and the lymphatics. As a result of experience in 130 patients, these same authors have found that the most satisfactory dosage was two millicuries per gram of tissue, with an upper limit of 150 millicuries total dose. Follow-up studies have shown negative biopsies in a significant number of patients, following this form of therapy. Clinical arrest of the disease was obtained in 48 of 100 cases which have been followed.

Mackay, (1956), discussed in some detail a technic he used in intracavity irradiation of bladder tumors. The author prefers the use of radioactive solutions injected into the bladder, or into an intravesical thin rubber bag, rather than a solitary central source of irradiation. He has treated 20 patients with radioactive colloidal gold injected directly into the bladder for a total dose of 6000 to 7000 beta r. and 600 to 700 gamma r. in 5 to 10 weeks without severe bladder reaction. Mackay is experimenting also with radioactive bromine which, like radioactive gold, he found did not give severe late reaction.

Nelson describes eight cases of bladder carcinoma in each of which Au^{198} was injected into the tumor tissue at the rate of 1 millicurie per cc. of tissue at 1-cm. intervals. Exposure for this procedure was by means of a suprapubic cystotomy or, in small lesions, by cystoscopic control. The author feels that Au^{198} is as effective as radium, radon, or roentgen therapy, and he indicates that, in his hands, it is easier to administer than the latter mentioned modalities of treatment.

Ellis and Oliver selected radioactive colloidal gold for purposes of delivering beta irradiation to bladder papillomata. It was estimated that about 3 millicuries in about 100 cc. of saline, retained for 2 or 3 hours, would deliver a dose of about 3000 beta r. to the bladder epithelium. Accordingly, a patient with hematuria, resulting from a multiplicity of papillomata covering the entire bladder surface, was given such a dose of Au^{198} through a Foley catheter. This was left in place for $2\frac{1}{2}$ hours. The fluid was then drained and the bladder was washed eight times. This treatment was repeated in 2 months, delivering a dose of 2400 r. to the bladder wall. Six weeks following the last treatment, the only residual papillomata seen were in a ring about the internal urethral meatus, where the Foley catheter bag prevented contact of the solution with the mucosa. These were treated locally with Co^{60} sources arranged in a Foley balloon, giving a dose of

3000 r. at a source epithelial distance of one cm. The patient is now well and symptom free, for 15 months. The measurements immediately afterward and about 24 hours after treatment revealed less than 0.5% of Au[198] to be retained in the bladder. No activity was detected elsewhere in the body.

Smithers, Wallace and Trott, (1956), historically reviewed the radioisotopic approach for treating carcinoma of the bladder, pointing out that in their own hospital experience there have been five phases carried out in the development of intracavity irradiation of the bladder. In the first phase, they used radioactive sodium in a single application; in the second phase, they changed to radioactive bromine in a single application; in the third phase, bromine was used in three divided doses at weekly intervals; in the fourth phase, bromine was used by a protracted, slow, continuous treatment; in the fifth phase, they have been using radioactive colloidal gold to fill the bladder directly, without employing any bag. They have used the Ellis and Oliver technique in treating bladder lesions with radioactive gold. Smithers, et al., have also used radioactive gold-grain implantations for treating cancer of the bladder.

It would appear from the foregoing studies on the use of radioactive gold that the potential uses of this radioisotope are many. Radiation therapy of tumors has largely been developed on an empirical basis and it is obvious that empiricism in the early phases of the use of such isotopes as radioactive gold is involved in the development of the clinical use of the isotope. Further evaluation, with more adequate estimates of dosage tolerance, will aid in furthering the use of the gold radioisotope.

20.9 Bromine

There are a number of radioactive isotopes of bromine. From the biologic point of view the most valuable is bromine (Br[82]) with a half life of 35.9 hours. This is a negative beta-emitter with a maximum energy of 0.46 mev. Each beta disintegration is associated with gamma rays some in cascade, with energies ranging from 0.55 to 2 mev. With this isotope dibromo derivatives of "trypanblue" have been made. The dye combines rapidly with plasma and tissue proteins. By this means it has been found that the dye tends to be distributed as follows: (1) retention in the blood stream, as against lymph, urine and cerebrospinal fluid; (2) accumulation in areas of inflammation and about neoplasms, being picked up by the cells of the reticulo-endothelial system; (3) storage in the tubular epithelium of the kidneys. Labeled bromine can be introduced into many of the analine dyes for biologic tracer work. Some of the dyes so treated are ortho-toluidine and Evans blue.

Bromine[82] in solution has been used in treating carcinoma of the bladder.

The isotope is introduced into a rubber bag placed intravesically by a complicated bit of equipment. About 0.3 millicuries per cc. in a volume of 150 cc. will deliver a dose of 2000 gamma r. at the surface of the balloon in about 2 days. The beta ray dose is about one quarter of the gamma ray dose. Smithers, et al., have preferred Br^{82} and Na^{24} over Co^{60} in treating superficial diffuse bladder lesions, since the use of short-lived material avoids the risk of extended time of contamination. (See under "Gold".) Twenty-three cases have been treated, by the three dose technic. The criteria for selection of cases included: those patients with generalized disease of the bladder mucosa with multicentric distribution; no clinical, radiological or histological evidence of spread of the disease into the muscle. The clinical results as reported would indicate control of the disease in some of the cases for more than 3 years. Cystectomy was performed on some of the patients where the radiation did not successfully control the disease.

20.10 Sodium

Sodium has two principal radioactive isotopes, sodium^{22} and sodium^{24}. Radioactive sodium^{22} emits positrons and gamma radiation, shows K capture and has a half life of 2.6 yrs. Sodium^{24} emits both penetrating negative beta rays with maximum energy of 1.390 mev and gamma radiation with energies of 1.37 and 2.75 mev emitted in cascade and has a half life of 15 hours. Sodium is uniformly distributed throughout extracellular fluids in amimals and man and passes readily through a capillary membrane in either direction. When radioactive sodium is administered orally or parenterally, it rapidly makes its appearance throughout the body. The penetrating radiations emitted from the radioactive sodium can be readily demonstrated by a Geiger counter on the body surface.

Radioactive sodium has not been used extensively in therapy because of its generalized distribution in the body and lack of concentration in the regions of rapid growth or cell division.

Hamilton and Stone in 1937 reported the first two leukemia patients who received radiosodium treatment. After two weeks the results were found unfavorable and further attempts to utilize the radiosodium in therapy were abandoned by these investigators. Radiosodium, as labeled sodium chloride, has been used in the treatment of chronic leukemia by Thygesen, Videboek and Villaume (1944). They observed favorable results in 7 cases of chronic lymphatic leukemia but did not follow the patients for an appreciable length of time. Evans and Quimby (1946) reported the effect of radioactive sodium on normal and leukemic mice and suggested that this form of therapy might prove comparable to total body x-ray radiation. Evans, Lenz, Donlon and LeMay (1948) reported the use of sodium (Na^{24}) in the treatment of 31 patients having a variety of neoplastic conditions. The radioactive material was administered by mouth as a solution of sodium chloride, diluted to less than 1 per cent, and was followed by an equal volume of water in order to rinse the mouth and dissipate the radioactive material in this area. The first treatment was considered a test dose and did not exceed 180 μc. per kilogram of body weight. Blood counts at frequent intervals and before each treatment regulated the frequency and amount of treatment to be given. Excretion studies revealed that the amount of radiosodium excreted was less than 10 per cent of the administered dose. Therapy varied with the condition to be treated, averaging from 20 to 40 mc. total dosage at each administration. One patient received up to 576 mc., the dosage being distributed over a period of 353 days.

These authors concluded: that radioactive sodium is an effective means of giving protracted whole body irradiation; that in a few individuals the radiosodium had produced good results; and that the method appeared to be adaptable to chronic myelogenous leukemia, chronic lymphatic leukemia, polycythemia vera and other radiosensitive generalized diseases. The authors, however, concluded that radiosodium therapy is not good when the disease is acute, when the radioresistance of the abnormal cells is high and when the hematopoietic system is already damaged. They emphasized that the data were too few and the follow-ups too early to submit a final evaluation of the radiosodium therapy, and pointed out that its use was limited to laboratories near the source of supply.

Walton and others have used Na^{24} (sodium chloride solutions) in a spherical rubber bag to treat bladder tumors. These tumors were classed as pre-malignant or malignant in a large area of mucosa without demonstrable spread to a depth of more than a few millimeters. After biopsy the bag is inserted into the bladder, through the urethra in the female, but a perineal urethrotomy is necessary in the male. The patient is carried from the cystoscopic room to the isotopic laboratory where an opaque medium is first placed in the bag for radiographic evidence of leaks in the system and to determine the amount of fluid comfortably tolerated by the patient. The bag is emptied and then from 300 to 400 millicuries of Na^{24} in some 150 cc. might be used in a typical case.

In general the treatment is well tolerated. Doses of up to 3000 r. of gamma radiation have been given. In using Na^{24} there will be, in addition, approximately 1.4 times this dose due to beta rays at the surface of the bag. At two mm. this becomes negligible. Early results have encouraged the investigator to continue the method but Br^{82} will be substituted for Na^{24}.

It would seem that the short half life of radiosodium, the source of supply, the intensity of the emanations and the necessary frequent handling of such emanations by professional personnel would preclude its use on a large scale for clinical therapeutic application.

20.10.1 *Radiosodium as a Tracer.* The usefulness of radiosodium as a tracer isotope is evident from a review of the literature.

Studies with sodium[24] have been directed toward the determination of the mode and time of normal uptake, distribution and excretion of sodium in animals. Sodium injected into man has been found to come to equilibrium in 9 to 12 hours. Initially, the spread is rapid for approximately 3 hours to a volume of fluid representing about one-fourth of the body weight. Some investigators have suggested that this represents the extracellular fluid volume. Sodium[24] has had wide application in studies of vascular and cellular permeability. The role of the mammalian adrenal in sodium metabolism has also been investigated with radioactive sodium.

Because of the longer half life of sodium[22], much longer terminal experiments can be carried out, but so far it has had relatively little application.

Kaltreiter and his associates have used radioactive sodium in determining the volume of the extracellular fluid in the body. The sodium was administered intravenously. Some hours later a sample of blood plasma was obtained and the concentration of the radioactive substance measured. During the experimental period the urine was saved and the amount of the test substance lost in it was determined. The amount remaining in the body (the amount administered minus the amount excreted) divided by the amount per unit volume in the serum gave the volume of fluid in which it was dissolved. The investigators found that about 21 per cent of body weight was "sodium space" extracellular fluid, of which 15 per cent was the plasma and 85 per cent interstitial fluid. Repeated studies on the same individuals checked well. In patients with serous effusions, concentration of radiosodium in pleural and ascitic fluid was essentially the same as in the blood serum. In such patients the volume of extra fluid was found to be included in the extracellular fluid as determined by the use of radioactive sodium. This was determined by comparing the readings from the abnormal extracellular fluid with normal readings for an individual of essentially the same weight.

Flexner and his associates have determined the extracellular and total body water of human newborns by means of radiosodium and deuterium tracer materials. The radioactive sodium chloride was dissolved in water containing deuterium oxide and the solution was injected into the scalp veins of infants. After two and one-half to three hours blood was drawn from the internal jugular vein. A portion of the plasma was assayed for radioactivity and the deuterium present was obtained from the water content of the blood, using vacuum distillation. By using either tracer an

average for total body water of 74.6 per cent of body weight was obtained
for three infants studied. An average of 43.5 per cent was estimated for
extracellular water. When the extracellular water content of newborns is
compared with adults, it is found that a ratio of 1.7 between infants and
adults is present. It would appear that growth is accompanied by a shift
from extracellular fluid to intracellular fluid.

Aikawa made simultaneous determinations of the radiosodium and thiocyanate spaces and showed that following injection, the Na^{24} and the
thiocyanate ions disappear from the blood serum rapidly and at practically
the same rate up to the third hour. After the third hour, the rate of disappearance of the sodium from the blood stream is at a slower rate.

After determinations were carried out on a variety of diseases it appeared
that the thiocyanate ion for practical purposes measures a volume of fluid
comparable to that measured by the radiosodium ion in determining the
extracellular space. The author felt that both methods should be employed
in critical investigations because the results obtained by the two methods
vary more widely in diseased than in normal states.

Hubbard, Preston and Ross used radiosodium to determine the velocity
of blood flow in infants and young children. The material was injected into
one antecubital vein and the time of its arrival at the opposite hand was
determined by a Geiger counter. The results were quite variable but were
as satisfactory as results by other methods.

Smith and Quimby, in studying patients suffering from peripheral vascular disease, injected radioactive sodium into an antecubital vein and observed the time of arrival in the sole of the foot. A portable, shielded Geiger
counter was used as the detector. No correlation between the clinical condition and the circulation time could be established, but the authors were
able to plot curves showing the increase in the counting rate with time, as
the equilibrium of radiosodium concentration was built up between plasma
and extracellular fluid. It was found that the shape of this curve could be
correlated with the clinical condition.

In studies by Veall on the "build up curve" of Na^{24} injected intravenously
and diffusing into the extravascular tissue fluid as outlined by Smith and
Quimby, it was not possible to obtain consistent results on the same individual. In addition, he indicated that no clear distinction could be drawn
between normal and diseased subjects. Changes in environmental temperature were held mainly responsible for these difficulties.

In a recent study by Mufson, Quimby and Smith, the vasodilating effect
of certain drugs in vascular disease have been studied by measuring the
circulation time. The authors studied patients with scleroderma, obliterative arteriosclerotic disease, non-specific arteritis and thromboangiitis ob-

literans. Radiosodium was used to measure changes in circulation time. Histamine, when given intravenously in the circulation time test, proved an effective means of finding optimum speed of injection, and by iontophoresis or given intravenously caused a definite rise in the curve. Build up curves were not affected by 5 per cent sodium chloride or papaverine.

Prinzmetal et al. made studies of the passage of sodium[24] in the blood through the heart. They have used the method successfully in differentiating heart disease and functional conditions and also have established heart disease in individuals in which it had not been previously suspected.

Cooper and his associates have developed a new approach to the question of circulating time. These investigators injected sodium[24] intramuscularly and determined the rate of clearance of the isotope from the muscle. It is to be pointed out that the objective was to determine the rate of mobilization of the sodium ion by the local circulation within the muscle. Kety also used a similar method by injecting five microcuries of sodium[24] in .5 to 1.0 cc. of isotonic sodium chloride solution into the gastrocnemius muscle of human subjects. The injection was made at a depth of about two centimeters within the muscle structure. Counts were made by placing the Geiger-Müller counter next to the calf, directed over the site of the injection. By these methods it was found that the rate of clearance followed a simple exponential curve. When a tourniquet was placed above the knee, there was a sharp reduction of the sodium clearance. Release of the tourniquet after 10 minutes produced a clearance rate more than twice that of normal. Exercise of the muscle also was accompanied by a considerable increase in the clearance rate between normal subjects and patients with diseases of the peripheral vascular system. Patients with arteriosclerosis showed a diminished clearance rate. In patients with thrombophlebitis, hyperthyroidism, and hypertension, the investigators noted an increase in the clearance rate. In edematous extremities the clearance rate was well below normal.

Semple, McDonald and Ekins used the method of Kety to determine whether the clearance rate of Na^{24} from muscle would measure blood flow directly. The Na^{24} was injected intramuscularly followed by serial counts with the Geiger-Müller counter. The slope of the exponential curve is the quantitative measure of the total ability of the local circulation to remove and supply freely diffusible substances. In such studies on subjects with peripheral vascular disease and on normal subjects the curves fell within the same range, thus indicating the method is unsatisfactory for estimating the effect of therapy on peripheral vascular disease. It appears from the available evidence that there is no fixed relation between blood flow and Na^{24} clearance.

Haigh and Reiss in Na^{24} tracer investigations on brain function in mental patients, using a multiple channel rate of counting meter, made some interesting observations.

The concentration of Na^{24} in the feet increased slowly, but in different areas of the head the counting rate went up more rapidly. In addition, there were remarkable differences in the uptake of Na^{24} in different parts of the head. Differences in the uptake due to the skull bones, brain circulation and the intracellular brain space are still to be determined. There were noted, however, alterations in Na^{24} concentration, due to postural changes in the patients. Further work is indicated to establish whether certain brain phenomena may find explanation by the study of circulation rates in the brain.

Fox and Keston showed, in humans with severe burns, that the increase in "sodium space" extracellular fluid, together with the disappearance of sodium from the urine, was due to the sodium being withdrawn from normal equilibrium in extracellular fluid. In one case they demonstrated with the Geiger counter that radioactive sodium was concentrated within a burned region as compared with its distribution in the corresponding part of the uninjured limb.

Burcher, Reaser and Cronvich have been able to show in congestive heart failure that sodium turnover and excretion ceased to follow normal patterns. They also showed that in normal individuals 32 per cent of the total plasma sodium diffuses out of the blood every minute and, of course, under equilibrium conditions an equal amount diffuses back in.

Thompson, Quimby and Smith, in an investigation of mechanical methods of artificial respiration, proved that the resuscitative procedures did circulate the blood and that passive diffusion played no significant part.

Quimby and Smith have also studied utilization of penicillin by the body with the aid of radioactive sodium. Patients received a known amount of radioactive sodium by means of a nebulizer and inhaled for a specific amount of time. Exhaled air was then conducted through a series of condensers and precipitators. At the end of the experiments the nebulizer and all parts of the exhaled air system were washed. The washings were also measured for radioactive sodium. The subjects were then removed to a separate room for the counts which were made over the upper esophagus, the sternum, and the lateral lung high under the axillae. It was found that the radioactive material extended to the outer part of the lung and that equilibrium was reached in about one-half hour. The uptake of the radioactive sodium was increased by the addition of 10 per cent glycol to the solution. When warmth and humidity were maintained during the inhalation of the sodium^{24} mixture, the uptake of the radioisotope was increased.

Boldrey and Low-Beer have studied the rate of appearance and concentration of radioactive sodium chloride in cerebrospinal fluid. They observed by using 250 microcuries of radioactive sodium chloride intravenously in a 5 year old patient with a complete block between the ventricles and the spinal subarachnoid space that radioactivity was first detected in both fluids about 5 minutes after the administration of the radioisotope. The concentration of the isotope in the ventricular fluid was greater for a period up to 85 minutes after injection. Following this, the radioactivity of the spinal fluid became greater than that of the ventricular fluid. Further studies are to be made in an attempt to determine whether the cerebrospinal fluid is produced only by the choroid plexus of the ventricles, or whether the subarachnoid lining contributes to the production of spinal fluid.

Experiments with Na^{24} in the dog show that there is not only a flow of cerebrospinal fluid from the cerebrum toward the cervical spine, but also that there is a second type of flow from the lumbar region toward the cervical region. Eichler and Linder believe that the finding proves that some of the cerebrospinal fluid is formed in the lining of the spinal canal.

Flexner and his associates have made a study of the sodium transfer of the unit weight of placenta at various stages of gestation. Several animal species, including man, have been studied. The rate of transfer was expressed as milligrams of sodium transfer by hour per gram of placenta. It appears to be characteristic for each morphological type of placenta studied. The number of cell layers between the maternal and fetal circulation affect the rate of transfer. The overall increase from 10 weeks to 38 weeks is given as about seven times.

Brown and Veall in a study of the localization of the placental site by means of radiosodium were able to successfully locate the placenta in 31 out of 34 cases. The findings were substantiated by caesarian section or by other means. The method depends on the fact that the placenta represents a local accumulation of blood and that for the first few minutes after injection, Na^{24} is still mainly confined to the blood plasma. The time available for measurements is limited to two or three minutes. At present the test cannot be used to exclude the possibility of placenta praevia, though a positive indication is significant.

Cox and Chalmers, by the use of Na^{24} injected intravenously just before the time of delivery, concluded that an active uterine circulation persists for the first few minutes of the third stage of labor. This was determined by comparing Na^{24} concentration in placental blood, taken at the end of the third stage of labor, with that of cord blood taken at delivery. These authors also established, by Na^{24} tracer technics, that anomalous plasma concentration curves are observed in some toxemia cases, and that, with such plasma changes, there is a diminished rate of Na^{24} transfer across the placenta.

Kunkel and Schmermund, by injecting radioactive saline in the skin and subcutaneous tissues and using both beta and gamma ray Geiger counters simultaneously, found that the clearance rates for cutaneous and subcutaneous tissues vary widely. The beta ray decay curve of intracutaneous radioactive skin wheals did not follow an exponential law.

20.11 Potassium

The isotope of potassium available for tracer work is potassium (K^{42}) with a half life of 12.5 hours. Potassium (K^{42}) emits very high energy negative beta particles with maximum energies of 2.0 and 3.5 mev. Gamma rays of 1.5 and 0.32 mev. also appear to be present. It should be noted in passing that natural potassium is radioactive because of the presence of K^{40}. The exchange of potassium (K^{42}) with the potassium of the body has been investigated in several laboratories. The uptake of potassium is fairly slow as compared with sodium. A fasting human subject absorbs 17 per cent of administered radiopotassium in the first half hour, while in the same interval 58 per cent of the ingested radiosodium is taken up (three times as much). A noticeable difference in the behavior in sodium and potassium has been observed, in that corpuscular potassium and plasma potassium equilibrated potassium (K^{42}) slowly, both in chemical experiments and in the living animal, whereas intracellular and extracellular sodium came to equilibrium at a more rapid rate.

When radiopotassium is injected into the circulation of an animal, the liver and kidney absorption is rapid, muscle tissue intermediate, and erythrocytes and brain tissue uptake is slow. It has been shown that in the normal red cell, the potassium has an affinity of the cell of about 20 times that of the plasma, and when the red cell is injured there is a tendency for the loss of potassium, which is exchanged for sodium. The reciprocal exchange of potassium for sodium has also been observed in anoxic nervous tissues, and also occurs in hepatic cells and the leukocytes. It is thus apparent that specific failure for potassium affinity by cells is a sign of injury.

Because radiopotassium K^{42} has a high specific energy for beta and gamma emission, and a short half life, it has been used for tagging erythrocytes in blood volume determinations. The radiopotassium was incubated with 10 mls of heparinized blood and the tagged blood cells used to determine blood volume. The method has the advantage of being accurate and safe.

R. I. Dorfman, has described a method for determining small amounts of desoxycorticosterone with adrenalectomized rats, using radiopotassium The rate at which potassium accumulates in cells is a function of the desoxycorticosterone. Adrenalin serves to increase blood glucose and plasma potassium, whereas, insulin decreases plasma glucose and potassium.

These are important in the clinical management of potassium disturbances, and it is important to bear in mind the potassium glucose levels in the plasma. Increased utilization of glucose by muscle tissue is accompanied by increased uptake of potassium. In the nervous tissue both glutamic acid and glucose are required for increased uptake of potassium. It is becoming increasingly evident that potassium is lost from the nerve during excitation.

Bauer and Associates have compared K^{42} with Na^{24} and I^{131} in a clinical study to determine the differences in rate of absorption from subcutaneous tissues by needle injection and jet injection (hypospray). The absorption rate was determined by counting directly over the area of injection. "Half-time" readings were compared, i.e., the time when the activity readings in the injection site dropped by one-half. The results obtained by needle injection were variable as compared with the jet injection test. K^{42} readings were identical with those where Na^{24} and I^{131} had been injected.

Several investigators have reported that radioactive potassium is concentrated in some malignant tumors comparable to radioactive phosphorus.

There are advantages in the use of K^{42} over that of P^{32}, such as the more energetic beta particle and penetrating gamma ray for detection purposes both inside and outside the body, as well as a more rapid uptake in the tumor. The disadvantages include the short half-life of the material and the lack of precise localization due to the more penetrating beta particles. Potassium tends to concentrate rapidly in muscle, thus making an adjacent tumor difficult to identify and delimit.

Nathanson, Baker and Silverstone have used K^{42} in 80 patients with histologically proved benign and malignant breast tumors. K^{42} was injected into patients intravenously (500 microcuries). Measurements at fifteen minutes after injection proved to be the optimal time. Increased activity was found over all malignant tumors, except in five cases. No increased activity was noted over benign or inflammatory lesions. The authors believed the procedure might be worthwhile in evaluating chemotherapeutic measures or radiation therapy results, by comparison between pre- and post-therapy scanning of the tumor-bearing area.

Susen, Small and Moore found K^{42} localization a successful method for localizing brain tumors above the tentorium, but the high concentration of isotope in the muscles closer to the scintillation counter interfered with tumor identification measurements below the tentorium. The short half-life of the isotope has been a great drawback and has limited the further clinical exploration of K^{42}.

20.12 Calcium and Strontium (See also par. 12.6)

Radioactive calcium (Ca^{45}) has beta emissions with peak intensity of 0.25 mev which makes this isotope difficult to use in tracer studies. The

TABLE III

Distribution of Radioactive Calcium in Tissues of Rat at End of 69 Hours

TISSUE	CONTENTS PER GM. OF DRY WEIGHT
Bones	2.23
Teeth	2.75
Blood serum	0.094
Muscle	0.017
Skin and hair	0.060
Stomach	0.015
Small intestine	0.060
Large intestine	0.060
Liver	0.017
Kidney	0.013
Spleen	0.042
Heart	0.089
Lung	0.067
Testes	0.012

low intensity of the emanations, together with its wide concentration in bone, detracts from the usefulness of radioactive calcium as a therapeutic agent. Furthermore, although a product of the n, p reaction in the pile and also of the cyclotron, radioactive calcium (Ca^{45}) is limited in supply. It has a relatively long half life of 160 days, bespeaking a hazard for personnel and in clinical use. Ashing of all biological material for proper radioisotopic assay is necessary in animal experimentation with radioactive calcium.

Radioactive strontium, an alkaline earth metal, is a chemical analogue of calcium and is readily available. Strontium (Sr^{89}) has a half life of fifty-four days and emits beta rays with an energy maximum of 1.5 mev. It is thus more easily detected than calcium (Ca^{45}) and has been found more suitable for biological investigations. There is, however, a biochemical difference between the two elements; while strontium is capable of replacing calcium to a considerable extent in the bones, Shipley and his associates have pointed out that this mineral cannot replace calcium in the formation of normal bone. It seems necessary, therefore, to evaluate both calcium (Ca^{45}) and strontium (Sr^{89}) in tracer studies of bone, utilizing the combined results to further unravel the mysteries of bone metabolism.

Campbell and Greenberg administered 5 cc. of a 5 per cent solution of calcium lactate prepared from calcium (Ca^{45}) to an adult male rat maintained on a normal diet. Excretion by urine and feces was measured for 69 hours, showing an absorption of 89.2 per cent and a total of 10.8 per cent passed in the feces. At the end of this time 65.6 per cent of the oral dose had appeared in the urine, leaving 23.6 per cent in the animal at the time of sacrifice. Nearly 60 per cent was excreted in the first ten hours, and the blood level reached a peak two hours after ingestion and returned to normal in about four hours after ingestion.

The distribution of retained calcium in the tissues is shown above. The greatest amount was retained in the bones and teeth.

Pecher measured the uptake of calcium (Ca^{45}) and strontium (Sr^{89}) along with phosphorus (P^{32}) 24 hours following intravenous administration to mice. The Ca^{45} and Sr^{89} were administered as the lactate. Fifty-eight per cent of the Ca^{45} (average of 30 mice) and 33 per cent of the Sr^{89} (average of 35 mice) were recovered from the skeleton after 24 hours.

For comparison, radiophosphorus was administered intravenously to five mice. The tissue distribution at the end of 24 hours is shown in Table IV. The uptake of calcium was similar to, but greater than, the uptake of strontium.

After the injection of calcium and strontium lactate intravenously, the skeletal concentration reached a maximum in eight hours. When the same materials were given by stomach tube, 13 to 30 per cent of the Ca^{45} was found in the skeleton at the end of 48 hours, and 6 to 14 per cent of the strontium. The skeletal uptake was three times as great after intravenous injection as it was by oral administration.

In regard to the distribution within the skeleton, more radioactive calcium is found in cancellous than in cortical bone, and more is found in the epiphysis than in the diaphysis. In growing animals, the concentration is particularly high at the epiphyseal line. Two weeks after an experimental fracture, the healing bone contained more than four times as much as the control bone (1.7 per cent compared to 0.4 per cent). With radioactive strontium, no significant difference in skeletal uptake was found when using the chloride, lactate and gluconate salts.

Radioautographic studies of deposition of calcium in the cranium, teeth and mandible of the growing rat, by Jarbak and his associates, reveals that the maximum deposition of calcium is found in the sutures between the bones of the skull, in the mandibular condyle, in the walls of the pulp chambers of the incisor teeth and in the cementum of the molars. These are the active areas of calcium deposition in the formation of new bone and teeth. The periosteum on the inner and outer tables of the membranous bones reveals concentration of calcium to a lesser extent. Least uptake is noted in the enamel of the molar teeth. The technic of administration of Ca^{45} utilized intraperitoneal injection of Ca^{45} as calcium chloride, giving 5 microcuries per 100 gm. of body weight. The animals were sacrificed 1 week after injection and processed for radioautography.

Tracer experiments have established the fact that much of the calcium in the feces is from unabsorbed foodstuffs. In the first three days after being

TABLE IV

TISSUES	PER GM. OF WET WT. % Ca^{45}	PER GM. OF WET WT. % Sr^{89}	PER GM. OF WET WT. % P^{32}
Bone	22.0	12.0	5.2
Muscles	0.33	0.17	1.4
Skin and hair	0.20	0.15	0.75
G-I tract	0.36	0.23	1.3
Liver	0.12	0.07	3.0
Other viscera	0.23	0.13	2.1
Fat	0.00	0.00	

absorbed, material is excreted largely by way of the urine, not by the feces. Some calcium, however, finds its way into the intestinal tract via the bile and pancreatic excretions. After the third day, excretion in urine and feces is about equal.

Studies have been made on rickets using as tracers: P^{32}, Ca^{45} and Sr^{89}. These studies reveal that there is no inability on the part of the rachitic patient to absorb phosphate. There is reduced absorption, however, if the phosphate is administered along with food, rather than in the postabsorptive condition. With labeled strontium, the skeletal uptake on oral administration in rachitic animals is practically doubled when vitamin D is given with the calcium or strontium. When the material is injected, far more calcium is concentrated in the skeleton than when it is fed by mouth. Again, vitamin D doubles the amount concentrated in the skeleton. These studies indicate that vitamin D not only aids in the absorption of calcium from the gastro-intestinal tract but also aids in its deposition in bone (Copp and Greenberg).

As indicated in the previous chapter, vitamin D also aids in the uptake of PO_4 by the bones as against the soft tissues, and decreases PO_4 excretion by the intestines.

When radioactive calcium is given to pregnant mice, the maximum uptake is in the skeleton; the activity in the uterus and soft tissues is low, as measured by the Geiger counter. In the last few days of pregnancy, calcium is lost to the fetus and the newborn mice may have in their bodies two to three times as much activity as remains in the mother's skeleton. When offspring with no radioactivity are nursed by radioactive mothers, radioactive calcium rapidly appears in the offspring. Anywhere from 10 to 20 per cent of radioactive strontium, two days after intravenous administration, can be recovered from the milk of nursing mice or cattle.

Marshak and Byron studied the healing of bone lesions in the rat using Sr^{89} and P^{32}. The lesions were produced by a circular saw, the cuts being made through the tibia without completely destroying the continuity of

TABLE V

*Comparison of Transcapillary Rates Found in Various Animals, Showing Rates of
Exchange in Percentage of Plasma Ion Per Minute*

OBSERVER	TRACER ION	SUBJECT	TOTAL %
Flexner et al.	Sodium	Man	78
Gellhorn et al.	Sodium	Dog	56.6
Cowie et al.	Chlorine	Guinea pig	60
Burch et al.	Chlorine	Dog	102
Thomas et al.	Calcium	Adult rabbit	88 ± 36
	Calcium	Young rabbit	71 ± 12

the shaft. Both old and young rats were used. The normal bones showed a
higher percentage of uptake of P^{32} in young than in old rats. In the first
week of healing there was little difference of P^{32} uptake in young or old
rats. In the second week of healing, the lesions in the old rats had three
times as much P^{32} because of the greater quantity of osteoid tissue formed.
The uptake of P^{32} and strontium (Sr^{89}) was maximum between the eighth
and 12th days. The ratio of one to the other was the same in healing bone
as in normal bone. In the early stages of healing, relatively more phosphorus
and less strontium were taken up. The P^{32} uptake in early healing indicates
cellular proliferation. In later healing, the P^{32} and strontium uptake represent mineral deposition during ossification.

Isolated studies have been made on bone disease by Low-Beer and his
associates, which include bone atrophy and rickets. The study of a late
case of rickets indicated that the primary defect in that disease was not in
the absorption of the bone salts but in the failure of the ossification mechanism.

The group at Georgetown University Medical Center Radio-Isotope
Laboratory have been working on some general problems related to the
dynamics of calcium metabolism, the processes of normal and abnormal
bone formation and resorption *in vivo*. Thomas, Litovitz, Rubin and
Geschickter have reported on the determination and correlation of blood
disappearance rates, urinary excretion rates and bone uptake rates of radiocalcium[45] in normal young and adult rabbits. The blood disappearance data
obtained for calcium in the studies reported were very much like those
found by Burch, Threefoot and Ray for chloride in dogs and are somewhat
similar to the work reported by Flexner et al. for sodium in man and Gellhorn, Merrell and Rankin for sodium in dogs (Table V).

Using the equation given by Gellhorn et al. and also Burch et al., one
can calculate the proportion of the plasma calcium leaving the plasma per
unit time, if the concentration-time data fit the following equation.

$$C(t) = A_1 e^{-b_1 t} + A_2 e^{-b_2 t} + A_3 e^{-b_3 t} + A_4 e^{-b_4 t} \qquad (2a)$$

$$R_p = \frac{A_1 b_1 + A_2 b_2 + A_3 b_3 + A_4 b_4}{A_1 + A_2 + A_3 + A_4} \qquad (2b)$$

Where R_p is the proportion of the calcium leaving the plasma per unit time, and b is the rate constant of each term, and A is the compartment factor indicating percentage of the injected dose involved in each term.

Using these equations, R_p has been found to be 71 ± 12 per cent/minute in the adult and 88 ± 36 per cent in young rabbits. The difference between R_p for adult and young rabbits found is within the limit of experimental accuracy and probably is not significant. In other words about 80 per cent of the plasma calcium (measured as calcium[45]) leaves the plasma per minute. This is true for both the administered exogenous calcium at zero time and endogenous serum calcium at all times. Since it is known that in normal animals the serum calcium remains constant it must be true that an amount of calcium equal to approximately 80 per cent of the serum calcium is returning from the extravascular compartment per minute. Therefore, R_p represents the rate of exchange of serum calcium with extravascular calcium.

The uptake of calcium by the bones in younger animals was about twice as large as in the bones of adults. A rapid uptake occurred in both age groups in the first several hours. It is interesting to note that though the total percentage of uptake of calcium[45] in the bones in the young rabbits was twice that of the adults, the rate constant in the exponential term was the same in both age groups. This indicates that the time for a given percentage of the equilibrium value to be found in the femurs is independent of age although the equilibrium value itself obviously is age-dependent.

The urinary output of intravenously administered calcium[45] was plotted as a function of the time after its injection into young and adult rabbits. It was noted that in both age groups 50 per cent of the total urinary excretion measured occurred in the first 24 hours. The average output after 16 days for adult rabbits was over twice that of the young animals.

The percentage of excretion of radiocalcium in the feces of the two age groups was plotted. After 16 days, in both groups, 20 per cent excretion of the injected dose of calcium had occurred via the stool. The other animals managed to excrete 50 per cent of the eventual fecal excretion measured in the first day as compared to 6 days for a like excretion for the younger group.

Mathematical analysis of the blood disappearance curves obtained in the study indicated that four exponential terms are needed to represent the data. From the first two terms the rates of exchange of calcium between plasma and extravascular compartments were calculated and shown to be in good agreement with data previously obtained by others for other ions. Within the experimental accuracy these above rates were found to be the same in both young and adult rabbits. The third term in the blood disappearance equation has been correlated with the bone uptake of calcium. The bone uptake of radiocalcium in the young age group was greater than in the adult age group. Therefore, it has been shown that the third blood term for the disappearance of calcium is a measure of bone activity. The fourth term from the equations expressing blood disappearance rates has been correlated with the excretion of calcium via the urine and feces. This excretory output has been found to be an inverse function of the bone uptake of calcium.

From the study it was deduced that a mathematical analysis of blood disappearance data and excretion data for calcium can yield information regarding bone activity.

Jacobson has established the fact that protection of the spleen during the x-irradiation of mice has resulted in a lessened effect on the hematopoetic system, with an increasing number of survivors among the animals. Friedell and Salerno, noting this, postulated that it was possible the injury to the spleen and other areas of the reticuloendothelial system were of such an extent that doses ordinarily producing mild injury would evoke, instead, a severe depression of the blood-forming tissues. They were stimulated to study the lethal action of internally administered radioisotopes in animals from which the spleen had been removed. They were able to demonstrate an important role of the spleen in the potentiated lethal effect produced by internal emitters in rats. Friedell and Salerno had noted, further, that the protective effect of spleen shielding during exposure to x-rays had been much greater in the mouse than in the rat. They, therefore, proceeded with a group of experiments to ascertain whether the capacity of the spleen to alter survival is greater in the mouse than in the rat. Strontium[89] was selected rather than some of the other emitters which had been used previously, to irradiate the bone marrow of the mouse selectively. Distribution studies revealed that some 90 % of the retained Sr[89] was uniformly distributed in the skeleton 24 hours after injection. The skeletal retention was approximately 40 % of the injected dose, initially, and more than 30 % of this dose remained in the skeleton for more than 30 days. The soft tissues contained less than 2 % Sr[89] per 100 mg. initially, and this percentage dropped to 0.1 % after 2 weeks. Normal splenectomized mice, in groups of 20, received intraperitoneal injections of Sr[89]. The mortality data was collected at 30 and 55 days. The results showed that 4 microcuries of Sr[89] per gram of tissue given as a dose is not lethal to intact mice in 30 days, but is lethal to 90 % of the splenectomized animals. In humans, there appears to be no certain evidence that the hematopoetic system and the spleen are specifically related in normal individuals. In a number of pathological conditions, the spleen and the hematopoetic tissues seem to have a closer association. The precise mechanism of the spleen in supporting the hemato- poetic system following the potentiating lethal action of isotopes is not clear, and the mechanism of the altered response of the hematopoetic sys- tem to injury, produced by ionizing radiations, requires further research for a better understanding.

Engfeldt and Associates have made a series of studies of the localization of radioisotopes in bone tissue. In a series utilizing Sr^{90}, given to a mature dog intravenously and, with the use of radioautography, they showed a diffuse uptake of radiostrontium throughout the bones, with high concen- trations in the endosteal and periosteal layers and in a few of the Haversian systems. The bone slices which had been prepared for the radioautographic study were then examined micrographically, using a 30-kvp x-ray machine. The areas of high strontium localization corresponded to regions of low mineralization. Such localization is of importance from the viewpoint of the concentration of radioactive strontium where it is an item of concern in the distribution of the radioisotope in nuclear fission activities.

Lushbaugh, Storer and Hale, in a series of experiments using Sr^{90} as a beta source, have studied the changes which occur in acute radiodermatitis produced by beta irradiation, both from the standpoint of pathogenesis and repair. Sprague-Dawley rats were used. The strontium[90] source de- livered beta irradiation at the rate of 90 rep per second. When the skin re- ceived 14000 rep, regeneration of the epithelium and fibroplasia in the deep portion of the skin occurred, in from 15 to 20 days. In 36 days there was complete healing. Further studies by these investigators showed that the amount of fibroplastic activity was inversely proportional to the amount of irradiation. It was also noted that even doses totalling nearly one million rep failed to completely inhibit glycolytic activity of the skin immediately. The authors pointed out that the Aloe vera plant has been used efficaciously in the treatment of acute and chronic radiodermatitis. They made a care- fully controlled study using the irradiated skin of rabbits. The animals were irradiated locally on the back with 28000 rep and the reacting areas were either used as controls or treated with the fresh whole leaf of Aloe vera. It was found that the leaves hastened both the degenerative and the repara- tive phases of the lesion, so that an ulcer produced by the irradiation which would not heal in four months without treatment, healed completely in 2 months with application of the leaves.

Attempts have been made to use Ca^{45} in the treatment of malignant bone tumors. The material is of insufficient intensity and the tumors are too radioresistant. No symptomatic improvement has been noted.

Pecher and his colleagues have used Sr^{89} for primary malignancies of bone and metastases of carcinoma to bone. Strontium is selectively absorbed by bone, the Sr[89] being deposited with exchange of calcium. The primary osseous tumors (malignant) are radioresistant. The absorption by the bone is highly selective but both normal and malignant osseous tissue concentrate the isotope. As a result, the normal osseous structures are affected along with the malignant tissue. This lack of selectivity prevents the clinical use of Sr[89] as a therapeutic agent.

Pahaut and Govaerts report three cases of bone tumors in which radioactive strontium (Sr[89]) had been used in combination with external roentgen therapy as the method of treatment. A total of 30 grams of Sr[89]CO_3 was given orally at the rate of six tablets per day for 5 days. The concentration factors were calculated to be 12 % in the case of Ewing's Sarcoma, 7 % in a case of osteoblastic metastases, and 4 % in a case of Chondrosarcoma. These authors report no systemic damage was observed by administration of adequate dosage, and felt Sr[89] in combination with external roentgen therapy in certain cases of fast growing bone tumors was of value therapeutically.

Fitzgerald has observed Sr[89] localized in the callus of fractures of normal rats, but not in those with severe rickets. He also reports the production of osteogenic sarcoma following administration of Sr[89]. The tumors were thought to be caused by the preferential localization of the isotopes in collagenous tissues, as demonstrated by autography.

Friedell, Thomas and Krohmer (1950) have used radioactive strontium (Sr[90]) with a half life of 28 years and with beta ray emissions of 0.54 mev, in applicators for the treatment of certain diseases of the eye. They pointed out that the average mev is about 0.195, but that a daughter product, yttrium (Y[90]), has a half life of 64 hours and has beta ray emissions with a maximum of 2.27 mev and an average energy of 0.8 mev. Thus, the application of Sr[90], with its daughter product, compares favorably with the Treatment from this source is made by surface application. These authors, (1954), have made an evaluation of the clinical use of the Sr[90] beta ray applicator upon which they first reported in 1950. In their original paper, Friedell, Thomas and Krohmer indicated that a number of lesions were treated successfully with comparatively small doses. They have found since that, in order to affect most of the processes, considerably larger amounts of beta irradiation were necessary. Combining an estimate of the radiosensitivity of the corneal process and the fractionation of the radiation dose were emphasized as generally permitting the smallest practicable dosage levels. In corneal vascularization, the authors recommend a dose of 1800 reps per treatment at weekly intervals. This type of lesion was treated with varying dosages up to 12,000 rep, with the average dose in the order of 6000 rep. Immediately following keratoplasty, where re-invasion of blood vessels is often encountered, 1800 rep were recommended within 48 hours after operation, with repeated doses every two or three days until a maximum of 9000 rep had been given. The average dose, however, is considerably lower. In pterygia, only thin, newly formed lesions were considered for beta radiation therapy. The dosage delivered, in general, ranged up to 16,000 rep, with an average of 12,000 rep. Where beta radiation followed excision by surgery, the average dose was approximately 4,000 rep, delivered at the rate of 600 reps per treatment. In vernal catarrh, doses were delivered ranging from 1800 r. to 16,000 rep. This larger dose, the authors feel, is unnecessary if the follicles are removed surgically first. The postoperative incision may then be treated by beta irradiation in more modest doses.

Papillomas of the eyelid which are spread out along the margin and are rather extensive, according to the authors are best treated by beta irradiation. In eight cases the dosage ranged up to a total of 6000 rep, with good results. Single treatments of 1200 rep as unit dosage may be repeated at intervals up to the total dose of 6000 rep. Papillomas of the conjectivae seem somewhat more resistant to therapy. A dosage of 1800 rep repeated five or six times is recommended as sufficient. In hemangiomata of the eyelid, the authors have treated three such cases with doses ranging from 1300 to 3000 rep in one or two treatments. Unit doses of 1200 rep, repeated at monthly intervals once or twice, is also recommended. Epitheliomas, either squamous or basal cell type, are best treated by surgical excision, to be followed by irradiation, using the same principal of dosage as that noted above.

Lederman and Sinclair have developed a range of applicators with the basic shell made of Perspex. The isotope used is fission product Sr^{90}, with its daughter product, Y^{90}. The active foil, which is approximately 150 milligrams per square centimeter thick, is backed with silver in cases where irradiation in one direction is desired. The chief clinical conditions pointed out by Lederman, in which the beta irradiation is effectively used about the eyes, are corneal ulceration, stubborn forms of keratitis, corneal vascularization, spring catarrh and also certain limbal neoplasms. Treatment schedules vary with the disease. Lederman has treated corneal ulceration with a single dose between 500 and 1500 roentgens, repeated at weekly intervals for 3 or 4 weeks. In stubborn forms of keratitis, if x-ray therapy has failed, strontium[90] is used in doses of 500 r., given at weekly intervals, for 2 to 3 weeks. In corneal vascularization, he has used single doses of 1000 r., given at weekly intervals of 3 to 4 weeks, but states that, as experience increases, this range of treatment may require modification. In spring catarrh, doses of 500 r. are applied to the bulbar fornices at weekly intervals for three to four weeks.

Lederman, in a report from the Royal Marsden Hospital and Central Eye Hospital, London, reports on the treatment of melanoma about the eye, with strontium[90] shell. In limbal melanoma, doses are given at the rate of 2500 r. weekly for a total dose of from 10,000 to 15,000 r. Where cancerous melanosis requires irradiation of the entire conjunctival sac and both lids, gamma irradiation is used and the risk of cataract accepted.

Sklaroff reports the treatment of 10 cases of hemangioma by the use of a strontium[90] applicator, containing a 25 millicurie source which delivered 34.6 r. equivalent betas per second. Only lesions less than 2 mm. in thickness were considered suitable for this form of treatment. A dose of 500 reps resulted in disappearance of the lesion in two cases, with a good cosmetic result.

Lawrence and Wasserman reported 9 patients with multiple myeloma, treated with a combination of P^{32} and Sr^{89}. The dosage depended on the general condition of the patient and the hemogram. Radioactive phosphorus up to a total of 5 to 10 m.c. was suggested per course. The Sr^{89} when administered with the phosphorus was given in doses of 0.2 to 2 m.c. There was no evidence that the combination of radioactive phosphorus and strontium[89] proved more effective than P^{32} alone.

20.13 Sulfur

Sulfur is of great significance as an organic metabolite and has a definite role as an anion in the electrolytic balance of the body. Three isotopes available for radioactivity are: S^{31}, S^{35} and S^{37}. Sulfur (S^{31}) is a positron-emitter with a half life of 2.6 seconds. Sulfur (S^{35}) is a negative beta-ray-emitter, with maximum energy of about 0.167 mev, and a half life of 87 days; and sulfur (S^{37}) is a negative beta-gamma-emitter with a half life of 5 mins. Radioactive sulfur (S^{35}) is best suited for biochemical investigation and has been used in both plant and animal sulfur metabolism. Tarver and his associates have made a number of important contributions on the synthesis of sulfur-containing amino acids and the metabolism of both the sulfur-containing amino acids and of elemental sulfur in animals. Most of the sulfur used in their experiments was prepared by neutron bombardment of CCl_4. The radioactive sulfur was isolated as barium sulfate ($BaSo_4$). It was then converted to sulfide (BaS) by reduction with hydrogen at 1000°.

Methionine was synthesized by a modification of the Hill and Robson method. With the labeled methionine available, experiments were undertaken to show whether or not methionine sulfur could be converted to taurine sulfur by the dog and rat. By bile fistula studies in dogs and rats it was found that a small conversion of methionine sulfur to taurine sulfur occurred. Tissue was removed from the bile fistula rats and dogs as soon as possible after the animals were sacrificed.

It was found that the specific activity in the total sulfur fraction of the various organs was quite variable. The very high specific activity in the intestinal mucosa and pancreas, and the low specific activities in the muscular tissues were considered especially noteworthy. Sulfur[35] also concentrates in the tissues of the eye. The cornea and the structures of the anterior chamber appear to be the chief sites of localization. The question of the high activity in the intestinal muscle might have been due to contamination with mucosa. In the bile fistula rats, 56 per cent of the methionine sulfur was found to be incorporated into tissue protein. Further experiments proved that ingestion of sulfur as a sulfate in rats resulted in rapid excretion of the major portion. In later experiments Tarver et al. (1947) found that, in animals without a liver, as much or more of a labeled sulfur (S^{45}) amino acid is incorporated into the animal's protein as in the animal with a liver. This indicates that the liver is not essential for synthesis of protein in other tissues. It appears, therefore, that the best way to incorporate sulfur into the tissues, particularly the proteins, is via thio-amino acids such as methionine or cystine, and that using the sulfur label has demonstrated a rapid turnover of protein sulfur, verifying the dynamic state of body constituents.

Methionine with labeled sulfur, S^{45}, has been used to study the metabolism of the plasma proteins. Although it was found that the sulfur containing amino acids could be synthesized to proteins in the various tissues without the presence of liver, this proved not to be the case for the plasma proteins. If the plasma proteins are labeled with sulfur in a donor animal and then injected intravenously into dogs, the half-value of plasma is reached in the circulation in about 30 hours, due to its loss in the extravascular compartments. This loss of plasma was no more rapid in animals under shock, unless they were in the final critical stages. Following the initial rapid loss in the first 30 hours, a slower process takes place, and the labeled plasma proteins are absorbed by the metabolism of the various tissues to be replaced by unlabeled proteins from various tissues. The half-life of the remaining labeled plasma proteins is slightly more than 5 days in dogs. It is correspondingly less (1.5 days) in rats. Eventually an equilibrium point is reached when labeled sulfur reappears in the plasma proteins from labeled components arising from a breakdown of the tissue proteins. The smaller the animal the shorter the half life of its plasma proteins. Apparently the plasma globulin has a shorter half life than plasma albumin. However, some experiments with glycine N^{15} as a labeling agent for plasma proteins in the rabbit indicate that antibody globulins in the actively immunized animal have a longer half life of about 14 days, and that the immune globulin has the same half life as normal serum globulins. The labeled glycine was not synthesized into the globulin in passively immunized animals. These experiments raise the question regarding the source of long-lasting or persisting immunity since the globulins which constitute the instrument of immunization apparently must be continuously renewed in the immune animal every few weeks.

Wormall, (1955), in discussing the use of radioisotopes in immunity and the methods of labeling antigens and antibodies with radioisotopes, points out four procedures for labelling by isotopes. He indicates that iodination, phosphorylation, coupling, etc., is generally the method of choice. The introduction of I^{131} into the 3‑5‑diiodotyrosine groups by iodination, and of S^{35} by the reaction of mustard gas sulphone with the free amino groups, both give stable structures, but the phosphate groups formed by phosphorychloride are not firmly bound. Double labeling of the same protein with I^{131} and S^{35} has many advantages.

Kamen describes in detail an example of the use of labeled antibiotics by S^{35} in studying the biosynthesis and mechanism of action of these agents. The specific study on penicillin indicated in the preliminary results that the uptake of penicillin is dependent on its concentration in all organisms, but that sensitive strains, at lower concentrations, pick up more penicillin than do resistant strains. The labeled antibiotic made by a fermentation procedure growing the penicillin-producing mold in a lactose-glucose medium, with the addition of highly radioactive carrier-free $S^{35}O_4$, and lowering the sulfur content to 0.2 mg. per ml. to avoid excessive dilution of the label, was described by Kamen in considerable detail.

The tracer approach has been highly successful in its application to problems involving the structure and interaction of virus components with the host cell. Hershey and his collaborators produced radioactive phage T2 by growing bacteria in a viscerol-lactate medium, containing S^{35} labeled sulfate. The radioactive bacteria were then infected with the phage which became radioactive growing in the host cells. The phage particles were isolated by centrifugation. Hershey then ran suitable immunological tests to establish the radiochemical purity of the phage particles. Much insight has been developed as to the mechanism involved in the attachment of bacterophages, origins of virus material, and the development of virus in the host cell by tracer technics and utilization of appropriate methods for viral assay.

It has been shown by Gottschalk and Allen that radioactive sulfur of labeled sulfate fed to rats is fixed by the cartilage to be incorporated into chondroitin sulfuric acid. The other tissues of the rat retained S^{35} in small amounts for a shorter period. There is little exchange between inorganic sulfur and the sulfuric amino acids and proteins. For this reason S^{35} given as sulfate is nearly all excreted within 24 hours. In the ground substance of chondrosarcoma, as well as normal cartilage, there are sulfuric esters of polysaccharides. On the basis of these facts the authors thought that radioactive sulfur could be taken up selectively by neoplastic cartilage and hence they tried it in two cases of chondrosarcoma. The material used was radioactive sulfuric acid neutralized by sodium hydroxide. One millicurie per cc. was used and the first patient received 6.7 millicuries. Tissues were obtained by biopsy 65 hours later. The patient died 11 days later. The highest concentrations of the isotopes were found in the chondrosarcoma, and progressively small amounts were found in other tissues in this sequence: cartilage, bone marrow, spleen, kidney, skin, liver, bone, fat, muscle. Radioautographs indicated maximum concentration in the growing portion of the chondrosarcoma, and those containing abundant ground substance. The energy (av) of S^{35} was 0.055 mev. Because of the low activity, the administration of very large doses of S^{35} would be required to damage the chondrosarcoma.

When radioactive sulfur is injected into the rat, it can be demonstrated in the long bones within a few hours, particularly in the cartilage of the epiphyses. It is known that cartilage formation is a phase in the repair of fractures. Watson-Jones has pointed out that if a fracture is not immobilized, there is an increase in the amount of cartilage formed in the healing process. Osborne and Kowalewski, to verify this point of view, studied the uptake of radiosulfur in a fractured humerus in the rat and reported finding radioactive sulfur in the fractures of unsplinted rat humeri greater than that in splinted humeri. No histologic studies were performed, but the sulfur was precipitated out in the form of barium sulfate, following digestion of the organic material of the bone. The findings presented by these authors indicate that Watson-Jones' observation was correct.

20.14 Carbon

Radioactive carbon is generally considered to be the most valuable tool for the attack on the problems of organic synthesis because of carbon's wide distribution in the plant and animal kingdom. Radioactive carbon (C^{11}) is a positron-emitter with maximum energy of 0.96 mev (annihilation reaction). The hard quality of the radiation present, however, makes it relatively simple to assay this isotope, but its short life limits its usefulness as a carbon tracer. So far, it has had its most important use in tracer studies of photosynthesis and studies in plant and animal assimilation of carbon dioxide.

Since the production of radioisotopes by use of the chain-reaction piles, long-lived radiocarbon (C^{14}) has become reasonably abundant and promises to be extremely important in studying intermediary metabolism. Carbon (C^{14}) is a negative beta emitter, with upper energy levels of 0.158 mev; gamma radiation is not appreciable. The softness of the radiations poses a problem in tracing this radioactive substance. Special counting tubes and methods of preparation have been devised which give reasonably accurate indication of the isotopic concentration. Carbon (C^{14}) can be incorporated by appropriate syntheses into the carbon chains of organic compounds, including carbohydrates, fats, amino acids, antigens, hormones and a host of other biologic materials. Personnel protection from the volatile forms of radioactive carbon is a major problem in working with this isotope.

When the radioisotopes of carbon dioxide are used in the study of metabolic processes in the various forms of life, CO_2 is found to be not only a metabolic end product, but is also used to form other organic compounds. Carbon[14] makes possible the preparation of almost any carbon-labeled compound for tracer studies by means of a number of well-known procedures. The advantages of biosynthetic methods lie in the considerable versatility of living organisms and, especially, the mirco-organisms. Kamen has elaborated the present status of C^{14} as a useful tool in intermediate metabolism: (*Isotopic Tracers in Biology*, Academic Press, Inc., N. Y., 1957, Chapter X, "The Isotopes of Carbon".) He outlines biosyntheses of carbohydrates and of organic acids from CO_2, biosyntheses of higher fatty acids, biosyntheses of amino acids and biosyntheses of other compounds such as chlorophyll, carotenoids, glycerol, etc. Kamen also points out the importance of degradation methods using C^{14} for checking postulated degradation reactions. The Harvard group has studied the deposition of liver glycogen in the fasting rat with radiocarbon (C^{11}). From these studies it would seem that labeled carbon, introduced in the form of a particular carbohydrate intermediate (lactate feedings), should be expected to be partly diluted by unlabeled molecules of the same substance formed in the body and, by chemical transformation, distributed in a variety of other forms.

Conant and his colleagues have used carbon (C^{11}) to study sources of glycogen carbon. They found that the three carbon atoms of the lactate molecule were not the sole source of the carbon of the new liver glycogen. Buchanan and Hastings indicate that two paths of glycogen synthesis occur, one supplementary to the other. Under conditions where glycogen synthesis does not take place at a rapid rate and carbon dioxide assimilation reactions are not marked, glycogen formation may be the direct conversion of pyruviate into phosphopyruviate. In liver tissue, however, the incorporation of CO_2 may be the primary pathway where glycogen synthesis is rapid.

Greenberg, as quoted by Hevesy, studied the distribution of carbon (C^{14}) labeled tyrosine in rats and mice, both normal and tumor-bearing animals. He found, after intravenous injection of the substance, that C^{14} was rapidly incorporated into the protein of the various organs of each animal and was retained, to a considerable extent, after a period of three days. Intestinal mucosa, kidney, plasma proteins and liver had the highest carbon (C^{14}) concentrations. The tumor protein also showed a high activity and accounted for one-third to one-fourth of the total absorbed radioisotope.

The literature is replete with experiments on the interrelationships between proteins, fats and carbohydrate constituents in the animal body and indicates that the intermediate metabolism of rapid breakdown, resynthesis and interchange is more extensive than previous studies with stable isotopes have indicated. The addition of carbon (C^{14}) as part of the armamentarium of tracer work with carbon, i.e., stable carbon (C^{13}) and radioisotopic carbon (C^{11}), vastly extends the possibilities of biochemical studies.

A compendium of some of the important advances made by the use of radioisotopic carbon is found in the published papers read at the Ciba Foundation Conferences (1951) on "Isotopes in Biochemistry", G. E. W. Wolstenholmes, Chief Editor.

At this conference Leblond reported on the metabolism of estrone, progesterone and desoxycorticosterone acetate labeled with C^{14}. It was found that the blood level remained high for periods up to 144 hours after injection, and the major portion of the hormones was excreted in the bile and in the urine. The blood level remained up long after the hormones had disappeared from organs and tissues. About 6.5 per cent of the hormone was metabolized to water and CO_2 and excreted by the lungs. The hormones could not be identified within the cells of the sex organs.

Hammarsten studied the rate of protein turnover for different stages of regeneration in rat liver after partial hepatectomy, measuring the rate of glycine incorporated into protein. The glycine was labeled with N^{15} and C^{14}. Partial hepatectomy was performed on a series of rats, each group of which received the same amount of isotopes during the same period before death. The glycine was fairly well distributed in the protein molecule, and the content of the isotope of glycine isolated from the protein was used as a measure of protein turnover. This rate of protein turnover in turn was used as an indicator of tissue regeneration. These experiments showed that the maximum rate for the uptake of all nitrogenous compounds in cell nuclei and cytoplasm appeared in about 30 hours after partial hepatectomy. This protein turnover tended to fall sharply as measured by glycine after 48 to 60 hours, and it returned to approximately normal levels at the end of a week.

From the clinical standpoint the long half-life of carbon[14] requires that it be handled as carefully as radium. The isotope is most often supplied as $BaCO_3$, an insoluble compound. This must be handled with extreme care when appreciable quantities are present, to prevent rubbing it into the skin or inhaling it in large amounts. In tracer work, the isotope is most often encountered as CO_2 or CO_3. Experiments with $BaCO_3$ indicate that

C^{14} is eliminated quite rapidly and that solid $BaCO_3$ is less dangerous than might be expected. The loss of C^{14} is rapid because of exchange with lung CO_2 induced in the moist environment of the lung. Ingestion of C^{14} as the material used in the synthesis of vital cell structures may be seriously hazardous.

Clinical applications of C^{14} in tracer work are slowly accumulating. The following are examples of this approach:

Barclay, Ebert, LeRoy and Manthei and Roth have studied the distribution and excretion of radioactive isoniazid in tuberculous patients. Carbon[14]-labeled isoniazid was administered in single doses as high as 430 microcuries. In one individual, a second tracer dose was given so that there was a total combined dosage of 860 microcuries of C^{14}. The authors point out that this fell within the dosage range now considered to be safe, employing a safety factor of approximately 10. Studies were conducted on three patients. One individual had active pulmonary tuberculosis; another tuberculous adenitis; and a third had a tuberculous pleural effusion. The drug and metabolites were largely excreted in the urine. From 75 % to 92 % was recovered from the urine in 24 hours. Feces contained less than 1 %, and minute amounts were found in the form of CO_2 from the lungs. Surgery was performed on all three patients within a few hours after the labeled drug was given. Peak blood levels and plasma levels were reached at the end of the first hour. They ranged from 2.8 to 3.5 micrograms per milliliter of blood. Normal lung tissue and skin contained roughly 1.79 micrograms of isoniazid per gram of tissue. Normal muscle, fat and bone contained 1.5, 0.78 and 0.61 micrograms per gram of tissue, respectively. The capsule of the tuberculous lesion contained 1.88 micrograms of the drug per gram of tissue. It is interesting to note that the caseous material in the tuberculous lesion contained 1.04 micrograms per gram of tissue. Similar findings were noted in the capsule of tuberculous lymph node and the caseous material within the node. The pleural fluid in one patient contained 1.65 micrograms per cc. at $2\frac{1}{2}$ hours.

De Paepe and Ficq utilized uterine cervical biopsies incubated for 1, 3 and 5 hours with C^{14}-labeled adenine and phenylalanine for fixation, staining and treating with nuclear emulsion. This work was predicated upon the desire to study the metabolism of nucleic acids and proteins in the cervical epithelium and to make autoradiographic studies of normal and neoplastic tissues. The authors observed that, with normal tissue, adenine is first incorporated mainly in the basal and parabasal cell layer, but after three hours is uniformly distributed. Phenylalanine is localized in the intermediary cells at all times and is concentrated in the nucleolus. It was suggested by this study with C^{14} that the correspondence between the nucleic acids in the basal layer and the proteins in the parabasal layer indicates the relation of the nucleic acids to protein synthesis. Before treating carcinoma of the cervix by irradiation, the radioactivity by this particular experimental technique was greater than normal, with considerable variability between regions of the same section and different cell types. After treatment, incorporation of adenine was diminished in most instances. The authors feel that this method permits the study of the individual surviving cancer cells, and that the inhibition of nucleic acid and protein metabolism may be related to the malignancy of the tumor and so provide a guide to radiation sensitivity.

Okita, Kelsey, Talso, Smith and Geiling have made studies on renal excretion of radioactive carbon-labeled digitoxin in human subjects with cardiac failure. They used radioactive C^{14} in labeling the digitoxin and the renal excretion rate was studied, using an extremely sensitive isotope tracer technique. In these studies there was a marked initial excretion of digitoxin during the first two days, followed by a gradual leveling off of the excretion after about the fifth day. Most of the C^{14} from the labeled drug was eliminated in the form of metabolic products, while only 6% to 10% of the original drug was excreted as unchanged digitoxin. A minute amount of unchanged digitoxin was detected in the urine for as long as 40 days after administration of a single dose of radioactive digitoxin, while C^{14}-labeled compounds could be detected up to the 74th day. In human beings, the major route of excretion of digitoxin seems to be through the kidneys and not by way of the liver and gastrointestinal tract. Sixty per cent to eighty per cent was eliminated through this route, either in the form of unchanged digitoxin or its metabolic products. In some animals, however, the major route of digitoxin excretion seems to be through the gastrointestinal tract. Rats, (digitoxin-resistant animals), appear to excrete most of the drug through the gastrointestinal tract, while cats, (digitoxin-sensitive animals), excreted about equally between the renal and gastrointestinal systems. The authors suggest the possibility that the more sensitive the animal species is to digitoxin, the more likely it will be to excrete a larger portion of the drug through the kidneys.

Tyrosine containing C^{14} localizes in "melanosarcomatous" tissue but has no therapeutic value, since the uptake both in the thyroid and adrenals is high. Carbon C^{14} stilbamidine is taken up by meylomata, but the uptake in liver is much greater. Recent studies of autoimmunization indicate that it may be possible to deliver a radiation dose to tumors by radioactive antibodies, (Lawrence and Tobias, 1956).

20.15 Gallium

The studies of Dudley and his colleagues on the physiological characteristics of gallium have shown that this element is an avid bone-seeker, and have created considerable interest in the possibility that a new tool for the study of bone metabolism has been found. More recent studies have indicated that it may be used as a diagnostic method and deserves investigation as a method of therapy in bone tumors.

Gallium (Ga^{72}) has a half-life of 14.1 hours, and emits negative beta rays, with a maximum energy of 3.17 mev, and gamma rays with a maximum energy of 3.35 mev. Extensive studies have been made by Dudley and his co-workers on the toxic effects of stable gallium to provide a basis for evaluating the effects of carrier gallium when radioactive isotopes of this element are administered. These investigators have found that gallium citrate is more suitable as a means of administering soluble gallium to experimental animals than is gallium lactate. It is not absorbed from the gastro-intestinal tract, and it produces no significant effect when fed to rats over a period of weeks. The toxicity (LD^{50}, 10 days) of gallium citrate on a basis of one milligram of gallium per kilogram of body weight for dogs and goats was 10 to 15 milligrams per kilogram of weight. Toxic doses of gallium citrate in the rabbit resulted in marked kidney changes with an uncompensated acidosis and insignificant changes in the serum sodium and potassium levels.

The toxicity of the carrier gallium limited the radiation dosage of Ga^{72} in five species of animals so that the only effect of radiation observed was a transitory reduction in leukocytes. The degree and duration of leukopenia varied with the dose (2.3 to 9 mc.) and species. Repeated injections of gallium citrate in dogs and rabbits revealed the element to be a cumulative poison for which no tolerance was developed. In the dog, repeated injections produced an exfoliative dermatitis which often appeared several weeks after the stoppage of the injections. The rat tolerated some ten times more gallium citrate than the dog indicating a distinct species difference. Man probably fits somewhere between the two species.

In 1950 Dudley et al. carried out clinical tracer studies with gallium[72] but indicated that the toxicity of the drug prevented therapeutic trial. They suggested that if Ga^{72} could be concentrated by removal of the inactive Ga^{71} by electromagnetic means before administration, therapeutic doses might be given without approaching the toxic concentration of gallium.

Properly controlled gallium citrate offers a satisfactory medium for the administration of soluble gallium and gives rapid localization of this substance in osteoid structures. Studies of the distribution of the gallium citrate in the rat, rabbit, and dog indicate that only the bone and kidneys received large amounts of the element. The other soft tissues received no significant concentration. A series of animals injected with from 0.9 to 1.1 millicuries of gallium citrate (Ga^{72}) per kilogram showed that 44.6 per cent of the injected dose was excreted in the urine in sixteen hours after injection, while 40.2 per cent was deposited in the bone. In general, the greater the quantity of gallium excreted, the less is deposited in the bone. The greatest disadvantage to the use of gallium citrate (Ga⁷²), when employed for tracer studies or in therapeutic amounts, is the possible radiation injury produced in the kidneys, as the radioisotope is concentrated and excreted by these organs. In addition, stable gallium compounds at toxic levels produce renal changes.

Munn, Dudley et al. have described a method for the separation of gallium from the urine and found in the rabbit and dog that intravenous injection resulted in an urinary excretion of gallium citrate comparable with animals similarly treated by subcutaneous injection of the isotope. In 60 patients, the urinary excretion of gallium during the first 24 hours after intravenous injection varied widely (4–78 %). No correlation was observed between the clinical manifestations and the rate or amount of gallium excreted. In man the initial excretion rate was high and reached a low level in 18 hours. The blood levels fell rapidly after intravenous injection and approached a low value within 6 hours.

King et al. used three patients, one having multiple myeloma, one having osteogenic sarcoma and one having Hodgkin's disease in studying the gallium, urinary excretion rates given at the end of 96 hours (Table VI).

The urinary excretion rate was affected by the size of the dose of the stable metal. The fecal excretion was less than 1 %.

Dudley and his associates have shown that radioactive gallium in young rabbits is found principally at the epiphyseal junctions of the long bones

TABLE VI

Urinary Excretion of Gallium by the Human

PATIENT NO.	DIAGNOSIS	ISOTOPE DOSE		METAL DOSE		PERCENTAGE OF INITIAL DOSE EXCRETED IN 96 HR
		mc	mc/kg	mg	mg/kg	
1	Osteogenic sarcoma	1.00	—	5	—	26
		22.5	0.86	90	2.81	47
		52.0	1.62	185	5.75	40
		46.3	1.45	180	5.60	46
		49.0	1.53	166	5.19	40
		1.00	—	5	—	6
2	Multiple myeloma	8.00	0.14	105	1.90	18
		49.90	0.92	166	3.07	22
3	Hodgkin's disease	1.00	—	5	—	37
		20.00	0.34	107	1.78	37
		51.50	0.83	200	3.33	48

in eight hours. This is the region of greatest osteogenic activity. In older animals, the trabecular bone showed the greatest activity, while the periodontal tissues of both age groups exhibited an especial affinity for the injected gallium. A dog weighing 8 kilograms, which was found to have a spontaneous osteoclastic lesion of the foreleg, was given a single subcutaneous injection of 0.5 millicuries of gallium lactate (Ga^{72}) per kilogram of body weight. In twenty-four to forty-eight hours, Geiger counter readings indicated 33 to 39 per cent higher radioactivity over the osteoid lesion than over the same area on the opposite normal leg. There were no hematological changes noted in a period of forty-five days.

King and Perkinson in distribution studies of Ga^{72} injected as an acid solution of gallium chloride into the tail vein of the Wistar rat found that the uptake of gallium was greatest in the kidney, liver and spleen. The blood plasma showed a rapid fall of gallium. The erythrocytes did not appear to pick up any of the element. The liver and spleen showed an early uptake within the first day, then there was a decrease in gallium content with a later rise. The kidney showed a similar pattern of uptake except the later rise appeared within 48 hours. The teeth, skeleton and trachea presented an early rise in gallium level at about 12 hours, then a decrease in level with a more gradual rise up to 96 hours. The teeth, which in the young rat are probably the site of the most intense osteogenic activity, had the highest activity of radiogallium. At the end of four days the greatest deposition of gallium per total organ was the skeleton and next the liver. The possibility of gallium acting as a protein precipitant and the colloid thus formed being picked up by the reticulo-endothelial system was mentioned.

Mulry and Dudley, in clinical studies at the Bethesda Naval Hospital, found that there was a differential radioactivity of gallium (Ga^{72}) in bones as compared with surrounding soft parts. These investigators used Geiger-counting techniques applied to the skin surface for the localization of radioactive gallium (Ga^{72}) in bone. They found that intravenous tracer doses of gallium (Ga^{72}) were selectively concentrated in both osteogenic and osteolytic bone lesions in fifteen of eighteen patients with primary and malignant metastatic bone tumors. Early metastases to bone were identified before changes were apparent by roentgenogram.

Lang in 1951 reported that only two attempts had been made thus far to treat therapeutically patients having bone malignancies. The meager information derived from the study of these two cases indicated that radiogallium at least has a palliative effect in prolonging life, and in relieving bone pain and other distressing symptoms.

Bruner indicates that the Oak Ridge Institute of Nuclear Studies in a 16 months intensive study with Ga^{72} against primary and metastatic osteo-

genic sarcoma has proven essentially negative. They have turned to research with another gallium isotope Ga[67] which is hoped will retain the
bone-seeking property of the element. It has a desirable radiation spectrum,
longer half-life and can be produced carrier free. The potential value of
treating bone malignancies by radioactive gallium remains sub judice.

Brucer, Andrews and Bruner in a study of Gallium[72] at the Oak Ridge
Institute of Nuclear Studies, (1953), came to the conclusion, after two years
of investigation, that the isotope is not a therapeutic agent in cancer of
bone for the following reasons: (1) lack of uniformity of concentration of
Ga[72] within the tumor; (2) because of the short half-life of the isotope, there
is a relatively high concentration of the drug developing in the tissues after
most of the activity has been expended; and (3) the undesirable total body
irradiation effects which become prominent at subtherapeutic dose levels.
The authors also point out the well known chemical toxicity of Gallium.

Behrens points out the toxicity of Gallium and cites the difficulties in
obtaining an effective concentration for therapy. He indicates, however,
that if it ever becomes possible to obtain Ga[72] sufficiently free of its stable
isotope, there may be more favorable results from its use. He also points
out the possible use of Ga[67] with a 78-hour half-life and with gamma ray
energies of 0.09–0.88 mev. plus x-rays.

Bruner, Hayes and Perkinson investigated Ga[67] by injecting the carrier
free isotope intravenously into white rats. The animals were sacrificed from
one to 20 days after injection. The urine and feces contributed equally to
a 39 % excretion for the first five days. The femur had a differential absorption ratio about 0.75 that of the spleen, while the liver lost much of the Ga[67]
activity it had picked up initially. The results proved to be significantly
different from previous studies with Ga[72]. The investigators found that
stable Ga[69] may have to be added to carrier free Ga[67] preparations in order
to secure the high differential concentrations of radioisotopes in or around
osteogenic neoplasms. The carrier free pattern occurred when the dose of
the carrier was below 0.25 milligrams of gallium per kilogram.

Dudley, Markowitz and Mitchell have shown that the concentration
gradient of Ga[72] citrate between normal muscle and bone is of the order of
1 to 50, while the ratio between normal and proliferating bone is approximately 1 to 4. They have found 2 millicuries of Ga[72], given intravenously,
to be most effective, followed after 48 hours by the appropriate scanning
procedures. Regional blood supply seems to account for discrepancies in
considering false positive and negative findings. The present scanning technique of the authors has only a limited usefulness as a diagnostic procedure
for malignant and benign lesions of bone. A correlation between stages of
bone healing and Ga[72] concentration in fractures suggests that Ga[72] tracer

study techniques may deserve a place in the investigation of the metabolism of healing bone lesions.

20.16 Mercury

Mercury has two essentially useful radioisotopes, $_{80}Hg^{203}$ with a half life of 48 days, emitting negative beta electrons of 0.21 mev and gamma rays of 0.28 mev. $_{80}Hg^{205}$ is often included in studies with radiomercury ($_{80}Hg^{203}$) because of the mass uncertainty still present concerning the status of the mercury isotope. (Hg^{205} is presently characterized by half life of 5.2 m, B^- 1.4 and 1.6 and γ 0.2 mev.) The second radioisotope is Hg^{197} with two isomers of 25 and 65 hours half-life each. The 25-hour half life radiomercury emits 0.134, 0.13 and 0.28 gamma radiation while the 65-hour half life radioisotope emits 0.077 and 0.191 gamma rays and K x-ray (au). Both show K capture. Studies with mercury have largely dealt with tracer work and chemotherapeutic studies, rather than with the use of the metal as a radiotherapeutic agent. Ray, Birch, et al., have studied the distribution of radiomercury, ($Hg^{203, 205}$) in edema fluid, ascitic fluid, pleural fluid, bile, saliva, gastric juice, cerebrospinal fluid, sweat and erythrocytes following intravenous administration of a single dose of a mercurial diuretic. No measurable quantities entered the cerebrospinal fluid, sweat, gastric juice and erythroperitoneal and pleural fluids. Relatively high concentrations were found in the bile. Ray, Threefoot, Birch, and associates, in a study of radioactivated "Mercurhydrin" found an interesting rate of regressions by measuring the radioactivity in blood samples withdrawn from individuals who had been injected with 2 cc. of the diuretic. At first the regression was rapid, apparently due to mechanical mixing of the tracer in the plasma. A second rate was noted which represented filling of potential mercury spaces; and a third rate was noted which reflected the elimination of mercury from the body, principally via the urine.

Kelly, Svedberg and Harp, in a study of the pharmacologic properties of mercurial diuretics also used "Mercurhydrin" prepared with radiomercury ($Hg^{203, 205}$).

Mercury was observed to pass across a cantharides blister membrane in a predictable manner. Studies on control patients were contrasted with those on patients with cardiac disease. No significant differences in transfer of mercury across the membrane were noted in patients with congestive heart failure and in control subjects. The results offered suggestive evidence of physiologically effective binding of mercury to plasma proteins.

20.17 Iridium

Freundlich, Haybittle and Quick have investigated the possibility of

74 day iridium (Ir^{192}) as a source of gamma rays for teletherapeutic units. An output of about 11 r per minute at 8 cm. focal skin distance is obtained from a unit weighing approximately 50 pounds, but which has sufficient lead protection to make pneumatic control unnecessary. The iridium (Ir^{192}) source decays by about 25 per cent per month and emits a gamma cascade of 0.14 to 1.16 mev. They have pointed out that, in a comparative study of energy absorption, the divergence between iridium and radium gamma rays is very small, in striking contrast with 200 kv. roentgen rays.

Mitchell has installed a unit utilizing radioiridium as a gamma ray source in teletherapy in the University of Cambridge. From the known physical factors available, he indicates an assumption that the biologically equivalent dose of radioiridium gamma radiation is 1.2 times the dose of filtered 220 kv. roentgen therapy under comparable conditions.

In 1954, Freundlich and Haybittle make a further report on an improved Iridium[192] teletherapy unit situated at Addenbrooke's Hospital, Cambridge, England. They describe the output of this new unit as 27.5 r. per minute at 9 cm. source skin distance; or 14 r. per minute at 13 cm. source skin distance. The mean energy of the gamma rays emitted is 400 kv. They report that central axis depth dose curves of a 7 cm. diameter field, when treated at 25 cm. source skin distance, compare favorably with those of roentgen rays of 1.5 mm. copper half-value layer, using a similar size field at a focus skin distance of 50 cm. The authors feel that the possibilities of wider use of Iridium[192] are worthy of consideration until sufficient quantities of cesium will be ready at Oak Ridge for construction of larger teletherapy units.

20.18 Ruthenium

Of all elements found in the fission process, ruthenium (Ru^{106}) is the source of the highest energy beta particles. Ruthenium, itself, emits only a weak beta ray with an energy of 0.039 mev., but the immediate daughter element, *rhodium* (Rh^{106}), with a half life of 30 seconds, decays to stable palladium by the emission of beta particles with an end point of 3.53 mev. Associated with this are gamma radiations, some occurring in a cascade of 0.87–2.66 and others of 0.5 and 0.6 mev. Cara investigated radioruthenium from the standpoint of its use in plaques as surface applicators. With unfiltered ruthenium (Ru^{106}) in contact with a phantom, it was found that the greatest energy dose was near the surface within the first millimeter. Simple filtration alone only slightly improved the depth dose and should be kept at a minimum. A clinical applicator of plexiglass, with gold foil and aluminum foil as a filter was constructed. The clinical application of the isotope was not discussed.

20.19 Astatine (all isotopes radioactive)

Astatine (At^{211}) decays by emitting alpha particles of 5.9 and 7.43 mev., γ and K, L x-rays. It has a 7.5 hour half life and must be produced by an accelerator. Bruner points out that it appears to behave as a halogen and biologically to follow the distribution of iodine, particularly the thyroid gland. It has been used in a limited number of persons with encouraging results and the isotope has been recovered from the thyroglobulin isolated from treated animals.

20.20 Hafnium

Hafnium, with eight radioactive isotopes, has produced an unexpected special localization which may prove of considerable value. Hf^{175} has a 70-day half life and emits gamma radiations of 0.34 to 0.43 mev. Hf^{181} has a half life of 46 days and emits negative beta radiation of 0.41 mev. and gamma radiations of 0.13 to 0.6 mev. Studies have shown by autoradiography that the zona glomerulosa of the adrenal cortex has a high specific preferential localization of radiohafnium (Hf^{181}). Brucer indicates that most of the hafnium compounds so far studied in animals have shown far greater deposits in the liver and spleen than in the adrenals, but that the proportional deposition can be changed by altering the compound. If the specificity of the adrenal localization can be enhanced, hafnium can become a useful isotope.

20.21 Fluorine

A few studies have been carried out with fluorine (F^{18} with 1.87 hr. half life) on the uptake of fluorine in bone and teeth. (β^+ emitter 0.65 mev.).

20.22 Rubidium

Rubidium is present in tracer amounts as an ion in vertebrate body fluids. Rb^{86} has been utilized in a few studies on the behavior of rubidium in biological systems. In the dog it closely resembles potassium in distribution after intravenous injection. It has also been suggested that rubidium may actually replace potassium in the nutrition of certain bacteria. It is a $\beta \ \gamma$ emitter.

20.23 Cesium

Cesium has a number of radioactive isotopes, two of which have a considerable half-life. Cs^{134} has a half-life of 2.3 years and emits beta radiations of 0.065 along with a gamma cascade of 0.47–1.37 and others of 0.6 and 0.8 mev. Cs^{137} has a half-life of 30 years and emits beta radiations of 0.52 and 1.2 mev. and gamma rays of 0.66. This gamma radiation is about the equivalent of 1 mev. x-ray therapy, the discrepancy resulting from the fact that 1 mev. peak voltage from the x-ray machine is higher than the mean effective voltage. In considering the use of fission products for teletherapy, Cesium[137] and Cerium[144] offer promise of usefulness. Difficulties of extraction of active material suitable for therapy sources from fission products has been a real problem. The lower output curie of Cesium[137]—(0.34 rhm/curie), —as compared to much higher specific activities for Cobalt[60], requires a source strength at least three or four times greater than that of Cobalt[60] for a given roentgen output. The higher activity sources required in teletherapy give rise to handling and shielding difficulties on a scale not ordinarily encountered.

Brucer, in a report before the Subcommittee on Research and Development of the joint Committee on Atomic Energy, Congress of the United States, (84th Congress), in 1956 indicated that two machines had been made for Cesium[137] sources. These are located in Oak Ridge, Tennessee and in Southampton, England. He stated that England is making about thirty Cesium[137] sources and that the United States is preparing to make additional sources.

Abersold, (1956) stated that there were two Cesium units in this country. He pointed out that Cesium[137] offered some advantages over Co[60] as a teletherapy source, chiefly because of its much longer half-life—(30 years vs. 5.2 years) and the reduced amount of heavy material needed to shield its less penetrating gamma rays—(0.66 mev. vs. 1.17–1.33 mev.) Abersold also spoke of the shortage of Cesium[137], but indicated that facilities can be developed to extract from fission wastes millions of curies per year of Cesium[137] and other fission products. The specific activity obtainable, however, has a definite limit which is less than that obtainable with Cobalt[60].

Comas and Brucer (1957) have reported their first impressions of therapy with cesium-137 using a kilocurie teletherapy machine at the Medical Division of the Oak Ridge Institute of Nuclear Studies. The machine consists essentially of a shielded 1,500-curie cesium-137 source that is capable of movement in four directions—tilt, vertical, horizontal, and circular. A detailed discussion is given of the complex mechanical and electronic set-up. Very short collimator-skin distances can be used in setting up stationary portals. In rotational therapy, however, they could seldom allow a gap of less than 10–15 cm. Most patients were treated with a distance of 29 cm. C.S.D. Rectangular fields were obtained by using a lead insert up to a maximum field of 12 cm. in diameter at a distance of 60 cm. from the source to the center of rotation. The relatively large size of the cesium-137 source (3 cm. in diameter) created an extensive penumbra that limited the "concentrating" effects of a moving source or a multiple portal arrangement. The skin reactions were similar to those observed with cobalt-60, except that in the case of cobalt the reactions usually occurred later. The erythema created by Cs^{137} was usually observed with a skin dose of approximately 2000 roentgens around the third or fourth week of treatment. The authors report that 11 patients have been treated within the past year and that it is too early to appraise results in terms of survival rates. From the preliminary indications, it would appear that one can give a higher dose without reference to excessive skin reaction comparable with cobalt therapy, except about the mouth and pharynx where there was noted no difference in timing, intensity, and character as compared with the reactions of 250-kvp x-ray therapy or cobalt therapy. Because of its abundance in the present atomic energy operations being carried on in this country, investigations are well under way to utilize cesium as a substitute for radium sources of energy.

20.24 Yttrium

Yttrium^{90} is a pure beta emitter with a maximum energy of 2.27 mev., and a maximum tissue range of 1.1 cm. Its half-life is 64 hours. The material is simple to prepare and to administer. It requires only moderate shielding and presents no problems to nursing and medical personnel. Localization of Y^{90} in the pleural and peritoneal cavity in the presence of sufficient Yttrium carrier is probably due to the formation of colloids of Yttrium with the constituents of the fluid in the pleural or peritoneal cavity, (principally with the proteins). The small amount of Yttrium^{90} which slowly escapes from the injected cavity into the circulation presents no significant danger to the patient, since the radioactivity decreases rapidly due to the 64 hour half-life of this isotope. Localization of Y^{90} on the serosal surfaces of the injected cavities has been experimentally noted by Kyker and also Andrews, et al.

Siegel, Hart, Brothers and Spencer have introduced tracer or therapeutic doses of Y^{90}, with 100 to 200 mg. of stable Yttrium as a carrier, into the pleural or peritoneal cavity of 40 patients with cancerous effusion. The solutions used were prepared from Yttrium oxide irradiated in the reactor at Brookhaven National Laboratory. After the administration of Y^{90} to the patients, samples of blood and daily urine and fecal collections were radioassayed, in some cases for as long as 19 days. It can be concluded from the data that no significant radioactivity was present in the blood at any time and that the excretions were very low. The low uptake in the liver and the skeleton is in agreement with the data on localization of the isotope in the injected cavity. Eight of sixteen patients appeared to have derived benefit from the therapy. Six of these required no further thoracenteses during a follow-up period of at least as long as the pre-treatment period of observation, which ranged from one to several months. Patients received from 10 to 40 or more millicuries of Y^{90}. No side reactions attributable to stable Yttrium were noted. No symptoms of radiation sickness were observed and no depression of the hematopoetic system was detected. In several instances, transient chest pain was noted after the installation of Yttrium. The advantages of this intracavity therapy listed by the investigators are: favorable radiation characteristics of the isotope; the increased safety for the patient and personnel; and, it would appear, that the palliative results are such that this modality of treatment may find its place in the management of the late cancer cases.

Bulkley, Cooper and O'Conor have utilized radioactive Yttrium chloride with carrier isotope to study its effects on the prostate of dogs. The radioactive Yttrium chloride solution was distributed through the lobes of the prostate in 19 mongrel dogs by injection from a shielded syringe. Animals were sacrificed, beginning after 1 week, to obtain tissues for radioactive assay. The Yttrium chloride injected contained Y^{90} with a specific activity of 1 millicurie per 1 mg. used. Microscopically, Yttrium chloride caused an acute radiation reaction, characterized by hemorrhage and necrosis. Some specimens demonstrated spread beneath the capsule, rather than through the parenchyma. Urinary excretion of Y^{90}, following intraprostatic injection, did not differ significantly from that observed in radioactive colloidal gold. Apparently, a considerable amount of the radioyttrium enters the urethra and bladder at the time of injection, or shortly thereafter, with continuing excretion during the second 24 hours. The liver was the only organ which contained more than 1 % of the activity, and the content was half that found in studies with radiogold or radioactive chromic phosphate. The remainder of the isotope apparently left the prostate along the lymphatic channels to regional lymph nodes, or by direct extension along the fascial planes of the pelvis. The greater retention within the prostate itself and the wider distribution in the regional lymphatics suggests that radioyttrium offers advantages over radiogold and radioactive chromic phosphate in the treatment of carcinoma of the prostate.

Fitzgerald reports Y^{90} as causing osteogenic sarcoma in animals following its administration. The tumors were thought to be caused by the preferential localization of the isotope in collagenous tissues as demonstrated by autography.

Einhorn, Larsson and Ragnhult have investigated Y^{90} with regard to possible use in the bladder in the treatment of papillomatous villi. Solutions of the radioactive salt, Yttrium chloride, formed in the presence of urine a precipitate of Yttrium phosphate which dissolved only in strong acid mixtures. This precipitation was prevented by the use of one of several chelating agents. After installation of the radioisotope through catheters into the bladders of four patients for periods of 1.5 to 2.5 hours, approximately

100 % of the amount of Y^{90} injected was recovered in three patients, when the bladders were emptied and washed out. In the fourth patient, some leakage occurred around the catheter and only 80 % of the Y^{90} was recovered. Blood samples and 24-hour urine specimens showed detectable, but extremely low, measures of radioactive material. Possibility of the use of Y^{90} in treating bladder tumors will need further investigation before it is acceptable as a method of therapy.

Boysen and Campbell have utilized Y^{90} spheres in a technic for producing predictable subcortical lesions in the brains of laboratory animals.

20.25 Bismuth

Bismuth^{206} is a cyclotron-produced isotope. It decays by K capture and a complex gamma spectrum. Bismuth^{206} has a mean energy of 0.75 mev., and the half-life is 6.4 days.

This isotope is reported by Van Der Werff as having been used for local infiltration of tumors. Its advantage is pointed out as an absence of beta rays, which reduces high dose concentrations locally and also intravenously, when used for diseases of the reticuloendothelial system. When given intravenously, the bismuth-activated charcoal particles are taken up by cells of the reticulo-endothelial system, especially in the liver, spleen and lymph nodes. The leucocyte count shows a smaller reduction than with P^{32} or Au^{198}. There is a loss of 35 % of the isotope by urinary excretion in the first 12 days. Van Der Werff reports two aleukemic leukemia patients treated with Bi^{206} living after 2 years. He reports eight cases of Hodgkin's disease, treated during the past 4 years, living without recurrence.

20.26 Chromium

Chromium^{51} is a gamma ray emitter with a mean energy of 0.32 ($\sim$8 %) mev. The isotope has a half-life of 27 days and also shows K capture.

The clinical application of Cr^{51} as a diagnostic tool is gaining ground rapidly, and a wide range of studies has been implemented through the use of the isotope by tagging the red blood cells.

Reilly, French, et al., hold that Cr^{51} is superior to other radioactive isotopes in making blood volume determinations. This contention is based upon its physical properties and ease of application. The radioiron method requires donor red blood cells and, therefore, is not so easily carried out as the other method. The localized radiation effect of P^{32} is greater than Cr^{51} which emits mainly gamma irradiation. In addition the Cr^{51} as the isotope for use in tagging cells is more stable and is constant for at least 24 hours, as opposed to about 60 minutes for P^{32}. The chromium is bound to the protein portion of the hemoglobin. The simplicity of the whole blood volume determination method is discussed. A blood sample is drawn, tagged with

Cr^{51}, injected, and then total counts per second per cc. of the injected material are compared to counts per second per cc. of the withdrawn blood after the Cr^{51} injection. The degree of dilution indicates the patient's blood volume. These investigators have made whole blood volume studies in normal patients and on patients with cardiac disease, with and without evidence of heart failure.

Reilly, Helwig, et al., made blood volume measurements in carcinoma, using the same Cr^{51} red-blood-cells-tagging method.

Kurtz and Tivey have emphasized the stability of the binding of Cr^{51} with red blood cells and that, due to this fact, only the intravascular space is measured. They further indicated that Cr^{51} makes possible repeated blood volume studies over a 24 hour period from a single injection.

Difficulties in assay arising from the soft radiation emitted by Cr^{51} can be minimized by use of scintillation detectors.

Apt and Pollycove have used Fe^{59} and Cr^{51} to study anemias associated with renal pathology.

Korst et al. have produced evidence that there are two types of acquired hemolytic anemia, as indicated by the splenic trapping. This phenomenon can be demonstrated by scintillation counting over the liver and spleen at intervals after transfusion. The authors feel that when such "trapping" is observed, the patient is a better candidate for splenectomy than when there is an absence of this phenomenon.

Quimby states that the comparison of red cell survival, measured simultaneously by radiochromium activity and by the method of selective adglutination, indicates that the rate of Cr^{51} elution from labelled erythrocytes is about 1 per cent per day. None of the chromium thus removed appears to be utilized. Chromium tagging, therefore, makes it possible to follow red cells throughout their lifetime.

Necheles, et al., using this technic, arrived at the half-life of a normal individual's cells as being 35 days. While this is shorter than the half-life obtained by the agglutination technique, because of chromium elution, it offers an adequate baseline for comparison with diseased states and the effects of treatment.

REFERENCES

Manganese

BURNETT, WM. T., JR., BIGELOW, ROBERT R., KIMBALL, ALLYN W., AND SHEPPARD, CHARLES W.: Radiomanganese Studies on the Mouse, Rat and Pancreatic Fistula Dog. *Am. J. Physiol., 168:* 620 (March) 1952.

COMAR, C. L.: Radioisotopes in Nutritional Trace Element Studies. *Nucleonics, 3(4):* 30, 1948.

GREENBERG, D. M., AND CAMPBELL, W. W.: Studies in Mineral Metabolism with the

Aid of Induced Radioactive Isotopes. IV. Manganese. *Proc. Nat. Acad. Sc., 26:* 448, 1940.

GREENBERG, D. M., COPP, D. H., AND CUTHBERTSON, E. M.: Studies in Mineral Metabolism with the Aid of Artificial Radioactive Isotopes; Distribution and Excretion, Particularly by Way of Bile, Iron, Cobalt and Manganese. *J. Biol. Chem., 147:* 749, 1943.

HAHN, P. F., AND SHEPPARD, C. W.: Selective Radiation Obtained by the Intravenous Administration of Colloidal Radioactive Isotopes in Diseases of the Lymphoid System. *South. M. J., 39:* 558, 1946.

MAYNARD, L. A., AND LOOSLI, J. K.: Mineral Nutrition. *Ann. Rev. Biochem., 12:* 251, 1943.

McCANCE, R. A., AND WIDDOWSON, E. M.: Mineral Metabolism. *Ann. Rev. Biochem., 13:* 315, 1944.

MOHAMED, M. S., AND GREENBERG, D. M.: A Tracer Study with Mn^{56} on Chicks with Perosis Produced by a Synthetic Manganese-deficient Diet. *Proc. Soc. Exper. Biol. & Med., 54:* 197, 1943.

MOTLEY, L.: Some Observations on the Use of Radioactive Isotopes in Therapy. *Memphis M. J., 23:* 135, 1948.

SHEPPARD, C. W., AND HAHN, P. F.: Retention and Excretion of Manganese Dioxide Dispersions Administered Intravenously to Humans. *South. M. J., 39:* 562, 1946.

SHEPPARD, C. W., ET AL.: Studies of the Distribution of Intravenously Administered Colloidal Sols of Manganese Dioxide and Gold in Human Beings and Dogs Using Radioactive Isotopes. *J. Lab. & Clin. Med., 32:* 274, 1947.

VON OETTINGEN, W. F.: Manganese: Its Distribution, Pharmacology and Health Hazards. *Physiol. Rev., 15:* 175, 1935.

Iron

AUSTONI, M. E., AND GREENBERG, D. M.: Studies in Iron Metabolism with the Aid of Its Artificial Radioactive Isotope; Absorption, Excretion and Distribution of Iron in Rat on Normal and Iron-deficient Diets. *J. Biol. Chem., 134:* 27, 1940.

AUSTONI, M. E., RABINOVITCH, A., AND GREENBERG, D. M.: Iron Content of Tissues of Normal, Anemic and Iron-enriched Rats Freed from Blood by Viviperfusion. *J. Biol. Chem., 134:* 17, 1940.

CHAPIN, M. A., AND ROSS, J. F.: The Determination of the True Cell Volume by a Dye Dilution, by Protein Dilution, and with Radioactive Iron. The Error of the Centrifuge Hematocrit. *Am. J. Physiol., 137:* 447, 1942.

CRUZ, W. O., HAHN, P. F., AND BALE, W. F.: Hemoglobin Radioactive Iron Liberated by Erythrocyte Destruction (Acetylphenylhydrazine) Promptly Reutilized to Form New Hemoglobin. *Am. J. Physiol., 135:* 595, 1942.

EMLINGER, P. J., HUFF, R. L., TOBIAS, C. A. AND LAWRENCE, J. H.: Iron turnover abnormalities in patients having anemia: serial blood and in vivo tissue studies with Fe^{59}. *Acta haemat. 9:* 73, 1953.

FINCH, C. A., GIBSON, J. G. II., PEACOCK, W. C. AND FLUHARTY, R. G.: Iron metabolism. Utilization of intravenous radioactive iron. *Blood 4:* 905, 1949.

GERRITSEN, T., HEINZ, H. J. AND STAFFORD, G. H.: Estimation of blood loss in hookworm infestation with Fe^{59}: Preliminary report. *Science 119:* 412, 1954.

HAHN, P. F.: The Use of Radioisotopes in the Study of Iron and Hemoglobin Metabolism and the Physiology of the Erythrocyte, in *Advances in Biological and Medical Physics.* New York: Academic Press, Inc., 1948, p. 287.

HAHN, P. F., AND WHIPPLE, G. H.: Iron Metabolism; Its Absorption, Storage and Utilization in Experimental Anemia. *Am. J. M. Sc., 191:* 24, 1936.

HAHN, P. F., BALE, W. F., AND BALFOUR, W. M.: Radioactive Iron Used to Study Red Blood Cells over Long Periods; the Constancy of the Total Blood Volume in the Dog. *Am. J. Physiol., 135:* 600, 1941.

HAHN, P. F., et al.: Radioactive Iron and Its Excretion in Urine, Bile and Feces. *J. Exper. Med., 70:* 443, 1939.

HAHN, P. F., ET AL.: The Utilization of Iron and the Rapidity of Hemoglobin Formation in Anemia due to Blood Loss. *J. Exper. Med., 71:* 731, 1940.

HAHN, P. F., ET AL.: Radioactive Iron Absorption by Gastro-intestinal Tract. *J. Exper. Med., 78:* 169, 1943.

HAHN, P. F., ET AL.: Ferritin: Conversion of Inorganic and Hemoglobin Iron into Ferritin Iron in the Animal Body. Storage Function of Ferritin Iron as Shown by Radioactive and Magnetic Measurements. *J. Biol. Chem., 150:* 407, 1943.

HAHN, P. F., ET AL.: Peritoneal Absorption. Red Cells Labelled by Radioiron Hemoglobin More Promptly from the Peritoneal Cavity into the Circulation. *J. Exp. Med., 80:* 77, 1944.

HAHN, P. F., WELLS, E. B., AND MENEELY, G. R.: The Circulating Red Cell Mass in Polycythemia Vera as Determined by Red Blood Cells Tagged with the Radioactive Isotope of Iron. *Southern Med. Jr., 43:* 947, Nov. 1950.

HEVESY, H.: Radioactive Indicators; Their Application in Biochemistry, in *Animal Physiology and Pathology.* New York: Interscience Publishers, Inc., 1948, p. 167.

KAMEN, M. D.: Isotopes of Importance in Biology; Iron, in *Radioactive Tracers in Biology.* New York: Academic Press, Inc., 1947, p. 237.

QUIMBY, E. H.: Isotope studies of blood flow and blood cells. *Am. J. Roentgenol. 75:* 1068, 1957.

SHEMIN, D., AND RITTENBERG, D.: Biological Utilization of Glycine for the Synthesis of the Protoporphyrin of Hemoglobin. *J. Biol. Chem., 166:* 620–627, 1946.

WASSERMAN, L. R., RASHKOFF, I. A., LEAVITT, D., MAYER, J. AND PORT, S.: Rate of removal of radioactive iron from plasma—index of erythropoiesis. *J. Clin. Invest. 31:* 32, 1952.

Copper

BRADT, H., ET AL.: K Capture and Positron Emission of Cu^{61} and Cu^{64}. *Helvet. phys· acta, 18:* 252, 1945.

BROWNELL, G. L. AND SWEET, W. H.: Localization of brain tumors with positron emitters. *Nucleonics 11:* 40, 1953.

COULSON, E. J., REMINGTON, R. E., AND LYNCH, K. M.: Studies in the Metabolism of Copper. Bureau Fish, Invest., Report No. 23, Washington, 1934.

CUNNINGHAM, I. J.: Some Biochemical and Physiological Aspects of Copper in Animal Nutrition. *Biochem. J., 25:* 1267, 1931.

SCHULTZE, M. O., AND SIMMONS, S. J.: Use of Radioactive Copper in Studies on Nutritional Anemia in Rats. *J. Biol. Chem., 142:* 97, 1942.

SWEET, W. H.: The uses of nuclear disintegration in the diagnosis and treatment of brain tumor. *New England J. Med.* 245: 875, 1951.

WRENN, F. R., JR. AND GOOD, M. L.: The use of radioisotopes for the localization of brain tumors. *North Carolina M. J. 13:* 231, 1952.

WRENN, F. R., JR., GOOD, M. L., AND HANDLER, P.: The use of positron-emitting radioisotopes for the localization of brain tumors. *Science, 113:* May 4, 1951.

YOSHIKAWA, H., HAHN, P. F., AND BALE, W. F.: Form of Combination of Radioactive Iron and Copper in Plasma Following Ingestion. *Proc. Soc. Exper. Biol. & Med., 49:* 285, 1942.

YOSHIKAWA, H., HAHN, P. F., AND BALE, W. F.: Red Cell and Plasma Radioactive Copper in Normal and Anemic Dogs. *J. Exper. Med., 75:* 489, 1942.

Cobalt

BARCROFT, J.: *Respiratory Function of Blood.* London: Cambridge University Press, 1928.

BECKER, J., AND SCHEER, K. F.: Radiocobalt as a plastic preparation for radiation therapy. *Strahlentherapie, 85:* 581, 1951.

BRAESTRUP, C. B. AND MOONEY, R. T.: Cobalt-60 protection design. *Radiology 65:* 884, 1955.

CALLENDER, S. T., TURNBULL, A. AND WAKISAKA, G.: Estimation of intrinsic factor of Castle by use of radioactive vitamin B_{12} . *Brit. M. J. 1:* 10, 1954.

CALLENDINE, G. W., JR., MORTON, J. L., AND MYERS, W. G.: Physical considerations in applying cobalt[60] to cancer therapy. *Nucleonics, 7(6):* 63, 1950.

COMAR, E. J., DAVIS, G. K., AND TAYLOR, R. F.: Cobalt Metabolism Studies: Radioactive Cobalt Procedures with Rats and Cattle. *Arch. Biochem., 9:* 149, 1946.

COPP, D. H., AND GREENBERG, D. M.: Studies in Mineral Metabolism with the Aid of Artificial Radioactive Isotopes. *Proc. Natl. Acad. Sc. U. S., 27:* 153, 1941.

EVANS. R. D., AND EVANS, R. O.: Studies of self absorption in gamma ray sources. *Modern Phys., 20:* 305, 1948.

FEDORUK, S. O., JOHNS, H. E. AND WATSON, T. H.: Isodose distributions for A 1100 Curie cobalt[60] unit. *Radiology 60:* 348, 1953.

FLETCHER, G. A.: Teletherapy with cobalt. Chapter 19 in: *Therapeutic Use of Artificial Radioisotopes.* (P. F. HAHN, ed.) New York: Wiley, 1956.

GLASS, G. B. J., PACK, G. T. AND MERSHEIMER, W. L.: Uptake of radioactive vitamin B_{12} by the liver in patients with total and subtotal gastrectomy. *Gastroenterology, 29:* 666, 1955.

GRIMMETT, L. G.: A 1000-Curie cobalt[60] irradiator. *Texas Reports on Biology and Medicine, 8:* 443, 1950.

GRIMMETT, L. G., KERMAN, H. D., BRUCER, M., FLETCHER, G. H. AND RICHARDSON, J. E.: Design and construction of a multicurie cobalt teletherapy unit; preliminary report. *Radiology 59:* 19, 1952.

HALE, W. M. AND STONER, R. D.: The effect of cobalt-60 gamma radiation on passive immunity. *Yale J. Biol. & Med. 25:* 326, 1953.

HINMAN, F., JR., SCHULTE, J. W. AND LOW-BEER, B. V. A.: Further experience with intracavity radiocobalt for bladder tumors. *J. Urol. 73:* 285, 1955.

JAMES, A. G., WILLIAMS, R. D., AND MORTON, J. L.: The use of radioactive cobalt in non-resectable head and neck cancer. *Cancer, 4:* 1333, 1951.

JAMES, A. G., WILLIAMS, R. D., AND MORTON, J. L.: Radioactive cobalt as an adjunct to cancer surgery. *Surg., 30:* 95, 1951.

JOHANSON, C. E., OSTLING, G., AND GASSTROM, R. V.: Treatment of uterine cancer with radioactive cobalt. *Acta Radiol., 36:* 324, 1951.

JOHNS, H. E.: Physical characteristics of the radiation in cobalt[60] beam therapy. *J. Canad. A. Radiologists, 5:* 2, 1952.

KLAYMAN, M. I. AND BRANDBORG, L.: Clinical application of Co[60]-labeled vitamin B_{12} urine test. *New England J. Med. 253:* 808, 1955.

LAWRENCE, J. H.: The clinical use of radioisotopes. *Bull., New York Acad. Med., 26:* 639, 1950.

Low-Beer, B. V. A.: *The clinical use of radioactive isotopes*, pp. 336–349, Charles C. Thomas, Publisher, Springfield, Ill., 1950.

Mayor, G.: The radiocobalt in the treatment of malignant tumors of the bladder. *Schwliz. Med. Wchnschr. 84:* 510, 1954.

Morton, J. L., Callendine, G. W., Jr., and Myers, Wm. G.: Radioactive cobalt[60] in plastic tubing for interstitial radiation therapy. *Radiology, 56:* 553, 1951.

Myers, W. G.: Applications of artificial radioactive isotopes in therapy. I. Cobalt[60] *Am. J. Roentgenol., 60:* 816, 1948.

Nettleship, A., and Kerekes, E.: Comparative effects of Cobalt[60] and radium when implanted interstitially in the skin of rabbits. *Am. J. Roent., 68:* 89, 1952.

Parr, W., O'Neill, T. and Krebs, A.: A study of the x-irradiation protection afforded by cobalt. *Science 117:* 155, 1953.

Richardson, J. E., Kerman, H. and Brucer, M.: Skin dose from a cobalt[60] teletherapy unit. *Radiology 63:* 25, 1954.

Sheline, G. E., Chaikoff, I. L., and Montgomery, M. L.: Elimination of Administered Cobalt in Pancreatic Juice and Bile of Dog, as Measured with its Radioactive Isotopes. *Am. J. Physiol., 145:* 285, 1946.

Smith, I. H.: Cobalt[60] beam therapy; some influences and advantages. *J. Canad. A. Radiologists 3:* 16, 1952.

Smith, I. H.: Cobalt[60] beam therapy; some impressions after 5 years. *Canad. M. A. J. 77:* 289, 1957.

Vermooten, V.: Use of radioactive cobalt (Co[60]) in nylon sutures in treatment of carcinoma of bladder: preliminary report. *J. Urol. 73:* 280, 1955.

von Haam, E., Hendricks, C. H., and Morton, T. L.: Cytological studies on patients with carcinoma of the cervix treated with Co[60]. *Cancer Research, 12:* 303, 1952.

Wakely, J.: Carcinoma of the cervix: Treatment with radioactive cobalt. *South African M. J., 25:* 523, 1951.

Watson, T. A.: The clinical possibilities of the cobalt beam unit. *J. Canad. A. Radiologists 3:* 7, 1952.

Wilson, C. W.: Radiocobalt (Co[60]) as a therapeutic alternative to radium. *Am. J. Roentgenol., 65:* 726, 1951.

Zinc

Banks, T. E., Tupper, R. L. F., and Wormall, A.: 1. The determination of zinc[65] in tissues. 2. The fate of injected zinc carbonate and phosphate and a zinc dithizone complex. *Biochemical J., 47:* 466, 1950.

Cohn, E. J., et al.: Studies in Physical Chemistry of Insulin. I. The Solubility and Dielectric Properties of Insulin and Its Crystallization with Radioactive Zinc. *Science, 90:* 183, 1939.

Dougherty, E. C., and Lawrence, J. H.: Heavy and Radioactive Isotopes in Medicine, in *Advances in Biological and Medical Physics*. New York: Academic Press, Inc., 1948, vol. 1, p. 28.

Heath, J. C., and Liquier-Milward, J.: Distribution and function of zinc in normal and malignant tissues; uptake and distribution of Zn[65] in tissues. *Biochmica et Biophysica Acta, 5:* 404, 1950.

Hevesy, G.: *Radioactive Indicators*. New York: Interscience Publishers, 1948, p. 185.

Kamen, M. D.: *Radioactive Tracers in Biology*. New York: Academic Press, Inc., 1947, p. 244.

Montgomery, M. L., Sheline, G. E., and Chaikoff, I. L.: Elimination of Administered Zinc in Pancreatic Juice, Duodenal Juice, and Bile of Dog as Measured by Its Radioactive Isotope (Zn[65]). *J. Exper. Med.*, *78:* 151, 1943.

MULLER, J. H.: Donnees Experimentales et Cliniques de l'Emploi d'Isotopes Radioactifs Artificiels dans un fot de Radio Therapie Localisee. *Schweiz. Med. Wchschr.*, *77:* 236, 1947.

MULLER, J. H.: Intraperitoneal application of radioactive colloids, Chapter 13 in: *Therapeutic Use of Artificial Radioisotopes* (P. F. HAHN, ed.). New York: Wiley, 1956.

MULLER, J. H., AND ROSSIER, P. H.: A new method for the treatment of cancer of the lungs by means of artificial radioactivity (Zn[65] and Au[198]); first experimental and clinical studies. *Acta radiol, 35:* 449, 1951.

SHELINE, G. E., ET AL.: Studies on the Metabolism of Zinc with the Aid of its Radioactive Isotope; Excretion of Administered Zinc in Urine and Feces. *J. Biol. Chem., 147:* 409, 1943.

SHELINE, G. E., ET AL.: Studies on the Metabolism of Zinc with the Aid of its Radioactive Isotope; Distribution of Administered Radioactive Zinc in Tissues of Mice and Dogs. *J. Biol. Chem., 149:* 139, 1943.

Arsenic

BENDA, P., DAVID, M. AND CONSTANS, J.: Arsenic radioactif[76] as et détection préopératoire des tumeurs cérébrales. *Rev. Neurol., 89:* 101, 1953.

DOUGHERTY, E. C.: Arsenic, *Isotopic Tracers and Nuclear Radiations*, p. 533. William E. Siri, McGraw-Hill Book Co., Inc. New York, 1949.

DUCOFF, H. S., NEAL, W. B., STRAUBE, R. L., JACOBSON, L. O., AND BRUES, A. M.: Biological studies with arsenic [76]. II. Secretion and tissue localization. *Proc. Soc. Exper. Biol. and Med., 69:* 548, 1948.

DUPONT, O., ARIEL, I., AND WARREN, S. L.: The distribution of radioactive arsenic in the normal and tumor-bearing (Brown-Pearce) rabbit. *Am. J. Syphilis, Gonorrhea, Venereal Diseases, 26:* 96, 1942.

DUPONT, O., ARIEL, I., AND WARREN, S.: Conference on Applied Nuclear Physics, Massachusetts Inst. Tech. *J. Applied Phys.*, April, 1941.

IRVINE, J. W., JR.: *J. Phys. Chem., 46:* 910, 1942.

GRIFFON, H., AND BARBAUD, J.: A meethod which can be used in toxicology for the detection of arsenic in hair, by the study of the radioactivity of this element induced in situ. *Ann. Pharm. Fr., 9:* 545, 1951.

LAWTON, A. H., NESS, A. T., BRADY, F. J., AND COWIE, D. B.: Distribution of radioactive arsenic following intraperitoneal injection of sodium arsenite into cotton rats injected with litomosoides carinii. *Science, 102:* 120, 1945.

LOWRY, O. H., HUNTER, F. T., KIP, A. F., AND IRVINE, J. W., JR.: Radioactive tracer studies on arsenic injected as potassium arsenite. II. Chemical distribution in tissues. *J. Pharmacol. Exptl. Therap., 76:* 221, 1942.

MALLET, L.: Use of arsenic[76], the radioisotope, in the treatment of certain malignant skin diseases. *J. de Radiol. et d'Electricite Med., 32:* 506, 1951.

MALLET, L., MARCHAL, G., AND DUHAMEL, G.: Radioactive arsenic in the treatment of Hodgkin's disease and mycosis fungoides. *Acta Haematol., 7:* 27, 1952.

WALINDER, G.: Colloidal $AS_2{}^{76}S_3$. Its production and possible use in the treatment of papillomatosis of the urinary bladder. *Acta radiol. 44:* 521, 1955.

Antimony

BRADY, F. J., ET AL.: Localization of Trivalent Radioactive Antimony Following

Intravenous Administration to Dogs Infected with *Dirofilaria Immitis*. *Am. J. Trop. Med.*, *25:* 103, 1945.

COWIE, D. B., ET AL.: Localization of Radioactive Antimony Following Multiple Daily Injections to a Dog Infected with *Dirofilaria immitis*. *J. Washington Acad. Sc.*, *35:* 195, 1945.

CULBERTSON, J. T., ROSE, H. M., AND GONZALEZ, O. J.: Chemotherapy of Human Filariasis by the Administration of Neostibosan. *Am. J. Trop. Med.*, *25:* 271, 1945.

Gold

A *Manual, The properties and experimental use of radioactive colloidal gold*[198], Abbott Laboratories, Chicago, August, 1951.

ALLEN, W. M., SHERMAN, A. I. AND ARNESON, A. N.: Carcinoma of the cervix; results obtained from the irradiation of the parametrium with radioactive colloidal gold. *Am. J. Obst. & Gynec. 68:* 1433, 1954.

BARROW, J., TULLIS, J. L., AND CHAMBERS, F. W.: Effect of total body x-radiation, antistine and pyribenzamine on the phagocytic function of the reticuloendothelial system in rabbits injected intravenously with colloidal gold. Naval Med. Research Inst., Report No. 24 Project NM007039, 1949.

BERG, H. F.: Localization of radioactivity of colloidal gold[198]; preliminary report, *Arch. Surg.*, *63:* 545, 1951.

BERG, H. F., CHRISTOPHERSON, W. M., ISAACS, A. M. AND BRYANT, J. R.: Localization of radioactivity in regional lymph nodes. *A. M. A. Arch. Surg. 67:* 228, 1953.

BERG, H. F., ISAACS, A. M. AND CHRISTOPHERSON, W. M.: Localization of radioactivity in the urinary bladder and the regional lymph nodes. *J. Urol. 72:* 382, 1954.

BLOCK, WALTER D., BUCHANAN, O. H., AND FREYBERG, R. H.: Metabolism toxicity and manner of action of gold compounds used in the treatment of arthritis. V. A comparative study of the rate of absorption, the retention and the rate of excretion of gold administered in different compounds. *J. Pharmacol. & Exper. Therap.*, *82:* 391–398, 1944.

BURSTONE, M. S.: Effect of radioactive colloidal gold on the development of oral structures of the mouth. *Arch. Path.*, *50:* 419, 1950.

CLARK, T. H.: Radioactive colloidal gold in the treatment of neoplastic effusions. *Quart. Bull. Northwestern Univ. M. School 26:* 98, 1952.

DOUGHERTY, E. C., AND LAWRENCE, J. H.: Heavy and Radioactive Isotopes in Medicine, in *Advances in Biological and Medical Physics*. New York: Academic Press, Inc., 1948, p. 39.

ELLIS, F. AND OLIVER, R.: Treatment of papilloma of bladder with radioactive colloidal gold Au[198]. *Brit. M. J. 1:* 136, 1955.

FLOCKS, R. H., ELKINS, H. B. AND CULP, D.: Treatment of carcinoma of the prostate by interstitial injection of Au[198]: studies in problem of distribution. *J. Urol. 77:* 505, 1957.

FLOCKS, R. H., KERR, H. D., ELKINS, H. B. AND CULP, D. A.: The treatment of carcinoma of the prostate by interstitial radiation with radioactive gold (Au[198]): A follow-up report. *J. Urol. 71:* 628, 1954.

GOLDIE, H., AND HAHN, P. F.: Distribution and effect of colloidal radioactive gold in peritoneal fluid containing free sarcoma 37 cells. *Proc. Soc. Exper. Biol. & Med.*, *74:* 638–642, 1950.

HAHN, P. F., ED.: A manual of artificial radioisotope therapy. New York: Academic Press, 1951.

HAHN, P. F. AND CAROTHERS, E. L.: Lymphatic drainage following intrabronchial instillation of silver coated radioactive gold colloids in theraputic quantities. *J. Thoracic Surg. 25:* 265, 1953.

HAHN, P. F.: Silver coated radioactive colloids as adjuncts in the surgical treatment of bronchiogenic tumor. Chapter 17 in: *Theraputic Use of Artificial Radioisotopes* (P. F. HAHN, ed.). New York: Wiley, 1956.

HAHN, P. F.: Tumor Therapy by Direct Infiltration of Radioactive Colloidal Metallic Gold. *Fed. Proc., 7:* 271, 1948.

HAHN, P. F., AND CAROTHERS, E. L.: Radioactive metallic gold colloids coated with silver and their distribution in the lung and its lymphatics following intrapulmonary administration; Therapeutic implications in primary lung and bronchiogenic tumors. *Brit. J. Cancer, 5:* 400, 1951.

HAHN, P. F., AND CAROTHERS, E. L.: Use of radioactive colloidal metallic gold in the treatment of malignancies. *Nucleonics, 6:* 54, 1950.

HAHN, P. F., CAROTHERS, E. L., HILLIARD, G. W., BERNARD, L. AND JACKSON, M.: Treatment of chronic leukemias by intravenously administered radioactive colloids. Chapter 8 in: *Therapeutic Use of Artificial Radioisotopes* (P. F. HAHN, ed.). New York: Wiley, 1956.

HAHN, P. F., JACKSON, M. A., AND GOLDIE, H.: Liver cirrhosis with ascites, induced in dogs by chronic massive hepatic irradiation with radioactive colloidal gold. *Science, 114:* 1951.

HAHN, P. F., MILLER, L. L., ROBSCHEIT-ROBBINS, F. S., BALE, W. F., AND WHIPPLE, G. H.: Peritoneal absorption; red cells labeled by radio-iron hemoglobin move promptly from peritoneal cavity into the circulation. *J. Exper. Med., 80:* 77–82, 1944.

HAHN, P. F., AND SHEPPARD, C. W.: Selective Radiation Obtained by the Intravenous Administration of Colloidal Radioactive Isotopes in Diseases of the Lymphoid System. *South. M. J., 39:* 558, 1946.

HAHN, P. F., AND SHEPPARD, C. W.: The therapeutic use of radioactive elements in malignancy. *Ann. Internal. Med., 28:* 598, 1948.

HAHN, P. F., SKIPPER, H. E., CAROTHERS, E. L., AND BERNARD, L. J.: The effect of radioactive colloidal metallic gold in the treatment of "acute" AK-4 leukemia in mice. *Cancer, 4:* 634, 1951.

HAHN, P. F., AND WHIPPLE, G. H.: II. Iron metabolism. Its absorption, storage and utilization in experimental anemia. *Am. J. Med. Sci., 191:* 24, 1936.

HAHN, P. F., ET AL.: Direct Infiltration of Radioactive Isotopes as a Means of Delivering Ionizing Radiation to Discrete Tissues. *J. Lab. & Clin. Med., 32:* 1442, 1947.

HEVESY, G.: *Radioactive Indicators.* New York: Interscience Press, Inc., 1948, p. 184.

JENTZEN, A., AND WENGER, P.: Distribution of colloidal radioactive gold in organisms after intra-peritoneal injection. *Clin. Chir., 5:* 425, 1950.

JNANANDA, S.: Radioactive isotope of gold, $_{79}Au^{198}$ and low energy range of its spectrum. *Physical Review, 70:* 812–814, 1946.

JONES, H. B., WROBEL, C. J., AND LYONS, W. R.: A method of distributing beta radiation to the reticulo-endothelial system and adjacent tissues. *J. Clin. Invest., 23:* 783, 1944.

KARNOFSKY, D. A., BURCHENAL, J. H., ORMSLEE, R. A., CORNMAN, I., AND RHOADS, C. P.: *Approaches to tumor chemotherapy.* Amer. Assn. Advancement Sci., p. 293, 1947.

KERR, H. D., FLOCKS, R. H., ELKINS, H. B., CULP, D. AND EVANS, T. C.: Follow-up study of one hundred cases of carcinoma of the prostate treated with radioactive gold. *Radiology 64:* 637, 1955.

KING, E. R., SPICER, D. W., DOWDA, W. F., BENDER, M. A., AND NOEL, W. E.: The use of radioactive colloidal gold (Au¹⁹⁸) in pleural effusions and ascites associated with malignancy. *The Am. J. Roent., 68:* 413, 1952.

MACKAY, N. R.: Tolerance of the bladder to intracavity irradiation. *J. Urol. 76:* 396, 1956.

MATUSKA, R. H., HAHN, P. F., CARLSON, R. I., AUERBACH, S. H. AND MENEELY, G. R.: The lymphatic drainage of silver coated radioactive gold colloid following intra-thoracic administration to pneumonectomized dogs. *J. Thoracic Surg. 30:* 525, 1955.

MENEELY, G. R., KORY, R. C., AUERBACH, S. H., AND HAHN, P. F.: Distribution of radioactive colloidal gold following intra-pulmonary administration. *Fed. Proc., 10:* 365, 1951.

MULLER, J. H.: Further development of treatment of peritoneal and pleural metastases from ovarian carcinoma with radioactive gold. *Gynaecologia, 129:* 289, 1950 Basel.

MULLER, J. H.: Internal tumor therapy with artificial radioactive isotopes. In: "Artificial Radioactive Isotopes" in: *Physiology, Diagnostic Medicine and Therapy.* Springer ed. (1953) p. 746.

MULLER, J. H.: Intraperitoneal application of radioactive colloids, Chapter 13 in: *Theraputic Use of Artificial Radioisotopes* (P. F. HAHN, ed.). New York: Wiley, 1956.

MULLER, J. H., AND ROSSIER, P. H.: New method for treatment of cancer of the lungs by means of artificial radioactivity (Zn⁶³ and Au¹⁹⁸). *Acta Radiol., 35:* 449, 1951.

NEISON, C. M.: Use of radioactive gold in the treatment of carcinoma of the bladder: Report of eight cases. *South. Med. J. 48:* 245, 1955.

REMOLD, F., SIEGERT, A. AND STAMM, H.: Treatment of peritoneal and pleural carcinomatosis from ovarian carcinoma with radioactive gold, Au¹⁹⁸. *Strahlentherapie 94:* 367, 1954.

ROUSER, G.: Preparation of Radioactive Gold Colloids for Use in the Therapy of Malignancies. *Fed. Proc., 7:* 279, 1948.

SHEPPARD, C. W., GOODELL, J. P. B., AND HAHN, P. F.: Colloidal Gold Containing the Radioactive Isotope Au¹⁹⁸ in the Selective Internal Radiation Therapy of Diseases of the Lymphoid System. *J. Lab. & Clin. Med., 32:* 1437, 1947.

SHEPPARD, C. W., AND HAHN, P. F.: The Use of Colloidal Radioactive Gold in Medical Therapy. *Federation Proc., 6:* 399, 1947.

SHEPPARD, C. W., JORDON, G., AND HAHN, P. F.: Disappearance of isotopically labeled gold colloids from the circulation of the dog. *Am. J. Physiol., 164:* 345, 1951.

SHEPPARD, C. W., ET AL.: Studies of the Distribution of Intravenously Administered Colloidal Sols of Manganese Dioxide and Gold in Human Beings and Dogs Using Radioactive Isotopes. *J. Lab. & Clin. Med., 32:* 274, 1947.

SHERMAN, A. I., BONEBRAKE, M., AND ALLEN, W. M.: The application of radioactive colloidal gold in the treatment of pelvic cancer. *Am. J. Roent., 66:* 624, 1951.

SHERMAN, A. I., NOLAN, J. F., AND ALLEN, W. M.: Experimental application of radioactive colloidal gold in the treatment of pelvic cancer. *Am. J. Roent., 64:* 75, 1950.

SMITHERS, D. W., WALLACE, D. M. AND TROTT, N. G.: The use of radioactive isotopes in the treatment of patients with bladder tumors. Chapter 15 in: *Therapeutic Use of Artificial Radioisotopes* (P. F. HAHN, ed.). New York: Wiley, 1956.

TABERN, D. L., GLEASON, G. I., AND LEITNER, R. G.: Apparatus for administration of colloidal gold[198]. *Nucleonics, 10:* 63, 1952.

TALAIRACH, J., RUGGIERO, G., ABOULKER, J. AND DAVID, M. H.: A new method of treatment of inoperable brain tumors by stereotoxic implantation of radioactive gold—A preliminary report. *Brit. J. Radiol. 28:* 62, 1955.

WILLIAMS, G. Z., STANTON, A. C., JAMISON, R. M., AND WILLIAMS, J. T., R. N.: The distribution of radioactive gold colloid in rats, mice and transplanted mouse tumors. *Southern Medical Journal, 43:* 1031–1038, 1950.

WISH, L., FURTH, J., SHEPPARD, C. W., AND STOREY, R. H.: Disappearance rate of tagged substances from the circulation of roentgen irradiated animals. *Am. J. Roent., 67:* 628, 1952.

Radiogold

ANDREWS, G. A.: Status of radiogold therapy. *Nucleonics, 10:* 48, 1952.

HAIGLER, M. L., AND WILLIAMS, G. Z.: Failure of placenta to pass radioactive gold. *Cancer Research, 12:* 268, 1952.

HARSHA, W. N.: Uses of radioactive gold colloid in therapy and palliation of neoplastic disease. *Western J. Surg., 59:* 358, 1951.

KENT, E. M., AND MOSES, C.: Radioactive isotopes in the palliative management of carcinomatosis of the pleura. *J. Thoracic Surg., 22:* 503, 1951.

KOLETSKY, S., AND GUSTAFSON, G.: Liver damage in rats from radioactive colloidal gold. *Lab. Investigation, 1:* 312, 1952.

MULLER, J. H., AND HELD, H. E.: On the direct infiltration of malignant tumors and areas of neoplastic spread with radioactive colloidal gold (Au[198]) during surgery. *Gynaecologia, 131:* 385, 1951.

MYERS, W. G., COLMERY, B. H., JR.: Radioactive gold[198] in gold seeds for cancer therapy. *Cancer Research, 12:* 285, 1952.

WILLIAMS, G. Z.: Effect of methyl-4-dimethylaminoazobenzene and radiogold on rat liver. *Cancer Research, 12:* 309, 1952.

WILLIAMS, G. Z., AND WILLIAMS, J. T.: Effect of radiogold colloid on the growth of HS-1 ascites tumor in mice. *Cancer Research, 12:* 309, 1952.

Bromine

FINE, J., AND SELIGMAN, A. M.: Traumatic Shock; Study of Problem of "Lost Plasma" in Hemorrhagic Shock by Use of Radioactive Protein. *J. Clin. Investigation, 22:* 285, 1943.

Sodium

AIKAWA, J. K.: The significance of the radiosodium space in human disease. *South Med. J., 44:* 654, 1951.

ANDERSON, E., AND JOSEPH, M.: Urinary excretion of radioactive Na and K in adrenalectomized rats with and without salt. *Proc. Soc. Exptl. Biol. Med., 40:* 347–350, 1939.

ANDERSON, E., JOSEPH, M., AND EVANS, H. M.: The use of radio-sodium and radiopotassium in the study of adrenal physiology. *J. Applied Physics, 12:* 316, 1941.

ANDERSON, E., JOSEPH, M., AND HERRING, V.: Salt after adrenalectomy. II. Urinary excretion of radioactive Na and K in adrenalectomized rats given various levels of salt. *Proc. Soc. Exptl. Biol. Med., 44:* 482–485, 1940.

COOPER, F. W., ELKIN, D. C., SHEA, P. C., JR., AND DENNIS, E. W.: The study of peripheral vascular disease with radioactive isotopes. *Surg. Gynec. and Obst., 88:* 711, 1949.

COPE, O., COHN, W. E., AND BRENIZER, A. G., JR.: Gastric secretion. II. Absorption of radioactive sodium from pouches of the body and antrum of the stomach of the dog. *J. Clin. Invest., 22:* 103–110, 1943.

COX, L. W. AND CHALMERS, T. A.: The effect of pre-eclamptic toxaemia on the exchange of sodium in the body and the transfer of sodium across the placenta, measured by Na^{24} tracer methods. *J. Obst. & Gynaec. Brit. Empire 60:* 214, 1953.

COX, L. W. AND CHALMERS, T. A.: The transfer of sodium to the placental blood during the third stage of labor determined by Na^{24} tracer methods. *J. Obst. & Gynaec. Brit. Empire 60:* 226, 1953.

EICHLER, O., AND LINDER, F.: Formation of cerebrospinal fluid in the lumbar space shown by radioactive sodium. *Klin. Wchnschr., 29:* 9, 1951.

EISENMAN, A. J., OTT, L., SMITH, P. K., AND WINKLER, A. W.: A study of the permeability of human erythrocytes to potassium, sodium, and inorganic phosphate by the use of radioactive isotopes. *J. Biol. Chem., 135:* 165–173, 1940.

EVANS, T. C., AND QUIMBY, E. H.: Studies on Effects of Radioactive Sodium and of Roentgen Rays on Normal and Leukemic Mice. *Am. J. Roentgenol., 55:* 55, 1946.

EVANS, T. C., ET AL.: Effects of Radioactive Sodium on Leukemia and Allied Diseases. *Am. J. Roentgenol., 59:* 469, 1948.

FLEXNER, L. B., AND GELLHORN, A.: The comparative physiology of placental transfer. *Am. J. Obstet. Gynecol., 43:* 965–974, 1942.

FLEXNER, L. B., AND GELLHORN, A.: The transfer of water and sodium to the amniotic fluid of the guinea pig. *Am. J. Physiol., 136:* 757–761, 1942.

FLEXNER, L. B., AND POHL, H. A.: Transfer of Radioactive Sodium across the Placenta of the Guinea Pig. *Am. J. Physiol., 132:* 594, 1941.

FLEXNER, L. B., AND POHL, H. A.: Transfer of radioactive sodium across the placenta of the cat. *Proc. Soc. Exptl. Biol. Med., 44:* 345–346, 1940.

FLEXNER, L. B., AND POHL, H. A.: The transfer of radioactive sodium across the placenta of the rabbit. *Am. J. Physiol., 134:* 344–349, 1941.

FLEXNER, L. B., AND POHL, H. A.: The transfer of radioactive sodium across the placenta of the white rat. *J. Cellular Comp. Physiol., 18:* 49–59, 1941.

FLEXNER, L. B., AND ROBERTS, R. B.: The measurement of placental permeability with radioactive sodium; the relation of placental permeability to fetal size in the rat. *Am. J. Physiol., 128:* 154–158, 1939.

FLEXNER, L. B., WILDER, W. S., PROCTOR, N. K., COWIE, D. B., VOSBURGH, G. J., AND HELLMAN, L. M.: The estimation of extracellular and total body water in the newborn human infant with radioactive sodium and deuterium oxide. *J. Pediat., 30:* 413–415, 1947.

FOX, C., AND KESTON, A.: The Mechanism of Shock from Burns and Trauma Traced with Radiosodium. *Surg. Gynec. & Obst., 80:* 561, 1945.

GELLHORN, A., FLEXNER, L. B., AND HELLMAN, L. M.: The transfer of sodium across the human placenta. Preliminary report. *Am. J. Obstet. Gynecol., 46:* 688–672, 1943.

GELLHORN, A., FLEXNER, L. B., AND POHL, H. A.: The transfer of radioactive sodium across the placenta of the sow. *J. Cellular Comp. Physiol., 18:* 393–400, 1941.

GELLHORN, A., MERRELL, M., AND RANKIN, R. M.: The rate of transcapillary exchange of sodium in normal and shocked dogs. *Am. J. Physiol., 142:* 407–427, 1944.

GREENBERG, D. M., CAMPBELL, W. W., AND MURAYAMA, M.: Studies in mineral metabolism with the aid of artificial radioactive isotopes. V. Absorption, excretion and distribution of labeled sodium in rats maintained on normal and low sodium diets. *J. Biol. Chem.*, *136:* 35–46, 1940.

GREENBERG, D. M., AIRD, R. B., BOELTER, M. D. D., CAMPBELL, W. W., COHN, W. E., AND MURAYAMA, M. M.: A study with radioactive isotopes of the permeability of blood-cerebrospinal fluid barrier to ions. *Am. J. Physiol.*, *140:* 47–64, 1944.

HAHN, L., HEVESY, G., AND REBBE, O. H.: Do the potassium ions inside the muscle cells and blood corpuscles exchange with those present in the plasma? *Biochem. J.*, *33:* 1549–1558, 1939.

HAIGH, C. P., AND REISS, M.: Some applications of I^{131} and Na^{24} to clinical diagnoses. *Brit. J. Radiol.*, *23:* 534, 1950.

HAMILTON, J. G.: The Rates of Absorption of Radiosodium in Normal Human Subjects. *Proc. Natl. Acad. Sc.*, *23:* 521, 1937.

HAMILTON, J. G., AND STONE, R. S.: The Intravenous and Intraduodenal Administration of Radiosodium. *Radiology, 28:* 78, 1937.

HAMILTON, J. G., AND STONE, R. S.: Excretion of Radiosodium Following Intravenous Administration in Man. *Proc. Soc. Exper. Biol. & Med., 35:* 595, 1937.

HEPPEL, L. A.: The diffusion of radioactive sodium into the muscles of potassium-deprived rats. *Am. J. Physiol.*, *128:* 449–454, 1940.

HODGE, H. C., KOSS, W. F., GINN, J. T., FALKENHEIM, M., GAVETT, E., FOWLER, R. C., THOMAS, I., BONNER, J. F., AND DESSAUER, G.: The nature of the insoluble sodium of bone. The absorption of sodium at forty degrees by bone, dentin, enamel, and hydroxyapatite as shown by the radioactive isotope. *J. Biol. Chem., 148:* 321–331, 1943.

HUBBARD, J. P., PRESTON, W. N., AND ROSS, R. A.: The velocity of blood flow in infants and young children determined by radioactive sodium. *J. Clin. Invest., 21:* 613–617, 1942.

KALTREITER, M., ET AL.: Determination of the Volume of the Extracellular Fluid of the Body with Radioactive Sodium. *J. Exper. Med., 74:* 569, 1941.

KAMEN, M. D.: Alkali Metal and Alkaline Earth Tracers in *Radioactive Tracers in Biology.* New York: Academic Press, Inc., 1947, p. 213.

KETZ, S. S.: Measurement of regional circulation by the local clearance of radioactive sodium. *Am. Heart J., 38:* 321, 1949.

KINSEY, V. E., GRANT, W. M., COGAN, D. G., LIVINGOOD, J. J., AND CURTIS, B. R.: Sodium, chloride and phosphorus movement and the eye. *Arch. Ophthalmol. (Chicago), 27:* 1126–1131, 1942.

KOSS, W. F., AND GINN, J. T.: Distribution of sodium in the teeth and bones of dogs as shown by the radioactive isotope. *J. Dental Research, 20:* 465–470, 1941.

KUNKEL, H. A. AND SCHMERMUND, H. J.: Clearance studies with Na^{24} in the skin and in the subcutaneous tissues. *Klin. Wchnschr. 31:* 380, 1953.

LEVI, E. J., AND LEWISON, E. F.: Venous velocity in the leg measured with radioactive sodium. *Bull. Johns Hopkins Hosp., 86:* 370, 1950.

LOW-BEER, B. V. A.: *The clinical use of radioisotopes,* pp. 187–207, Charles C. Thomas, Publisher, Springfield, Ill. 1950.

MANERY, J. F., AND BALE, W. F.: The penetration of radioactive sodium and phosphorus into the extra- and intracellular phases of tissues. *Am. J. Physiol., 132:* 215–231, 1941.

MONTGOMERY, M. L., SHELINE, C. E., AND CHAIKOFF, I. L.: Elimination of sodium in pancreatic juice as measured by radioactive sodium. *Am. J. Physiol., 131:* 578–583, 1941.

MUFSON, I., QUIMBY, E. H., AND SMITH, B. C.: Use of radioactive sodium as a guide to the efficacy of drugs used in treatment of diseases of the peripheral vascular system. *Am. J. Med., 4:* 73, 1948.

POHL, H. A., AND FLEXNER, L. B.: Transfer of Radioactive Sodium across the Placenta of the Cat. *J. Biol. Chem., 139:* 163, 1941.

POMMERENKE, W. T., AND HAHN, P. F.: Secretion of radioactive sodium in human milk. *Proc. Soc. Exptl. Biol. Med., 52:* 223–224, 1943.

PRINZMETAL, M., CORDAY, E., SPRITZLER, R., AND FLEIG, W.: Radiocardiography and its clinical applications. *J.A.M.A., 139:* 617, 1949.

QUIMBY, E. H.: Radioactive Sodium as a Tool in Medical Research. *Am. J. Radiol., 58:* 741, 1947.

QUIMBY, E. H.: Radiosodium, a Diagnostic Tool. *Nucleonics, 1:* 2, 1947.

QUIMBY, E. H., AND SMITH, B. C.: Tracer studies with radioactive sodium in patients with peripheral vascular disease. *Science, 100:* 175–177, 1944.

REASER, P. B., AND BURCH, G. E.: Radiosodium tracer studies in congestive heart failure. *Proc. Soc. Exptl. Biol. Med., 63:* 543–546, 1946.

SEMPLE, R., MCDONALD, L., AND EKINS, R. P.: Radioactive sodium (Na^{24}) in the measurement of local blood flow. *Am. Heart J., 41:* 803, 1951.

SMITH, B. C., AND QUIMBY, E. H.: The Use of Radioactive Sodium in Studies of Circulation in Patients with Peripheral Vascular Diseases; Preliminary Report. *Surg., Gynec. & Obst., 79:* 142, 1944.

SMITH, B. C., AND QUIMBY, E. H.: The Use of Radioactive Sodium as a Tracer in the Study of Peripheral Vascular Disease. *Radiology, 45:* 335, 1945.

SMITH, B. C., AND QUIMBY, E. H.: The Use of Radioactive Sodium in the Study of Peripheral Vascular Disease. *Ann. Surg., 125:* 360–371, 1947.

SOHRNE, G.: Diagnostic use of radioactive common salt. *Acta Radiol., 26:* 279–284, 1945.

THOMPSON, S., QUIMBY, E. H., AND SMITH, B.: Radioactive Sodium as an Agent for Demonstrating the Effect of Pulmonary Resuscitative Procedures upon the Circulation. *Surg., Gynec. & Obst., 83:* 387, 1946.

THYGESEN, J. C., VIDEBOEK, A., AND VILLAUME, I.: Treatment of Leukemia with Artificial Radioactive Sodium. *Acta radiol., 25:* 305, 1944.

VEALL, N.: I. Some general problems in connection with the measurement of radioactivity in patients. *Brit. J. Radiol., 23:* 527, 1950.

VISSCHER, M. B., AND CARR, C. W.: The rate of entrance of radiosodium into the aqueous humor and cerebrospinal fluid. *Am. J. Physiol., 142:* 27–31, 1944.

VISSCHER, M. B., VARCO, R. H., CARR, C. W., DEAN, R. B., AND ERICKSON, D.: Sodium ion movement between the intestinal lumen and blood. *Am. J. Physiol., 141:* 488–505, 1944.

WALTON, R. J.: Therapeutic uses of radioisotopes in the royal cancer hospital. *Brit. J. Radiol., 23:* 559, 1950.

WINKLER, A. W., EISENMAN, A. J., AND SMITH, P. K.: The use of radioactive isotopes in studies of the permeability of the human erythrocyte. *J. Applied Phys., 12:* 349, 1941.

WINKLER, A. W., ELKINTON, J. R., AND EISENMAN, A. J.: Comparison of sulfocyanate with radioactive chloride and sodium in measurement of extracellular fluid. *Am. J. Physiol., 139:* 239–246, 1943.

Potassium

BAUER, FRANZ K., CASSEN, BENEDICT, YOUTCHEFF, ELSIE AND SHOOP, LUCILLE: Jet injection of radioisotopes; A clinical study comparing needle and jet injection of I^{131}, K^{42} and Na^{24}. *Am. J. M. Sc. 225:* 374, 1953.

FENN, W. O., ET AL.: Exchange of Radioactive Potassium with Body Potassium. *Am. J. Physiol., 135:* 149, 1941.

HEVESY, G.: Potassium Interchange in the Human Body. *Acta physiol. scandinav., 3:* 123, 1942.

LOCKSLEY, H. B., SWEET, W. H., POWSNER, H. J. AND DOW, E.: Suitability of tumor-bearing mice for predicting relative usefulness of isotopes in brain tumors; comparative clinical and laboratory study in localization and treatment of brain tumors with P^{32}, Na^{24}, K^{42} and sodium borate. *A. M. A. Arch. Neurol. & Psychiat., 71:* 684, 1954.

NATHANSON, I. T., BAKER, W. H. AND SELVERSTONE, B.: Radioactive potassium (K^{42}) in the study of benign and malignant breast tumors. (Abstr.) *Proc. Am. A. Cancer Res. 1:* 40, 1953.

SEAMAN, W. B., TER-POGOSSIAN, M. M. AND SCHWARTZ, H. G.: Localization of intra-cranial neoplasms with radioactive isotopes. *Radiology, 62:* 30, 1954.

SELVERSTONE, B., SWEET, W. H. AND IRETON, R. J.: Radioactive Potassium, A New Isotope for Brain Tumor Localization. Surgical Forum: Proceedings of the Forum Sessions, Thirty-sixth Clinical Congress of the American College of Surgeons, Boston, Mass., October, 1950. W. B. Saunders Company, Philadelphia, pp. 371–375, 1951.

SELVERSTONE, B. AND WHITE, J. C.: Evaluation of the radioactive mapping technic in the surgery of brain tumors. *Ann. Surg., 134:* 387, 1951.

SUSEN, A. F., SMALL, W. T. AND MOORE, F. D.: Studies on the External Diagnostic Localization of Brain Lesions Using Radioactive Potassium. Surgical Forum: Proceedings of the Forum Sessions, Thirty-sixth Clinical Congress of the American College of Surgeons, Boston, Massachusetts, October, 1950. W. B. Saunders Company, Philadelphia, pp. 362–368, 1951.

Calcium and Strontium

ARMSTRONG, W. D., AND BARNUM, C. P.: Concurrent use of Radioisotopes of Calcium and Phosphorus in the Study of Metabolism of Calcified Tissues. *J. Biol. Chem., 172:* 199, 1948.

BELLIN, J. AND LASZLO, D.: Metabolism and removal of Ca^{45} in man. *Science 117:* 331, 1953.

BURCH, G. E., THREEFOOT, S. A., AND RAY, C. T.: Rates of turnover and biologic decay of chloride and chloride space in the dog determined with the long-life isotope, Cl^{36}, *J. Lab. & Clin. Med., 35:* 331, 1950.

CAMPBELL, W. W., AND GREENBERG, D. M.: Studies in Calcium Metabolism with the Aid of its Induced Radioactive Isotope. *Proc. Nat. Acad. Sc., 26:* 176, 1940.

COPP, D. H., and GREENBERG, D. M.: Studies on Bone Fracture Healing. I. Effects of Vitamins A and D. *J. Nutrition, 29:* 261, 1945.

ENGFELDT, B., BJÖRNERSTEDT, R., CLEMEDSON, C. J. AND ENGSTROM, A.: A preliminary study of the in vivo in vitro uptake of Sr^{90} in bone tissue and the osseous localization of radioactive fission products from atomic explosions. *Acta Orthop. Scandinav. 24:* 101, 1954.

ERF, L. A., AND PECHER, CHARLES: Secretion of radiostrontium in milk of two cows following intravenous administration. *Proc. Soc. Exper. Biol. and Med., 45:* 762–764, 1940.

EVANS, F. G., CARLBAUGH, C. C., AND LEBOW, M.: An apparatus for measuring bone density by means of radioactive strontium (Sr⁹⁰). *Science, 114:* 182, 1951.

FITZGERALD, P. J.: Radioautography in cancer. *Cancer 5:* 166, 1952.

FRIEDELL, H. L., THOMAS, C. I. AND KROHMER, J. S.: An evaluation of the clinical use of a strontium 90 beta-ray applicator with a review of the underlying principles. *Am. J. Roentgenol. 71:* 25, 1954.

FRIEDELL, H. L., THOMAS, C. I., AND KROHMER, J. S.: Beta-ray application to the eye. With the description of an applicator utilizing Sr⁹⁰ and its clinical use. *Am. J. Ophth., 33:* 525–535, 1950.

FRIEDELL, H. L. AND SALERNO, P. R.: Synergistic effect of radioisotopes used in combination. Chapter 6 in: *Theraputic Use of Artificial Radioisotopes* (P. F. HAHN, ed.). New York: Wiley, 1956.

GREENBERG, D. M.: Studies in Mineral Metabolism with the Aid of Artificial Radioactive Isotopes. Tracer Experiments with Radioactive Calcium and Strontium on the Mechanism of Vitamin D Action in Rachitic Rats. *J. Biol. Chem., 157:* 99, 1945.

JARBAK, J. R., KAMINS, M. M. AND VEHE, K. L.: Radioautographic study of the deposition of calcium in the cranium, teeth and mandible. *J. Am. Dent. A. 47:* 639, 1953.

LAWRENCE, J. H., AND WASSERMAN, L. R.: Multiple myeloma; a study of 24 patients treated with radioactive isotopes (P³² and Sr⁸⁹). *Ann. Int. Med., 33:* 41, 1950.

LEDERMAN, M.: Some applications of radioactive isotopes in ophthalmology. *Brit. J. Radiol. 29:* 1, 1956.

LEDERMAN, M. AND SINCLAIR, W. K.: Radioactive isotopes for beta- and gamma-ray applicators, Chapter 16 in: *Theraputic Use of Artificial Radioisotopes* (P. F HAHN, ed.). New York: Wiley, 1956.

LUSHBAUGH, C. C. AND HALE, D. B.: Experimental acute radiodermatitis following beta irradiation. IV. Changes in respiration and glycolysis. *Cancer 6:* 686, 1953.

LUSHBAUGH, C. C. AND HALE, D. B.: Experimental acute radiodermatitis following beta irradiation. V. Histopathological study of the mode of action of therapy with Aloe vera. *Cancer 6:* 690, 1953.

LUSHBAUGH, C. C., STORER, J. B. AND HALE, D. B.: Experimental acute radiodermatitis following beta irradiation. I. Its pathogenesis and repair. *Cancer 6:* 671, 1953.

LUSHBAUGH, C. C. AND STORER, J. B.: Experimental acute radiodermatitis following beta irradiation. II. The inhibition of fibroplasia. *Cancer 6:* 678, 1953.

MARSHAK, A., AND BRYON, R. L.: A Method for Studying Healing of Bone. *J. Bone & Joint Surg., 27:* 95, 1945.

PAHAUT, J. E. AND GOVAERTS, J.: Use of radioactive strontium Sr⁸⁹ in treatment of cancer. *J. radiol. et electrol. 37:* 164, 1956.

PECHER, C.: Biological Investigations with Radioactive Calcium and Strontium. *Proc. Soc. Exper. Biol. & Med., 46:* 86, 1941.

PECHER, CHARLES: Biological investigations with radioactive calcium and strontium. Preliminary report on the use of radioactive strontium in the treatment of metastatic bone cancer. *Univ. California Publ. Pharmacol., 2:* 117–150, 1942.

PECHER, C., AND PECHER, J.: Radiocalcium and Radiostrontium Metabolism in Pregnant Mice. *Proc. Soc. Exper. Biol. & Med., 46:* 91, 1941.

SHIPLEY, P. G., PARK, E. A., McCOLLUM, E. V., SIMMONDS, NINA, AND KINNEY, E. M.: Studies on experimental rickets. XX. The efforts of strontium administration on the histological structure of the growing bones. *Bull. Johns Hopkins Hosp., 33:* 216–220, 1922.

SKLAROFF, D. M.: Treatment of hemangiomas with strontium-90 beta-ray applicator. *Radiology 68:* 87, 1957.

SMITH, M. E.: The Role of Boron in Plant Metabolism. I. Boron in Relation to the Absorption and Solubility of Calcium. *Australian J. Exper. Biol. & M. Sc., 22:* 257, 1944.

THOMAS, R. O., LITOVITZ, T. A., RUBIN, M. I., AND GESCHICKTER, C. F.: Dynamics of calcium metabolism: Time distribution of intravenously administered radiocalcium. *Am. J. Physiol., 169:* 568, 1952.

Sulfur

BORSOOK, H., ET AL.: The Course of Thiamin Metabolism in Man as Indicated by the Use of Radioactive Sulfur. *Proc. Natl. Acad. Sc., 26:* 412, 1940.

DOUGHERTY, E. C., AND LAWRENCE, J. H.: Heavy and Radioactive Isotopes in Clinical and Experimental Medicine, in *Advances in Biological and Medical Physics*. New York: Academic Press, Inc., 1948, vol. 1, p. 34.

GOTTSCHALK, R. G., AND ALLEN, H. C., JR., Uptake of Radioactive Sulphur by Chondrosarcoma in Man. *Proc. Soc. Exptl. Biol. Med., 80:* 334, June 1952.

HENDRICKS, R. H., ET AL.: Measurement of the Activity of Radiosulfur in Barium Sulfate. *J. Phys. Chem., 47:* 469, 1943.

HERSHEY, A. D.: An upper limit to the protein content of germinal substance of bacteriophages. *Virology 1:* 108, 1955.

HERSHEY, A. D.: Conservation of nucleic acids during bacterial growth. *J. Gen. Physiol. 38:* 145, 1954.

HERSHEY, A. D.: Nucleic acid economy in bacteria infected with bacteriophage T2; phage precursor nucleic acid. *J. Gen. Physiol. 37:* 1, 1953.

HERSHEY, A. D. AND CHASE, M.: Independent functions of viral protein and nucleic acid in growth of bacteriophage. *J. Gen. Physiol. 36:* 39, 1952.

KAMEN, M. D.: *Isotopic Tracers in Biology.* New York: Acad. Press, 1957, Ch. 8, p. 352.

HILL, E. M., AND ROBSON, W.: A New Synthesis of Methionine and a Scheme Relating Certain a-Amino Acids. *Biochem. J., 30:* 248, 1936.

KAMEN, M. D.: *Radioactive Tracers in Biology.* New York: Academic Press, Inc., 1947, p. 201.

LAWRENCE, JOHN A., AND HAMILTON, JOS. G., *Advances in Biologic and Medical Physics*, Vol. II, page 301, 1951.

OSBORNE, J. C. AND KOWALEWSKI, K.: The uptake of radiosulfur in the fractured humerus in the rat. *Surg., Gynec. & Obst. 103:* 38, 1956.

TARVER, H., AND SCHMIDT, C. L. A.: The Conversion of Methionine to Cystine: Experiments with Radioactive Sulfur (S^{35}). *J. Biol. Chem., 130:* 67, 1939.

TARVER, H., AND SCHMIDT, C. L. A.: Radioactive Sulfur Studies; Synthesis of Methionine; Conversion of Methionine Sulfur to Taurine Sulfur in Dogs and Rats; Distribution of Sulfur in the Proteins of Animals Fed Sulfur or Methionine. Experiments *in vitro* with Sulfur and Hydrogen Sulfide. *J. Biol. Chem., 146:* 69, 1942.

WORMALL, A.: The use of radioisotopes in immunology. *Brit. J. Radiol. 28:* 33, 1955.

Carbon

ALLEN, M. B., AND RUBEN, S.: Tracer Studies with Radioactive Carbon and Hydrogen. The Synthesis and Oxidation of Fumaric Acid. *J. Am. Chem. Soc., 64:* 948, 1942.

BARKER, H. A., AND KAMEN, M. D.: Carbon Dioxide Utilization in the Synthesis of Acetic Acid by *Clostridium thermoaceticum. Proc. Nat. Acad. Sc., 31:* 219, 1945.

BARKER, H. A., KAMEN, M. D., AND HAAS, V.: Carbon Dioxide Utilization in the Synthesis of Acetic and Butyric Acids by *Butyribacterium rettgeri. Proc. Nat. Acad. Sc., 31:* 355, 1945.

BARKER, H. A., KAMEN, M. D., AND BORNSTEIN, B. T.: The Synthesis of Butyric and Caproic Acids from Ethanol and Acetic Acid by *Clostridium kluyveri. Proc. Nat. Acad. Sc., 31:* 373, 1945.

BARKER, H. A., RUBEN, S., AND KAMEN, M. D.: The Reduction of Radioactive Carbon Dioxide by Methane-producing Bacteria. *Proc. Nat. Acad. Sc., 26:* 426, 1940.

BARCLAY, W. R., EBERT, R. H., LEROY, G. V., MANTHEI, R. W. AND ROTH, L. J.: Distribution and excretion of radioactive isoniazid in tuberculous patients. *J. A. M. A. 151:* 1384, 1953.

BUCHANAN, J. M., AND HASTINGS, A. B.: The Use of Isotopically Marked Carbon in the Study of Intermediary Metabolism. *Physiol. Rev., 26:* 120, 1946.

BUCHANAN, J. M. HASTINGS, A. B., AND NESBETT, F. B.: The role of Carboxyl-labeled Acetic, Propionic, and Butyric Acids in Liver Glycogen Formation. *J. Biol. Chem., 150:* 413, 1943.

CONANT, J. B., ET AL.: Metabolism of Lactic Acid Containing Radioactive Carboxyl Carbon. *J. Biol. Chem., 137:* 557, 1941.

DePAEPE, J. C. AND FICQ, A.: A preliminary study of the metabolism of the nucleic acids and proteins in the cervical epithelium: Autoradiographic study of normal and neoplastic tissues. *Brit. J. Radiol. 30:* 141, 1957.

KAMEN, M. D.: *Isotopic Tracers in Biology.* (Chapter X, The isotopes of carbon) p. 293–338, New York: Acad. Press, 1957.

KAMEN, M. D.: *Radioactive Tracers in Biology.* New York: Academic Press, Inc., 1947, pp. 148, 168.

LAWRENCE, J. H. AND TOBIAS, C. A.: Radioactive isotopes and nuclear radiations in treatment of cancer. *Cancer. Res. 16:* 185, 1956.

OKITA, G. T., KELSEY, F. E., TALSO, P. J., SMITH, L. B. AND GEILING, E. M. K.: Studies on the renal excretion of radioactive digitoxin in human subjects with cardiac failure. *Circulation 7:* 161, 1953.

RUBEN, S., KAMEN, M. D., AND HASSID, W. Z.: Photosynthesis with Radioactive Carbon. II. Chemical Properties of the Intermediates. *J. Am. Chem. Soc., 62:* 3443, 1940.

SOLOMON, A. K., ET AL.: The Participation of Carbon Dioxide in the Carbohydrate Cycle. *J. Biol. Chem., 140:* 171, 1941.

VENNESLAND, B.: Nitrogen and Carbon Isotopes: Their Application *in vivo* to the Study of the Animal Organism in *Advances in Biological and Medical Physics.* New York: Academic Press, Inc., 1948, vol. 1, p. 45.

Gallium

ANDREWS, G. A., ROOT, S. W. AND KERMAN, H. D.: Study of gallium[72]. VI. Clinical studies with gallium[72]. *Radiology 61:* 570, 1953.

BEHRENS, C. F.: Recent advances in radioisotope therapy. *Southern M. J. 46:* 1155, 1953.

BRUCER, M., ANDREWS, G. A. AND BRUNER, H. D.: A study of gallium[72]; summary and conclusions. *Radiology 61:* 534, 1953.

Brucer, M., Andrews, G. A., Rehbock, D. J., Root, S. W., and Gray, J.: A study of gallium[72]. VIII. Autopsy studies of distribution of gallium[72]. *Radiology 61:* 590, 1953.

Brucer, M. and Bruner, H. D.: A study of gallium[72]. I. Physics and radiation characteristics of gallium[72]. *Radiology 6:* 537, 1953.

Bruner, H. D.: Problems with newer isotopes being investigated. *Nucleonics, 10:* 49, 1952.

Bruner, H. D., Cooper, B. M. and Rehbock, D. J.: A study of gallium[72]. IV. Toxicity of gallium citrate in dogs and rats. *Radiology 61:* 550, 1953.

Bruner, H. D., Hayes, R. L. and Perkinson, J. D., Jr.: A study of gallium[72]. X. Preliminary data on gallium[67]. *Radiology 61:* 602, 1953.

Dudley, H. C.: Biological Significance of Radiogallium. (To be published.)

Dudley, H. C.: *Photofluormetric Determination of Gallium in Tissues.* Naval Medical Research Institute, Nat. Naval Medical Center, Bethesda, Md. Project NM 011 013, Report No. 1, Jan., 1948.

Dudley, H. C.: Determination of gallium in biological materials. *J. Pharmacol. and Exper. Therapeutics, 95:* 482–486, 1949.

Dudley, H. C.: Preparation of gallium citrate. *J. Am. Chem. Soc., 72:* 3822, 1950.

Dudley, H. C., and Garzoli, R. F.: *Preparation and Properties of Gallium Lactate.* Naval Medical Research Institute, Nat. Naval Medical Center, Bethesda, Md., Project NM 011 013, Report No. II, May, 1948.

Dudley, H. C., and Levine, M. D.: Studies of the toxic action of gallium. *J. Pharmacol. and Exper. Therapeutics, 95:* 487–493, 1949.

Dudley, H. C., Louviere, L. J., and Shaw, J. C.: Effects of injection of radiogallium, NM 007081.06.10, The Naval Medical Research Institute, National Naval Medical Center, Bethesda, Maryland, Sept. 15, 1951.

Dudley, H. C., and Maddox, G. E.: Deposition of radiogallium (Ga[72]) in skeletal tissues. *J. Pharmacol. and Exper. Therapeutics, 96:* 224–227, 1949.

Dudley, H. C., Henry, K. E., and Lindsley, B. F.: Studies of the toxic action of gallium II. *J. Pharmacol. and Exper. Therapeutics, 98:* 409–417, 1950.

Dudley, H. C., Imirie, G. W., Jr., and Istock, J. T.: Deposition of radiogallium (Ga[72]) in proliferating tissues. *Radiology, 55:* 571–578, 1950.

Dudley, H. C., Maddox, G. E., and LaRue, H. C.: Studies of the metabolism of gallium. *J. Pharmacol. and Exper. Therapeutics, 96:* 135–138, 1949.

Dudley, H. C., Markowitz, H. A. and Mitchell, T. G.: Studies on the localization of radioactive gallium (Ga[72]) in bone lesions. *J. Bone & Joint Surg. 38A:* 627, 1957.

Dudley, H. C., Munn, J. I., and Henry, K. E.: Studies of the metabolism of gallium, II. *J. Pharmacol. and Exper. Therapeutics, 98:* 105–110, 1950.

Einecke, E.: Salt-like Compounds of Gallium. *Chemie., 55:* 40, 1942.

King, E. R., and Perkinson, J. D.: Preliminary distribution studies of Ga[72] in the wistar rat. *Texas Reports on Biology and Medicine, 8:* 443, 1950.

King, E. R., Perkinson, J. D., Jr., Bruner, H. D., and Gray, J.: Excretion of gallium by the rat and man. *Science, 113:* 555, 1951.

Lang, F. R.: Study of the use of radioactive gallium in medicine. *Ann. Int. Med., 35:* 1237, 1951.

Meek, S. F., Harrold, G. C., and McCord, C. P.: Toxicity of gallium. *Indust. Med. 12:* 7, 1943.

Mulry, W. C., and Dudley, H. C.: Radiogallium as a diagnostic agent in bone tumors. *J. Lab. and Clin. Med., 37:* 239, 1951.

Mulry, W. C., and Dudley, H. C.: Studies of radiogallium as a diagnostic agent in bone tumors, Project N.M. 007 081.06.09, Naval Medical Research Institute, National Naval Medical Center, Bethesda, Maryland, March 1, 1951.

MUNN, J. I., DUDLEY, H. C., WALTERS, N. H., AND MORRER, H. H.: The urinary excretion of gallium, N.M. 007 081.06.11, Naval Medical Research Inst., National Naval Medical Center, Bethesda, Maryland, Dec. 17, 1951.

NEOGI, P., AND NAUDI, S. K.: New Compounds of Gallium I. *J. Indian Chem. Soc.*, *13:* 399, 1936.

PERKINSON, J. D., JR., ELDRIDGE, J. S. AND COOPER, B. M.: A study of gallium[72]. II. Gallium chemistry of biological interest. *Radiology 61:* 543, 1953.

RABUTEAU, A.: Recherches sur les effets des sel a de gallium. *Compt. rend. Soc. de biol., 5:* 310, 1883.

SANDELL, E. B.: Determination of Gallium in Silicate Rocks. *Analyt. Chem., 19:* 63, 1947.

SCHWARZ, L., AND SICKLE, F.: Über gallium. *Arch. Hyg., 100:* 143, 1928.

SWIFT, E. H.: New method for the separation of gallium from other elements. *J. Am. Chem. Soc., 46:* 2375, 1924.

Yttrium

ANDREWS, G. A., KYKER, G. C., KNISELEY, R. M. AND PALMER, E. L.: Preliminary studies of yttrium-90 in man, Abstracted, *Proc. Am. Assoc. Cancer Research 2:* 1, 1955.

BOYESEN, S. AND CAMPBELL, J. B.: Stereotoxic implantation of calibrated Pd^{109} and Y^{90} spheres: A technique for producing predictable subcortical lesions in the brains of laboratory animals. *Yale J. Biol. & Med. 28:* 216, 1955.

BULKLEY, G. J., COOPER, J. A. D. AND O'CONOR, V. J.: Intraprostatic injection of radioactive yttrium chloride in the dog. *Surg., Gynec. & Obst. 100:* 405, 1955.

EINHORN, J., LARSSON, L. G. AND RAGNHULT, I.: Radioactive yttrium (Y^{90}) as a possible adjunct in the treatment of papillomatosis of the urinary bladder. *Acta radiol. 43:* 298, 1955.

FITZGERALD, P. J.: Radioautography in cancer. *Cancer 5:* 166, 1952.

KYKER, G. C.: The distribution of interstitial and intracavitary injections of certain radiochemical preparations of medical interest. *Bol. Asoc. Med. Puerto Rico 46:* 362, 1954.

SIEGEL, E. P., HART, H. E., BROTHERS, M. E., SPENCER, H. AND LOSZLO, D.: Radioyttrium (Y^{90}) for the palliative treatment of effusions due to malignancy. *J. A. M. A. 161:* 499, 1956.

Chromium

ABAJIAN, J., JR., BRAZELL, E., MILLS, E. L. AND PETERSON, O. S., JR.: Blood volume studies utilizing the radiochromium 51 method and its application to anesthesiology. *Anesthesiology 16:* 733, 1955.

APT, L. AND POLLYCOVE, M.: The anemia of chronic renal disease. *Am. J. Dis. Children 90:* 633, 1955.

GIBSON, JOHN, G. II. AND SCHEITLIN, W. A.: A method employing radioactive chromium for assaying the viability of human erythrocytes returned to the circulation after refrigerated storage. *J. Lab. & Clin. Med. 46:* 679, 1955.

KORST, D. R., CLATANOFF, D. V. AND SCHILLING, R. F.: External scintillation counting over the liver and spleen after the transfusion of radioactive erythrocytes. *Clin. Res. Proc. 3:* 192, 1955.

KURTZ, M. M. AND TIVEY, H.: Use of radioactive chromium 51 as the erythrocyte tagging agent in determining blood volume and in vivo erythrocyte survival. *Am. J. Med. 19:* 299, 1955.

REILLY, W. A., FRENCH, R. M., LAU, F. Y. K., SCOTT, K. G. AND WHITE, W. E.: Whole blood volume determined by radiochromium-tagged red cells; comparative studies on normal and congestive heart failure patients. *Circulation 9:* 571, 1954.

REILLY, W. A., HELWIG, H. L. AND SCOTT, K. G.: Blood volume measurements in cancer using the Cr[51] red blood cell tagging method. *Cancer 9:* 273, 1956.

STOHLMAN, F., JR. AND SCHNEIDERMAN, M. A.: Application of the Cr[51] technique to the study of experimental hemolysis in the dog. *J. Lab. & Clin. Med. 47:* 72, 1956.

STRUMIA, M. M., TAYLOR, L., SAMPLE, A. B., COLWELL, L. S. AND DUGAN, A.: Uses and limitations of survival studies of erythrocytes tagged with Cr[51]. *Blood 10:* 429, 1955.

WENNESLAND, R.: Intra- and extra-vascular distribution of carbon monoxide (Co and radioactive chromium 51) in blood volume determination. *Am. J. Med. 19:* 287, 1955.

Miscellaneous isotopes

ABERSOLD, P. C.: Radioisotopes as sources of gamma rays for therapy. *Am. J. Roentgenol. 70:* 126, 1953.

ABERSOLD, P. C.: The development of nuclear medicine. *Am. J. Roentgenol. 75:* 1027, 1956.

Atomic Energy Commission: Announcements of the isotopes division: Isotopes for teletherapy. *Isotopics, 2:* No. 4, 2, 1952.

BRUCER, MARSHALL: Therapeutic potentialities of radioisotopes. *The Merck Report, 61:* 9, 1952.

BRUCER, M. H.: Statement of Medical Division, Oak Ridge Institute of Nuclear Studies, Oak Ridge, Tenn., Progress Report on Atomic Energy Research page 229, U. S. Gov. Printing Press, Washington, 1956.

BRUCER, M.: An automatic controlled pattern cesium 137 teletherapy machine. *Am. J. Roentgenol. 75:* 49–55, January 1956.

CARA, D. J.: Factors determining depth dose distribution from a ruthenium plague. *Texas Reports on Biol. and Med., 8:* 471, 1950.

COMAS, F. AND BRUCER, M.: First impressions of therapy with cesium 137. *Radiology 69:* 231, August 1957.

COPELAND, M. M.: Evaluation of radioisotopes as an adjunct to surgical diagnosis and therapy. *J. Bone & Joint Surg. 33A:* 1021, 1951.

FREUNDLICH, H. F. AND HAYBITTLE, J. L.: An improved iridium-192 teletherapy unit, *Acta. radiol. 39:* 231, 1953.

FREUNDLICH, H. F., HAYBITTLE, J. L., AND QUICK, R. S.: Radio-iridium teletherapy. *Acta. Radiol., 34:* 115, 1950.

GREEN, D. T., ERRINGTON, R. F., BOYD, F. C. AND HOPKINS, N. J.: Production of multicurie gamma-ray teletherapy sources. *Nucleonics 11:* 29, 1953.

GREENBERG, D. M., AIRD, R. B., BOELTER, M. D. D., CAMPBELL, W. W., COHN, W. E., AND MURAYAMA, M. M.: A study with radioactive isotopes of the permeability of blood-cerebrospinal fluid barrier to ions. *Am. J. Physiol., 140:* 47–64 (1943).

KELLY, F. J., SVEDBERG, A. H., AND HARP, V. C., JR.: The transfer of radioactive mercury across a membrane produced by application of cantharides to the skin of man. *J. Clin. Investigation, 29:* 988, 1950.

KING, E. R.: Practical radioisotope therapy. *Medical Annals of D. C. 24:* 652, 1955.

MITCHELL, J. S.: Practical aspects of radioactive isotopes in relation to medical treatment. *Brit. M. J.*, Vol. II, 747, 1951.

RAY, C. T., BURCH, G. E., THREEFOOT, S. A., AND KELLY, F. J.: The distribution of radiomercury of a mercurial diuretic in some of the body fluids of man. *Am. J. of Med. Sc.*, *220:* 160, 1950.

SMITHERS, D. W., WALLACE, D. M. AND TROTT, N. G.: The use of radioisotopes in the treatment of patients with bladder tumors. Chapter 15 in: *Theraputic Use of Artificial Radioisotopes* (P. F. HAHN, ed.). New York: Wiley, 1956.

STOUT, P. R.: Applications of radioactive K, Rb, Na, P, and Br to studies of the mineral nutrition of higher plants. *J. Applied. Phys.*, *12:* 327, 1941.

VAN DER WERFF, J.Th.: Bi^{206} a pure gamma-emitter for therapy. *J. belge de radiol.* *39:* 134, 1956.

VOLKER, J. F., HODGE, H. C., WILSON, H. J., AND VAN VOORHIS, S. N.: The absorption of fluorides by enamel, dentin, bone, and hydroxyapatite as shown by the radioactive isotope. *J. Biol. Chem.*, *134:* 543–548, 1940.

VOLKER, J. F., SOGNNAES, R. F., AND BIBBY, B. G.: Studies on the distribution of radioactive fluoride in the bones and teeth of experimental animals. *Am. J. Physiol.*, *132:* 707–712, 1941.

WILLIAMS, M. M. D. AND CHILDS, D. S., JR.: Diagnostic tests that depend on radio-isotope localization. *Am. J. Roentgenol.* *75:* 1040, 1956.

WILLS, J. H.: Secretion of intravenously injected fluorine in the submaxillary saliva of cats. *J. Dental Research*, *19:* 585–590, 1940.

21 ▸

The Design and Operation of Medical Radioisotope Laboratories

GORDON C. BELL, B.S., M.S. AND W. S. MAXFIELD, M.D.

21.0 Introduction and Main Features

Radioisotopes have attained an important place as valuable tools in medical research, diagnosis and therapy. However, many hospitals and medical groups still lack a radioactive isotope laboratory due mainly to the lack of trained personnel and the high cost of equipment. Nevertheless, the number of radioisotope laboratories is constantly increasing because of the demand for the useful tests they make possible.

The requirements for space, equipment and personnel vary greatly with the volume and type of work to be performed. Since most laboratories are established initially to do diagnostic studies, an adequately equipped laboratory for such studies will be the main feature of this discussion. Therapeutic applications usually involve I^{131}, P^{32} and occasionally Au^{198}. Modifications needed to deal with these will be noted.

Essentially, the establishment and operation of a radioisotope laboratory can be divided into five categories:
1. Design and construction
2. Equipment required
3. License for use of radioisotopes
4. Personnel
5. Operation

21.1 Design and Construction

The diagnostic laboratory is usually divided into two areas, the counting area and one for the preparation of doses to be administered and for storage. Most commonly two separate rooms are used but one large room may suffice.

The counting area should be located away from the storage space of large amounts of radioactive materials (over 10 mc); also away from diagnostic and therapeutic x-ray units to avoid an elevated background counting rate. If proper location of this room is not possible, it may be lined with lead to the degree necessary to reduce the background rate

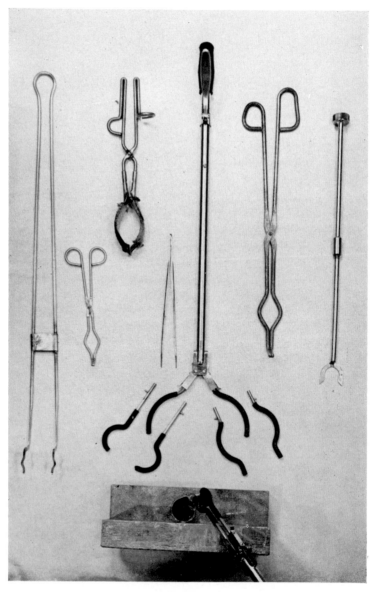

FIG. 1. Commercially available tongs, with lead bricks and beakers

to normal (normal range depenent upon equipment used). It is obvious that this means of reducing background activity is not as desirable as the location of the counting room. If the background is high despite precautions, then the material from which the room is constructed should be surveyed for radioactivity.

The counting room should be air-conditioned since the equipment functions most accurately at a near constant temperature and humidity.

A separate electrical supply line, preferably from a constant voltage supply transformer, should be used for the counting equipment.

Finally, location should be governed by accessibility for in-patients, out-patients and the preparation room. Adequate space for the anticipated work load (minimum 10 x 15 ft.) must be provided and the probable future expansion of the laboratory considered. This is especially true if scanning procedures may be anticipated, since this equipment requires much space. Often a separate room is set aside for this purpose.

Furniture for the counting room should include a stout table for general

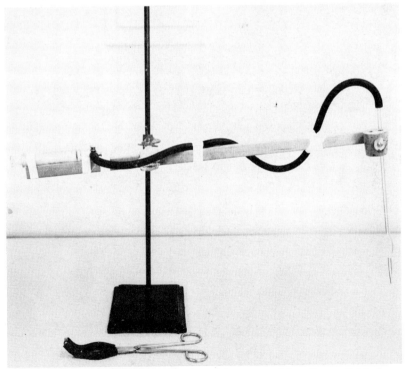

Fig. 2. Remote control pipet. Constructed from material easily available to most laboratories. In the foreground is a pair of short handling tongs made by placing rubber (or plastic) tubing over the ends of crucible tongs.

work and the support of a "well" type scintillation counter. Some laboratories have found it advantageous to use a counter-height working area with the scaler raised above the bench top. All top surfaces should be of non-porous materials (stainless steel or formica). Floor covering should also be of non-porous material such as synthetic tile or linoleum laid over two (2) layers of tar paper. These precautions are needed to maintain the meticulous cleanliness required in the counting room.

The requirements for the preparation and storage area have been simplified in recent years by the availability of capsulated, precalibrated tracer and therapeutic doses. Nevertheless, a storage vault or "corral" is still necessary. It may be made of 2-inch lead bricks supported on a strong table and enclosing a minimum space of 1 x 2 ft. with a non-porous surface. The floor should also have a non-porous covering. A stainless steel sink is necessary for cleaning equipment and waste disposal. If bulk dosage bottles are to be used or ashing of samples carried out, a fume hood is necessary; also

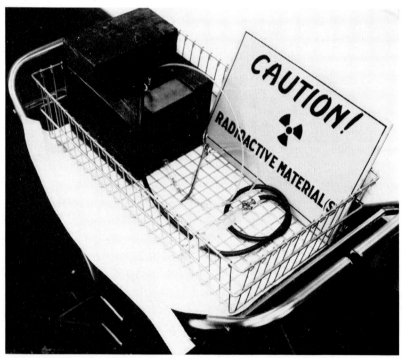

FIG. 3. Strong cart with cave of 2-inch-thick lead bricks. For transport of Au[198] or other "hot" sources. The bottom of the cave is shielded and absorbent paper extends beneath the lead cave. Radiation sign should always be used when activity is present.

if heating, boiling or evaporation of radioactive fluids is performed or dusty radioactive materials handled. The air circulation for the hood should be approximately 100 cu.ft. per minute. Suction type ventilation should be employed with the blower at the end of the flue so as to preclude contamination if a leak in the flue should develop. The outlet should be well away from any open windows in immediate or adjacent buildings. If practicable, it is well to place this outlet on top of the building in such location that the prevailing winds will drive the fumes from the vicinity of the buildings. When radioactive fumes are vented within a densely populated city it may prove necessary to employ a suitable dust filter or an electrical precipitator in the exhaust stack.

Therapeutic doses of Au^{198}, P^{32} and I^{131} can be safely stored in a vault made of 2-inch lead bricks. I^{131} and P^{32} may be administered in the laboratory, using handling tongs and 2 remote control pipettes. Au^{198} should be administered on the ward or in a separate room other than the laboratory itself. Transportation of the Au^{198} may be effected by use of a stout cart with a lead box or enclosure (Fig. 3).

21.2 Equipment

Minimum equipment for a moderate sized hospital should include:

Scaler, 1, designed for use with scintillation and GM detectors
Scintillation probe, 1, equipped with 1 inch crystal which can be fitted into a well shield
Well type shield, 1, to fit scintillation detector
Stand for scintillation detector, 1
Rate meter, 1
GM tubes, 2
Shield for GM tubes, 1
Portable survey meters, 2; low to moderate range; moderate to high range for therapy cases
Collimator for scintillation detector, 1
Aluminum filters
Lead bricks, 30
Remote control pipetor, 1.
Handling tongs, 2 (one long and one short)
Radioactivity signs
Absorbent paper
Refrigerator
Centrifuge
Sterilizer
Chair or table for counts on thyroid patients
Desk and chair
File cabinet
Glassware:
 Assorted pipettes, 1, 3, 5 and 10 cc.

Flasks, 25, 500 and 1,000 cc.
Syringes, 1, 2, 5, 10, 20 and 30 cc.
Needles
Can opener, wall type
Electroscope, 1
Standard sources of radioactivity
Film badges
Pocket dosimeters and charger
Test tube rack, stainless steel
Waste container for "hot" waste, stainless steel with cover
Bags for waste, grocery type
Incubator for Cr^{51} tagging
(*Ed. Note:* A scintiscanner will prove of great value if much localization work is to be done)

For the equipment described above the outlay is likely to be between $4,000 and $5,000. One should price the equipment desired in the particular locality in which it is to be purchased and used, to obtain accurate estimates.

In the case of smaller hospitals and medical groups, the matter of equipment and, indeed, whether or not to set up an isotope laboratory at all, may well depend on the amount of thyroid work. If nothing but radioiodine tracer studies are contemplated the main equipment requisite consists of a scintillation detector, a scaler and a suitable chair with head-rest along with some minor incidentals; cost about $2,500 in 1958.

Additional equipment is highly desirable. It comprises a second scaler and "well" type scintillation counter. These allow for substitution in case of equipment failure, and greater efficiency. It cannot be stressed too strongly that all detecting equipment and scalers should have connectors which permit of interchange.

Since failure of equipment should always be anticipated an important factor in purchasing counting equipment is the availability of repair facilities.

If liver function and cardiac output studies are to be performed, a recording ammeter will be needed. Again, the present trend is toward the use of pulse height analysis in counting, thus making at least one single channel analyser desirable. If Cr^{51} and Fe^{59} are used simultaneously for hematological studies an analyser is an essential.

When ordering glassware and needles, it must be remembered that a considerable part of this equipment will not be available for use because it will be in storage to permit of decontamination by radioactive decay. Therefore the quantity ordered should be several times the amount needed for ordinary use. The substitution of disposable plastic test tubes, when practicable, cuts down the possibility of contamination and eases the problem of cleaning glassware.

Equipment for the radioisotope laboratory should not be mixed with that for general medical use. A separate sterilizer should be provided in the radioisotope laboratory to prevent this.

An essential piece of equipment often overlooked, is a can-opener for opening sealed radioisotope shipment containers. It should be of wall-mounted type.

Readily available appliances can be adapted: (1) Short handle tongs, by slipping rubber or plastic tubing over the ends of crucible tongs. (2) Wooden cones for measuring; by making the large end the same diameter as the collimator, the detector may be automatically centered on the source when the distance is measured. (3) Cafeteria trays lined with absorbent paper serve to contain accidental spills and so provide excellent working surfaces. Decontamination is thereby made much easier. (4) Combination of ring stand with test tube clamp, syringe, three-way stop cock, cork-stopper, rubber tubing and a piece of wood, makes an excellent remote control pipette.

Many useful ideas for the establishment and operation of an isotope laboratory can be obtained by visiting as many actively functioning laboratories as possible. Each laboratory will usually exemplify some novel and practical ideas.

21.3 License

In granting licenses for the medical use of radioisotopes, the Atomic Energy Commission recognizes two types of programs, viz., Institutional Medical Radioisotope Programs and Individual Practice Medical Programs. Application forms are the same for both programs:

1. AEC Form 313—Application for Byproduct Material License.
2. AEC Form 313a—Supplement for human use.
3. AEC Form 313b—Supplement b to Form 313, for the use of sealed sources.
4. Preceptor statement for the physician using isotopes. This should be filed upon completion of training, with the AEC. It will be permanently filed for future use.

Both types of program require the individual who uses radioisotopes on human subjects to be a licensed physician with basic radioisotope training and active personal experience in the medical applications of those radioisotopes to be used in his laboratory. However, since an institutional program calls for an isotope committee, the qualifications for the physician who actually administers the radioisotopes need not be so high as when the medical user is solely responsible. An isotope committee must be composed of at least the following: Internist (or hematologist); pathologist, therapeutic radiologist and person experienced in the assay of radioisotopes and cognizant of the requirements for protection of laboratory personnel from ionizing radiations (10 CFR 20).

21.4 Personnel

The physician who supervises the laboratory must, as noted above, meet the requirements of the AEC. If an isotope committee is not formed, then physicians with special training in hematology (or internal medicine), pathology and radiology along with a radiation physicist should be available as consultants especially if radioisotope therapy is undertaken.

Technicians, of course, will require special training. These must not be under the age of 18 and pregnant women should not be employed. Those with a background in x-ray or laboratory technics can learn the technics readily. However, any conscientious person of average intelligence can be trained under adequate supervision. Meticulous attention to detail is vital. There are now schools for training radioisotope technicians but the supply of graduates is short. There is at present no registry board for radioisotope technicians such as we now have for x-ray or laboratory technicians.

It must be stressed that the hazards of working with radioisotopes are not to be treated lightly. Only personnel thoroughly trained in work with radioactive materials, including technics and measurement, should be employed in any responsible capacity. Training of technicians may be by special courses or by serving an apprenticeship under properly qualified personnel.

One technician will ordinarily suffice for the work of a small diagnostic laboratory. However, the work load usually increases rapidly so that a second technician is apt to be required.

A nurse is not a necessity in the isotope laboratory, but nurses should be made cognizant of the applications of radioisotopes and the inherent problems associated with their use. This is especially true for the therapeutic applications.

Routine cleaning of an isotope laboratory is usually carried out by the janitors of the building. The meaning and significance of the radiation signs must be taught them. Also, it must be emphasized that their cleaning jobs involve no hazard as long as strict attention to the caution signs is given.

21.5 Operation of the Laboratory

21.5.1 *Administration*

Records to be kept include application forms and licenses plus:
(a) Isotopes ordered

(b) Isotopes received (with calibration bulk uncalibrated shipment)
(c) Isotopes dispensed (account for total volume of each shipment)
(d) Patients' log
(e) Monitoring record for laboratory
(f) Personnel film badge and dosimeter readings
(g) Results of CBC and physicals on employees
(h) Daily record of operation of various scalers and detectors (back grounds and patient data)
(i) Proceedings of isotope committee meetings
(j) Patient charts
    (1) Studies performed with results
    (2) Therapy
    (3) History and physical
    (4) Follow-up

Additional forms required are:
    (a) Work sheets for each study
    (b) Calibration sheets.
    (d) Distribution sheet
    (e) Request for study to be performed
    (f) Therapy monitoring forms
    (g) Autopsy forms

Instructions: Inform the patient as to the amount of time each visit to the laboratory will require so as to allow the patient to arrange for care of children and other obligations. As an aid in smooth operation or the laboratory, medical personnel who order the work should be given a list of procedures available, indications, limitations, and information relative to the scheduling of work. Forms should be provided for submission prior to the scheduling of all patients. This precaution prevents error and confusion. In addition call for the use of the patient's full name in marking samples and other data in tests.

21.5.2 *Radiological Safety.* This is discussed in other chapters and as regards radioisotopes, more particularly in Chapter 12. A few notes on waste disposal are nevertheless considered appropriate here.

Disposal of radioactive waste is one of the greatest but most neglected problems in radioisotope work. The present prevailing recommendations as regards medical usage, are that, in almost all cases, the radioisotopes can be emptied into the main sewage system with generous flushing. The tolerable level is 10 mc/1,000,000 gallons of water through the sewage system per day. For disposal of large quantities of radioactivity, a constant drip technique should be used so that the radioactive material is discharged into the sewer over a 6–8-hour period. It is advisable to trace out the sewage pipes from the laboratory to the main line. These pipes should be monitored from time to time since "hot" areas may develop in dependent parts of the system.

Highly radioactive material such as urine from a patient treated with I^{131} for carcinoma of the thyroid and fluid containing Au^{198} should be allowed to decay before discharge into the sewage system. For more specific details see: N.B.S. Handbook #48.

21.5.3 *Radioactive Contamination.* In addition to the hazards of internal and external personnel radiation already described, there are also experimental hazards; for example, every piece of apparatus which has contained radioactive material will retain a fraction which is difficult to remove. The apparatus is thereby contaminated and small portions of this radioactive contamination will be lost to succeeding solutions with which the contaminated surface comes in contact.

Studies by research workers in various laboratories have shown that glass apparatus which has held high level radioactive materials retains a sufficient amount of activity to jeopardize results in tracer studies, no matter how intense the cleaning method. It has been suggested that the glassware be kept segregated as to type and level of radioactivity after once being used.

The use of materials possessing a smooth surface that can easily be decontaminated e.g., stainless steel and formica, is to be desired. Rounded corners in hood trays and sinks are advisable to avoid places where radioactivity can accumulate.

Special consideration must be given to the half life of the radioisotopes used. It has been our experience that a person working with an isotope of short half life (a few days or less), often becomes careless, since he feels that any contamination suffered will be gone after a short period of time. This situation should not be allowed to exist, since there are some short-lived isotopes which, if handled carelessly, are dangerous.

REFERENCES (See also Chapter 12)

COLEMAN, H. S. (Editor): Laboratory Design. National Research Council Report, Part III, Chapter 7 (Myron B. Hawkins, U. S. A. E. C.), New York: Reinhold.

FIELDS, T. AND SEED, L., *Clinical Use of Radioisotopes; A Manual of Technique.* Chicago, Ill.: Yr. Bk. Pub.

National Bureau of Standards Handbook #48, Control and Removal of Radioactive Contamination in Laboratories: Govt. Printing Office, Washington 25, D. C.

National Bureau of Standards Handbook #49, Recommendations for Waste Disposal of P^{32} and I^{131} for Medical Users: Govt. Printing Office, Wash., 25, D. C.

22A

Clinical Radioisotope Techniques

E. R. KING, CAPTAIN (MC) U. S. NAVY

22A.1 Introduction

In the average clinical radioisotope laboratory by far the majority of all procedures involve diagnostic radioisotope tests. In our own laboratory at least 95 % of the work load falls under the above headings and 5 % or less is of a therapeutic nature. Despite these facts the average individual still regards the medical application of the by-products of the Nuclear Age as being predominantly that of the treatment of cancer. Nothing can be further from the truth.

Consequently this chapter will deal with the laboratory methods of diagnostic applications of radioisotopes. Therapeutic procedures will be discussed in the section on dosimetry as will radiation dosage determination resulting from diagnostic studies.

Before any type of clinical diagnostic procedure is performed the technique should be firmly established and practiced. "Normal values" have been given after each description, but it should be emphasized that these are for the Radioisotope Laboratory of the U. S. Naval Hospital, Bethesda, Maryland, and not necessarily for any other laboratory.

22A.1.1 *Types of Study.* The discussion will therefore be divided into:

(1) Studies involving the isotope dilution principle.

(2) Function studies.

(3) Localization studies.

(4) Combined studies including hematological studies.

It will be limited to procedures which are generally accepted as being routine at the time of the writing of this Chapter, in the summer of 1957.

22A.2 Isotope Dilution Studies

These studies are based upon a simple dilution formula, the same type that is used in various colorimetric dye tests. The basis of the test is that

if a known amount of radioactivity in a known volume of liquid is placed
in an unknown greater volume of liquid, the same amount of radioactivity
will still be present but will be diluted in direct proportion to the increase
in the volume of dilutent compared with the original known volume. Thus:
$V_1Q_1 = V_2Q_2$ where
V_1 is the known volume of fluid containing Q_1, the known radioactivity
in this volume, Q_2 is the determined radioactivity of the unknown volume
per unit volume, V_2 is the unknown volume.

Usually the unit of volume is milliliters and the unit of radioactivity is
counts per minute, corrected for background. This formula becomes
$V_2 = \dfrac{V_1Q_1}{Q_2}$, or, the unknown volume equals total radioactivity injected
divided by radioactivity of 1 ml of unknown volume.

22A.2.1 This simple formula can be transposed into a method for determining the various fluid volumes of the body, or even the turnover of various electrolytes. The basic formula is always used with pertinent factors
substituted depending upon which fluid space is to be studied.

22A.2.2 *Blood Volume Determination.* These studies have been performed
for many years utilizing various dyes and radioisotopic labels as dilutents.
At present the Cr^{51} erythrocyte labeling technique appears most practical
(Fig. 1).

22A.2.2.1 *Methodology of Cr^{51} blood volume (washed cell technique).*

1. Place 30 μc of Cr^{51} as sterile $Na_2Cr^{51}O_4$ in a sterile vacuum tube containing 0.1 ml of heparin (1 ml = 1000 units or 10 mg).

2. Draw 15 ml of blood from the patient without stasis, and place the
blood in the sterile dose tube using aseptic technic.

3. Incubate the blood for 45 minutes at 37°C, inverting the tube about
every fifteen (15) minutes.

4. Centrifuge the blood at 3000 rpm for 15 minutes. Withdraw the plasma
using aseptic technic.

5. Reconstitute the blood to the original volume with cold isotonic saline.
Centrifuge as before.

6. Withdraw the supernatant fluid and repeat above steps (4, 5) for a
total of three washings. The final reconstituted volume should equal 15
to 15.5 ml.

7. Inject intravenously 6 ml of this reconstituted, washed suspension
of red cells in the patient.

8. Twenty minutes later withdraw without stasis 10 ml of blood from
the opposite arm (or leg) of the patient.

9. Perform duplicate hematocrits on this sample, using Wintrobe tubes,
and centrifuging at 3000 rpm for 30 minutes. Correct the hematocrit by
the factor 0.96, to account for the trapped plasma.

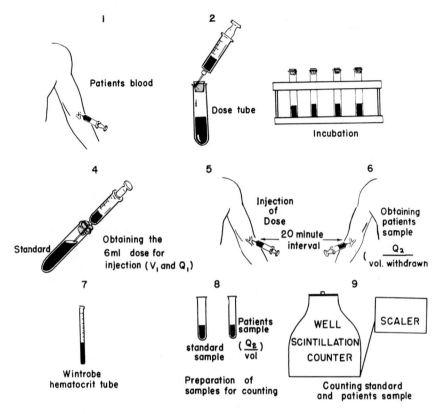

**DIAGRAM OF AN
ISOTOPIC DILUTION STUDY**
(Blood volume determination)
$V_2 = $ unknown volume $= \dfrac{V_1 Q_1}{Q_2}$

Fig. 1

10. Count duplicate 3-ml samples of this whole blood (step 8) in a well-type scintillation counter.

11. Dilute 3 ml of the original suspension of washed RBC's (step 6) to 1000 ml with water, in a 1000 ml volumetric flask. This is the "standard".

12. Count duplicate 3-ml samples of this standard in a well-type scintillation counter.

13. Total Blood Volume =

$$\frac{cc/m \text{ of 1 ml of standard} \times \text{dil. factor} \times \text{vol. inj.}}{cc/m \text{ of 1 ml of patient's whole blood}}$$

14. Total Red Cell Volume = TBV × corrected hematrocrit.

22A.2.2.2 The only disadvantage of this method is that some length of time is required for washing prior to reinjection into the patient and the resultant withdrawal of the diluted sample. Another technic whereby excess hexavalent chromium[51] ($Na_2Cr^{51}O_4$) obtained from Abbott Radiopharmaceuticals is reduced to trivalent chromium is also used. This is performed by the addition of ascorbic acid after an appropriate incubation period.

22A.2.2.3 *Methodology of Cr^{51} blood volume (ascorbic acid reduction technic).* 1, 2, and 3 same as in previously described technic.

4. Add 50 mg sterile ascorbic acid (1 cc of 5% solution). Invert the tube gently several times to mix the contents thoroughly. The ascorbic acid reduces the free, hexavalent, (anionic) chromium, that has not entered red blood cells, to the trivalent (cationic form) of chromium. The trivalent chromium does not tag the red blood cells, but temporarily labels the plasma albumin.

5. Prepare duplicate samples of this blood (4) for hematocrit determinations.

6. Inject intravenously six (6) ml of this labeled whole blood.

7. After 20 minutes, withdraw 15 ml of whole blood, without stasis, from the opposite arm (or leg). Prepare duplicate 3-ml samples for counting.

8. Prepare duplicate samples of this blood (7) for hematocrit determinations.

9. Centrifuge samples (5) and (8) for 30 minutes at 3000 rpm to obtain the hematocrits. The average values for the paired samples are corrected for trapped plasma by multiplying by the factor .96.

10. Prepare a 3-ml sample for counting from the patient's whole blood remaining in the original tube (4). This is the whole blood standard, which may have to be diluted if the counting rate is too high.

11. Centrifuge patient's blood (7) and the remaining standard blood (4) at 3000 rpm for 15 minutes. Use a sufficient quantity of each blood specimen to produce at least 3 ml of plasma.

12. Count the whole blood standard samples (10), plasma standard sample (11), patient's whole blood (7), and patient's plasma samples (11) for a length of time sufficient to reduce error due to randomness to a minimum consistant with economy of time.

13. Total Blood Volume =

$$\frac{6\,[\text{cc/m whole blood st'd} - (\text{cc/m plas. std. } (1 - \text{c/stand. hct.})]}{\text{cc/m pat. whole blood} - (\text{cc/m pat. plas. } (1 - \text{c/sample hct})}$$

Red Cell Volume = TBV × c/hct
Plasma Volume = TBV × 1 − c/hct
c/hct. = hematocrit corrected for trapped plasma.

22A.2.2.4 The trivalent Cr^{51}, after reduction by the ascorbic acid, cannot enter the erythrocyte, but labels the plasma. Thus the labeled blood can be injected much earlier allowing patient's requiring emergency surgery to be released for this surgery an hour or so earlier. However, the plasma and red cells must be separated after withdrawal from the patient and the total time required is not shortened by this procedure.

22A.2.2.5 *Normal values for blood volumes obtained by Cr^{51}-labeled erythrocytes.*

> Total red cell volume—27–32 ml/kg
> Plasma volume—30–40 ml/kg
> Total blood volume—57–72 ml/kg

22A.2.3 *Extracellular Fluid Space Determination.* Here, again, many substances both stable and radioactive have been used in an attempt to determine the volume of this important fluid space. This fluid which bathes the cells of our body has been described as most like the sea water in which the original one celled organism thrived.

Only one method will be described, that of utilizing $S^{35}O_4$, and obtaining the sulphate space. It is felt that the sulphate space most nearly resembles the extracellular fluid space of the body.

22A.2.3.1 *Methodology of extracellular fluid space* $(S^{35}O_4)$.

1. 300 μc of carrier free radiosulfate in a volume of 6 ml of sterile saline is injected intravenously into the patient. At the same time that the dose is prepared, a standard is also prepared by diluting an additional 300 μc of the radiosulfate to 1000 ml of plasma. The "standard" dose is measured with the same syringe that is to be used for injecting into the patient.

2. Twenty (20) minutes after the injection 10 ml of blood is withdrawn from the patient. No-anticoagulant is added to the blood.

3. The whole blood is centrifuged for 15 minutes at 3000 rpm. The serum is pipetted from the test tube.

4. 3 ml of the serum counted in the gas flow counter or a liquid scintillation counter, (a thin end-window Geiger Counter may be used).

5. 3 ml of the "standard" are counted in the same manner.

6. Extracellular fluid space =

$$\frac{\text{Standard cc/m} \times 1000 \times 0.804}{\text{cc/m serum}}$$

$$\% \text{ Body Weight} = \frac{\text{Total volume of extracellular fluid space}}{\text{Body weight in kilograms}}$$

22A.2.3.2 Normal extracellular fluid space is 16–20% of the total body weight.

22A.2.4 *Total Body Water Determinations.* This method involves diluting a suitable material, stable or radioactive into the body water pool. The ideal material would be water itself, and thus "heavy water" (D_2O) or tritiated water (H_2O plus H_2^3O) are used. The latter is radioactive but requires special counting equipment due to a weak beta emission. Abbott Radiopharmaceuticals has produced an iodinated antipyrine (I^{131}-4-iodo-antipyrine) which can be used for these studies.

22A.2.4.1 *Methodology of I^{131}-4 iodoantipyrine total body water determination.*

1. Inject 30–40 μc I^{131} as sterile 4-iodoantipyrine diluted to a total volume of 6 ml with saline.

2. Withdraw 15 ml samples of blood at 3, 4 and 5 hours.

3. Prepare a standard by diluting an amount equivalent to injected I^{131} antipyrine. Dilute to 1000 ml in a volumetric flask.

4. Count duplicate 3-ml samples of standard, and duplicate 3-ml samples of serum from blood samples (2).

5. Calculations.

1. Plot serum sample activity as a function of time on semi-log paper extrapolating to time zero.

2. Solve formula.

$$\text{TBW} = \frac{\text{Dose in ml} \times \text{dil. factor} \times \text{spec. act. of stand.}}{\text{Corr. spec. activity serum extrapolated to zero time}}$$

22A.3 Function Studies

Two function studies have been accepted as routine clinical radioisotope procedures. These are of the thyroid and pancreas. Two tests are under evaluation, those of liver function and of kidney function. The former will probably not be of great clinical value except as an overall test of liver function.

22A.3.1 *Thyroid Function.* Various methods using I^{131} have been tried to study the function of the thyroid. These are:

(1) The thyroid uptake. Different time factors have been used but the most widely accepted is the 24-hour uptake, or the percent of the dose in the gland 24 hours after it was administered.

(2) The Conversion Ratio. This determines the amount of radioiodine in the blood that is converted to protein bound radioiodine. This conversion is presumed to be performed in the thyroid gland.

(3) Saliva-PBI-I^{131} Ratio. This indirectly determines the fraction of free radioiodine allowed to remain in the blood by measuring the amount excreted in the saliva.

Other methods are used in various clinics but the methods described are those routinely utilized in our laboratory. Again it should be emphasized that the technics, once established, should be adhered to most rigidly and with no alterations or exceptions.

22A.3.1.1 *Methodology of the 24-hour I^{131} uptake.*

1. If a full battery of thyroid studies are to be performed, 100 microcuries of I^{131} are given orally in distilled water, to the fasting patient. The cup is rinsed twice, and the patient drinks the rinse water. If only a 24 hour uptake is to be performed the dose is reduced to 10 microcuries.

2. A standard is prepared in identical fashion, and placed in a 50 ml volumetric flask.

3. 24 hours later, the standard is placed 10 inches from the tip of the non-collimated scintillation probe, and a three minute count taken, background corrected; this is repeated. (A $\frac{1}{8}''$ lead shield is placed over the end of the scintillation probe).

4. The patient is seated in a chair with a firm head rest. The tip of the scintillation probe is placed 10 inches from the isthmus of the thyroid. Counts are taken as in para. 3.

5. $$\frac{\text{Counts over thyroid} - \text{background} \times 100}{\text{Counts from standard} - \text{background}} = \text{uptake in per cent}$$

22A.3.1.1.2 In this laboratory, the following *values* in per cent are considered within the normal range.

Hypothyroid   0–15 per cent
Euthyroid   15–45 per cent
Hyperthyroid   Above 45 per cent

Exogenous sources of iodine (inorganic iodine, dyes, containing iodine etc) and thyroid hormone will interfere with the 24 hour uptake.

22A.3.1.1.3 *Methodology for the Conversion Ratio.* This has been performed by precipitating the protein bound iodine or by separating the inorganic serum I^{131} by ion exchange. Our laboratory has studied four methods and now employs the following:

1. Count 2 ml of serum.

2. Using a polyethylene ion exchange column, stopper the bottle with a piece of Abbott Filter Paper. Pour in 3 ml of Amberlite, Chloride Form, resin, allow liquid to drain off, (Caution: use column immediately, before drying takes place). Do not disturb column after packing.

3. By means of tape attach column above test tube, leaving a small air hole.

4. Pour serum into the exchange column. Rinse serum tube with 2 ml distilled water, and pour this into column. Rerinse with 1 ml of distilled water, allow to sit for 5 minutes, then expel remaining fluid into test tube

be means of air from a tight fitting rubber bulb. Count the liquid (effluent) in the test tube.

5. $$\frac{\text{Counts/min. effluent} \times 100}{\text{counts/min. serum}} = \text{PBI}^{131} \text{ conversion ratio}$$

1.3.2.1 *Normal values of PBI conversion ratio.*

Hypothyroid   0–10   per cent
Euthyroid   10–40 per cent
Hyperthyroid   40–100 per cent

22A.3.1.3 *Methodology of saliva-PBI ratio.*

1. Count 3 ml of saliva in well-type scintillation counter. The free-flowing saliva is collected within a period of 15 minutes without stimulation.

2. Count 3 ml of the effluent, which is the protein bound iodine of the serum, prepared by the ion exchange method previously described.

3. $$\frac{\text{Counts/minute saliva} - \text{background}}{\text{Counts per minute effluent} - \text{background}} = \text{Saliva} - \text{PBI Ratio}$$

22A.3.1.3.1 *Normal values of saliva-PBI ratio.*

Hypothyroid   300 and up
Euthyroid   50 to 299
Hyperthyroid   Under 50

22A.3.2 *Liver Function Tests.* Rose bengal is an organic dye that is handled by the liver similarly to bromsulfalein. The polygonal cells remove the dye from the blood stream and it is excreted via the bile into the gastrointestinal tract. Abbott's have labeled Rose Bengal with a tight I^{131} bond.

This labeled dye is used to study the gross function of the liver by means of external counting with a scintillation crystal probe.

22A.3.2.1 *Methodology of liver function test.*

1. The patient is placed in the supine position.

2. The collimated scintillation probe connected to the recorder via the counting rate meter, is positioned on the right antero-lateral aspect of the chest wall, over the upper portion of the liver, as determined by percussion, and directed cephalad, away from the gall bladder region.

3. 10–25 μc of Rose Bengal I^{131} is injected intravenously. Simultaneously the recorder is started and the time of injection marked on the graph. The volume of the dose should be 2–5 ml and the injection should be completed in 1 minute.

4. Recording of the uptake and excretion portion of the curve is made for a period of not less than 30 minutes and generally not more than sixty minutes.

5. *Note:* Adjust the pen recorder to zero prior to injection of the Rose Bengal. This establishes a reproducible base line.

22A.3.2.2 *Interpretation.* The peak in the normal is reached in 20–30 minutes. Then a gradual decline in the curve is noted. This denotes excretion of the I^{131} Rose Bengal in the biliary system. Each laboratory must determine its own "normal curve" (Fig. 2).

Blockage of the biliary system does not allow a fall of the curve. Hepatitis and cirrhosis will give gradients of flattened curves.

22A.3.3 *Pancreatic Function Tests.* This procedure tests for the presence of lipase in the gut, secreted by the exocrine glands of the pancreas. The test performed at the U. S. Naval Hospital, Bethesda, Maryland uses a fat, triolein, labeled with I^{131}. Our method involves the radioassay of the I^{131} in the feces, which indicates either a failure of lipase action on the fat, or a malabsorptive state of the gut. Other clinics make direct blood radioassays in order to determine the lipase enzymatic activity.

22A.3.4.1 *Methodology of the pancreatic function test.*

1. The patient drinks a suspension of 10 drops of Lugol's solution and approximately 1/20 ounce activated charcoal in 60 cc of water. The Lugol's solution is to prevent the uptake of radioiodine by the thyroid gland, and the charcoal acts as an indicator to mark the completion of passage of the material through the digestive tract.

2. After washing down the above drink with water, the patient drinks

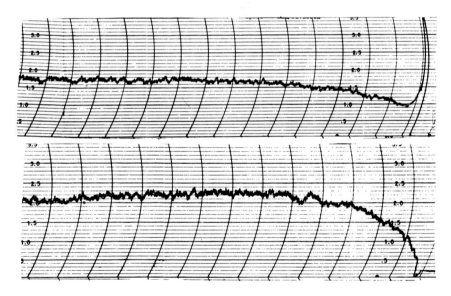

FIG. 2. Rose Bengal-I^{131} liver function curve. The curve reads from right to left with a speed of 4 minutes per division. Dose is 15 microcuries of Rose Bengal-I^{131}. The bottom scan is normal with a 20-minute peak and a 40-minute fall off. The top patient had extensive liver metastases. This curve is lower and has less fall off.

the triolein I[131] in a carrier composed of peanut oil-emulsifying agent-water. Twenty-five microcuries of triolein I[131] are made up in the carrier, so that the final volume is 1 cc/kg of body weight. Make a duplicate, to be used as a standard, in the same way. The carrier is composed of 200 cc peanut oil, 200 cc of water, 15 cc Tween-80 (emulsifying agent).

3. Save the cup from which the patient drank the triolein I[131], it contains residual counts that will have to be subtracted from the standard.

4. All stools are saved after the fatty mixture is ingested until all of the charcoal marker appears. Collect specimens in 1 quart leakproof containers, refrigerate standard to prevent deterioration of the fat. It is of the utmost importance that no urine contaminates the stool. This point must be repeatedly stressed to the patient and the nursing staff.

5. If desired, urine and blood specimens can be collected, to follow iodine uptake and excretion.

6. Standard is placed in the same type of container as used for collecting stool, water added to top, and it is thoroughly mixed. After getting 3-minute background, count the standard, stool sample and cup which contained the fatty mixture. Use a sodium-iodide-thallium activated scintillation crystal counter, and place the container 15 cm from the probe.

7. $$\frac{\text{Corrected c/m of the stool} \times 100}{\text{Corrected c/m standard} - \text{cc/m of the cup}} = \% \text{ excretion in stool}$$

22A.3.4.2 The normal value is 0–2.6% of the administered dose in the stools of the period required for complete transport through the gut. Elevated values are found in various pancreatic diseases, obstruction of the pancreatic ducts, etc. Also elevated values are found in defects of intestinal absorption.

22A.3.5 *Measurement of Cardiac Output.* This involves measuring a quantity of an I[131]-labeled compound, usually human serum albumin, that leaves that heart per unit time. Other gamma ray emitting radioisotopes may be used, however.

22A.3.5.1 *Methodology of cardiac output.*

1. After the patient's height and weight are recorded he is placed in the supine position and allowed to rest for 5 minutes.

2. A non-collimated scintillation probe is placed at skin distance between the 2nd and 3rd rib at the left parasternal border. (It is possible to better localize the ascending aorta by fluoroscoping the patient and marking the position).

3. A dose of 25–30 μc of RISA is injected into the left or right brachial vein as rapidly as possible. Use not more than 2 cc of solution. The patient's pulse should be taken immediately prior to injection.

4. Using a short time response counting rate meter and a suitable re-

corder, a 1-minute recording is made starting at the time of injection. The recorder is then turned off.

5. Do not disturb the equipment. After ten minutes take an additional one minute recording. This is the final level, or C_f (Fig. 3).

6. A 10-ml sample of venous blood can be withdrawn from the opposite arm for the blood volume determination. (However, we routinely perform a blood volume by the Cr^{51} tagging method instead of using the RISA and count the Cr^{51} by pulse height analysis.)

7. Calculations:

C_f = The equilibrium counting rate (average count rate after 10 min.).

Cav   = Average counting rate under the primary curve (including the extrapolated portion). This is obtained from the one minute count postinjection.

60   = Conversion factor, seconds to minutes.

T   = Total time, in seconds, under primary curve.

C. O. = Cardiac output.

A   = Area under known portion of primary curve.

B   = Area under extrapolated portion of primary curve.

B. V. = Blood volume.

Note: Area of A + B divided by T in seconds = Cav

The area may be obtained by (1) planimeter (2) averaging (3) counting the squares of the graph paper.

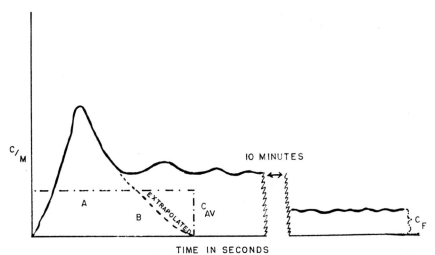

TIME IN SECONDS

FIG. 3. Cardiac output curve. A reproduced curve reading from left to right. The formula utilizing data from this curve is presented in the text.

$$\text{C. O. (cc/min.)} = \frac{C_f \times \text{B. V.} \times 60}{C_{av} \times \text{T (in seconds)}}$$

$$C_{av} = \frac{A + B}{\text{T (in seconds)}}$$

$$\text{C. O. (L/min.)} = \frac{\text{C. O. (cc/min.)}}{1000}$$

$$\text{Stroke volume} = \frac{\text{C. O. (cc/min.)}}{\text{Pulse rate}}$$

$$\text{Cardiac Index} = \frac{\text{C. O. L/min.}}{\text{Body surface (meters}^2)}$$

22A.3.5.2 *Normal values for our laboratory.*
Cardiac output—3,000–7,000 cc/min. 3–7 l/min.
Stroke volume—50–120 cc
Cardiac index—3 plus or minus .8 L/min/m²

22A.3.6 *Kidney Function Tests.* This study is under evaluation but, like the liver function test, promises to be a good gross determination of the overall functional ability of one kidney when compared with the other. The test utilizing Diodrast I¹³¹ administration at present appears to be most promising so this is the technique that will be described.

22A.3.6.1 *Methodology of kidney function tests.*

1. Diodrast, with a specific activity of 31 μc/ml is used as the test agent.

2. The patient is in a sitting position with two scintillation probes placed against his back and directed caudally toward the kidney region. The kidneys are also located by either radiographic or fluoroscopic examinations and are marked on the skin.

3. A dose of 1 μc/3 kg body weight of the above preparation is injected, intravenously, after dilution with normal saline to 31 μc/ml.

4. The probes which have been placed over the kidney region are connected to counting rate meters and compatible recorders. A continuous 30-minute record of each kidney's excretion rate is obtained.

22A.3.6.2 In the normal the curve reaches a peak 3–5 minutes after administration of the labeled dye and falls off sharply. If the curve for one kidney does not peak it represents malfunction. If the curve peaks and does not fall off it may represent a delay in the excretion of the urine due to a urethral obstruction.

22A.4 Localization Studies

When radioisotopes became available for clinical use a large number of tests were studied in an effort to diagnose and localize malignant tumors. Most of these studies were proven inadequate; however, there are a few that have become accepted as valid procedures.

With the increasing use of more sensitive detection equipment employing pulse height analysis, large crystals and better collimation it may be that some of the tests that were discarded as impractical will actually prove of value.

22A.4.1 *Brain Tumor Localization.* This has been the most popular of all tumor localization procedures. Various technics are still in use; using manual or automatic scanning, photoscanning, and positron detection. Iodine[131]-labeled human serum albumin (RISA of Abbott Radiopharmaceuticals) is used in many clinics by applying one of the above technical counting methods. Positron emitters such as As[74] and Cu[64] are also used. We will describe two different methods that have been studied at the U. S. Naval Hospital, Bethesda, Maryland.

22A.4.1.1 *Methodology of brain tumor localization by a manual scan using RISA.*

1. 200–300 μc of RISA is injected intravenously 24 hours prior to the examination. (The scan may be performed at 1 hour, if desired.)

2. Symmetrical contralateral points are counted for a time sufficient to give a statistical accuracy of plus or minus 3%.

3. Six points are counted on the frontal area of the skull and 12 points are counted on each side of the skull.

4. The scintillation probe is positioned at a 90 degree angle to the sagittal plane of the skull for the lateral counts and as close to the skin as feasible. It is important that all counts are made at the same distance from the skin to prevent erroneous results.

5. The corrected counts at each point on one side of the head are divided by the counts at the corresponding point of the other side to obtain a plus or minus percentage uptake.

6. Points to be counted:

a. For the side counts the distance from the frontal to the occipital portion of the skull in centimeters divided by 3 to obtain the lateral interval between the side counts.

b. For the frontal counts the width of the head in centimeters is divided by 2 to obtain the lateral interval of the points counted.

A maximum of 5% of the iodine contained in the RISA may be assimilated by the thyroid gland. In order to prevent assimilation of this iodine, 15 drops of potassium iodide as Lugol's solution is administered 3 times a day for 24 hours prior to the survey.

22A.4.1.1.1 This method uses a rectangular coordinate method of plotting in order to indicate areas of increased "localization" in the brain (Fig. 4).

The same type of study may be performed by an automatic scanner when a print of the patient's head is obtained.

22A.4.1.2 *Methodology of positron scintiscanning.*

1. As^{74} or Cu^{64} is administered intravenously. The dose of As^{74} is in the region of 30 µc/kg body weight, and it is given by syringe as $As^{74}Cl_3$ or as sodium arsenite[74]. Cu^{64} versenate is administered by slow intravenous drip in 5 % dextrose in order to eliminate chance of blood calcium removal by excess versene. The dose of Cu^{64} is about 50 µc/kg. Either isotope may be used depending upon its availability.

2. One hour later the patient is carefully positioned on the positron scintiscanner and the asymmetrical scale is balanced with the probes opposite the facial musculature. The scanning takes about 45 minutes and the patient should not move during this procedure. If As^{74} is used the scan is repeated the next day. In certain instances it will be wise to repeat the entire procedure.

22A.4.2.1 Evidently there is no difference in the results between As^{74} and the Cu^{64} scans. However, As^{74}, because of its longer half-life, delivers a total body irradiation dose of 10 r, while Cu^{64} delivers a dose of less than 1 r. As^{74} is cyclotron produced and is difficult to obtain. Cu^{64} is obtained from the nuclear reactor by the (n, gamma) reaction but its short-half-life makes it rather impractical to use any distance from a nuclear reactor.

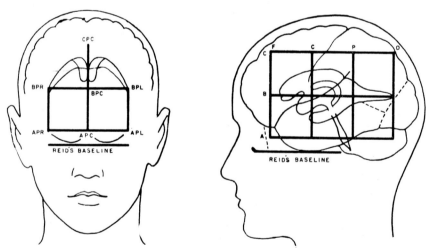

FIG. 4. The brain tumor study using radioactive iodinated serum albumin. This plot demonstrates the intersects at which points the counts are made.

Thus the debits cancel out the credits in each instance. Our laboratory uses either As^{74} and Cu^{64} whichever we happen to have available, when a brain scan is requested.

22A.4.1.2.2 This study requires a special type of scanner obtainable from the Baird Atomic Instrument Company of Cambridge, Massachusetts (Figs. 5 and 6).

22A.4.2 *Eye Tumor Localization.* Radiophosphorus[32] is used in this study with a small, thin end window, Geiger probe that is placed against the eye. A thin needle Geiger probe is also available that passes behind the globe after opening the conjunctival sac.

22A.4.2.1 *Methodology of eye scan.*

1. 300 μc of P^{32} is injected intravenously.

2. Manual scans with an appropriate Geiger probe (obtained from Nuclear of Chicago) over each quadrant of the unaffected eye and each quadrant of the affected eye. The eye is anesthetized with a suitable agent.

3. Counts are obtained at 1 hour, 24 hours and 48 hours following injection.

4. Results are plotted on rectangular coordinate paper. If a tumor is present there will be a higher counting rate level over the tumor when compared with non-tumerous area. This rate will be maintained over the 48 hour period (Fig. 7).

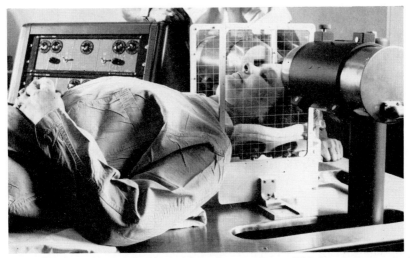

FIG. 5. Brain tumor localization with positron emitters. This is a positron scinti-scanner with a coincidence circuit. Radioactive arsenic (As^{74}) or copper (Cu^{64}) is used.

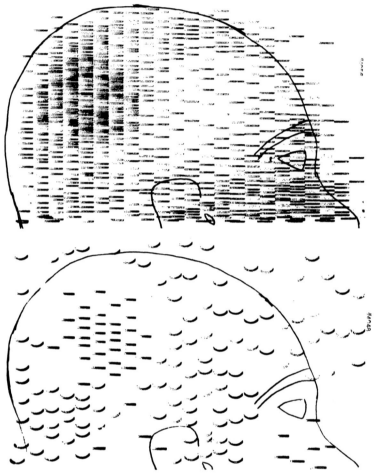

FIG. 6. A positron scintiscan using a tracer dose of As[74]. The top view is the symmetrical scan demonstrating a differential increase of As[74] in the posterior parietal region. The bottom view is the asymmetrical scan which, by the straight marks, localizes the tumor to the left of the midline. This patient was proven to have a glioma at that site.

5. Other areas than the above listed quadrants may be counted if indicated, providing similar areas are counted over the unaffected eye for comparison.

6. The thin probe may be passed behind both eyes for comparison, or may be used at time of surgery to estimate the extent of the tumor.

22A.4.3 *Liver Metastasis Localization.* Several materials have been utilized in an attempt to localize liver metastases. Of these the most promising utilizes the dye, Rose Bengal, which is labeled with I[131].

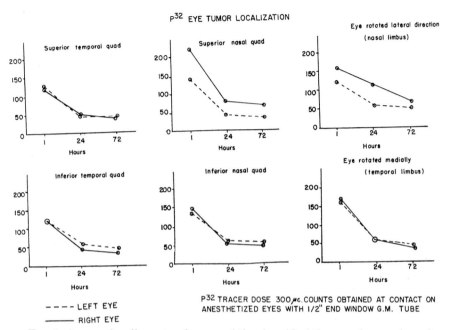

P³² EYE TUMOR LOCALIZATION

- - - - LEFT EYE
——— RIGHT EYE

P³² TRACER DOSE 300 μc. COUNTS OBTAINED AT CONTACT ON
ANESTHETIZED EYES WITH 1/2" END WINDOW G.M. TUBE

FIG. 7. A case of malignant melanoma of the choroid of the superior nasal quadrant of the right eye, adjacent to the limbus. An increase in localization of the P³² is demonstrated at this site.

22A.4.3.1 *Methodology of Rose Bengal I¹³¹ liver metastases localization.*

1. The patient is placed in the supine position and 3 μc per kilogram/body weight of Rose Bengal I¹³¹ is injected intravenously at a rate of about 10 cc/min.

2. Ten minutes after the injection a trial scan of the liver is made by running the scintillation probe from the third anterior intercostal space on the right side in the mid-clavicular line to the level of the crest of the ileum. The superior and inferior borders of the liver are thus determined by noting the counting rate of activity.

3. Adjustment of the spectrometer is made so that the 0.364 mev gamma of the I¹³¹ is recorded and other energy radiation is not recorded. Thus a favorable ratio of the primary radiation to scatter radiation and background will be achieved and the scan will clearly outline functioning liver tissue.

4. The scan is begun 2 cm above the percussable upper limit of the liver in the anterior right axillary line and is continued to the left mid-clavicular line and distally to a level 2 cm below the lower palpable border of the liver.

5. Scanning time should not exceed 90 minutes, preferably 60 minutes

or less, as after one hour there is appreciable decrease of activity within the liver due to excretion of Rose Bengal.

6. A counting rate of 600–800 counts per minute is considered desirable for which a speed of 10 inches per minute and a scaling factor of 10 is generally selected.

7. Negative areas within the liver represent tissue other than functioning liver.

8. A defect for the xyphoid process is noted in its usual position.

9. A defect for the cardiac impression on the superior border of the left lobe of the liver is noted.

10. A "positive nodule" or mass is noted in the gall bladder region due to concentration of Rose Bengal I^{131} in the gall bladder.

22A.4.3.2 Rose Bengal is selectively removed from the blood stream by the polygonal cells of the liver. The biliary system collects the dye and it is finally eliminated from the body via the feces. By flooding the liver with Rose Bengal I^{131} an external count of the activity within the liver is possible. By use of proper collimation and a spectrometer, to eliminate soft scatter and background, a small area of liver tissue can be analyzed for activity and the result recorded on the printing mechanism. Metastatic tumors in the liver, cysts, or other masses not containing functioning liver will not be recorded and on the scan presents a "cold" area. The final record of the scan demonstrates the outline of the liver with masses over 1.5 cm in diameter in the left lobe and over 2.5 cm in diameter in the right lobe reproduced as areas of no uptake of Rose Bengal I^{131}. By varying the depth of focus of the collimation it is possible to scan various planes within the liver (Fig. 8a, 8b).

After intravenous injection of Rose Bengal I^{131} the level of activity in the liver rapidly raises to a peak within 20–30 minutes. Eight minutes following injection at least 50 % of the Rose Bengal has been removed from the blood stream. Since there is no dye re-absorbed from the G.I. tract, the biological half-life of Rose Bengal I^{131} is a matter of a few hours. Dosage used is 2.5–3 $\mu c/kg$ of body weight. There is no toxicity due to stable dye as only 1–2 mg of the dye are required per patient. Satisfactory liver visualization in children under 4 years of age has been obtained with 50 μc of Rose Bengal.

22A.4.3.3 A manually operated probe may be used if no automatic scanner and printer are available.

22A.5 Hematological Studies

22A.5.1 *The use of $B_{12}Co^{60}$ in diagnostic pernicious anemia (Schilling test).*

1. $B_{12}Co^{60}$ containing 0.5 μc of Co^{60} as radiocyanocobalimin and 0.75 μg

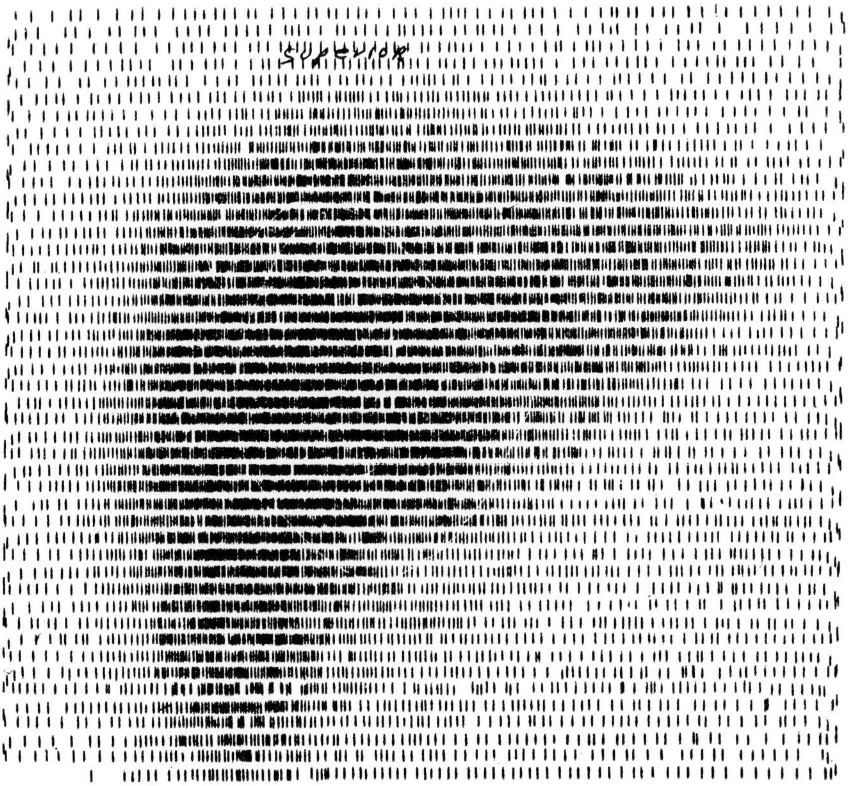

Fig. 8a. A Rose Bengal Liver scan on a normal patient. The dose was 300 microcuries of Rose Bengal-I[131] intravenously by slow drip.

of B_{12} is administered to a fasting patient with an empty urinary bladder.

2. Two hours later a "flushing dose" of B_{12} in the form of 1.0 mgm of Bevidox, crystalline, is administered subcutaneously.

3. The urine is collected for the next 24 hours, and returned to the laboratory. An aliquot of the urine is counted, and the per cent of the total dose excreted is determined:

$$\frac{\text{cc/m of 1 ml of urine} \times \text{volume of urine} \times 100}{\text{cc/m of 1 ml of standard} \times \text{dilution factor}} = \% \text{ Excreted}$$

Normal range: 13–15 % of dose administered is excreted in urine in first 24 hours. If less than 10 % is excreted the examination is repeated in 2 days with the following change in procedure.

4. Intrinsic factor (30 mg) is given orally with dose of $B_{12}Co^{60}$ (radio-cyanocobalimin). The flushing dose of 1 mg of Bevidox is administered as before, and the urine is collected.

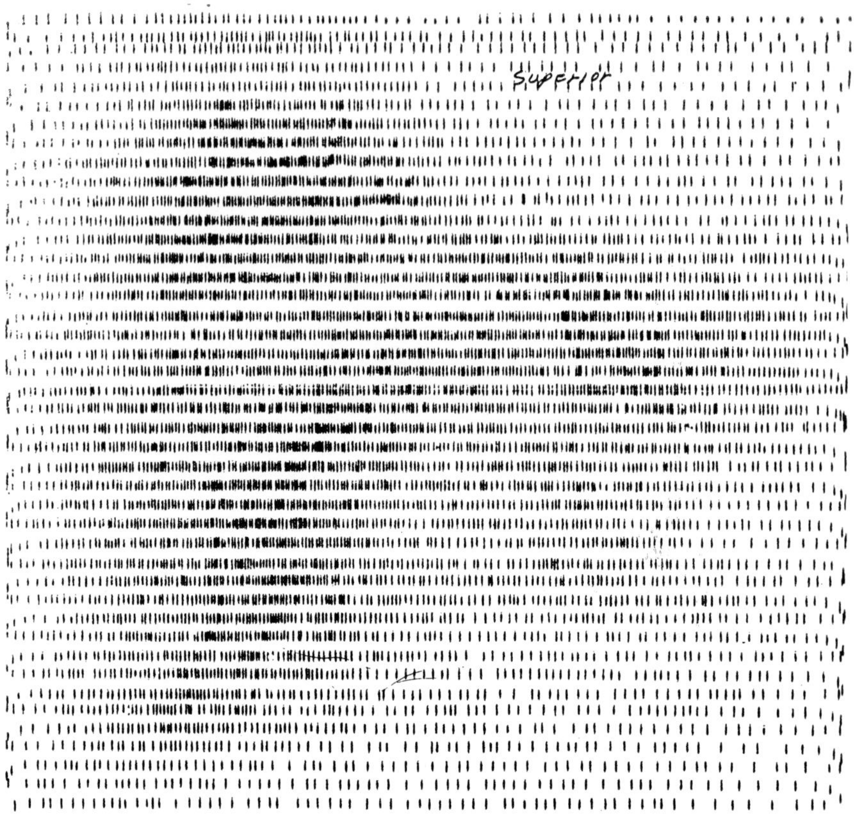

FIG. 8b. A Rose Bengal liver scan on a patient with multiple metastases to the liver. The scattered areas of decreased uptakes represent metastases.

5. If the excretion of the $B_{12}Co^{60}$ has risen to approximately normal levels its results indicate a lack of intrinsic factor and the diagnosis of pernicious anemia is probable.

6. If the percentage of the administered dose of $B_{12}Co^{60}$ does not rise after intrinsic factor, a defect in the upper gastrointestinal tract is likely, and this is often of the malabsorption syndrome type (Fig. 9).

7. Failure to collect urine voided during the 24 hour period is a source of error. Patients should be questioned to ascertain if urine collection was complete. Chronic renal disease may also alter the urinary excretion rate of $B_{12}Co^{60}$.

22A.5.1.2 Pernicious anemia patients, even in remission, do not absorb B_{12} in the absence of intrinsic factor.

After the oral administration of $B_{12}Co^{60}$ and a subcutaneously injected

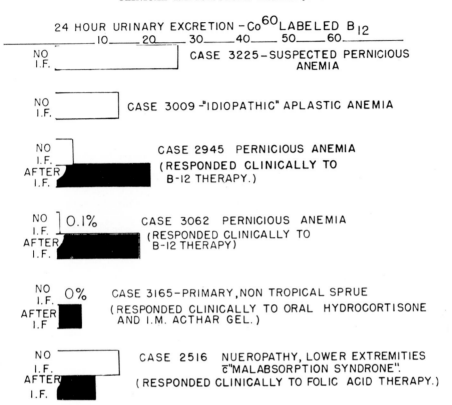

FIG. 9. The Schilling Test—$B_{12}Co^{60}$ dose: 0.15 μc Co^{60} in 0.75 μgm B_{12} ; flushing dose: 1 mgm B_{12} ; intrinsic factor dose: 30 mg. The white bars represent percentage 24 hour urinary excretion of $B_{12}Co^{60}$ without intrinsic factor, while the black bars represent the excretion after intrinsic factor.

"flushing dose" of Bevidox, the normal person will excrete 13–15 % of the dose of Co^{60} in the first 24 hour urinary excretion. Patients with intrinsic factor defects or a gastrointestinal malabsorption syndrome excrete less than 3 % of the dose in urine during the first 24 hour postinjection period. In the latter group of cases the test is repeated with an adequate dose of intrinsic factor. If the excreted amount of Co^{60} does not rise to normal levels, it is possible that the patient has a malabsorption syndrome.

22A.5.3 *Iron*[59] *Studies.* The use of Fe^{59} to study the metabolism of iron and the rate of production of the red blood cell can be combined with the red blood cell survival study if a medical gamma ray spectrometer is available. The method described is for the combined study of Cr^{51}-labeled erythrocyte survival and Fe^{59} utilization. If Fe^{59} studies alone are to be performed, the sections referring to Cr^{51} should be deleted.

22A.5.3.1 *Methodology of Fe^{59} and Cr^{51} combined studies.*

1. 50 ml of blood is drawn from the patient and distributed as follows:

20 ml into a heparinized tube for Cr^{51} labeling.

20 ml into a heparinized tube for Fe^{59} labeling.

10 ml into a tube without anticoagulant for serum iron determination.

2. 150 μc of Cr^{51} is used to label the red blood cell by wash-cell technic as has been described previously (2.2.1).

3. The 20-ml sample for Fe^{59} labeling is centrifuged, the plasma drawn off under sterile technic, and 50 μc of Fe^{59} as ferrous citrate is added to plasma. The plasma is incubated for at least 20 minutes at room temperature.

4. The Cr^{51}-labeled red cells are injected (6 ml) and the remainder of the labeled cells are retained as a standard.

5. Twenty minutes later a 10-ml sample of the patient's blood is withdrawn without stasis. This sample is used to determine the blood volume as described previously (2.2.1).

6. Immediately following withdrawal of the sample for the blood volume, 6 ml of the Fe^{59}-labeled plasma is injected. The remainder of labeled plasma is retained as a standard.

7. At the following intervals of time, 10 minutes, one-half hour, 2 hours and 3 hours, 10 ml of blood are withdrawn. The plasma alone is counted for Fe^{59} from the aforementioned specimens in a scintillation well counter.

8. Four hours following injection 20 ml of blood is withdrawn and separated into a plasma and red cell fraction. The plasma is counted as in the above samples, for Fe^{59} activity, the red blood cells are retained, and counted for Cr^{51} and for Fe^{59} activity.

9. The plasma activity for all counts is plotted in c/m vs time elapsed and the resultant curve is the plasma disappearance curve, from which the plasma iron disappearance half time (PDT½) is obtained. This is plotted on semi-log paper.

10. The red blood cells of the 4-hour 20-ml volume sample are reconstituted to volume and after one wash are counted for both Cr^{51} and Fe^{59} using pulse height analysis. The Cr^{51} activity is considered 100% survival on the RBC survival curve. The Fe^{59} activity is considered the first point of the curve for the Fe^{59} utilization by erythrocytes. A hematrocrit is determined from each blood sample (Fig. 10a).

11. At each of the above time intervals an in vivo count of the liver, spleen and sacrum (bone marrow) is obtained by using a scintillation probe and pulse height analysis (Fig. 10b).

12. Whole blood samples and in vivo counting are then performed on days 2, 4, 6, 9, 12, 15, 21, 28 and 35, following injection. The schedule should be observed as well as possible. Counts of the red cells for Cr^{51} and Fe^{59}

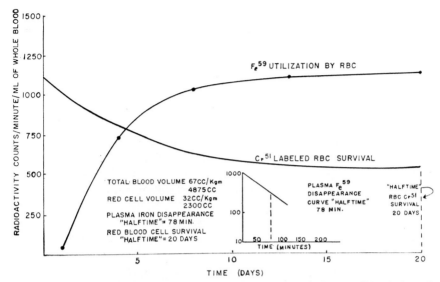

Fig. 10a. Erythrokinetic studies. Simultaneous Fe59 and Cr51 studies of the red blood cell demonstrating rates of red cell production and destruction as well as Fe59 turnover in a normal case.

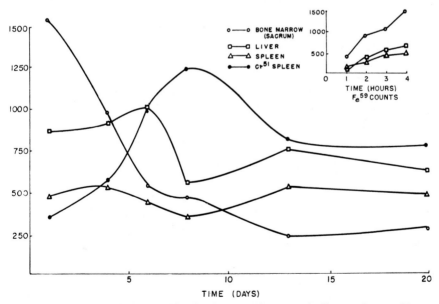

Fig. 10b. Erythrokinetic studies. In vivo counting over the liver, spleen and bone marrow (sacrum). Both Fe59 and Cr51 were counted over the spleen. These curves are typical of a normal case.

and a hematocrit are performed on each sample of whole blood. It should be noted that the activity of both radioisotopes are in the erythrocyte. The hematocrits are used to correct for changes in the red blood cell volume. The Cr^{51} determinations are used to construct the survival curve and the Fe^{59} determinations are used to construct the Fe^{59} utilization curve.

13. The Cr^{51} red cell activity (for 1 ml of whole blood) from the 4 hour and succeeding samples (after correction for radioactive decay) is plotted vs time on semi-log paper. The half-time of RBC survival is obtained.

14. The Fe^{59} red cell activity (for 1 ml of whole blood) from the 4 hour and succeeding samples (after correction for radioactive decay) is plotted vs time on rectangular coordinate paper. The curve for the red cell uptake of Fe^{59} is obtained. The percentage of the total amount of Fe^{59} injected which is in the cells is noted.

15. The activities of the in vivo counts of the liver, spleen, and bone marrow are plotted vs time on rectangular coordinate paper. The values plotted are corrected for radioactive decay and for the radioactivity in the blood at the time the in vivo determinations were performed. The latter correction utilizes this formula:

$$c/m^c = c/m^s - \frac{(c/m^d \times bld^{act})}{bld^o}$$

c/m^s = Activity of the in vivo count at any time.

c/m^o = Activity of the in vivo count at 10 min. (time 0).

c/m^c = Corrected activity. (value to be plotted).

bld^{act} = Activity of 1 ml of whole blood drawn at same time in vivo counts were made.

bld^o = Activity of 1 ml of whole blood drawn 10 minutes after injection (time 0).

Here again, each laboratory should determine its own "normal" values and curves.

22B ▸

Radiation Dosimetry

LT. T. G. MITCHELL, MSC, USN AND CAPT. E. R. KING, MC, USN

22B.1 Introduction

In the present treatment of the dosimetry of radioactive isotopes of the elements, an unsophisticated introductory approach to dosimetry will be attempted, the advanced worker being referred to other works on dosimetry listed at the end of this chapter (1–3).

A question, which often comes to the mind of many, is the actual necessity or value of determination of radiation dosimetry. Is radiation dosimetry really worth the effort, or is it sufficient to use radioactive nuclides on an empirical basis as is done presently with many other medicaments? If one is interested merely in the production of a desired clinical result, for example, the reduction in activity of hyperfunctioning thyroid tissue, it matters little to the clinician whether the absorption of 5000 rads or 10,000 rads due to ionizing radiation is necessary to produce this result. On the other hand, if one is interested in the underlying causes for the difference in response of tissue to ionizing radiation, then one must necessarily be concerned with radiation dosimetry.

Radiation dosimetry requires not only considerable time and effort on the part of the physician and/or physicist, but also may necessitate great inconvenience on the part of out-patients if it is necessary for them to return at frequent intervals, as is often the case. For this reason, the tendency is for some physicians to treat patients with small doses of radioactive materials until the desired effect is achieved. This method is not without merits when one considers the many uncontrollable variables involved in radiation dosimetry calculation.

The point to be made is that even when the quantity of radioactive material to be given is calculated on the basis of a dose of ionizing radiation sufficient to produce a desired result, the result may not ensue, and further radioisotope administration may be necessary. Conversely, the effect of a single dose in μc or mc, calculated to be optimal for the production of a desired result may be in excess of that necessary to produce the desired result.

Radiation dosimetry is of unquestionable value in many cases, several of which are: (1) determination of the quantity of administered radioisotope which will produce radiation levels not in excess of the weekly maximum permissible exposure as listed in NBS Handbooks 52 and 59 (4); (2) determination of blood levels of radioactive isotopes which will produce reduction in numbers of formed elements; (3) estimation of relative biological effects of various energies and types of radiation.

22B.2 Factors Affecting Radiation Dosage

Many variables are involved in determination of radiation dosimetry· Some of the variables which may be open to choice by the clinician, esti‾ mable or easily determinable, include the following:

22B2.1 *The Radioisotope Itself.** Of the elements normally found in the body, radioisotopes of suitably long half-lives and radiation characteristics exist for all elements excepting nitrogen and oxygen. The availability of any particular radionuclide will depend on the availability of a feasible method of production which is not economically prohibitive. The choice of a particular radioisotope will depend on the use to which the investigator wishes to put it. For example, if one were interested in repeat studies on the thyroid gland at daily intervals, he may find it more convenient to use a short-lived radioisotope of Iodine such as I^{128} or I^{132} rather than the longer-lived I^{131}; on the other hand, if one were interested in the rate of turnover of Iodine in the thyroid gland over a period extending from days to weeks, then I^{131} would be the radioisotope of choice. Of those elements having more than one available radioisotope we may list as examples, iron, Fe^{55} ($T\frac{1}{2} = 2.9$ years) and Fe^{59} ($T\frac{1}{2} = 45$ days); chlorine, Cl^{36} ($T\frac{1}{2} = 3.1 \times 10^5$ years) and Cl^{38} ($T\frac{1}{2} = 37.3$ min.); iodine, I^{128} ($T\frac{1}{2} = 25$ min.), I^{130} ($T\frac{1}{2} = 12.6$ hr.), I^{131} ($T\frac{1}{2} = 8$ days), I^{132} ($T\frac{1}{2} = 2.3$ hr.).

One may choose the element which he desires to use depending on the function to be performed. For example, for blood volume determinations one may use P^{32}, K^{42}, Cr^{51}, Fe^{55}, Fe^{59} or I^{131} to mention but a few which have been used for this purpose. For intracavitary administration Colloidal Gold (Au^{198}), Chromic Phosphate (P^{32}) or Yttrium (Y^{90}) have found widespread usage, each having its particular advantages and disadvantages.

22B2.2 *The Effective Half-Life.* Whenever a radioactive isotope of an element is deposited in tissue it will continue to undergo radioactive decay in accordance with its characteristic half-life. If there were no metabolic

---

* Table II, page 619 lists those in frequent use, Table III, page 621 some less frequently used.

turnover of a radioisotope in tissue, the change in activity of the isotope in that tissue would be a function of the rate of decay of the radioisotope. In this restricted case the effective half-life of the isotope would be equal to the physical half-life of the isotope. Conversely, if one had a stable isotope or a radioisotope of extremely long half-life, such that there was no apparent change in activity during the period of observation, and one observed the change in the amount of this isotope present in tissues as a function of time, he would note that the isotope would leave the tissue at a rate characteristic of the metabolic half-life of the element. In this restricted case, the effective half-life of the radioactive isotope would be equal to the metabolic half-life of the element.

The physical half-life of a radioactive isotope is a concept which has real meaning; it indicates the time during which an original quantity of radioactive atoms disintegrate to one-half the original value, independent of any extraneous factors. If one plots the logarithm of activity as a function of time a straight line will necessarily result, the slope of which is equal to the decay constant.

The metabolic half-life, however, is an approximation and is not constant for a particular organ-element combination except under closely controlled conditions for short periods of time. It will be found, that depending on changes of the metabolic state of the tissue in question, a log plot of quantity of element present as a function of time will not necessarily follow a straight line.

Since the effective half-life concept is based on the metabolic as well as the physical half-life of an isotope it appears that the effective half-life will not be constant, but in general it is assumed to be so.

The quantity of radioisotope Q_t present at any time t will be proportional to the original amount present, Q_o at $t =$ zero, the time elapsed, $t - t_o$, and the decay constant λ according to the following equation:

$$Q_t = Q_o \, e^{-(0.693t/T_{\frac{1}{2}}p)}$$

and

$$Q_t = Q_o \, e^{-(0.693t/T_{\frac{1}{2}}m)}$$

combining

$$Q_t = Q_o \, e^{-(0.693t/T_{\frac{1}{2}}p)} \, e^{-(0.693t/T_{\frac{1}{2}}m)}$$

also

$$Q_t = Q_o \, e^{-(0.693t/T_{\frac{1}{2}}\mathrm{eff})}$$

therefore

$$Q_o \, e^{-(0.693t/T_{\frac{1}{2}}\mathrm{eff})} = Q_o \, e^{-(0.693t/T_{\frac{1}{2}}p)} \, e^{-(0.693t/T_{\frac{1}{2}}m)}$$

$$e^{-(0.693t/T_{\frac{1}{2}}\mathrm{eff})} = e^{-(0.693t/T_{\frac{1}{2}}p)+(0.693t/T_{\frac{1}{2}}m)}$$

Taking natural log on both sides

$$-\frac{0.693t}{T\frac{1}{2}\mathrm{eff}} = -\frac{0.693t}{T\frac{1}{2}p} - \frac{0.693t}{T\frac{1}{2}m}$$

Dividing through by $-0.693t$

$$\frac{1}{T\frac{1}{2}\mathrm{eff}} = \frac{1}{T\frac{1}{2}p} + \frac{1}{T\frac{1}{2}m} \quad\text{or}\quad T\frac{1}{2}\mathrm{eff} = \frac{T\frac{1}{2}p \times T\frac{1}{2}m}{T\frac{1}{2}p + T\frac{1}{2}m}$$

In practice, the effective half-life may be estimated when the physical half-life of the isotope and metabolic half-life of the element are known. A direct method for determination of the effective half-life is to determine the activity of the tissue periodically, plot the log of specific activity as a function of time and graphically determine the half-life. Effective half-lives for radioactive isotopes localized in tissues, such as iodine[131] in the thyroid gland, may be estimated by serial in-vivo counting under identical geometrical conditions, the log of activity detected being plotted as a function of time and effective half-life determined graphically. The graphic method requires that counts be made over a period of time equal to several half-lives for best results. A quick approximation may be made by making two counts with a known interval of time between counts, utilizing the following formula:

$$T\frac{1}{2}\mathrm{eff} = \frac{0.693(t_2 - t_1)}{\ln C_1 - \ln C_2}$$

where $C_1 =$ counts at time t_1
$C_2 =$ counts at time t_2

Where a constant effective half-life is not obtainable, some idea of the average life of the radioactive isotope in the tissue may be estimated by plotting activity as a function of time on linear paper, the area under the curve being determined planimetrically or graphically, and the average life then estimated. This method finds use primarily in determining radiation dosage after a dose of radioactive material has been given.

A basic assumption in the use of the effective half-life in pretreatment radiation dosimetry is that the effective half-life of a therapeutic dose will be the same as that for a tracer dose. The validity of this assumption will depend on the amount of radiation damage to the tissue in both cases, and on the specific activity of the tracer and therapy dose.

22B.2.3 *The Decay Scheme.* Complete decay schemes have not been determined for all radioactive isotopes, and it is reasonable to assume that minor revisions may be made periodically. Depending on the decay scheme which one chooses to use, different radiation doses will be calculable for the same radioactive isotope. Even so, for most radioactive isotopes clinically useful, the differences in the decay schemes currently being used would not make much more than a few per cent error in estimation of radiation dosage. Accurate calibration of radioactive isotopes is dependent on the presently accepted decay schemes (5). An inherent error of several per cent may be found in any calibration in addition to the incidental error of perhaps 3 per cent which may be introduced by systematic errors in preparation of the material for standardization, counting errors, etc.

22B.2.4 *Retention In Tissue.* That portion of an administered radioactive isotope which remains in tissue and decays exerts the greatest effect on that tissue. Retention in tissue may be estimated by in-vivo counting, as in the case of the thyroid glands or by sampling the tissue, as with blood or urine to estimate total body retention.

It may not be feasible to use in-vivo or tissue sampling methods to estimate retention of an isotope in some cases. Recourse may then be had to the data of NBS Handbook 52, tables 3 and 4 for estimation of the uptake of various radioactive isotopes by body tissues.* This data is dependent on the chemical form of the element which is added to a biological system, not only on the element to which the radioactive isotope belongs.

22B.2.5 *Specific Activity.* Depending on the method of production and preparation, one may have radioactive isotopes of different specific activities. Specific activity may not be a critical factor in some applications of radioactive isotopes but in others it is of paramount importance. This is true in tracer studies as well as therapeutic applications.

Specific activity may be stated in terms of radioactivity per unit mass of the element, or in terms of radioactivity per unit mass of the particular isotope of an element. For example, the specific activity of P^{32} in terms of the isotope P^{32} is given by

$$A = \lambda N$$

$$= \frac{0.693}{14.3d \times 86,400 \text{ sec/day}} \times \frac{6.02 \times 10^{23} \times 1 \text{ gram}}{32}$$

$$A = 1.06 \times 10^{16} \text{ dis/sec/gm}$$

$$= 2.9 \times 10^{5} \text{ curies/gm}$$

This is the specific activity of carrier-free P^{32}. One method of production of carrier-free P^{32} is by deuteron bombardment of Si^{30} in a cyclotron.

To separate P^{32} from the silicon target it may be necessary to add a small amount of inert P^{31} as "carrier". The specific activity of the resultant P^{32}

* This data also available in Table I, Chapter 12, this text.

in terms of radioactivity per unit mass of the element would depend on the amount of "carrier" added.

P^{32} produced by thermal neutron activation of P^{31}, is not carrier-free, its specific activity being dependent on the flux of the neutron source, the cross section of the P^{31} nucleus for thermal neutron capture and the duration of irradiation. Maximum specific activity would be achieved after an irradiation time equal to approximately 7 half-lives of the resultant P^{32} (>99% saturation).

Specific activity at any time $= \sigma f N (1 - e^{-\lambda t})$

where σ = thermal neutron capture cross section in cm²

   f = thermal neutron flux in neutrons/cm²-sec

   N = number of target atoms/gram

$(1 - e^{-\lambda t})$ = fraction of saturation activity

With presently available sources, radiative capture of thermal neutrons leads to a maximum specific activity given approximately by,

$$A = \overset{f}{10^{13}} \times \underset{31}{\overset{N}{6.02 \times 10^{23}}} \times \overset{\sigma}{0.3 \times 10^{-24}} \times \overset{(1 - e^{-\lambda t})}{1}$$

$A = 5.8 \times 10^{10}$ dis/sec

$A = 1.6$ curies/gram Phosphorus

$= 0.625$ grams/curie

The specific activity of P^{32} produced in this manner is not as high as that previously outlined. A dose of 1 mc of P^{32} of this specific activity would result in administration of only 0.625 mg of Phosphorus. Carrier-free P^{32} is produced commercially by irradiation of S^{32} with fast neutrons, S^{32} (n, p) P^{32}.

Specific activity is a problem when one has a low flux source of neutrons; where the thermal neutron capture cross section of the target atoms is small, or the time of irradiation is short with respect to the half-life of the radio-nuclide produced.

With low specific activity material, the toxicity of the element may become a greater problem than that of radiation dosage. Commercially available radioactive isotopes are ordinarily produced in high specific activity, therefore, the user need not fear chemical toxicity unless the radioactive materials are produced under conditions outlined in the preceding paragraph.

Specific activity will determine the distribution of an administered radioisotope in the body. For example, higher specific activity I^{131} leads to higher thyroid uptakes than low specific activity I^{131}. This is due to "saturation" of the gland with elemental Iodine at low specific activity. Hence the necessity of using carrier-free material for uptake studies to determine dosage, and the necessity of using carrier-free material to achieve a high degree of uptake in the gland when a therapeutic dose is administered.

22B.3 Dosimetry of Clinically Administered Radioisotopes

22B.3.1.1 Radioactive isotopes have been used for over 30 years as indicators to determine the fate of an element introduced into a biological system. The use of radioactive isotopes as tracers is based on the premise that biological systems are unable to differentiate between radioactive and stable isotopes of the same element. For elements of low Z number, principally for carbon and below, there is, however, considerable difference between the masses of radioactive and stable isotopes, and between different stable isotopes of the same element. For example, the most common isotope of hydrogen, protium, has a mass of approximately one atomic mass unit while the other stable isotope of hydrogen, deuterium, has a mass of approximately two atomic mass units. A difference in the rates of utilization of water containing deuterium (heavy water) and ordinary water may be noted due to this mass effect. The radioactive isotope of hydrogen, tritium, has a mass of approximately three atomic mass units, therefore, a difference may be noted in utilization of tritiated water in comparison to ordinary water. This is an isotope effect and not related to the fact that tritium is also radioactive.

22B.3.1.2 Radioactive isotopes may be used as indicators provided another criterion is fulfilled, that is, there must be no effect on the utilization of the isotope due to radiation. For example, if one were to attempt to determine something of the metabolism of iodine and gave a tracer dose of 1 uc of carrier free I^{131} to a patient the normal physiology of the gland would not be disturbed by the minimal radiation dose. However, if one were to give a therapy dose of 10 mc carrier-free I^{131} instead, the radiation effect may be such as to destroy all or part of the gland's function, leading to rapid release of I^{131} from the gland in comparison to that noted with the smaller dose. This would be a radiation effect.

22B.3.1.3 A third effect noted when using radioactive isotopes as tracers is a chemical effect. This effect is noted where the specific activity of a radioactive material is so low that quantities of the element administered with the radioactive isotope are in excess of those usually found in the system. For example, if one compares the incorporation of Fe in red cells using high specific activity Fe^{59} and low specific activity Fe^{59} he would note in the former case a higher percentage iron incorporation than in the latter case.

22B.3.2.1 *Clinical dosimetry of externally administered radiation from* *radioisotopes.* Portable units designed for radiography in the field have been developed utilizing the gamma rays from radioactive Thuluim, Tm^{170}, to produce the radiographic effect. The dosimetric problems associated with radiographic apparatus, using radioactive isotopes as the source of ionizing radiation, are similar to those associated with conventional roentgenographic apparatus.

22B.3.2.2 Radium^{226}, Cesium^{137}, and Cobalt^{60} have all been used as external sources of radiation for therapy. The dosimetric problems associated with these instruments are similar to those associated with conventional super-voltage roentgen-ray apparatus (6).

22B.3.2.3 External sources of radioactive isotopes applied directly to the skin could conceivably include any radioactive isotope of convenient half-life and suitable radiation characteristics. P^{32} solution, soaked up in blotting paper, has been used in the past (7). Problems of dosimetry for such external sources have been treated adequately by Rossi and Ellis (8). One source of danger inherent in the application of sources of radiation directly to the skin is the possibility of absorption of the radioactive material through the intact or broken skin. To avoid this, it is necessary to place a thin layer of matter, impervious to the radioactive material, between the source of radiation and the skin.

22B.3.2.4 The development of sealed sources of beta emitting radionuclides such as the Sr^{90}-Y^{90} ophthalmologic beta ray applicator precludes the necessity for extensive radiation dosimetry calculations (9). These instruments are generally calibrated by the manufacturer with an extrapolation chamber. The instrument is supplied with the surface dosage rate given in roentgens equivalent physical (rep) per second. Sources are currently available with dosage rates in the range 25–40 rep/sec. Depth dose curves are also supplied with these instruments.

22B.3.3.1 *Clinical dosimetry of interstitial and intracavitary administered radioisotopes.* Implantation technics utilizing artificial radioactive isotopes are similar to those in current use with radon or radium with the added advantage that there is greater flexibility in the shapes and sizes of the artificially radioactive sources available. Notable among these are the use of Cobalt^{60} needles, tubes and wires, as well as the glass and plastic vehicles developed by Dudley (10) for the interstitial implantation of Au^{198}, Y^{90} or other short-lived radionuclides. Iridium^{192} is gaining interest as a source of both temporary and permanent interstitial radiation therapy.

22B.3.3.2 Interstitial injection of radioactive colloidal gold (Au^{198}), radioactive colloidal chromic phosphate (P^{32}) and other radioactive isotopes is generally done on an empirical basis or by following technics empirically derived by others. The uncertainties in diffusion of radioactive material throughout the injected tissue, non-uniform concentration and inability to estimate the rate of removal of the isotope from the tissue make pretreatment radiation dosimetry very elusive.

22B.3.3.3 Intracavitary administrations of radiocolloids of Au^{198}, P^{22} (as chromic phosphate) and Y^{90} have been used to control accumulation of abdominal and/or pleural fluid, as a palliative procedure.

The usual doses for these are:

	Au^{198}	P^{32}	Y^{90}
Intrapleural	75–100	5–15	5–15
Intra-abdominal	100–150	10–25	10–25

Systemic Administration.

22B.3.4.1 *Clinical dosimetry of internally administered radioisotopes.* This brief discussion will be limited to therapeutic applications of radioisotopes.

22B.3.4.1.1 *Iodine*[131]. This radioisotope is used for treatment of several conditions. In treating hyperthyroidism of the diffuse type, an initial dose of about 5 mc is usually administered orally. This is an arbitrary treatment method and is not based upon the gland weight. The patient is re-evaluated in about 3 months and quite often is still toxic. In such an instance a smaller dose of from 1–2 mc is administered by the oral route. Usually this is sufficient although occasionally another small dose will be required three months later when the patient is seen again. The scientific approach is to deliver a pre-determined radiation dose to the thyroid. A dose in the order of 8,000–10,000 rads is required for remission of the disease. This dose is calculated by a formula presented in paragraph 20.6 of this chapter. Our group does not believe it is possible to accurately determine the thyroid weight and prefers to use the arbitrary method of giving small doses of iodine[131]. Certain cardiac conditions are also treated with this radioisotope, and in these cases an initial dose is 10 mc, and the patient is retreated until he becomes hypothyroid. Iodine[131] is used in treating certain types of metastatic carcinoma of the thyroid. Here the doses are in the order of 100 mc, orally, and are repeated at 3–4-month intervals until the metastases "pick up" no more iodine, or the bone marrow becomes depressed.

22B.3.4.1.2 *Phosphorus*[32]. This isotope may be given orally, or intravenously. In treating chronic leukemias, our laboratory administers 1 mc of phosphorus[32] at weekly intervals until the total white blood cell count drops below 30,000 per cubic millimeter. In treating polycythemia vera, we give 3–4 mc and re-evaluate the patient in 4 months. At this time we may give another 2–3 mc. Radiophosphorus is also used to treat bone metastases from carcinoma of the breast or of the prostate. This therapy includes intravenous phosphorus[32] and male sex hormones orally. A dose of 1 mc of radiophosphorus is administered daily for a total of 7–12 days. This treatment is used in demonstrating phosphorus[32] localization in the lesions by a tracer dose and a scanning procedure.

22B.3.4.1.3 Several other radioisotopes have been used internally but only iodine[131] and phosphorus[32] are generally accepted. In the above discussion, one should realize that many variations in dosage schedules are observed in different clinics. The dosages mentioned are the ones used in most cases treated at our clinic.

22B.4 Determination of Radiation Tissue Dose from Radioisotopes

Generally, radioactive materials may be administered systemically either orally or intravenously depending on the physical or chemical form in which the radioactive material is administered and the distribution desired.

In addition to those variables listed above, there are certain factors not easily estimable about which some supposition must be made.

22B.4.1 *Tissue Weight.* The weight of tissues may be estimated on the basis of the weight of the patient's body in accordance with the data calculated and listed in several places for the "standard man" (11). Unfortunately for the clinician, all men are not "standard", having greatly variable amounts of adipose tissue. Attempts to estimate organ or tissue weight by palpation are subject to human error. Scanning with a suitable detector an area containing localized radioactivity may be helpful in estimating organ weight if this scanning is performed in two planes, at right angles to each other. Scanning in one plane only is not a reliable method of estimation.

The error in estimation of gland weight, even something readily accessible, such as the thyroid gland, is probably accurate to only plus or minus 25% at best. Estimation of gland weight may be the greatest source of error in estimating dosimetry.

22B.4.2 *Uniform Distribution in Tissue.* For purposes of estimation of radiation dosage, it is generally assumed that the radioisotope is uniformly distributed throughout a tissue whose dimensions are large with respect to the range of beta particles. This assumption is not as important a consideration in gamma ray dosimetry due to the great range of gamma rays in tissue.

A uniform distribution is not always necessary to produce the best result. A non-uniform distribution may be best in some cases. For example, in treatment of hyperthyroidism, cells functioning to the greatest extent may take up iodine[131], be preferentially irradiated, leaving cells with normal activity to carry on normal thyroid function. From the standpoint of the dosimetrist, a uniform distribution is desirable, making calculation simple, but from the clinical standpoint, non-uniform distribution may be best.

22B.4.3 *The Average Dose.* A dose calculated for a tissue will be an average dose, calculated for some representative point in the tissue. For tissues whose dimensions are large with respect to the range of beta particles the dose at the surface will be less than that at the center of the gland. The surface dose is about equal to one half the dose at a depth in tissue equal to or greater than the range of the most energetic beta particles emanating from the radionuclide.

The average dose is generally calculated for the center of the tissue for beta particle dosimetry in large tissues, and for gamma rays is either calculated for the center of the tissue or organ, or at a point equidistant from center and surface which more nearly represents the average gamma ray dose.

22B.4.4 *Energy Absorption.* For beta particle dosimetry the assumption is made that the energy dissipated in a tissue is equal to the energy absorbed by that tissue. This is true, except at the boundaries of the tissue where equilibrium of dissipation and absorption of energy is not attained.

This assumption is not true for gamma ray dosimetry and for this reason efforts have been made to determine the amount of energy absorbed as a function of the size of tissue and the absorption coefficient of the gamma rays.

22B.4.5 *g Factor.** It is assumed that the g factor can be approximated for tissues, organs, and bodies by assuming that these tissues, organs, and bodies have symmetrical forms which may be approximated by simple geometrical models, generally spheres or cylinders.

g factors have been calculated for various sizes and shapes of models, by several investigators (12, 13), and such a table of average *g* factors is listed. See Table I.

The *g* factor for a point in a body is determined by calculating the contribution of radiation from every other point in the volume, allowing for reduction in intensity due to the inverse square law, as well as absorption of the radiation.

For example, the radiation intensity at a point P at the center of a sphere due to radiation from a point S, is given by

$$I_p = \frac{I_o e^{-ud}}{d^2}$$

Where I_p = radiation intensity at point P

I_o = radiation intensity at unit distance from the point source S.

u = the "true" linear absorption coefficient

d = the distance between points P and S

* Geometrical Factor.

TABLE I*

Average Geometrical Factor, $\bar{g}$, for γ-Ray Emitter Uniformly Distributed in Total Body Tissues

WEIGHT OF PATIENT, KG	HEIGHT OF PATIENT, CM						
	200	190	180	170	160	150	140
100	138	139	142	145	147	150	154
90	134	136	138	140	143	146	148
80	129	130	131	134	136	139	141
70	123	124	125	126	129	131	135
60	117	118	119	120	122	125	128
50	112	113	114	116	117	119	122
40	102	104	105	106	108	109	110

Average Geometrical Factor, $\bar{g}$, for Cylinders Containing a Uniformly Distributed γ-Ray Emitter

LENGTH OF CYLINDER, CM	RADIUS OF CYLINDER, CM							
	3	5	10	15	20	25	30	35
2	17.5	22.1	30.3	34.0	36.2	37.5	38.6	39.3
5	22.3	31.8	47.7	56.4	61.6	65.2	67.9	70.5
10	25.1	38.1	61.3	76.1	86.5	93.4	98.4	103
20	25.7	40.5	68.9	89.8	105	117	126	133
30	25.9	41.0	71.3	94.6	112	126	137	146
40	25.9	41.3	72.4	96.5	116	131	143	153
60	26.0	41.6	73.0	97.8	118	134	148	159
80	26.0	41.6	73.3	98.4	119	135	150	161
100	26.0	41.6	73.3	98.5	119	136	150	162

* From "Radiation Dosimetry", page 858, HINE AND BROWNELL, Courtesy of Academic Press, N. Y.

more simply, $g = \dfrac{e^{-ud}}{d^2}$

Where the source of radiation is uniformly distributed throughout the tissue, the dosage to the point P from all other points in the volume may be found by evaluating the integral

$$\int \frac{e^{-ud}}{d^2}\, dv$$

For the simplest geometric forms, the following approximations are given:

Center of sphere of radius d

$$g = \frac{4\pi}{u} (1 - e^{-ud}) \cong 4\pi\, d$$

Surface of sphere of radius d

$$g = \frac{2\pi}{u} (1 - e^{-ud}) \cong 2\pi\, d$$

22B.4.6 *Absorption Coefficient.* The true linear absorption coefficient of gamma radiation is dependent on the atomic number of the absorber and the energy of the radiation. In the range of energies from approximately 150 kev to 2 mev the energy absorbed per gram of tissue per roentgen is relatively independent of the atomic number of the tissue. For example, at 150 kev the energy absorption in ergs/gm-r is 95.3 for fat (effective Z number = 5.92) and 94.5 for bone (effective Z number = 13.8). At 2 mev the energy absorbed in ergs/gm-r is 95.8 and 84.5 for fat and bone, respectively, compared to 83.8 ergs/gm-r for air at these energies.

In general, for gamma ray dosimetry, the assumption is made that the soft tissues of the body are equivalent to water in density and have an average atomic number equal to air (14).

The energy absorption in ergs/gm-r for muscle varies from 95.3 to 96.8 (15) in the range .15–3 mev, and for this reason the approximation is made that the dose in roentgens to soft tissue is generally equal to the dose in rads.

For energies much less than .150 mev the energy absorption per gm-r in bone rises sharply to a maximum of approximately 480 ergs/gm-r at 10 kev and drops to a minimum of approximately 45 ergs/gm-r for fat at the same energy (16).

Energy absorption in the region .01–.15 mev is strongly dependent on energy of the gamma rays. Fortunately, many of the gamma rays from radioactive isotopes presently available have energies in the range .15–3 mev (17).

Extremely low energy gamma rays, as well as low energy characteristic radiation may be treated in a manner similar to that for beta radiation for purposes of dosimetry. This would apply only where the size of the tissues was large compared with the range of the gamma rays.

22B.4.7 *Rapid Localization In Tissue.* It is generally assumed that the maximum uptake of a radioisotope occurs within a very short time after administration. For I^{131}, and the thyroid gland, the maximum uptake in the gland may occur as early as several hours or as late as 2 days. The dose during the period of time prior to that at which maximum uptake occurs may be calculated by determining the average amount of I^{131} in the gland during this time, and using this in the dosage calculations. Where the effective half-life is long with respect to the time necessary to achieve maximum uptake in a tissue, the assumption that maximum uptake occurs spontaneously leads to over estimation of the dose. The magnitude of over-estimation will be dependent on the relative times.

22B.5 Units of Radiation Dosimetry (See 6.8)

22B5.1 *Rad.* The rad is the unit of absorbed radiation dose and is equal to the absorption of 100 ergs/gm of material regardless of energy of the incident radiation and the composition of the absorbing material.

22B.5.2 *Roentgen.* The roentgen has been defined (6.8) as an exposure dose of X or gamma radiation such that the associated corpuscular emission per .001293 grams of air produces, in air, ions carrying one electrostatic unit of quantity of electricity of either sign.

22B.6 Beta Particle Dosimetry

If the assumptions previously referred to are valid and one can determine effective half-life of a radioisotope in a tissue and its concentration in the tissue at the same time, one can calculate the absorbed dose in the tissue.

If the size of the tissue is large with respect to the range of the beta particles, the beta particle energy dissipated per unit mass of tissue will be equal to the beta particle energy absorbed. Calculation of beta particle energy dissipated consequently leads directly to absorbed dose.

If the total number of atoms of a radioactive isotope present is given by N_0, and λ is its decay constant, then activity A, would be given by $A = N_0\lambda$.

Knowing A and λ, N_0 is seen to be equal to $\dfrac{A \times 1}{\lambda}$, and is therefore equal to $A \times$ average life, provided the units of decay constant and average life are comparable. If A is given as disintegrations per second then average life must be given in seconds. The total number of atoms which will disintegrate per microcurie per gram of tissue can then be estimated from

$$3.7 \times 10^4 \times 8.64 \times 10^4 \times T\tfrac{1}{2} \text{ eff} \times 1.443$$

$$\text{d/s/uc} \qquad \text{Sec/day} \qquad \text{Ave. Life in days}$$

$$N_0 = 4.61 \times 10^9 \times T\tfrac{1}{2} \text{ eff in days} = \text{Atoms Dis/}\mu\text{c–gm.}$$

Assuming 1 beta particle of average energy per disintegration, this also gives the number of beta particles/gram for complete decay.

If the average beta particle energy, $\bar{E}_B$, is given in million electron volts,

TABLE II*

Radiological Data of Frequently Used Radioisotopes

RADIOISOTOPE	RADIATION EMITTED	HALF-LIFE	AVERAGE β-RAY ENERGY, $\bar{E}_\beta$, mev	Kβ, gm-rad/μcd	POINT SOURCE γ-RAY DOSE-RATE CONSTANT, Γ, cm²-r/mc-hr
H³	β^-	12.26 years	0.0055	—	0
C¹⁴	β^-	5600 years	0.049	—	0
Na²⁴	β^-, γ	15.0 hours	0.55	25	18.4
P³²	β^-	14.5 days	0.69	730	0
S³⁵	β^-	87 days	0.049	315	0
K⁴²	β^-, γ	12.5 hours	1.45	55	1.50
Ca⁴⁵	β^-	160 days	0.076	920	0
Cr⁵¹	E. C., γ	27 days	0.0049	10	0.18
Fe⁵⁹	β^-, γ	45 days	0.120	410	6.13
Co⁶⁰	β^-, γ	5.2 years	0.094	—	12.8
Sr⁹⁰ + Y⁹⁰	β^-	28 years	0.20 + 0.93	—	0
I¹³¹	β^-, γ	8.0 days	0.187	110	2.18
Cs¹³⁷	β^-, γ	30 years	0.23	—	3.2
Au¹⁹⁸	β^-, γ	2.70 days	0.331	66	2.35
Radium²²⁶	Secondary electrons, γ	1620 years	—	—	8.4 ± 0.2 (0.5mmPt)

I¹³¹: The conversion electrons have an energy of about 8 kev per disintegration. This energy is included in the value given for $\bar{E}_\beta$.

Cs¹³⁷: The conversion electrons have an energy of about 50 kev per disintegration. This energy is included in the value given for $\bar{E}_\beta$. The computation of Γ is based on $0.92/(1 + \alpha K) = 0.84$ γ-ray escaping per disintegration.

Au¹⁹⁸: The conversion electrons have an energy of about 11 kev per disintegration. This energy is included in the value given for $\bar{E}_\beta$. The computation of Γ is based on $1/(1 + \alpha K) = 0.97$ γ-ray per disintegration of energy 0.412 mev.

then the energy dissipated during complete decay of the radioactive atoms would be

$$D_B = 4.61 \times 10^9 \times T\tfrac{1}{2} \text{ eff} \times \bar{E}_B \text{ mev} \times 1.6 \times 10^{-6} \text{ ergs/mev}$$

ergs/gram for complete decay

Since the RAD equals 100 ergs/gram, the beta dose in rads/gm is given by

$$D_B = 73.8 \times T\tfrac{1}{2} \text{ eff} \times \bar{E}_B \times C$$

days   mev μc/gm

22B.7 Gamma Ray Dosimetry

A basic concept used in gamma ray dosimetry is that of the dosage rate at unit distance from a point source of radioactive material. This is symbolized by Γ, whose dimensions are roentgens/mc-hr. at 1 centimeter from a point source, unshielded.

* "From Radiation Dosimetry." See Footnote page 621.

Γ may be calculated according to the following formula:

$$3.7 \times 10^7 \times 3600 \times \frac{\Sigma(f\gamma \times E\gamma \times u_1)}{4\pi r^2 \times 6.77 \times 10^4 \text{mev/cc/r}}$$

Where: $f\gamma$ = fraction of atoms decaying which leads to a gamma ray of a particular energy,

$E\gamma$ = gamma ray energy in mev

u_1 = "true" linear absorption coefficient in air

$4\pi r^2$ = area of a sphere.

For example, Γ may be simply calculated for Fe^{59}.

$f\gamma$	$E\gamma$ mev	u_1 cm-1	$f\gamma \times E\gamma \times u_1$
.43	1.289	3.18×10^{-5}	1.76×10^{-5}
.57	1.098	3.26×10^{-5}	2.04×10^{-5}
.03	.191	3.2×10^{-5}	$.02 \times 10^{-5}$
		$\Sigma \; (f\gamma \times E\gamma \times u_1)$	3.82×10^{-5}

$$= \frac{3.7 \times 10^7 \times 3600 \times 3.82 \times 10^{-5}}{4 \times 3.14 \times 6.77 \times 10^4} = 6 \, \text{r/mc-hr at 1 cm from a point source.}$$

The total dose of gamma radiation delivered to a point during complete decay of a gamma emitting radionuclide can be computed from Γ, if the average life, the distance from source to point of measurement, and the quantity of radioactive isotope present is known. Dose to any point within a tissue, which has a gamma-emitting radionuclide homogeneously distributed throughout it, may also be calculated if the concentration and the "g" factor are known.

Γ = r/mc-hr. If concentration is expressed in $\mu c/gm$ then this may be reduced to $10^{-3} \, r/\mu c$-hr.

Γ multiplied by the average life (effective) in hours enables one to determine the total dose delivered to a point during complete decay of a radionuclide.

i.e. $d\gamma = \Gamma \times \mu c$ Present Initially $\times 10^{-3} \times T\frac{1}{2}$ days $\times 24 \times 1.443$

$d\gamma = \Gamma \times \mu c$ Present Initially $\times T\frac{1}{2}$ eff in days $\times .0346$.

If one introduces C for concentration, in $\mu c/gram$ of tissue, and the geometry factor, "g", the total gamma ray dose would be:

$D\gamma = \Gamma \times C \times T\frac{1}{2}$ eff in days $\times .0346 \times g$ roentgens/gram.

The total dose due to beta and gamma, assuming that 1 roentgen/gram is approximately equal to 1 rad/gram, will be the sum of the individual beta particle and gamma ray dose.

$$D \text{ Total} = D_B + D_\gamma$$

$$D_B = 73.8 \times T\frac{1}{2} \times C \times \bar{E}_B$$

$$D_\gamma = .0346 \times T\frac{1}{2} \times C \times \Gamma \times g$$

$$D_{B+\gamma} = T\frac{1}{2} \times C \, (73.8\bar{E}_B + .0346\Gamma g) \text{ rads.}$$

TABLE III*

Radiological Data of Less Frequently Used Radioisotopes

RADIOISOTOPE	RADIATION EMITTED	HALF-LIFE	AVERAGE β-RAY ENERGY, $\bar{E}_\beta$, mev	$K\beta$, gm-rad/μcd	POINT SOURCE γ-RAY DOSE-RATE CONSTANT, Γ, cm²-r/mc-hr
Be⁷	E. C., γ	53 days	0.00005	0.2	0.30
Na²²	β^+, E. C., γ	2.6 years	0.19	—	11
Cl³⁶	β^-	3.1 × 10⁵ years	0.26	—	0
Sc⁴⁶	β^-, γ	85 days	0.12	750	11
V⁴⁸	β^+, E. C., γ	16.2 days	0.14	170	10
Mn⁵²	β^+, E. C., γ	5.7 days	0.072	30	19
Fe⁵⁵	E. C.	2.9 years	0.0059	—	0
Mn⁵⁴	E. C., γ	300 days	0.0054	116	4.6
Ni⁶³	β^-	80 years	0.018	—	0
Cu⁶⁴	β^+, β^-, E. C., γ	12.8 hours	0.13	5.1	1.1
Zn⁶⁵	β^+, E. C., γ	245 days	0.01	180	2.7
As⁷⁴	β^-, β^+, γ	17 days	0.37	480	5.1
As⁷⁶	β^-, γ	26.7 hours	1.14	94	3.1
Rb⁸⁶	β^-, γ	18.6 days	0.67	906	0.51
Sr⁸⁹	β^-	54 days	0.56	2200	0
Sn¹¹³	E. C., γ	112 days	0.004	33	(2.2 + 1.3)
Sb¹²⁴	β^-, γ	60 days	0.35	1550	9.8
I¹³⁰	β^-, γ	12.6 hours	0.285	11	12
I¹³²	β^-, γ	2.3 hours	0.49	3.1	11.8
Cs¹³⁴	β^-, γ	2.3 years	0.116	—	8.0
La¹⁴⁰	β^-, γ	40.2 hours	0.54	66	12
Tm¹⁷⁰	β^-, γ	129 days	0.32	3000	0.01
Au¹⁹⁹	β^-, γ	3.15 days	0.13	30	0.42
Hg¹⁹⁷	E. C., γ	2.71 days	0.06	12	(0.4)
Hg²⁰³	β^-, γ	48 days	0.10	350	1.2
Tl²⁰⁴	β^-, E. C.	4.1 years	0.24	—	(0.007)

Tm¹⁷⁰: The conversion electrons have an energy of about 10 kev, which is included in the value of $\bar{E}_\beta$.

Au¹⁹⁹: The conversion electrons have an energy of about 50 kev, which is included in $\bar{E}_\beta$.

Hg²⁰³: The conversion electrons have an energy of about 50 kev, which is included in $\bar{E}_\beta$.

* Tables II and III from "Radiation Dosimetry", pages 898, 900–901, HINE AND BROWNELL, Courtesy of Academic Press, N. Y.

22B.8 Cumulative Dose

The dose calculated for any period of time less than that necessary for complete decay to occur is based on the fact that the dose delivered is proportional to the number of atoms which have decayed.

If N_o = the number of atoms present at t_o, the number of atoms present at any future time, t would be equal to

$$N_o e^{-\lambda t}$$

The number of atoms which had decayed would then be equal to

$$N_o - N_o e^{-\lambda t}$$

or

$$N_o(1 - e^{-\lambda t})$$

N_o is the total number of atoms initially present, therefore, the fraction decayed at any time is equal to $1 - e^{-\lambda t}$. The fractional dose delivered at any time is similarly equal to $1 - e^{-\lambda t}$, or $(1 - e^{-.693t/T_{\frac{1}{2}}})$ rads

Cumulative beta particle dose may be expressed as

$$D_B \text{ (Cumulative)} = 73.8 \times T_{\frac{1}{2}} \times E_B \times C \times (1 - e^{-.693t/T_{\frac{1}{2}}}) \text{ rads}$$

$$D\gamma \text{ (Cumulative)} = .0346 \times T_{\frac{1}{2}} \times C \times \Gamma \times g \times (1 - e^{-.693t/T_{\frac{1}{2}}}) \text{ rads}$$

$$D_{B+\gamma} \text{ (Cumulative)} = T_{\frac{1}{2}} \times C \, (73.8 \, \bar{E}_B$$
$$+ .0346 \, \Gamma \, g) \times (1 - e^{-.693t/T_{\frac{1}{2}}}) \text{ rads}$$

Where $T_{\frac{1}{2}}$ is effective half-life in days.

22B.9 The Average Life

The average life is defined as that period of time during which all atoms of a radionuclide would decay, provided that they decayed at the initial rate of decay. It is also defined as the average lifetime of the radioactive atoms present. Computation of the average life is fairly direct.

$$\text{Ave. life} = \frac{1}{\lambda}$$

For example: If $\lambda = 10^{-6} \text{ Sec}^{-1}$, then average life would

$$= \frac{1}{10^{-6} \text{ Sec}^{-1}} = 10^6 \text{ sec.}$$

But λ also equals $\dfrac{.693}{T_{\frac{1}{2}}}$

$$\therefore \text{Ave. Life} = \frac{1}{\lambda} = \frac{1}{.693/T_{\frac{1}{2}}} = \frac{T_{\frac{1}{2}}}{.693} = T_{\frac{1}{2}} \times 1.443$$

Example:

Calculate the total dose due to both beta and gamma radiation to an individual who has received a tracer dose of 200 μc NA^{24} intravenously. Weight of subject = 70 kg, height, 67″. Data:

$$\text{Physical } T\tfrac{1}{2} \ Na^{24} \ = \ 15.0 \text{ hrs.}$$

$$\text{Effective } T\tfrac{1}{2} \ Na^{24} \ = \ .6 \text{ days}$$

$$E_\beta \text{ maximum } = \ 1.39 \text{ mev}$$

$$\bar{E}_\beta \ = \ .55 \text{ mev}$$

$$\Gamma \ = \ 18.4 \text{ r/mc-hr at } 1 \text{ cm}$$

Average g for 170 cm tall, 70 kg individual = 126

$$D_{B+\gamma} \ = \ T\tfrac{1}{2} \times C \times (73.8 \ \bar{E}_B + .0346 \Gamma g) \text{ rads.}$$

$$D_{B+\gamma} \ = \ .6 \times \frac{200}{70,000} \times (73.8 \times .55 + .0346 \times 18.4 \times 126)$$

$$D_{B+\gamma} \ = \ .208 \text{ rads}$$

What is the dose delivered during the first day?

$$D_{B+\gamma} \text{ first day } = \ .208 \times (1 - e^{-.693 \times 1/.6})$$

$$= \ .208 \times .685 = .142 \text{ rads first day.}$$

What contribution to the total dose is due to beta? To Gamma?

$$D_B \ = \ 73.8 \times T\tfrac{1}{2} \times C \times \bar{E}_B$$

$$D_B \ = \ 73.8 \times .6 \times \frac{200}{70,000} \times .55$$

$$D_B \ = \ .070 \text{ rads}$$

$$D_\gamma \ = \ .0346 \times T\tfrac{1}{2} \times C \times \Gamma \times g$$

$$D_\gamma \ = \ .0346 \times .6 \times \frac{200}{70,000} \times 18.4 \times 126$$

$$D_\gamma \ = \ .138 \text{ rads}$$

REFERENCES*

1. HINE, G. J. AND BROWNELL, G. L.: *Radiation Dosimetry*. New York: Acad. Press, 1956.
2. GLASSER, O., QUIMBY, E. H., TAYLOR, L. S. AND WEATHERWAX, J. L.: *Physical Foundations of Radiology*. New York: Hoeber, 2nd Ed., 1954.
3. YALOW, A. A.: Chapter 3, *Therapeutic Use of Artificial Radioisotopes*, edited by HAHN, P. F. New York: Wiley, 1956.
4. U. S. Department of Commerce, National Bureau of Standards Handbook 52, 20 March 1953. Maximum permissible amounts of radioisotopes in the human body and maximum permissible concentrations in air and water.

* See also Chapter 12.

5. Radiological Health Handbook, Edited by KINSMAN, S., U. S. Department of Health, Education and Welfare, Robert A. Taft Sanitary Engineering Center, Cincinnati, Ohio; January 1957.

6. BRAESTRUP, C. B.: Teletherapy, Chapter 43 in ORO-125. *Radioisotopes in Medicine*, Edited by ANDREWS, G.; A., BRUCER, M. and ANDERSON, E. B., Medical Division, Oak Ridge Institute of Nuclear Studies, September 1953.

7. LOW-BEER, B. V. A.: *The Clinical Use of Radioactive Isotopes.* Springfield, Ill.: Thomas, 1950. pp. 173–178 and pp. 309–317.

8. ROSSI, H. H. AND ELLIS, R. H., JR.: Calculations for distributed sources of beta radiation. *Am. J. Roentgenol. 67:* 980, 1952.

9. Tracerlab Strontium Medical Applicator, Tracerlog ⚹28, July 1950, Tracerlab, Inc., Waltham, Massachusetts.

10. DUDLEY, H. C. AND MITCHELL, T. G.: A study of methods for interstitial implantation of radioactive materials. *Am. J. Roentgenol. V. LXXV:* No. 6, June 1956.

11. HINE, G. J. AND BROWNELL, G. L.: Radiation dosimetry, p. 907, Table VII, Some characteristics of the standard man from recommendations of the International Commission on Radiological Protection. *Brit. J. Radiol.* Supp. 6, 1955.

12. *Ibid.* p. 858, Tables V and VI.

13. SIRI, W. E. *Isotopic Tracers and Nuclear Radiations.* New York: McGraw-Hill, 1949, p. 435.

14. HINE, G. J. AND BROWNELL, G. L.: *Radiation Dosimetry*, Table III, p. 16.

15. *Ibid.* Table VI p. 88.

16. *Ibid.* Fig. 21, p. 90.

17. FANO, U., U. S. Department of Commerce, NBS, Circular 499, and supplements "Nuclear Data".

18. U. S. Department of Commerce, NBS, Handbook 62. Report of the International Commission on Radiological Units and Measurements (ICRU), 1956.

23▸

Oral Effects of Radiation and Features of Importance in Dentistry

JAMES A. ENGLISH, B.S., D.D.S., M.S., PhD.

23.1 Introduction

Roentgenography has become so well established as a means of diagnosis in the field of dentistry that a majority of practicing dentists have an x-ray machine available as a part of their equipment. Therapeutic use of radium and x-ray in the oral region is equally well established, but such therapy is usually administered in hospitals or clinics by professional teams specifically trained in this specialty. All people who are in any way engaged in the diagnostic or therapeutic use of x-ray or radioactive materials should be thoroughly familiar with the dangers involved (Stenstrom) and with any special considerations related to the anatomic area they are handling. The first purpose of this chapter is to review the basic principles of radiation phenomena that may be helpful to members of the dental profession in maintaining rational procedures in roentgenology. Secondly, we will re-examine oral and dental effects of radiation, and emphasize relationships that must be remembered by both the dentist and radiologist in order that they may cooperate for the best interests of the patient.

Early workers in roentgenology and the pioneers who explored the radio-active materials made fatal errors in handling these new discoveries because of lack of understanding. Similar accidents today are due to carelessness or unintelligent therapy (Daland). Because of our accumulated knowledge of radiobiology, and with the technologic progress that has provided us with modern, safe equipment, danger to the operator in carrying out therapeutic measures employing radioactive materials is reduced to a minimum (Failla), and there is no danger in x-ray therapy since the treatment room is vacated by the radiologist during the exposure of patient (Nuttall). In roentgenographic procedures, the relative exposure is exceedingly small compared to those of therapy. In dental roentgenography, for example, the peak electrical tension is only about 75 KV, whereas the milliamp.-second per film is from 50 to 200 (Files; Ennis; Santé). Thus damage to the operator can be accomplished only by grossly incorrect technique. Yet no system can render x-ray foolproof; the first protective measure is to eliminate people who are ignorant of electrical and radiation dangers (Barclay and Cox).

In order to prevent untoward damage to the patient by radiation, it is important that the radiotherapist have a clear understanding of possible secondary effects which may result from his treatment. It is no discredit to a therapeutic measure that there have been occasional rare or exceptional responses, but to the contrary, such effects may be utilized to an advantage when they are known to occur and subsequent administration of treatment regulated so as to capitalize on this knowledge (Ruppe and Lebourg). Sometimes side effects can be avoided by following certain precautions as, for example, placing a lead shield over a susceptible organ in the general area of a lesion to be irradiated. Developing teeth and jaws must be included among organs which are sensitive to irradiation and frequently can be protected. The treatment of such lesions as diffuse angiomata of the face in children by radiation does include a risk of damage to developing teeth and interference with normal growth of the mandibles (LaCronique, Beal, and Goudaert). If such damage cannot be prevented, it must be considered as a calculated risk prior to treatment.

Finally, even though no clinical application were to be made of an attained knowledge of radiation principles, an acquisition of this information is necessary in order to fully understand current trends in dental literature. The availability of artificially radioactivated substances in recent years has resulted in an increasing number of research applications in the dental field. The radioisotopes have served efficiently in providing much information on the distribution of various elements in teeth and in solving certain problems of metabolism (McCauley; Volker, Sognnaes, and Bibby; Koss and Ginn; English and Dudley; Pecher; Manley and Bale; Bartlestone). In a similar manner, the administration of measured amounts of x-ray irradiation under controlled conditions of animal experimentation has provided a tool of value in unravelling hidden mechanisms of physiology and pathology (English and Tullis).

23.2 Protective Measures

One could assume that professional graduates who have advanced far enough in their science to be using radiology as a diagnostic or therapeutic means would fully understand any hidden dangers that may be involved.

This is apparently not true, for there are on record many cases where physicians, dentists, and technicians have been inadvertently subjected to damaging doses of radiation in performing clinical procedures. The over-exposure to radiation may occur as a single large accidental dose or as intermittent exposures to smaller doses over a long period of time. In clinical dentistry, the latter is more likely, though it has been reported (Pfahler) that in at least one instance the dental machine was used for fluoroscopy in attempting to extricate metal foreign bodies from the hand, with disastrous results to both patient and doctor.

It is extremely important to remember that there is a cumulative effect to ionizing irradiation and that the tissues and organs can tolerate just so much without outward signs of damage (Goldsmith). Unfortunately, the resulting lesions are often discovered too late to serve as an adequate warning, for by the time there is an ulcerative dermatitis there may be sufficient damage to the involved tissues to retard healing. As a result of poor epithelization and local damage to the vascular system by the rays, these lesions tend to become chronic in character. This chronicity leads to thickening of the peripheral epithelium, downgrowth, and sometimes to carcinoma (Wolbach). Any such damage to the hands of the dentist will only occur as the result of faulty technique. Lesions such as described have occurred when the operator persistently has held the dental films in pa-tients' mouths during the exposure period. Because there was no pain involved or no apparent damage to his hands or to the patient, he believed he was doing himself no harm. It is because of the insidious and stealthy nature of radiation damage (Morgan) and the irreversibility of the injury done that constant warnings must be given. Frequently repeated exposures to relatively low doses constitute the greatest hazard in contemporary radiation work (Ingram). There is no antidote to such radiation injury (Chamberlain, Newell, Taylor, and Wyckoff) nor any reliable clinical sign which will serve as an adequate warning of overexposure.

There have been other late effects attributed to radiation in people who were exposed to small amounts of radiation over considerable periods of time. Important among these systemic consequences are leukopenia, ane-mia, leukemia, sterility and possibly other genetic changes (Henshaw; Hen-shaw and Hawkins; Nuttal). The significance of the relationship of blood changes and genetic changes in radiation workers has been questioned (Ellis; Barclay and Cox; Ingram; Glucksmann), and it is certainly true that such effects will not occur in radiographic procedures with very mod-erate precautions. The amount of scattered radiation in x-ray diagnostic procedures is not sufficient to damage the operator if he stands 2-½ feet from the center of field of radiation (5 feet in the case of fluoroscopy).

Even if the operator is in a direct line with the primary beam of the anti-cathode, 1 mm. of lead will provide adequate protection at 4 feet (Barclay and Cox).

23.2.1 *Detailed Protection Measures.* There are several precautionary measures which the dentist should follow in the interests of safety: (1) Never follow a technique which will require either himself or his technician to be directly exposed to the rays, (2) use the proper cones and filters that are provided with the equipment (Chamberlain), (3) when the amount of roentgenography is more than that incidental to an average practice, and particularly when a technician is spending a large portion of his time performing this service, provide a lead lined shield, booth or partition as an additional protection, (4) periodically check for leakage of radiation from the equipment by means of a dosimeter or by means of carrying a dental x-ray film packet partially covered by a metal shield, to be developed after a few days to observe evidence of a difference in the shielded and unshielded portions (Quimby).

23.3 The Effects of Irradiation on Teeth

As early as 1905 it was reported (Tribondeau and Recamer) that roentgenization could have an arresting effect on the development of the facial bones and particularly on the teeth. In this study the right anterior-lateral side of the face of a three day old cat was exposed for a 60 minute period (in 6 treatments over two weeks time) at a distance of 10 cm. The effects were noted on the exposed side of the face, whereas the opposite side was relatively unaffected.

In the early years following the discovery of radiation phenomena many clinicians went overboard in the extensive use they made of this form of treatment. As often happens with new remedies, treatment by radium and x-ray became a panacea. A few excerpts from the literature, beginning in 1914 (Levy), will illustrate this point.

Speaking of "Bequerel-rays", Levy says, "It has become an established therapy in general medicine, which has resulted in outstanding success in the different disciplines. One can speak today with justice of a radium therapy of total medicine. Dentistry has been somewhat late in considering radium treatment. . . . This is interesting to me . . . since it was Walkhoff (a dentist) who first established for Bequerel in 1900 the biological effects of radiation. Early in 1912 I introduced this therapy in dentistry . . . (and) indicated that radioactive substances may be very suitable to favorably influence oral disease, and recommended the use of radium emanation for inflammation of the oral cavity. Through the publications of Trauner, Warnekros, Levy, Leger-Dorez and Mamlok the scope of radium therapy has become significantly broadened. . . . For the technique of irradiating the mouth we need thin-walled, small glass tubes containing radium salts, or vulcanite tubes of radium, tubes of gold, silver, etc. . . . The manner of reaction of the oral mucous membrane follows in general the known rules for skin reaction to irradiation. . . . Favorable results are brought about in local inflammation, marginal gingivitis, and extensive gingivitis. Epuli, decubital ulceration, hornification and leucoplakia of the tongue showed themselves amenable to capsule irradiation. No lasting effect was observed with chronic alveolar pyorrhea. . . ."

In the ten year period following 1922 German and French investigators became aware of the damaging results of radiotherapy beyond the therapeutic effects intended. In 1925–27 Leist carried out some experimental studies with dogs and rats to determine the effect of x-ray and radium on developing teeth and observed a definite retarding effect in growth and eruption. His findings were verified shortly thereafter by another investigator (Herold). At about the same time there was a clinical observation of incomplete development of premolar teeth following irradiation (Herbst), that gave further evidence of the hazards of a too general use of radiotherapy about the mouth. In 1934 Ochsen gave a complete review of the various accounts of radiation damage which had appeared in German literature up to that time, which included not only damage to the teeth, but also to bone and soft tissue. He spoke of "galloping caries" in teeth which had been exposed simultaneously with swollen lymph glands and reported a case where teeth were loosened following x-ray treatment of fungus infection of hair follicles of the face. As clinical experience was gained by radiologists, techniques improved, more restriction of the field of exposure and magnitude of doses were imposed, and a tightening of the indications for radiologic treatment developed (Pordes; Rona).

23.3.1 *Pathogenesis and Nature of Dental Lesions.* With regard to the actual pathogenesis of changes observed in teeth following irradiation, probably a distinct separation should be made between developmental effects occurring in the growing teeth of children or experimental animals and those effects observed in exposed adult teeth. The early work of Leist, which has been corroborated (Herold; Ludin and Müller), points out that irradiation causes (1) damage to the odotoblasts within the teeth, (2) a reticular atrophy of the pulp tissue and (3) a cystic degeneration of the roots. The odontoblastic change may in part explain the failure in root development, dwarfed teeth, absence of teeth, and irregularities in tooth eruption that have been observed among radiotherapy patients (Bruce and Stafne). More recent animal experimentation has shown that x-ray irradiation will cause:

(1) Stoppage of growth of dentin (lengthwise) in rats' incisors locally

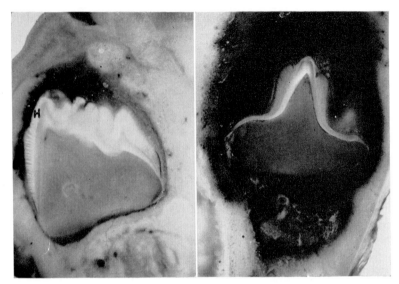

FIG. 1   FIG. 2

FIG. 1. Section through developing second molar tooth of swine (×3) unstained.

Section from swine exposed to 500r total body x-ray radiation to right side of body. Animal died, acute radiation sickness, 11 days after exposure. Note hypoplasia of enamel on occluso-buccal surface of tooth (H). Marked hemorrhage into dental crypt (black).

FIG. 2. Section through distal end, developing second molar tooth of swine (×3) unstained.

Section from swine exposed to 450 r total body x-ray radiation administered bilaterally. Animal died in 13 days with acute radiation sickness. Note massive hemorrhage into crypt of developing tooth, mandibular canal and marrow spaces (black). Hypoplasia of enamel over buccal incisal tip.

exposed to 4000 r.; and retardation in eruption of incisors exposed to 2000 r. and above (Weinreb, Schour, Medak, and Klauber).

(2) Enamel hypoplasia and retarded enamel dentin formation in rats' teeth, with total body irradiation of 375 r. and above (Dale).

(3) Disturbed enamel, dentin and bone formation, with distortion or destruction of odontoblasts and ameloblasts in mice with local doses of 1500 and 5000 r. (Burstone and Levy).

(4) Impeded growth and development, anodontia, and dwarfing of teeth and roots of teeth in 5 to 19 day old Syrian hamsters exposed locally to radon for 3 hours (Bruce).

(5) Marked enamel hypoplasia in developing teeth of swine exposed to total body irradiation above the 400 r. level (English and Tullis).

In adult teeth the lesions that appear following irradiation are not due to failure in the formation of tooth substance, but rather to a dissolving away of enamel or dentin in fully formed teeth. This is the so called "galloping caries" of Ochsen. There is a recent case reported (Marcello) that is typical, in which a 32 year old woman wished to have hair removed from her lip and chin. She received 24 treatments by a medical specialist in radiotherapy (4 treatments per week, 10–15 minutes each. Dosage not given). The dentist, who observed her teeth prior to radiation and found them sound, observed that very rapidly thereafter erosion of the enamel occurred, with exposure and sensitivity of the dentin. The facial hair was removed, but at the expense of damage to her teeth. In this situation, a lead shield placed in the buccal vestibule of the mouth would probably have satisfactorily protected the teeth.

Del Regato has described destruction of adult teeth as a frequent occurrence in those oral malignancies requiring radiotherapy. This destruction may involve the cervical portion of the teeth in a pattern similar to typical dental erosion. Sometimes, however, the occlusal and incisal surfaces are involved. The involved surfaces occasionally become blackened and the destruction may be severe enough to cause fracture of the teeth at their necks or marked occlusal attrition. In these patients who have excellent teeth at the beginning of a series of roentgen treatments, in from six months to four years following exposure, decay often begins which may eventually cause destruction of the teeth. There seem to be great variations in the time of beginning and conclusion of the destructive processes, and there may be severe pain or practically no pain. Inasmuch as the lesions of the teeth are usually accompanied by involvement of their supporting structures, the subjective symptoms of pain and a sense of elongation of the teeth may well be due to this latter involvement.

The cause of the destruction of adult teeth is not known, but it may be due to the lessened flow of saliva and a qualitative change in salivary secretion as a result of the roentgen rays penetrating the salivary glands (Del Regato; Ochsen). This secondary reaction, which changes the environment of the teeth, could well be a cause of the caries.

Regardless of the processes involved, it is important to know that teeth which are in the field of heavy irradiation may rapidly deteriorate. These teeth may also become loosened and infected as the result of radiation effects on the peridontium, Sharpey's fibers, and the surrounding bone (Leist). Calcification and bone formation may be disturbed and resorption, fibrosis, and actual necrosis of the bone may occur (Warren). The importance of these consequences will be brought out in a subsequent discussion of the effects of ionizing irradiation on the bone of the jaws.

The effect of radiation on ondontoblasts, resulting in their shrinkage or destruction, or only in re-arrangement, is not in conflict with similar cells elsewhere. This response in developing teeth is entirely in keeping with the inhibition of the growth of developing bone by a single exposure of roentgen ray of approximately half an erythema dose (Brooks and Hilstrom). It is well established that chondroblasts show histological damage with excess irradiation, that cartilage formation is disorganized and that bone formation is abnormal (Gates; Brooks and Hilstrom). In view of the parallel function of chrondroblasts, osteoblasts and odontoblasts, it is not strange that similar functional failure should result from degenerative effects on all three cell types due to excess irradiation. Similarity in the effects of irradiation on comparable cell types has been established (Loeb), and the morphological changes observed in dental tissues are in keeping with general reactions of the organism.

It should be clearly understood that the amount of roentgen irradiation required to initiate the destructive processes to teeth is far in excess of that which would be used in exposing several sets of dental roentgenograms. Experimental work has been done with rats, using roentgen exposure comparable to clinical doses which might be used in x-raying children's teeth (Smith). No ill effects have been found in growing or mature teeth when the exposure to roentgen rays is within that which would be used clinically for producing roentgenograms.

23.3.2 *The Effects of Irradiation on the Jaws.* The importance of the dentist having a knowledge of the effects of irradiation on the jaws lies in the necessity for adequate oral preparation prior to extensive roentgen or radium treatment. It is equally important that he understand the sequela or irradiation to these parts, under both favorable and unfavorable conditions. With this knowledge he will be prepared to cooperate with the radiologist and physician in diagnosing and caring for the patient who requires therapeutic irradiation or who has osteoradionecrosis as a result of occupational exposure.

In this day and age it is to be hoped that patients suffering from occupational exposure to roentgen rays or radioactive substances will be a rarity. This is indeed the case, for industrial regulations and a high standard of working conditions have eliminated most of the tragedies which were so publicized twenty-five to thirty years ago. With the advent of atomic energy and research with radioactive materials there are bound to be a few additional mistakes in the techniques of handling these powerful substances. Lack of understanding and carelessness have always taken their toll among scientists.

23.5 Effects of Radium

It was about 27 years after the discovery of naturally occurring radiations from certain ores that a dentist-physician discovered the disastrous effects of radioactive substances used in the manufacture of luminous dials for watches (Blum). It was observed that numerous girls employed in applying the luminous paint to watch dials suffered from a kind of necrosis of the jaws which was different from the osteomyelitis that resulted from simple infection. The litigation and newspaper publicity which followed the announcement that an occupational injury was the cause of the jaw necrosis and death of these girls, served to arouse the lawmakers into writing protective legislation and the scientists into making additional studies of the biological effects of irradiation.

It was found that the paint used by the dial painters contained about one milligram of a 20–30 per cent radium bearing substance for each 30–40 grams of zinc sulfide (Martland). However, the technique of painting which was used by the girls led them to point their brushes in their mouths and, as a result, they ingested toxic amounts of the substance over a long period of time. The detailed clinical and necropsy studies which were made of a large number of these tragic cases led to a better understanding of the disease (Martland, Conlon and Knef; Hoffman). The mechanisms of the disease and the clinical and pathological results are similar whether the radiations arise from radioactive substances or from the roentgen tube (Loeb). For this reason a single description will suffice.

Osteoradionecrosis of the jaw is a culmination of many individual effects of irradiation to the tissues which comprise this structure. The seriousness of the disease therefore depends not only on the magnitude of dose of irradiation, but also on variations which exist in certain of the tissues. It is in an understanding of these variations that we find our reward, for some of them are controllable.

Experience from early cases of occupational poisonings revealed that inflammation of the soft tissues of the mouth and Vincent's angina might occur as a result of irradiation (Martland). Of course, even here, there may be systemic factors, such as anemia or leukopenia, which add impetus to the direct effect of the rays on the mucous tissues.

The effects of irradiation on the periosteum are a swelling or thickening, together with hyalinization and vascular changes (Watson and Scarborough). Vascular damage, together with restricted lumina due to the swelling, result in a lessened blood supply to the cortical bone by way of the nutrient vessels. The blood vessels which supply the Haversian systems of bone are surrounded by non-expanding calcified material. As a result of this restriction the blood channels become smaller when the vessel walls or adventitious tissue become swollen due to radiation damage. It has been long recognized (Regaud) that the periosteum, and the bone itself, suffered not only from the effects of the primary irradiation, but that secondary rays were caused by reflection from the calcium of the bone.

It has been frequently observed that the mandible is more liable to necrosis than the maxilla (Stewart; Lawrence). The fact that the main supply of blood to the mandible comes from a single source at the posterior attachment of each half of the jaw, results in inadequate collateral blood supply in case this vessel is damaged. This is a contributing factor in necrosis. The most important reason however why osteoradionecrosis is more frequent in the mandible is because there is more frequent therapeutic irradiation of this area. This is due to the fact that malignant conditions occur more frequently in the lower jaw, tongue, lower lip, and neck as compared to the maxillary region.

The reaction of the bone tissue itself to irradiation is primarily a loss of vitality due to inadequate blood supply and to degenerative effects on the bone cells (Gates; Watson and Scarborough). This may occur without changing the general structure and appearance of the bone, and if the dose is not too great there need be no disabling effects (Woodward and Coley). However, when irradiation exceeds certain limits, there is permanent injury to the bone. The results depend upon several conditions of the surrounding tissues: on whether there is an ensuing invasion by bacteria, on whether pathological fractures occur, and on the general health of the individual.

It should be understood that the bone of the jaw is inherently no different from the other bones of the skeleton and the reason it is frequently involved by necrosis is because of collateral conditions (Ruppe and Lebourg). It was pointed out earlier that teeth frequently deteriorate as a result of irradiation and may thereby become infected. It is also true that a large percentage of patients who require therapeutic irradiation, because of oral malignancy, have a deplorable state of oral hygiene (Ehrlech). Because of the infection of teeth, it is readily seen that a pathway to infection of the bone exists. The combination of strangulation of the blood supply to the bone, the degenerative effects and loss of vitality of the bone itself, and the ready access of infection, are factors which provide the setting for osteoradionecrosis.

The difference between osteoradionecrosis and osteomyelitis is mainly one of tissue response. Because of the lack of vitality of irradiated bone, sequestration of the necrosed tissue is very slow. There may be slight demarcation between the normal bone and necrosed bone and the formation of an involucrum may not occur (Lawrence). Providing there is no ingress of infection, fibrous tissue may form around the sequestrum, and it helps to preserve anatomical form.

23.6 Preparation of Mouth for Heavy Dosage of Radiation

In the preparation of the mouth for radiologic treatment it is generally accepted (Daland; Watson and Scarborough; Stewart; Lawrence; Ehrlech; Kanthak; Colby) that the first duty of the dentist is to remove, as much as possible, all septic conditions which may exist in the mouth. Secondly, it is advisable that all teeth which lie in the direct path of radiation should be removed. If this is not done, and if they subsequently become infected as a result of radiation necrosis, or through natural causes, they cannot be removed without considerable danger of spreading infection, sloughing, extensive loss of tissue, trismus, emaciation and systemic reactions. Sometimes the malignancy is so located that one can construct a metal appliance which will serve to restrict the rays from reaching the teeth and bone. The use of intraoral treatment tubes, shields and filters (Daland; Quick) has served to protect many structures which formerly may have been destroyed.

Once the jaws have received a series of roentgen or radium treatments, surgical procedures should be delayed for at least two years (Daland). This will require any teeth which subsequently become infected to be treated by conservative and restorative means. If a necrotic condition of the bone occurs in spite of preventive measures, this too should be treated conservatively (LaDow). Attempts should not be made to remove sequestra until they can be lifted out with a forceps (Lawrence). In the meantime supportive measures should be taken to insure the highest degree of oral hygiene and general nutrition of the patient. Frequent irrigation of the involved area and occasionally feeding by means of a nasal tube are helpful (Watson and Scarborough). In certain cases, when there is an extreme amount of pain related to the necrotic process, it may be advisable to denervate the fifth nerve by means of an alcohol injection. If surgical procedures must be applied because of residual conditions or extreme infection, a radical removal to good vascular areas is recommended (Daland). The unfortunate situation is that usually the patients who require radical treatment are already emaciated, dehydrated, suffering from severe pain and infection, and in an elderly age group. For these reasons jaw resection is hazardous (Watson).

In the last analysis it may be seen that the understanding and ability of the dentist, who assists in treating the radiological patient, may be the deciding factor in the comfort and recovery of this patient. His advice and treatment of the patient, and the value of his consultation with the radiologist and physician will be in direct proportion to his knowledge, training and experience. His thoroughness in taking a complete history prior to surgical procedures may well prevent serious trouble in patients having had radiotherapy. If there is a history of such treatment, it is advisable to communicate with the radiotherapist to ascertain dosage administered, area treated and any relevant factors that will be of value in establishing a prognosis (Colby).

The foregoing material pertains to chronic changes in the bone of the jaws. There are acute effects appearing within a few days that are the same as occur in other bones of the body. Since this is covered in a previous chapter, it will suffice to mention here that gross hemorrhage occurs in the crypts of developing teeth, as well as in the mandibular canal and marrow spaces of animals exposed to total body radiation of about 400 r (English and Tullis). Fig. 2.

REFERENCES

1. BARCLAY, A. E. AND COX, S.: The radiation risks of the roentgenologist. An attempt to measure the quantity of roentgen rays used in diagnosis and to assess the dangers. *Am. J. Roentgen and Rad. Therapy, 19:* 551, 1928.
2. BARTLESTONE, H. J.: I[131] studies of enamel and dentine permeability *in vivo*. Paper presented at A.A.A.S. Cleveland meeting subsection on dentistry. Dec. 30, 1950.
3. BLUM, T.: Osteomyelitis of the Mandible and Maxilla. *J. Am. Dent. Assoc., 11:* 802, 1924.
4. BROOKS, B. AND HILLSTROM, H. T.: Effect of roentgen rays on bone growth and bone regeneration. *J. Am. Surg., 20:* 599, 1933.
5. BRUCE, K. W.: The effect of irradiation on the developing dental system of the Syrian hamster. *J. Dent. Research, 29:* 665, 1950 (abstract).
6. BRUCE, K. W. AND STAFNE, E. C.: Effects of irradiation on developing dental system as demonstrated by the roentgenogram. *J. Am. Dent. Assoc., 41:* 684, 1950.
7. BURSTONE, M. S. AND LEVY, B. M.: Effect of X-radiation on jaws of mice. *J. Dent. Research, 28:* 656, 1949 (Abstract).
8. CHAMBERLAIN, W. E.: Protection in diagnostic roentgenology; avoiding the dangers of X-ray exposure and high tension shock. *Radiology, 19:* 22, 1932.
9. CHAMBERLAIN, W. E., NEWELL, R. R., TAYLOR, L., AND WYCKOFF, H.: Radiation hygiene: hazards to physicians, patients, nurses and others from use of radioactive isotopes. Council on Physical Medicine. *J.A.M.A., 138:* 818, 1948.
10. COLBY, R. A.: Radiation effects on structure of the oral cavity: a review. *J. Am. Dent. Assoc., 29:* 1446, 1942.
11. DALAND, E. M.: Surgical treatment of post-irradiation necrosis. *Am. J. Roentgenol. & Rad. Therapy, 46:* 287, 1941.
12. DALE, P. B.: The Effect of x-rays on the rat incisor. *J. Dent. Research, 27:* 730, 1948 (abstract).
13. DEL REGATO, J. A.: Dental lesions observed after roentgen therapy in cancer of the buccal cavity, pharynx and larynx. *Am. J. Roentgen and Rad. Ther., 42:* 404, 1939.
14. EHRLECH, D. E.: Bone necrosis in intraoral cancer. *Arch. Phys. Therapy, 18:* 565, 1937.
15. ELLIS, F.: Medical Aspects of protection from ionizing radiations. *J. Brit. Radiology, 23: 28, 1950.*
16. ENGLISH, J. A. AND DUDLEY, H. C.: Distribution of radioactive gallium in the teeth and jaws of experimental animals. *J. Dent. Research, 29:* 93, 1950.
17. ENGLISH, J. A. AND TULLIS, J. L.: Oral manifestations of ionizing radiation. I. Oral lesions and effect on developing teeth of swine exposed to 2000 KV total body X-ray irradiation. *J. Dent. Research, 30:* 33, 1951.
18. ENNIS, L. M.: Dental Roentgenology, Ed. 2., Phila. Lea & Febiger, 1936.
19. FAILLA, G.: Radium Protection. *Radiology, 19:* 12, 1932.
20. FILES, G. W. (ed) (by Tech. Serv. Dept. G. E. Elect. X-ray Corp.): *Medical Radiographic Technic.* Springfield, 1949. Charles C Thomas, p. 338.

21. FLEMING, J. A. C.: Investigations into the degree of scattered radiation received by x-ray workers during routine diagnostic examinations in a military hospital department. *J. Brit. Radiology, 16:* 367, 1943.

22. GATES, O. in WARREN, S.: Effects of radiation on normal tissues XII. Effects on bone, cartilage and teeth. *Arch. Path., 35:* 323, 1943.

23. GLUCKSMANN, A.: Cytological aspects of protection from ionizing radiations. *J. Brit. Radiology, 23:* 41, 1950.

24. GOLDSMITH, N. R.: Dangers of culminative exposure to roentgen rays. *J. Am. Dent. Assoc., 34:* 290, Feb. 13, 1947.

25. HENSHAW, P. S. AND HAWKINS, J. W.: Incidence of leukemia in physicians. *J. Nat. Canc. Inst., 4:* 339, 1944.

26. HENSHAW, P. S.: Further problems in x-ray protection. II. Irradiation injury and the tolerance dose. *Radiology, 44:* 569, 1945.

27. HERBST, E.: Fehlgriffe in der Orthodonitie. *Fortscher Zahnheilk,* 855, 1927.

28. HEROLD, KURT: Röntgenstrahlenwirkung auf der wachsenden Hundekiefer. Experimentelle Untersuchungen unter Berücksichtigung der Organveränderungen. *Deutsche Monatsschrift für Zahnheilkunde, 49:* 97, 1931.

29. HOFFMAN, F. L.: Radium (Mesotherium) necrosis. *J.A.M.A., 85:* 961, 1925.

30. INGRAM, M.: Health hazards in radiation work, *Science, 111:* 103, 1950.

31. KANTHAK, F. F.: X-ray irradiation and osteonecrosis of the jaws. *J. Am. Dent. Assoc., 28:* 1925, 1941.

32. KOSS, W. F., AND GINN, J. T.: Distribution of sodium in the teeth and bones of dogs as shown by radioactive isotope. *J. Dent. Research 20:* 465, 1941.

33. LACRONIQUE, G., BÉAL, G., AND GOUDAERT, M.: Influence de la radiumthérapie sur la calcification des germes dentaires. *Rev. de Stomat., 48:* 541, 1947.

34. LOEB, L.: Effects of roentgen rays and radioactive substances on living cells and tissues. *J. Cancer Research, 7:* 229, 1922.

35. LADOW, C. S.: Osteoradionecrosis of the jaw. *Oral Surg., Oral Med., Oral Path., 3:* 582, 1950.

36. LAWRENCE, E. A.: Osteoradionecrosis of the mandible. *Am. J. Roentgen. and Rad. Therapy, 55:* 733, June 1946.

37. LEIST, M.: Über die Einwirkung der Röntgenstrahlen und des Radiums auf Zähne und Kiefer. *Strahlentherapie, 24:* 268, 1927.

38. LEIST, M.: Über den Einfluss der Röntgenstrahlen auf den wachsenden Zahn. *Wein. med. wchnschr., 75:* 2247, 1925.

39. LEVY, M.: Radiumtherapie in der Zahnheilkunde. *Strahlentherapie, 4:* 123, 1914.

40. LUDIN, M. AND MÜLLER, O.: Zahnveränderungen nach protrahiert-fractionierter Röntgenbestrahlung. *Strahlentherapie, 56:* 644, 1936.

41. MANLY, M. L., AND BALE, W. F. The metabolism of inorganic phosphorus or rat bones and teeth as indicated by the radioactive isotope. *J. Biol. Chem., 129:* 125, 1939.

42. MARCELLO, L.: Grave atrofia smalto da radioterapia. *Clinica Odontoiatrica, 3:* 60, 1948.

43. MARTLAND, H. S.: Occupational poisoning in manufacture of luminous watch dials. *J.A.M.A., 92:* 466 and 552, 1929.

44. MARTLAND, H. S., CONLON, P., AND KNEF, J. P.: Some unrecognized dangers in the use and handling of radioactive substances with special reference to the storage of insoluble products of radium and mesothorium, etc., in the reticuloendothelial system. *J.A.M.A., 85:* 1769, 1925.

45. MCCAULEY, H. B.: Significance of radioactive isotopes in dental research. *J. Am. Dent. Assoc., 29:* 1219, 1942.

46. MORGAN, K. Z.: Protection against radiation hazards and maximum allowable exposure values. *J. Indust. Hyg. and Toxical, 30:* 286, 1948.

47. MEDAK, H., SHOUR, I., KLAUBER, W. A., JR.: The Effect of x-ray irradiation on the eruption of the upper incisor of the albino rat. *J. Dent. Research, 28:* 633, 1949 (abstract).

48. NUTTALL, J. R.: The radiation hazards of radiotherapeutic staff. *J. Brit. Radiology, 23:* 35, 1950.

49. OCHSEN, H.: Über Röntgenstrahlen-schädigungen der an der Bildung der Mund-höhle beteiligten Hartsubstanzen. *Zschr. f. Stomat., 32:* 145, 1934.

50. QUICK, D.: Carcinoma of the lower jaw. *Am. J. Surg., 1:* 360, 1926.

51. PICHER, C.: Biological investigations with radioactive calcium and strontium. *Proc. Soc. Exper. Biol. and Med., 46:* 86, 1941.

52. PORDES, F.: Über Röntgenbehandlung entzündlicher Erkraukungen. Allegemeines und Spezielles. II Entzündungen in Bereich der Zähne und Kiefer. *Strahlentherapie, 24:* 77, 1927.

53. PFAHLER, G. E.: Danger of Injury to the dentist in roentgenography. *J. Am. Dent. Assoc., 26:* 949, 1939.

54. QUIMBY, E. H.: A method for the study of scattered and secondary radiation in x-ray and radium laboratories. *Radiology, 7:* 211, 1926.

55. RONA, A.: Über die Röntgentherapie entzündlicher Erkrankungen in der Stomotologie. *Strahlentherapie, 54:* 680, 1935.

56. REGAUD, C.: Sur la Necrose des Os Atteints par un Processus Cancéreux et Traités par les Radiations. *Compte rend. Soc. de biol., 87:* 427 and 629, 1922.

57. RUPPE, C. AND LEBOURG, L.: Apropos de deux cas ce necrose des maxillaries survenue a la suite d'un traitement par le thorium X. *Rev. de Stomat., 34:* 462, 1932.

58. SANTE, L. R.: Manual of Roentgenological Technique, Edwards Brothers Inc., Ann Arbor, Mich. 1949, p. 150.

59. SMITH, R. A.: Effect of Roentgen rays on developing teeth of Rats. *J. Am. Dent Assoc., 18:* 111, 1931.

60. STENSTROM, W.: Protection in x-ray therapy. *Radiology, 19:* 7, 1932.

61. STEWART, M. B.: Osteoradionecrosis and cancer of the head and neck. *Arch. Otolaryng., 38:* 403, 1943.

62. TRIBONDEAU AND RECAMIER.: Altérations des yeux et du squelette d'un chat nouveau-né par roentgenisation. *C. r. Soc. Biol., 58:* 1031, 1905.

63. VOLKER, J. F., SOGNNAES, R. F., AND BIBBLY, B. G.: Studies on the distribution of radioactive fluoride in the bones and teeth of experimental animals. *Am. J. Physiol., 132:* 707, 1941.

64. WATSON, W. L. AND SCARBOROUGH, J. E.: Osteoradionecrosis in intraoral cancer. *Am. J. Roentgenol. and Rad. Therapy, 40:* 524, 1938.

65. WATSON, W.: Discussion of paper by EHRLECH, D. E.: Bone Necrosis in intraoral cancer. *Arch. Phys. Therapy, 18:* 565, 1937.

66. WEINREB, M., SCHOUR, I., MEDAK, H., AND KLANBER, W. A., JR.: Effect of a single exposure to x-ray irradiation on the growth rate of dentin of the rat incisor. *J. Dent. Res., 28:* 633, 1949 (abstract).

67. WOLBACH, S. B.: Summary of the effects of repeated roentgen-ray exposures upon the human skin, antecedent to the formation of carcinoma. *Am. J. Roentgenol. and Rad. Therapy, 13:* 139, 1925.

68. WOODARD, H. Q. AND COLEY, B. L.: The correlation of tissue dose and clinical response in irradiation of bone tumors and of normal bone. *Am. J. of Roentg. and Rad. Therapy, 57:* 464, 1947.

24▸

Some Pertinent Results from Recent Research

SHIELDS WARREN, M.D. AND R. HAROLD DRAEGER, M.D.

24.1 Introduction

The advent of the chain-reacting pile within the past few years has made available a large number of artificial radioactive substances at a reasonable cost including isotopes of almost every element. This has resulted in an expansion of the field of radiobiology, unusually rapid in the history of science. The radioisotope as a scientific tool is of inestimable value in both physical and biologic sciences. Historically, it would be necessary to go back for several hundred years to find a discovery of comparable importance, such as the microscope.

24.2 Medical Aspects

The medical problems created by use of atomic energy fall into three categories; those associated with an atomic explosion, industrial hygiene problems which occur in plants and laboratories where fissionable materials are produced and handled, and the problems related to biomedical research.

Clinicians have long been faced with problems created by the use of radium and x-rays. Safe techniques have been developed and standards of permissible exposure established over the past fifty years. Industrial x-ray techniques have also been developed; however, these methods were not adequate to cope with the problems of large scale handling of uranium and plutonium. It was necessary, therefore, for the Manhattan District and the Atomic Energy Commission to develop a whole new field of industrial hygiene sometimes referred to as "health physics".

With the successful use of atomic weapons against Japan it has also become necessary to create a new branch of medical science concerned with the prevention and treatment of casualties peculiar to an atomic explosion. The effects of an atomic detonation are the result of the liberation of

enormous amounts of kinetic and radiant energy. The kinetic energy involves the motion of matter either as atomic particles or gross aggregates
in gas, liquid or solid state. The radiant energy which includes all wave
lengths of the electromagnetic spectrum from the infra-red to gamma rays
is usually divided into thermal and ionizing radiation. The thermal radiations include infra-red, visible and ultra-violet light, producing mostly heat
when absorbed, while shorter wave lengths produce mainly ionization.

The character of the biologic effects of an atomic explosion is directly
related to the form of energy dissipated, while the extent of injury depends
largely upon the amount of energy transferred or absorbed. Thus, it will
be seen that the kinetic energy is responsible for mechanical effects suitably
designated as blast injuries, thermal radiation may produce flashburns, while
ionizing radiation is the cause of radiation illness as discussed in Chapter 10.

The advance of atomic medicine has been so extensive that it would
require encyclopedic treatment to take up all aspects of the subject. We
will, therefore, attempt to draw attention to only a few of the more important items.

24.2.1 Fallout

Problems as well as benefits come from atomic energy. An aspect of both
weapons testing and industrial use of atomic energy that has concerned
thoughtful people throughout the world is radioactive fallout. This concern
has stimulated research which has greatly increased our knowledge of fallout.

An inevitable accompaniment of a nuclear detonation employing fission
and fusion processes is widespread distribution of radioactive substances,
a number of which are completely new to man such as Sr^{90} and I^{131}. Through
this scientific "cataclysm" these substances have been spread throughout
the world, from the stratosphere to the depths of the ocean, including every
form of life. In most instances the quantity is almost infinitesimal, however,
in areas of concentrated fallout the accompanying radiation may temporarily reach lethal levels for man or animals.

Fallout is of two main types; local, made up of the debris from the site
of the explosion, mixed with fission products, and distant, made of minute
particles derived from the nuclear reaction. If the fireball comes in contact
with the earth or sea there will be local fallout such as was experienced by
some of the Marshallese Islanders. If the fireball does not touch the earth
but does not ascend well into the stratosphere, the bulk of fission products
will be carried in a large cloud by winds and be deposited in a zone up to a
few hundred miles wide with heavier accumulation occurring in regions of
rain or snowfall. However, if the fireball ascends well up into the stratosphere most of the fission products will be widely distributed by the strato-

spheric winds. They will remain suspended for long periods of time and will gradually settle below the tropopause and then be largely brought down by rain or snow with some gradual settling of particles without the aid of precipitation. Therefore, fallout tends not to be uniform but rather to vary probably by a factor less than 10. Induced radioactivity from neutron flux depends on the neutron flux impinging upon the site of the explosion, will vary, and is negligible if the fireball does not come in close contact with the surface.

The materials of longer half-life obviously are of greater import than those of short except near the release point. Its long half-life and its strong tendency to accumulate in bone have made radioactive strontium perhaps the most significant component of fallout after an explosion, whereas, I^{131} tends to be the chief factor in a limited period of time after an explosion, melt-down or burnup.

Because of the complex interrelations of the biosphere, concentrations of radioactive substances can occur in one or another links of the food chain. Some of these concentrations are insignificant to man while others may be of importance, as for example, the contamination of fish from the Bikini lagoon or the potentially significant contamination of dairy products with I^{131} as a result of accidental release of fission products from the Windscale No. 1 pile recently. Fortunately, some of the more troublesome isotopes may be discriminated against in the food chain, for example, calcium is absorbed in preference to strontium by the gastrointestinal tract.

As a result of the widespread interest in fallout, a great deal more has been learned about the natural background of radiation to which man is exposed and its variations in different areas. These, while low throughout the country, vary widely. Thus, New York City has a level of 12.3 $\mu r/hr.$, Pittsburgh, Pennsylvania about 12 $\mu r/hr.$, Mt. Rushmore, South Dakota, 22 $\mu r/hr.$, Denver 16.6 to 22.4 $\mu r/hr.$, and Pike's Peak 38.6 $\mu r/hr.$

24.2.2 Body Counters

The development of total body scintillation counters is a significant advance in the accurate measurement of the body content of gamma emitters such as radium or cesium[137] and the determination of their biologic half-life. The Los Alamos counter is extremely sensitive with an accuracy of around .01 μc but cannot localize or differentiate gamma emitters while the Argonne counter which uses NaI crystals is capable of localization and can detect a particular gamma emitter in the presence of others.

24.3 Radioisotopes in Metabolic Studies

The use of radioisotopes in metabolic studies has now become a routine procedure. With the low level counting techniques now available, a number of procedures may be safely carried out upon man. Thus, significant advances have been made by Tolbert and his group in understanding the oxidation of glucose with the utilization of carbon[14] carrying on the chain of significant investigations undertaken by Hastings and his associates. The determination of uptake by the thyroid of microcurie quantities of I[131] has become a virtually routine method in estimation of thyroid activity. A further refinement has been the development of scanning the gland by means of scintillation counters so that foci of hypo- or hyperactivity can be distinguished from the bulk for the thyroid tissue. These refinements have added materially to our knowledge of thyroid function and malfunction. With the combination of radioactive carbon and tritium incorporated into different positions of the molecules, a large number of compounds can be followed and their metabolic pathways determined. As lag in recording time of the instruments available has been increasingly eliminated, radioactive isotopes of particularly short-lived substances such as sodium[24] have become of increasing value in the determination of circulation time.*

The use of tracer substances, particularly carbon[14] and hydrogen[3] has permitted a much greater understanding of intermediary metabolism. To pick out any one use for special mention is difficult. A number of compounds that have relatively short life in the metabolic chain have been discovered whose existence would have been impossible to detect by the means formerly available. Carbon[14] has also been of value in studies of protein synthesis. The use of tagged amino acids and study of their incorporation into the protein molecule not only has provided important data on the structure, but the rate appears to be a matter of minutes or possibly even of seconds.

Iron[59] has proved to be an important tool in the study of hemoglobin synthesis and also is of special use in studies of red blood cell production. For these reasons the obscure anemias can be more satisfactorily studied with its aid than by other techniques. Chromium 51 can also be used for red cell survival studies and for studies of total red cell volume just as in the case of the P^{32}-labeled cells but with marked advantage in counting technique, since chromium 51 is a gamma emitter. For the study of total red cell turnover, however, iron 59 is more satisfactory, giving a dynamic picture of the incorporation and release of iron with relation to hemoglobin and the red cells but in addition giving information as to tissue localization of the tagged iron.

Radioactive cobalt has been chiefly used therapeutically as an external source of radiation where it has virtually displaced radium. As a tracer substance it has proved of particular value incorporated into the B_{12} molecule serving as a means of determining intrinsic factor activity in the study

---

* The very short half lives of some of the isotopes of the noble gases must be considered as being of value for physiologic investigations.

of pernicious anemia. The test with cobalt 60-labeled B_{12} is probably the most accurate means of diagnosing pernicious anemia.

24.4 Neutrons in Medical Research

In the tissues of experimental animals, activation analysis (subjecting the whole animal or samples of tissue to neutron flux) has permitted subsequent determination of the amount and character of radioactivity induced in various elements. The radiation characteristics are adequately distinctive to permit an effective and accurate analysis of the elements present. This has been of appreciable value in determining the distribution in the body of many of the trace elements, for example, zinc and cobalt providing clues as to their probable significance. However, there are still technical difficulties and the method requires an adequate flux of neutrons.

24.5 Blast Injuries

Blast injuries are due to the explosive release of energy, whether from ordinary explosives or the atomic bomb. During an explosion much energy is converted to mechanical movement and appears as a pressure wave or flying missiles activated by that wave. It is convenient to designate as direct those injuries produced by the pressure wave and as indirect other harmful effects. The type of direct injury to the individual largely depends on the medium which transmits the pressure wave. If through air, water or solid structures: air blast, water blast or solid blast injuries are the result.

The majority of casualties in the case of an atomic bomb detonation in air is apt to be indirect blast injury. These injuries are qualitatively similar to those produced by ordinary bombs, except that they are likely to be complicated by flashburns and radiation illness. From the diverse nature of the mechanical injuries encountered it will be evident that direct protection of the individual is practically impossible. However, adequate disaster planning as discussed in Chapter 13 can do much to reduce these casualties.

The problem of direct air blast injury is largely academic due to the relatively high pressure zone in which these injuries occur, being practically within the area of total destruction. An individual so exposed would also likely receive several times the lethal dose of ionizing and thermal radiation. There appear to be no cases of direct air blast injury except ruptured ear drums reported from Hiroshima and Nagasaki.

The not uncommon vagaries in blast effect, such as noted in ships, are caused by either reflections of the blast wave or the so-called Mach effect, where the reflected shock front traveling more rapidly than the incident shock may at times overtake it so that the two shock fronts fuse and reinforce each other to form a single shock stronger than either alone. This Mach effect shows the same positive and negative phases as does an incident shock wave. Blast effects are further modified by irregularities in the terrain and variations in the weather, such as inversions.

The harmful effects of air or water pressure waves are largely exerted upon the air-containing portions of the body, i.e., the lungs and intestines. Thus an air pressure wave of 175 pounds peak pressure is apt to produce fatal pulmonary hemorrhage in man, while a water compression wave of 500 lbs. peak pressure is likely to produce fatal pulmonary hemorrhage or intestinal perforation (Zuckerman; Greaves, et al.; Draeger, Barr and Sager). Flexion waves in ships' structures, caused by an underwater explosion producing a deck movement of 25 feet per second terminal velocity, are likely to produce lower extremity fractures in individuals standing upon the surface accelerated (Barr, Draeger and Sager). Injuries of this type have been observed only in the case of torpedoes and depth charges, but atomic bomb injuries would no doubt be qualitatively similar.

24.6 Flashburns

The high temperature of an atomic bomb explosion results in intense thermal radiations of short duration which are capable of producing flashburns of the exposed skin at a considerable distance as compared with the flame burns of ordinary bombs which are due largely to contact with hot gases.

A 20-Kt. bomb explosion at about 1800 feet altitude produces temperature on the ground at the hypocenter probably between 3000° to 4000° C. The heat exceed 1600° C. as much as 4000 feet away.

It will be realized that flashburns in atomic bomb casualties may also be accompanied by burns of the ordinary type caused by fires started by blast effects as well as the intense thermal radiations. Burns of the exposed portions of the body were common at Hiroshima and Nagasaki and constituted the largest number of early casualties (Block). This was no doubt influenced by the warm August day and scant clothing worn by many of the populace. Tsuzuki says that 90 % of those who came for treatment in the first week did so because of burns. A number of clothing materials may ignite at these temperatures causing some burn from the clothing itself.

Considerable advances have been made in understanding the physical factors concerned in the production of skin burns. The contribution of flash burns to the total medical problem can be quite readily calculated. The time-intensity is an important factor. Thus, in a 1-Kt explosion a second degree burn will be caused by 4 calories/sq. cm. while in a 10 megaton explosion 7 calories/sq. cm. will be required to produce the same effect. With the smaller explosion the thermal energy is received within a few tenths of a second. With the larger explosion, however, it is received over a period of several seconds. Shadow producing objects between the fireball and the skin serve to protect the skin. As a rule, two separated layers of fairly heavy white clothing will afford a considerable degree of protection.

The differences between the atomic bomb flashburns and ordinary burns with respect to healing, infection, and mortality, are not well known for man. In animals, flashburns tend to produce a dry coagulated surface while contact burns are wet and edematous. Pearse has indicated that severe flashburns appear to destroy the stratum germinativum more uniformly, thus adversely affecting healing by destroying the epithelial islands of the hair follicles and skin appendages from which re-epithelization occurs. The flashburns are sharply outlined and show the effect of shadowing by clothing, extraneous objects or body contours. The rather marked localized pigmentation at the margin of the burned areas which occurred in many of the Japanese following the healing of flashburns is not clearly understood, but is probably a part of the healing phenomenon rather than specifically related to atomic bomb injuries.

24.6.1 *Keloids.* Hyperplastic scarring and keloid formation that frequently followed the burns are difficult to differentiate without both clinical and histologic study. At first these keloids were thought to be characteristic of atomic bomb thermal radiations in combination with gamma radiation. However, the occurrence of similar connective tissue response in flame burns suggests that malnutrition and inadequate treatment with prolonged healing due to secondary infection may have been factors. The tendency for the keloid formation to be most marked in the portions of burns which healed last also supports this contention. Some keloids developed following mechanical injury. It has also been suggested that there is a racial predisposition to keloids in the Japanese. The fact that many of the keloid or hyperplastic scars occurred in individuals who received little ionizing radiation may indicate that ionizing radiation was not an important factor in their formation. Spontaneous partial regression of the keloids has occurred in some of the patients.

24.7 Calculated Risk

A somewhat unfamiliar concept in ordinary medical practice is that of calculated risk. This type of exposure to noxious stimuli must often be assumed by military personnel in wartime or in a major emergency by civilian personnel in time of peace. The determination has been made as to the amount of harm that may come from one type of exposure as against another. For example, it might be better to take a small dose of radiation than to face the danger of a highly explosive shell exploding in the immediate vicinity or to be within range of a machine gun. We still have, unfortunately, a considerable area of ignorance as to the effects of small doses of radiation. In general, it can be said that doses of 100 r received within a short period of time may result in transient disability and some long-range injurious effect. Doses under 100 r do not ordinarily produce immediate effects, although there may be some degree of permanent damage resulting. A single dose of 25 r is not followed by demonstrable injury, and this has been adopted as an emergency permissible dose for civil defense and other emergency workers.

24.8 Genetic Effects

Atomic energy has provided an enormous stimulus to the advance of genetics. Muller demonstrated a generation ago the importance of ionizing radiation as a mutagenic agent. The studies of Neel, Russell, Carter and others have done much to clarify our understanding of the significance of radiation-induced mutations. The study of Neel and Schull of the offspring of the Hiroshima and Nagasaki survivors has demonstrated that in the first generation at least there is no significant increase in harmful mutations. On the other hand, the numbers of cases studied are too few to permit the assumption of absence of effect. Entirely aside from the findings with regard to the effect of radiation this study is of major importance as being probably the most detailed and extensive genetic study on man. It has already provided an excellent baseline for studies in human population genetics and will increase in value each year that it is carried on.

REFERENCES

Aub, J. C., et al.: Effects of Treatment on Radium and Calcium Metabolism in Human Body. *Ann. Int. Med.*, *11:* 1443–1463, 1938.

Barr, J. S., Draeger, R. H., and Sager, W. W.: Solid Blast Personnel Injury: A Clinical Study. *Mil. Surgeon, 98:* 1–12, 1946.

Block, M. A.: Considerations in the Study of Burns Sequelae in Atomic Bomb Survivors, Appendix 5, General Report Atomic Bomb Casualty Commission, Washinton, D. C.: National Research Council, 1947.

Cantril, S. T.: The Contributions of Biology to Radiation Therapy: Janeway Lecture, 1957. *Am. J. Roentgenol. 78:* 751–768, 1957.

Cantril, S. T. and Parker, H. M.: *The Tolerance Dose.* Manhattan District Declassified Document No. 1100; Date declassified 30 June 1947.

Committee on Atomic Casualties. National Research Council, Washington, D. C.: Genetic Effects of the Atomic Bombs in Hiroshima and Nagasaki. *Science, 106:* 331–333, 1947.

Cope, Oliver: *The Burn Problem, in U. S. Office of Scientific Research and Development.* Committee on Medical Research: Advances in Military Medicine. Boston: Little, Brown and Co., 1948, vol. 1, pp. 149–158.

Desjardins, A. U.: Action of Roentgen Rays and Radium on the Heart and Lungs. *Am. Jr. Roentgenol., 28:* 701, November 1932.

Draeger, R. H., Barr, J. S., and Sager, W. W.: Blast Injury. *J.A.M.A., 132:* 762–767, 1946.

ELLINGER, F.: *The Biologic Fundamentals of Radiation Therapy.* New York: Elsevier Publishing Co., 1941.

GLASSTONE, S.: *The Effects of Nuclear Weapons.* Book No. 1010. U. S. Atomic Energy Commission, June 1957.

GREAVES, FREDERICK C., ET AL.: An Experimental Study of Underwater Concussion. *U. S. Nav. M. Bull., 41:* 339–352, 1943.

HAMILTON, J. C.: *Metabolism of Carrier Free Fission Products in the Rat.* Manhattan District Declassified Document No. 1275; Date declassified, 26 Aug. 1947.

Hearings Before the Special Subcommittee on Radiation of the Joint Committee on Atomic Energy, Congress of the United States, on The Nature of Radioactive Fallout and Its Effect on Man (Two Parts). United States Government Printing Office, Washington, 1957.

LAWRENCE, J. H.: Proc. Internat. Conf. Peaceful Uses Atomic Energy. *10:* 142, 956. United Nations, New York.

LEA, D. E.: *Actions of Radiations on Living Cells.* New York: The Macmillan Co., 1947.

Medical Research Council. The Hazards to Man of Nuclear and Allied Radiations. June, 1956. Her Majesty's Stationery Office.

MIDDLESWORTH, L. V.: *Study of Plutonium Metabolism in Bone.* Manhattan District Declassified Document No. 1022; Date declassified 6 June 1947.

MULLER, H. J.: Artificial Transmutation of the Gene. *Science, 66:* 84–87, 1927.

National Bureau of Standards. Handbook 60. X-ray Protection. December 1, 1955.

National Bureau of Standards. Handbook 52. Maximum Permissible Amounts of Radioisotopes In The Human Body and Permissible Concentrations in Air and Water. March, 1953.

National Academy of Sciences, Washington. Publication 452, 1956.

NEEL, J. V. AND SCHULL, W. J.: The Effect of Exposure to the Atomic Bombs on Pregnancy Termination in Hiroshima and Nagasaki. National Academy of Sciences—National Research Council Washington, D. C., 1956.

OUGHTERSON, A. W. AND WARREN, S.: Medical Effects of the Atomic Bomb in Japan. Division 8, Vol. 8, National Nuclear Energy Series, Manhattan Project Technical Section, 1956.

PEARSE, H. E.: Personal communication.

ROSENTHAL, D. J. AND LAWRENCE, J. H.: *Ann. Rev. Med., 8:* 361, 1957.

SEIDLIN, S. M., MARINELLI, L. D., AND OSHRY, E.: *J.A.M.A., 132:* 838, 1946.

Tsuzuki General Report, Atomic Bomb Casualty Commission, Washington National Research Council, 1947, Appendix IX.

United Nations Official Records. A/3838. 1958.

ZUCKERMAN, S.: Experimental Study of Blast Injuries to the Lungs. *Lancet, 239:* 219–224, 1940.

Appendix I

Isotope Table

For convenience the stable and radioactive isotopes are listed separately. However when a naturally occurring isotope is radioactive, its mass number is also indicated under the stable isotopes. These isotopes are marked by asterisk.

Energy of radiation is indicated in Mev when known; when energy is unknown, a plus sign (+) is used.

Current tables show some discrepancies and it is to be expected that changes and additions will occur as more complete information becomes available. The table is substantially complete but may not contain all members of fission product chains.

For further and more detailed reference, see:

1. General Electric Research Laboratory Chart of the Nuclides, Apr. 1956, 4th Ed., G. E. Co., Schenectady 5, N. Y., Dept. 6–221.
2. Trilinear Chart of Nuclides 1956. Catalog No. Y3. At 7: 2N88/8. Govt. Printing Office, Wash. 25, D. C.
3. Kinsman and Simon: Radiological Health Handbook, Jan. 1957. U. S. Dept. of Health and Welfare, U. S. P. H. S.; U. S. Dept. of Commerce, Office of Technical Services, Wash., D. C.
4. Strominger, D., Hollander, J. M. and Seaborg, G. T.: Table of Isotopes. Review of Modern Physics, Vol. 3, Part 2, No. 2; April, 1958.

APPENDIX I, SYMBOLS USED IN TABLE

I. Radiations:
    α, alpha particles
    β^-, negative beta particles (electrons)
    β^+, positive beta particles (positrons)
    e^-, internal conversion electrons
    γ, gamma rays
    n, neutron
    p, proton
    X, x-ray

II. Time
    μs, microsecond
    s, second
    m, minute
    h, hour
    d, day
    y, year

III. Other

    A, mass number

    * naturally occurring or otherwise available radioisotope

    d, (after radiation energy), delayed emission

    I.T., isomeric transition by gamma emission (gamma ray may be absorbed by internal conversion)

    K or L, nuclear capture of orbital electron

    Parentheses (about energy figures), radioactivity from short-lived daughter nuclides

    σ, sigma, nuclear cross section for thermal neutron capture in "barns"

    S.F., spontaneous fission

    Z, atomic number

ALPHABETICAL LOCATION LIST OF ELEMENTS, SYMBOLS AND ATOMIC NUMBERS. APPENDIX I

Element	Symbol	Z	Element	Symbol	Z
Actinium	Ac	89	Holmium	Ho	67
Aluminum	Al	13	Hydrogen	H	1
Americium	Am	95	Indium	In	49
Antimony	Sb	51	Iodine	I	53
Argon	A	18	Iridium	Ir	77
Arsenic	As	33	Iron	Fe	26
Astatine	At	85	Krypton	Kr	36
Barium	Ba	56	Lanthanum	La	57
Berkelium	Bk	97	Lead	Pb	82
Beryllium	Be	4	Lithium	Li	3
Bismuth	Bi	83	Lutetium	Lu	71
Boron	B	5	Magnesium	Mg	12
Bromine	Br	35	Manganese	Mn	25
Cadmium	Cd	48	Mendelivium	Mv	101
Calcium	Ca	20	Mercury	Hg	80
Californium	Cf	98	Molybdenum	Mo	42
Carbon	C	6	Neodymium	Nd	60
Cerium	Ce	58	Neon	Ne	10
Cesium	Cs	55	Neptunium	Np	93
Chlorine	Cl	17	Nickel	Ni	28
Chromium	Cr	24	Niobium	Nb	41
Cobalt	Co	27	Nitrogen	N	7
Copper	Cu	29	Nobelium		102
Curium	Cm	96	Osmium	Os	76
Dysprosium	Dy	66	Oxygen	O	8
Einsteinium	E	99	Palladium	Pd	46
Emanation	Em	86	Phosphorus	P	15
Erbium	Er	69	Platinum	Pt	78
Europium	Eu	63	Plutonium	Pu	94
Fermium	Fm	100	Polonium	Po	84
Fluorine	F	9	Potassium	K	19
Francium	Fr	87	Praseodymium	Pr	59
Gadolinium	Gd	64	Promethium	Pm	61
Gallium	Ga	31	Protactinium	Pa	91
Germanium	Ge	32	Radium	Ra	88
Gold	Au	79	Rhenium	Re	75
Hafnium	Hf	72	Rhodium	Rh	45
Helium	He	2			

Rubidium	Rb	37	Thallium	Tl	81
Ruthenium	Ru	44	Thorium	Th	90
Samarium	Sa	62	Thulium	Tm	69
Scandium	Sc	21	Tin	Sn	50
Selenium	Se	34	Titanium	Ti	22
Silicon	Si	14	Tungsten: See Wolfram		
Silver	Ag	47	Uranium	U	92
Sodium	Na	11	Vanadium	V	23
Strontium	Sr	38	Wolfram	W	74
Sulphur	S	16	Xenon	Xe	54
Tantalum	Ta	73	Ytterbium	Yb	70
Technitium	Tc	43	Yttrium	Yt	39
Tellurium	Te	52	Zinc	Zn	30
Terbium	Tb	65	Zirconium	Zr	40

REVISION OF OLD TERMS

Old	New	Old	New
Actinium A	Po^{215}	Radium D	Pb^{210}
Actinium B	Pb^{211}	Radium E	Bi^{210}
Actinium C	Bi^{211}	Radium E''	Tl^{206}
Actinium C'	Po^{211}	Radium F	Po^{210}
Actinium C''	Tl^{207}	Radon	Em^{222}
Actinium K	Fr^{223}	Thorium A	Po^{216}
Actinium U	U^{235}	Thorium B	Pb^{212}
Actinium X	Ra^{223}	Thorium C	Bi^{212}
Actinon	Em^{219}	Thorium C'	Po^{212}
Ionium	Th^{230}	Thorium C''	Tl^{208}
Mesothorium$_1$	Ra^{228}	Thorium X	Ra^{224}
Mesothorium$_2$	Ac^{228}	Thoron	Em^{220}
Radioactinium	Th^{227}	Tungsten	$_{74}W$ (Wolfram)
Radiothorium	Th^{228}	Uranium I	U^{238}
Radium A	Po^{218}	Uranium II	U^{234}
Radium B	Pb^{214}	Uranium X_1	Th^{234}
Radium C	Bi^{214}	Uranium X_2	Pa^{234}
Radium C'	Po^{214}	Uranium Y	Th^{231}
Radium C''	Tl^{210}	Uranium Z	Pa^{234}

TABLE OF ISOTOPES

			NATURALLY OCCURRING ISOTOPES				RADIOACTIVE ISOTOPES						
Z	Name	Symbol	Atomic weight	A	σ Thermal	Abundance, %	A	Half life	Alpha α	Beta β	Positron β+	Gamma γ	Other
1	Hydrogen σ 0.33	H	1.008	1	0.33	99.985	3	12.26y	—	0.018	—	—	—
				2	0.00057	0.015							
2	Helium σ 0.007	He	4.003	3	5400	0.00013	5	2×10^{-21}s	+	—	—	—	n
				4	0	~100	6	0.82s	—	3.50	—	—	
3	Lithium σ 71	Li	6.940	6	950	7.5	5	$\sim 10^{-21}$s	3(2α)	—	—	—	p
				7	0.033	92.5	8	0.84s	+	13	—	—	
							9	0.17s	+(2α)	+	—	—	n
4	Beryllium σ 0.01	Be	9.013	9	0.01	100	7	53d	—	—	—	0.48	K
							8	$< 4 \times 10^{-15}$s	3(2α)	—	—	—	
							10	2.7×10^{6}y	—	0.56	—	—	
5	Boron σ 755	B	10.82	10	4020	18.8	8	0.5s	—	—	14	—	p
				11	<0.05	81.2	9	$> 3 \times 10^{-19}$s	9.0162(2α)	—	—	4.4	
							12	0.025s	—	13.4; 9.0	—	—	
6	Carbon σ 0.0032	C	12.011	12	0.0032	8.89	10	19s	—	—	1.9	0.72; 1.03	—
				13	0.0009	91.11	11	205m	—	—	0.96	—	—
				14*	$<10^{-6}$	Trace†	14*	5600y	—	0.158	—	—	
							15	2.3s	—	4.3; 9.8	—	5.3	
7	Nitrogen σ 1.9	N	14.008	14	1.8	99.63	12	0.012s	~4(3α)	—	16.7	—	—
				15	0.00002	0.37	13	10m	—	—	1.2	—	—
							16	7.4s	—	4; 10.4	—	6.13; 7.10; 2.7	
							17	4.14s	—	3.7	—	—	(n 1.0)
8	Oxygen σ <0.0002	O	16.000	16	<0.0002	99.759	14	72s	—	—	1.83	2.30	—
				17	0.5	0.037	15	2.1m	—	—	1.7	—	—
				18	0.00002	0.204	19	29s	—	3.2; 4.4	—	{0.197d; 1.37; 0.11}	

† C14 due to cosmic rays.

TABLE OF ISOTOPES—Continued

			NATURALLY OCCURRING ISOTOPES				RADIOACTIVE ISOTOPES						
Z	Name	Symbol	Atomic weight	A	σ Thermal	Abundance, %	A	Half life	Alpha α	Beta β	Positron β+	Gamma γ	Other
9	Fluorine σ 0.009	F	19.00	19	0.009	100	17	66s	—	—	1.75	—	—
							18	1.87h	—	—	0.65	—	—
							20	11s	—	5.42	—	1.63	—
							21	5s	—	+	—	—	—
10	Neon σ < 1	Ne	20.183	20	<1	90.8	18	1.6s	—	—	3.2	—	—
				21	<1	0.26	19	18.5s	—	—	2.2	—	—
				22	<1	8.9	23	40s	—	4.2; 3.8	—	0.44; 1.65	—
							24	3.4m	—	1.95; (~4.3)	—	—	—
11	Sodium σ 0.53	Na	22.991	23	0.53	100	20	0.3s	(>2)	—	2.50	—	—
							21	23s	—	—	0.54	—	—
							22	2.6y	—	—	+	1.28	K
							24	15h	—	1.39	—	2.753; 1.368	—
							25	60s	—	4.0; 2.6–3.4	—	(0.98; 0.53; 0.38, 1.6)	—
12	Magnesium σ 0.63	Mg	24.32	24	0.03	78.8	23	12s	—	—	3.0	—	—
				25	0.27	10.1	27	9.5m	—	1.75; 1.57	—	0.84; 1.02; 0.18	—
				26	0.03	11.1	28	21.3h	—	0.45	—	(0.032; 1.35; 0.95, 0.40)	—
13	Aluminum σ 0.23	Al	26.98	27		100	24	2.1s	(~2)	—	<8.5; 8.5	1.38–7.2	—
							25	7.3s	—	—	3.24	—	—
							26	6.5s	—	—	3.21	—	—
							26	~10^{6}y	—	—	1.2	1.82; 0.72; 2.9	—
							28	2.30m	—	2.87	—	1.78	—
							29	6.6m	—	2.5; 1.4	—	1.28; 2.43	—
14	Silicon σ 0.13	Si	28.09	28	0.1	92.17	26	1.7s	—	—	3.8	—	—
				29	0.3	4.71	27	4.4s	—	—	+	—	—
				30	0.11	3.12	31	2.62h	—	1.48	—	1.26	—
							32	~300y	—	0.1	—	—	—

Z	Element (σ)	Sym	At. wt	A	σ	% abund.	A	Half-life	(~3)				Decay
15	Phosphorus σ 0.2	P	30.975	31	0.20	100	28	0.28s	—	—	11; ~8	1.78; 2.6–7.6	—
							29	4.5s	—	—	3.94	1.28; 2.43	—
							30	2.5m	—	—	3.3	—	—
							32	14.5d	—	1.71	—	—	—
							33	2.5d	—	0.25	—	—	—
							34	12.4s	—	5.1; 3.2	—	2.1; 4.0	—
16	Sulphur σ 0.49	S	32.066	32	0.002	95	31	2.6s	—	—	4.4	—	—
				33	0.26	0.75	35	87d	—	0.167	—	—	—
				34	0.014	4.2	37	5.0m	—	1.6; 4.7	—	3.1	—
				36		0.017							
17	Chlorine σ 33	Cl	35.457	35	44	75.53	32	0.31s	(~3)	—	10; 8	2.2; 4.8	—
				37	0.005; 0.56	24.47	33	2.8s	—	—	4.2	2.82	—
							34	32.4m	—	—	2.5; 1.4	2.1; 1.1; 3.2	—
							34	1.5s	—	—	4.5	—	I.T. 0.14
							36	3.1 × 10⁵y	—	0.71	—	—	K
							38	1s	—	4.8; 1.1; 2 7	—	2.1; 1.6	I.T. 0.66
							38	37.3m	—	3.0; 1.7	—	0.3; 1.3	—
							39	55m	—	~7	—	1.46; 2.75; ~6	—
							40	1.4m	—	—	—	—	—
18	Argon σ 0.06	A	39.944	36	6	0.337	35	1.8s	—	—	4.95	1.22; 1.76	—
				38	0.8	0.063	37	35d	—	0.57	—	—	K; L
				40	0.53	99.6	39	260y	—	—	—	—	—
							41	1.82h	—	1.2; 2.49	—	0.129d	—
							42	>3.5y	—	+	—	—	—
19	Potassium σ 2.0	K	39.100	39	1.9	93.2	38	0.95s	—	—	5.1	2.1	—
				40*	70	0.0119	38	7.7m	—	—	2.7	1 46	—
				41	1.1	6.8	40*	1.3 × 10⁹y	—	1.33	—	1.5; 0.32	K
							42	12.5h	—	3.5; 2.0	—	0.62; 0.37	—
							43	22h	—	0.83; 0.24–1.84	—	1.1; 2.1; 2.5	—
							44	22m	—	4.9; 1.5	—	—	—
							45	34m	—	+	—	—	—

TABLE OF ISOTOPES—Continued

				NATURALLY OCCURRING ISOTOPES			RADIOACTIVE ISOTOPES						
Z	Name	Symbol	Atomic weight	A	σ Thermal	Abundance, %	A	Half life	Alpha α	Beta β	Positron β+	Gamma γ	Other
20	Calcium σ 0.43	Ca	40.08	40	0.2	96.9	39	1.0s	—	5.7	—	—	—
				42	40	0.64	41	1.1 × 10⁵y	—	—	—	—	K
				43		0.14	45	160d	—	0.25	—	—	—
				44	0.6	2.1	47	4.7d	—	0.7; 2.0	—	1.3; 0.81; 0.5	—
				46	0.3	0.0032	49	8.7m	—	2.0; 1.0	—	3.09; 4.05; 4.7	—
				48	1.1	0.18							
21	Scandium σ 23	Sc	44.96	45	10; 13	100	40	0.2s	—		9	—	—
							41	0.87s	—		5	—	—
							42	0.66s	—		~5	—	—
							43	3.9h	—		1.9; 0.82; 0.39	0.37; 0.62; 0.25 0.84	—
							44	2.4d	—		1.47	1.16; 2.54	I.T. 0.271; e⁻
							44	4.0h	—		—	—	K
							46	20s	—		—	1.12; 0.88	I.T. 0.14; e⁻
							46	85d	—	0.36	—	0.16	—
							47	3.4d	—	0.44; 0.6	—	1.32; 1.04; 0.99	—
							48	44h	—	0.64	—	—	—
							49	57m	—	2.0	—	1.6; 1.2	—
							50	1.7m	—	~3.5	—	—	—
22	Titanium σ 6	Ti	47.90	46	0.6	8.0	43	0.6s	—	—	+	—	—
				47	1.6	7.4	44	>20y	—	—	—	0.16	K
				48	7.8	73.8	45	3.08h	—	—	1.02	—	K
				49	1.8	5.5	51	5.8m	—	2.1; 1.5	—	0.32; 0.93; 0.61	—
				50	0.14	5.3							
23	Vanadium σ 4.9	V	50.95	50	~100	0.25	45	~1s	—		>6	—	K
				51	4.5	99.75	46	0.4s	—		1.89	—	K
							47	31m	—		0.69	—	—
							48	16.2d	—		+	0.99; 1.32; 2.23	—
							49	~1y	—		—	—	—
							52	3.77m	—	2.6	—	1.4	K
							53	2.0m	—	2.5	—	1.0	K
							54	55s	—	3.3	—	0.99; 0.84; 2.21	—

Z	Element (σ)	Symbol	At. wt.	Mass	σ	Abund. %	Half-life	α	β⁻	β⁺	γ	Decay type
24	Chromium σ 3.1	Cr	52.01	50	16	4.4						
				52	0.8	83.7						
				53	18	9.5						
				54	0.37	2.4						
				46			1.1s	—	—	+	—	—
				48			23h	—	—	—	0.32; 0.12	K; e⁻
				49			42m	—	—	1.54	0.15; 0.09; 0.06	e⁻
				51			27d	—	—	—	0.32	K
				55			3.6m	—	2.8	—	—	—
25	Manganese σ 13.3	Mn	54.94	55	13.3	100						
				50			0.28s	—	—	>6	—	—
				51			4.5m	—	—	2.2	—	—
				52			21m	—	—	2.7	1.4	I.T. 0.39
				52			5.7d	—	—	0.6	1.4; 0.9; 0.7	K
				53			~140y	—	—	—	—	I.T.?
				54			2m	—	+ or e⁻	—	—	K
				54			300d	—	—	—	0.84	K
				56			2.58h	—	2.8; 1.0; 0.7	—	0.85; 1.8; 2.1-3	—
				57			1.7m	—	2.6	—	0.117; 0.134; 0.069	—
26	Iron σ 2.5	Fe	55.85	54	2.2	5.9						
				56	2.6	91.6						
				57	2.4	2.2						
				58	0.9	0.33						
				52			8h	—	—	0.8; (2.7)	(1.4; 0.39)	K
				53			9m	—	—	2.6	0.37	K
				55			2.9y	—	—	—	—	—
				59			45d	—	0.46; 0.27; 1.56	—	1.1; 1.29; 0.19	—
				60			~3 × 10⁵y	—	+	—	(0.059)	—
				61			5.5m	—	+	—	—	—
27	Cobalt σ 37	Co	58.94	59	18; 19	100						
				54			0.18s	—	—	>7	0.93; 0.48-2.2	K; e⁻
				55			18h	—	—	1.5; 1.0	0.85; 1.2; 1.7-3.2	K
				56			77d	—	—	1.5	—	K; e⁻
				57			267d	—	—	0.48	0.123; 0.014d; 0.137	I.T. 0.25; e⁻
				58			9h	—	—	—	—	K
				58			71d	—	—	—	0.81; 1.64	I.T. 0.059
				60			10.5m	—	1.5	—	1.33	—
				60			5.2y	—	0.31	—	1.33; 1.17	K
				61			1.65h	—	1.22	—	0.07	—
				62			1.6m	—	+	—	+	—
				62			14m	—	2.8	—	1.2; 1.0	—

TABLE OF ISOTOPES—*Continued*

			NATURALLY OCCURRING ISOTOPES				RADIOACTIVE ISOTOPES						
Z	Name	Symbol	Atomic weight	A	σ Thermal	Abundance, %	A	Half life	Alpha α	Beta β	Positron β+	Gamma γ	Other
28	Nickel σ 4.6	Ni	58.71	58	4.3	68.0	56	6.4d	—	—	—	0.16; 0.85; 0.26–1.74	K
				60	2.6	26.2	57	36h	—	—	0.84	1.38; 1.91; 0.12	K
				61	2	1.1	59	8 × 10⁴y	—	—	—	—	K
				62	15	3.7	63	80y	—	0.063	—	—	—
				64	2	1.0	65	2.56h	—	2.1; 0.6; 1.0	—	1.5; 1.12; 0.37	—
							66	56h	—	0.3	—	—	—
29	Copper σ 3.7	Cu	63.54	63	4.4	69.0	58	9.5m	—	—	<0.7	—	—
				65	2.2	31.0	58	3s	—	—	~8	—	—
							59	81s	—	—	3.7	—	—
							60	24m	—	—	2.0; 3.0; 3.9	0.9; 1.3; 1.33; 1.76; 0.85; 2.1–4.0	K
							61	3.3h	—	—	1.22	0.28; 0.66; 1.22; 0.07	—
							62	9.9m	—	—	2.9	—	—
							64	12.8h	—	0.57	0.66	1.34	K
							66	5.1m	—	2.63; 1.59	—	1.04	—
							67	61h	—	0.40; 0.48; 0.58	—	0.182; 0.09; 0.092d	e⁻
							68	32s	—	3.0	—	+	—
30	Zinc σ 1.10	Zn	65.38	64	0.5	48.9	60	2.1m	—	—	—	→	Radiation?
				66		27.8	61	1.5m	—	—	5	—	K; e⁻
				67	109; 1	4.1	62	9h	—	—	0.66	0.041	K
				68	0.09	18.6	63	38m	—	—	2.36; 1.40	0.96; 1.9; 2.6	K
				70		0.63	65	245d	—	—	0.33	1.12	I.T. 0.44
							69	14h	—	0.9	—	—	—
							69	52m	—	1.5	—	0.4; 0.5; 0.6	—
							71	3h	—	2.4	—	0.51	—
							71	2.2m	—	0.3; 1.6	—	—	—
							72	49h	—	—	—	+	—

Z	Element (σ)	Sym	At. wt.	Stable A	σ	Abund. %	Radio. A	Half‑life	β⁻	β⁺ / part.	γ	Decay
31	Gallium σ 2.9	Ga	72.60	69	1.9	60.1						
				71	4.6	39.9						
							64	2.5m	—	~5	0.97–3.8	I.T. 0.052 —
							65	15m	—	2.5	0.09; 0.11	K —
							65	8m	—	2.2	{1.04; 2.75; 0.8–4.8}	K; e⁻
							66	9.4h	—	4.15	0.092; 0.18; 0.3; 0.09–0.88	K —
							67	78h	—	—	1.10	—
							68	68m	1.65	1.88; 0.78	1.04; 0.17	—
							70	21m	0.64–3.17	—	0.84; 0.6–3.35	—
							72	14.1h			0.69d	—
							73	5h	1.4	—	(0.054–0.013d)	—
32	Germanium σ 2.3	Ge	72.60	70	3.4	20.5						
				72	1.0	27.4						
				73	14	7.8						
				74	1.2; 0.5	36.5						
				76	0.15; 0.3	7.8						
							66	2.5h	—	?	0.17	K
							67	19m	—	3.4	—	K
							68	250d	—	—	—	K
							69	40h	—	1.21; 0.6	{1.2; 0.58; 0.87; 0.09–1.6}	K
							71	12d	—	—	0.013	I.T. 0.054; e⁻
							73	0.53s	1.18; 0.92	—	0.27; 0.07–0.63	I.T. 0.14; e⁻
							75	49s	2.9	—	0.21	I.T. 0.16
							75	82m	2.20	—	0.21–2.3	—
							77	52s	0.9	—	+	—
							77	12h				—
							78	86m				—
33	Arsenic σ 4.3	As	74.91	75	4.3	100						
							68	~7m	—	+	0.23	e⁻ —
							69	15m	—	2.9	1.1; 2.0	K —
							70	50m	—	1.4; 2.5	0.175; 0.023	K; e⁻
							71	62h	—	0.81	0.84; 0.69d; 1–3	I.T. 0.28
							72	26h	—	2.50; 3.34	(0.054; 0.013d)	—
							73	76d	—	—	0.6; 0.64	—
							74	17d	1.36; 0.72	0.93; 1.53	0.55; 1.19; 0.64	—
							75	0.018s	—	—	—	—
							76	26.7h	2.96; 2.41	—	1.4; 2.1	—
							77	39h	0.69	—	0.24; 0.52; 0.086; 0.16	—
							78	90m	4.1	—		—
							79	9m	2.3	—		—
							80	~36s	+	—	(0.096)	—

TABLE OF ISOTOPES—*Continued*

NATURALLY OCCURRING ISOTOPES							RADIOACTIVE ISOTOPES						
Z	Name	Symbol	Atomic weight	A	σ Thermal	Abundance, %	A	Half life	Alpha α	Beta β	Positron β⁺	Gamma γ	Other
34	Selenium σ 13	Se	78.96	74	40	0.93	70	44m	—	—	—	—	—
				76	0.7; 78	9.1	72	9.7d	—	—	+	—	K
				77	41	7.5	73	7.1h	—	—	1.29; 1.65	0.36; 0.066	—
				78	0.4	23.6	73	44m	—	—	1.7	—	—
				80	0.03; 0.5	49.9	75	127d	—	—	—	{0.27; 0.14; (0.28); 0.066-0.4}	K
							77	17s	—	—	—	—	I.T. 0.16
				82	0.05; 0.004	9.0	79	3.9m	—	0.16	—	—	I.T. 0.096; e⁻
							79	7 × 10⁴y	—	—	—	—	—
							81	57m	—	1.38	—	—	I.T. 0.103; e⁻
							81	18m	—	3.4	—	—	—
							83	69s	—	1.5	—	{0.04; 0.06; 0.18}	—
							83	25m	—		—	0.95	—
							84	~2 m	—	+	—	—	—
35	Bromine σ 6.6	Br	79.916	79	2.9; 8.5	50.6	74	36m	—	—	1.70	—	K
				81	2.6	49.4	75	1.6 h	—	—	3.57	0.6	K
							76	17h	—	—	0.34	1.2; 0.2-0.96;	K
							77	57h	—	—	—	{0.52; 0.086-1.0; (0.16)}	K
							78	6.4 m	—	—	2.4	0.05; 0.11	I.T.
							78	<6m	—	—	—	—	—
							80	4.6h	—	—	0.86	0.04	I.T. 0.05; e⁻
							80	18m	—	2.0; 1.4	—	0.62	—
							82	35.9h	—	0.46	—	{0.55; 0.77; 1.04; 0.6-2}	—
							83	2.3h	—	0.94	—	{0.051; (0.032-0.009)}	—
							84	32m	—	4.68	—	0.89; 1.9	—
							85	3.0m	—	2.5	—	—	—
							87	56s	—	2.6; 8.0	—	3; 2; 5.4	(n 0.3)
							88	16s	—	+	—	—	—
							89	4.5s	—	+	—	—	(n 0.5)

Z	Element	Symbol	At. wt.	Stable isotope	σ	Abundance %	Radioactive isotope	Half-life	α	β⁻	β⁺	γ	Radiation
36	Krypton σ 28	Kr	83.80	78	?; 2	0.35	76	10h	—	—	1.86; 1.67	0.28–0.40	K
				80	20	2.27	77	1.2h	—	—	—	{0.108; 0.131; 0.024; 0.149–0.87}	K
				82	40	11.6	79	55s	—	—	—	—	I.T. 0.13
				83	200	11.5	79	34h	—	—	0.60; 0.34	{0.26; 0.044; 0.08–0.83}	K; L
				84	0.1; 0.06	57.0	81	13s	—	—	—	—	I.T. 0.19
				86	0.08	17.3	81	2 × 10⁵y	—	—	—	—	K
							83	1.68h	—	—	—	0.009	I.T. 0.032
							85	4.4h	—	0.83	—	0.15	I.T. 0.31
							85	10.4y	—	0.67	—	0.52	—
							87	78m	—	3.8; 1.3; ~3.3	—	0.4; 2.57; 0.85	—
							88	2.8h	—	0.52; 2.7	—	{2.4; 0.19; 0.85; 0.028–2.2}	—
							89	3.2m	—	4.2; 2	—	+	—
							90	33s	—	3.2	—	+	—
							91	10s	—	3.6	—	+	—
							92	3s	—	+	—	—	—
							93	2s	—	+	—	—	—
							94	1s	—	+	—	—	—
							95	short	—	—	—	—	—
							97	~1s	—	—	—	—	—
37	Rubidium σ 0.7	Rb	85.48	85	0.05; 0.8	72.2	<81	8d	—	—	1.0	0.9; (0.19)	Rad. ?
				87*	0.14	27.8	81	4.7h	—	—	0.77	0.78; 0.32–1.46	—
							82	6.3h	—	—	—	—	—
							82	75s	—	—	3.2	0.52; (0.32–0.09)	K
							83	83d	—	—	—	0.23; 0.89	—
							84	21m	—	—	—	—	I.T. 0.23, 0.46:
							84	33d	—	0.4	1.7	0.89–1.9	K
							86	1m	—	—	—	—	I.T. 0.56
							86	18.6d	—	1.77; 0.7	—	1.08	—
							87*	4.3 × 10¹⁰y	—	0.27	—	—	—
							88	18m	—	5.2; 3.3; 2	—	{1.85; 0.91; 2.7; 1.39–4.9}	—

TABLE OF ISOTOPES—Continued

			NATURALLY OCCURRING ISOTOPES				RADIOACTIVE ISOTOPES						
Z	Name	Symbol	Atomic weight	A	σ Thermal	Abundance, %	A	Half life	Alpha α	Beta β	Positron β+	Gamma γ	Other
							89	15m	—	3.9	—	1.05; 0.25; 0.66; 1.26–2.12	—
							90	2.7m	—	5.7	—		—
							91	1.7m	—	4.6	—	+	—
							91	14m	—	3.0	—	+	—
							92	~80s	—	+	—		—
							93	short	—	+	—		—
							94	short	—	+	—		—
							95	short	—	+	—		—
							97	short	—				
38	Strontium σ 1.3	Sr	87.63	84	1	0.55	81	29m	—		+		e⁻
				86	1; ?	9.8	82	26d	—				K
				87	0.005	7.0	83	33h	—		(3.2)	0.04–0.16	K; e⁻
				88		82.7	85	70m	—		1.2	0.22	I.T. 0.007, 0.23;
							85	65d				0.51d	K
							87	2.8h					I.T. 0.39
							89	~10d					I.T.
							89	54d		1.48		(0.91)	—
							90	28y		0.54; (2.2)		+	—
							91	9.7h		0.61–2.67		(0.55); 0.65 – 1.41	—
							92	2.7h		~0.55		1.38	—
							93	7 m		+		—	—
							94	~2m		+		—	—
							95	short		+		—	—
							97	short				—	—
39	Yttrium σ 1.3	Y	89.92	89	1.3	100	82	70m	—	—	2	—	Radiation ?
							83	3.5h					K
							84	3.7h			2.0	+	Radiation ?
							85	5h	—				—
							86	15h			1.8; 1.2	1.93; 1.08; 0.18; 0.63	

Zirconium — Z = 40; Zr; σ 0.18; at. wt 91.22

Stable isotopes:

Mass no.	% abundance	σ
90	51.5	0.1
91	11.2	1.0
92	17.1	0.2
94	17.4	0.1
96	2.8	0.1

Radioactive isotopes:

Mass no.	Half-life	β⁻	β⁺	α	γ	Other
87	14h	—	0.7	—	0.48; (0.39)	I.T. 0.38; e⁻
87	80h	—	0.83	—	1.85; 0.91	—
88	105d	—	—	—	—	—
89	16s	2.27	—	—	—	I.T. 0.91
89	64h	—	—	—	1.19	e⁻
90	50m	1.54	—	—	0.94; 0.21-2.4	I.T. 0.55; e⁻
91	58d	3.6; 2.7; 1.3	—	—	0.7	—
92	3.5h	3.1	—	—	1.4	—
93	10h	5.4	—	—	—	—
94	17m	+	—	—	—	—
95	10m	+	—	—	—	—
97	short	—	—	—	—	—

Niobium — Z = 41; Nb; σ 1; at. wt 92.91

Stable isotopes:

Mass no.	% abundance	σ
93	100	1; ?

Radioactive isotopes:

Mass no.	Half-life	β⁻	β⁺	α	γ	Other
86	~17h	—	2.1	—	0.24	K
87	1.6h	—	—	—	0.6; 0.3	K
88	85d	—	0.9; 2.4	—	0.39d	K; e⁻
89	4.4m	—	0.9	—	1.5	I.T. 0.59
89	79h	—	—	—	(0.91)	K
90	0.8s	—	—	—	—	I.T.
93	9×10^5 y	0.063	—	—	(0.029)	—
95	65d	0.36; 0.39; 0.88	—	—	0.75; 0.72; (0.23)	e⁻
97	17h	1.91; (1.27)	—	—	(0.75; 0.66)	—
89	~2h	—	2.9	—	(0.59)	—
89	1.9h	—	—	—	—	I.T. 0.12; e⁻
90	24s	—	1.50	—	1.14; 2.23; 0.14	—
90	14.6h	—	—	—	1.19	I.T. 0.105; e⁻; K
91	62d	—	—	—	—	K
91	long	—	—	—	2.36	K
92	13h	—	—	—	0.93; 1.83; 0.90	K
92	10d	—	—	—	—	I.T. 0.029; e⁻
93	3.7y	1.3	—	—	0.9	I.T. 0.04; e⁻
94	6.6m	0.5	—	—	0.87; 0.7; 1.57	—
94	20,000y	—	—	—	0.76	I.T. 0.23; e⁻
95	84h	0.16	—	—	0.77; 0.22-1.19	—
96	35d	0.7; 0.4	—	—	—	I.T. 0.75; e⁻
97	23h	—	—	—	0.66	—
97	1m	1.27	—	—	—	—
98?	72m	+	—	—	—	—
98?	30m	3.2	—	—	—	—
99	2.5m	—	—	—	—	—

TABLE OF ISOTOPES—Continued

		NATURALLY OCCURRING ISOTOPES					RADIOACTIVE ISOTOPES						
Z	Name	Symbol	Atomic weight	A	σ Thermal	Abundance, %	A	Half life	Alpha α	Beta β	Positron β⁺	Gamma γ	Other
42	Molybdenum σ 2.5	Mo	95.95	92	0.006; ?	15.7	90	5.7h	—	—	1.2	0.25d; (0.12)	K; e⁻
				94		9.3	91	66s	—	—	2.45; 2.78; 3.99	1.54; 1.21	I.T. 0.65
				95	14.0	15.7	91	15.6m	—	—	3.44		
				96	1.0	16.5	93	6.9h	—	—	—	1.48; 0.69	I.T. 0.26; e⁻
				97	2.0	9.5	93	>2y	—	—	—	—	K
				98	0.13	23.8	99	67h	—	1.23; 0.45	—	(0.14); 0.74; 0.04; 0.78	—
				100	0.2	9.5	101	15m	—	1.1; 2.2	—	0.19; 0.96	—
							102	11m	—	1.0	—	—	—
							105	<2m	—	+	—	—	—
43	Technitium	Tc					92	4.3m	—	—	4.1	1.3	I.T. 0.39; e⁻;K
							93	44m	—	—	—	2.7	K
							93	2.7h	—	—	0.8; 0.6	1.3; 1.5; 2.0	K
							94	53m	—	—	2.41	0.87; 1.85; 3.3; 2.7	
							95	60d	—	—	0.6	0.2–1.0	I.T. 0.39; K
							95	20h	—	—	—	0.76; 1.1	K
							96	52m	—	—	+		I.T. 0.034; e⁻; K
							96	4.3d	—	—	—	0.84; 0.77; 0.81; 1.12	K
							97	91d	—	—	—	0.09	I.T. 0.99; e⁻
							97	~10⁵y	—	—	—	—	K
							98	~10⁴y	—	0.3	—	0.74; 0.65	I.T. 0.002,
							99	6.0h	—	—	—	0.14	0.14;2 e⁻
							99	2.1 × 10⁵y	—	0.29	—	—	—
							100	16s	—	2.8	—	0.54	—
							101	15m	—	1.2	—	0.3	—
							102	5s	—	4.0	—	—	—
							104?	3.8m	—		—	—	Rad. ?
							105	10m	—	+	—	—	—

44	Ruthenium σ 2.5	Ru	101.1	96	0.01	5.6	<94	0.9m	—	—	+	+	—
				98		1.9	94	1h	—	—	—	—	K
				99		12.7	95	98m	—	—	1.2	1.1	K
				100		12.7	97	2.9d	—	—	—	{0.22; 0.33; 0.57; 0.11	K; e^-
				101		17.0	103	40d	—	0.2; 0.13; 0.69	—	{(0.04); 0.5; 0.05; 0.61	—
				102	1.2	31.5							
				104	0.7	18.6	105	4.5h	—	1.15	—	0.73; (0.13)	—
							106	1y	—	0.04; (3.53)	—	(0.51; 0.62–2.4)	—
							107	4.5m	—	4.3	—	+	—
							108	$\sim$4m	—	+	—	—	—
45	Rhodium σ 150	Rh	102.91	103	12; 138	100	97	35m	—	—	+	—	—
							98	9m	—	—	3.3	0.65	—
							99	15d	—	—	+	0.353; 0.086	e^-
							99	4.5h	—	—	0.74	0.29	—
							100	21h	—	—	2.62	{0.53; 0.44; 0.03–2.4	K
							101	$\sim$5y	—	—	—	0.198	I.T.(?) 0.127
							101	4.5d	—	—	—	0.3; 0.15; 0.56	K; e^-
							102	220d	—	1.15	1.24	{0.48; 0.2; 1.17; 0.12–1.7	K
							103	54m	—	—	—	—	I.T. 0.4; e^-
							104	4.4m	—	+	—	0.055	I.T. 0.077; e^-
							104	42s	—	2.5	—	0.55; 1.24	—
							105	30s	—	—	—	—	I.T. 0.13; e^-
							105	36h	—	0.25; 0.56	—	0.31	—
							106	2h	—	$\sim$1.0	—	0.2–1.5	—
							106	30s	—	3.53	—	{0.51; 0.62; 0.87–2.66	—
							107	22m	—	1.2; $\sim$2.0	—	{0.31; 0.4; 0.1–0.7	—
							108	18s	—	$\sim$4	—	+	—
							109	<1h	———	———	———	——→	Rad. ?

TABLE OF ISOTOPES—Continued

				NATURALLY OCCURRING ISOTOPES			RADIOACTIVE ISOTOPES						
Z	Name	Symbol	Atomic weight	A	σ Thermal	Abundance, %	A	Half life	Alpha α	Beta β	Positron β+	Gamma γ	Other
46	Palladium σ 8	Pd	106.4	102	4.8	1.0	98	17m	—	—	+	0.13	—
				104		11.0	99	24m	—	—	—	0.081; 1.8(?)	K
				105		22.2	100	4d	—	—	—		K
				106		27.3	101	8h	—	—	0.5; 2.3(?)		K; e⁻
				108	0.07; 11	26.7	103	17d	—	—	—	(0.04); 0.053	I.T. 0.2; e⁻
				110	?; 0.4	11.8	105	23s	—	—	—	—	—
							107	7 × 10⁶y	—	0.04	—	—	—
							109	4.8m	—	1.0	—	—	I.T. 0.17; e⁻
							109	13.6h	—	—	—	(0.088)	—
							111	5.5h	—	+	—	0.16; 1.77	I.T.
							111	22m	—	2.14	—	0.38–0.73	—
							112	21h	—	0.28	—	0.018	—
							113	1.5m	—	+	—	—	—
47	Silver σ 60	Ag		107	30	51.4	102	16m	—		+	—	K; e⁻
				109	2; 82	48.6	103	1.1h	—	—	1.3	0.76; 0.55	—
							104	27m	—	—	2.7	0.55, 0.12	K
							105	40d	—	—	—	{0.34; 0.28; 0.064; 0.65; 0.16–0.44}	—
							106	24m	—	—	1.96; 1.45	0.51	K
							106	8.3d	—	—	—	0.51; 0.22–2.66	K
							107	44s	—	—	—	—	I.T. 0.093; e⁻
							108	2.3m	—	1.77	0.8	0.62; 0.43; 0.6	K
							109	40s	—	—	—	—	I.T.; e⁻
							110	270d	—	0.53; 0.1	—	{0.66; 0.89; 0.93–2}	I.T. 0.12
							110	24s	—	2.22; 2.88	—	0.66	—
							111	75s	—	—	—	—	I.T.
							111	7.5d	—	1.04; 0.7	—	0.34; 0.247d	—
							112	3.12h	—	3.5; 4.1; 2.7	—	{0.62; 1.39 1.1–2.8}	—
							113	5.3h	—	2.0	—	0.29	—
							114	2m	—	+	—	—	—
							115	21m	—	3	—	0.23	—

48	Cadmium	Cd	112.41	106	1	1.22	104	59m	—	—	—	0.067; 0.084; 0.124; 0.134	K
	σ 3300			108		0.88							
				110	0.20; ?	12.4	105	55m	—	—	1.69	0.025–2.32	K; e⁻
				111		12.8	107	6.7h	—	—	0.32	0.85; (0.094)	e⁻
				112	0.031; ?	24.0	109	1.3y	—	—	—	(0.087)	(e⁻); K; L
				113	27,000	12.3	111	49m	—	—	—	0.247d	I.T. 0.5; e⁻
				114	0.14; 1.1	28.8	113	5y	—	0.58	—	—	—
				116	1.4	7.6	115	43d	—	1.63	—	0.95; 0.45–1.28	—
							115	54h	—	1.11	—	0.52; (0.34)	—
							117	3.0h	—	—	—	—	I.T.
							117	50m	—	1.6; 3.0	—	1.3; 0.27–2.0	—
							118	∼30m	—	(4)	—	—	—
49	Indium	In	114.81				107	30m	—	—	2	+	—
	σ 190			113	61; 2	4.2	108	50m	—	—	2.3	—	e⁻
				115*	145; 52	95.8	109	43h	—	—	0.7	0.058; 0.2; 0.35; 0.43	K
							110	5.0h	—	—	—	0.66; 0.88; 0.94	I.T. 0.12; K
							110	66m	—	—	2.25	0.66d	K
							111	2.8d	—	—	—	0.247d; 0.172; 0.33; 0.09; (0.15)	K; e⁻
							112	21m	—	—	—	(0.15)	I.T.; e⁻
							112	2.5s	—	—	—	0.15	I.T.; e⁻
							112	14m	—	0.66	1.52	—	K
							113	1.73h	—	—	—	—	I.T. 0.39; e⁻
							114	49d	—	—	—	0.72; 0.56	I.T. 0.19; K
							114	72s	—	1.98	∼1	0.55–1.28	—
							115	4.5h	—	0.83	—	—	I.T. 0.33; e⁻
							115*	6×10^{14}y	—	0.6	—	—	—
							116	54m	—	1.0	—	1.27; 1.09; 2.1; 1.5	—
							116	13s	—	3.3	—	—	—
							117	1.9h	—	1.77; 1.61	—	0.16	I.T. 0.31
							117	1.1h	—	0.74	—	0.56; 0.16	—
							118	4.5m	—	1.5	—	+	—
							118	<1m	—	4	—	—	—
							119	18m	—	2.7	—	—	—

TABLE OF ISOTOPES—*Continued*

				NATURALLY OCCURRING ISOTOPES			RADIOACTIVE ISOTOPES						
Z	Name	Symbol	Atomic weight	A	σ Thermal	Abundance, %	A	Half life	Alpha α	Beta β	Positron β+	Gamma γ	Other
50	Tin σ 0.6	Sn	118.70	112	1.3	1.02	108	4h	—	—	—	—	K
				114		0.69	109	18m	—	—	+	0.073; 0.68	K
				115		0.38	110	4h	—	—	—	0.28	K
				116	0.006; ?	14.3	111	35m	—	—	1.51	—	K
				117		7.6	113	112d	—	—	—	0.26; (0.39)	K; L; e−
				118	0.01; ?	24.1	117	14d	—	—	—	0.162	I.T. 0.159;e−
				119		8.5	119	275d	—	—	—	0.024	I.T. 0.065; e−
				120	~0.001; 0.1	32.5	121	>1y	—	0.42	—	—	—
				122	0.001; 0.2	4.8	121	27h	—	0.38	—	—	—
				124	0.2;0.004	6.1	123	130d	—	1.42	—	0.15	—
							123	40m	—	1.26	—	0.33; 1.4	—
							125	9.5m	—	2.1	—	0.33–2.0	—
							125	10d	—	2.4	—	—	—
							126	50m	—	+	—	—	—
							127	1.5h	—	+	—	—	—
51	Antimony σ 5.5	Sb	121.76	121	7	57.0	116	15m	—	—	2.4	1.27; 0.9; 2.2	—
				123	(0.03; 0.0.3; 3.4)	43.0	116	60m	—	—	1.4	1.27; 0.9; 0.41	—
							117	2.8h	—	—	—	0.16;	e−; K
							118	3.5m	—	—	3.1	—	I.T. 0.11
							118	5.1h	—	—	0.7	0.26; 0.15	e− 0.2; K
							119	38h	—	—	—	0.024d	e−; K
							120	5.8d	—	—	—	1.18; 1.04; 0.2 / 0.09	e−; K
							120	17m	—	—	1.70	1.18	—
							122	3.5m	—	—	—	0.06	I.T. 0.075; e−
							122	2.8d	—	1.4; 1.98; 0.73	0.5	0.56; 0.7–1.2	K
							124	21m	—	+	—	—	I.T. 0.018; e−
							124	1.3m	—	3	—	—	I.T. 0.012; e−
							124	60d	—	2.31	—	0.6–2.11	—

52 Tellurium σ 4.6   Te   127.61

Stable isotopes

Mass	σ	Abundance %
120	<140	0.091
122	1; 2	2.5
123	400	0.88
124	5; 2	4.6
125	1.5	7.0
126	0.09; 0.8	18.7
128	0.016; 0.14	31.8
130	0.01; 0.2	34.4

Radioactive isotopes

Mass	Half-life	β	(β⁺)	γ	e⁻
125	2.7y	0.3; 0.12–0.62	—	0.035; 0.42; (0.11); 0.6	—
126	9h	1	—	0.07–0.9	—
126	28d	1.9	—	—	—
127	93h	0.86; 1.57; 1.11	—	0.67; 0.46; 0.24; 0.058–0.76	—
128	~1h	+	—	0.16–0.78	—
129	4.6h	0.92–1.7	—	0.19–0.76	—
130	10m	2.9	—	+	—
130	40m	+	—	—	—
131	22m	1.1	—	—	—
132	2m	+	—	—	—
133	4.1m	+	—	—	—
134	0.8m	+	—	—	—
116	~3h	—	(2.4)	—	—
117	2.5h	—	2.5	—	—
118	6.0d	—	(3.1)	—	K
119	16h	—	—	(0.11)	K; e⁻
119	4.5d	—	—	0.56	e⁻ 0.2, 0.5
121	150d	—	—	1.6	I.T. 0.082; e⁻
121	17d	—	—	0.213	e⁻; K
123	104d	—	—	0.57; 0.51	I.T. 0.088; e⁻
125	58d	—	—	0.159	I.T. 0.035 e⁻
127	110d	—	—	—	I.T. 0.008; e⁻
127	9.3h	0.68	—	—	—
129	33d	—	—	0.03; 0.45; 1.08	I.T. 0.106; e⁻
129	72m	1.46; 1.01	—	0.77; 0.05–1.2	—
131	30h	0.4–2.5	—	0.05–0.77	I.T. 0.18; e⁻
131	25m	2.1	—	0.23; 0.67–2.2	—
132	77h	0.22; (0.9–2.1)	—	—	—
133	63m	1.4; 2.4	—	0.6; 1.0	I.T. 0.4; e⁻
133	2m	+	—	—	—
134	44m	—	—	—	—

TABLE OF ISOTOPES—*Continued*

	NATURALLY OCCURRING ISOTOPES						RADIOACTIVE ISOTOPES						
Z	Name	Symbol	Atomic weight	A	σ Thermal	Abundance, %	A	Half life	Alpha α	Beta β	Positron β+	Gamma γ	Other
53	Iodine σ 6.3	I	126.91	127	6.3	100	119	18m	—	—	+	—	—
							120	→1.3h	—	—	4.0	—	—
							121	1.4h	—	—	1.13	0.213	—
							122	3.5m	—	—	3.12	—	—
							123	13h	—	—	—	0.159	K; e⁻
							124	4.5d	—	—	2.2	0.6; 1.7; 2.0; 0.7	K
							125	60d	—	—	—	0.035	K; L
							126	13.3d	—	0.87	1.11	0.38; 0.65; 1.4	K
							128	25m	—	2.12; 1.67	—	0.45; 0.54–0.98	K
							129	1.7 × 10⁷y	—	0.15	—	0.38	e⁻
							130	12.6h	—	1.02; 0.6	—	0.74; 0.66; 0.53; 0.41	—
							131	8.05d	—	0.61; 0.25–0.81	—	0.36; 0.08; 0.72	—
							132	2.3h	—	0.9–2.12	—	0.67; 0.78; 0.53–2.2	—
							133	21h	—	1.3; 0.4	—	0.53; 0.85; 1.4	—
							134	52m	—	1.5; 2.5	—	0.86; 1.1; 1.8	—
							135	6.7h	—	1.0; 0.5; 1.4	—	1.3; 1.8; 2.4; (0.52)	—
							136	86s	—	6.4; 5.0; 3.6	—	1.4; 2.8	—
							137	22s	—	+	—	—	—
							138	5.9s	—	+	—	—	—
							139	2.7s	—	+	—	—	—
54	Xenon σ 3.5	Xe	131.30	124		0.094	121	40m	—	—	+	0.096	K
				126		0.092	122	19h	—	—	—	0.18; 0.23	K
				128	<5	1.92	123	1.8h	—	—	(3.12)	0.15	I.T.
				129	45	26.4	125	55s	—	—	1.7	0.111	I.T. 0.075
				130	<5	4.1	125	18h	—	—	—	0.187; 0.243 0.056–0.46	K
				131	120	21.2							
				132	<5; 0.2	26.9	127	75s	—	—	+	0.125	I.T. 0.175
				134	<5; 0.2	10.4	127	36.4d	—	—	—	0.203; 0.057– 0.36	K

Z	Element	Symbol	At. wt.	Stable isotope (mass; %)			
55	Cesium σ 31	Cs	132.91	133; 100	133; 1.016; 31	136; 0.15	136; 8.9

Mass No.	Half-life	α	β⁻	β⁺	γ	Radiation / Decay
129	8d	—	—	—	0.04	I.T.; e⁻
131	12d	—	—	—	—	I.T. 0.164; e⁻
133	2.3d	—	0.35	—	0.081d	I.T. 0.233; e⁻
133	5.27d	—	—	—	—	e⁻
135	1.5m	—	0.91; 0.54	—	0.25d; 0.62; 0.37	I.T. 0.52; e⁻
135	9.2h	—	3.5	—	+	—
137	3.8m	—	2.4	—	0.42; 0.51; 1.8; 2.0	—
138	17m	—	+	—	—	—
139	41s	—	+	—	—	—
140	16s	—	+	—	—	—
141	3s	—	+	—	—	—
143	1s	—	+	—	—	—
144	~1s	—	+	—	—	—
123	6m	—	—	+	0.111	K
125	45m	—	—	2.05	0.38	K
126	1.6m	—	—	3.8	0.41; 0.125; 0.175–0.44	K
127	6.2h	—	—	1.06; 0.7	—	—
128	3.8m	—	—	3.0; 2.5; 1.5	0.13; 0.45; 0.98	K
129	31h	—	0.44	—	0.38; 0.56	K
130	30m	—	—	1.97	—	—
131	9.7d	—	—	—	0.67; 1.27; 1.1	K; L
132	6.2d	—	0.55	—	0.01d	K
134	3.1h	—	—	—	—	I.T. 0.13, 0.14; e⁻
134	2.3y	—	0.65	—	0.6; 0.8; 0.47–1.37	e⁻
135	2 × 10⁶y	—	0.21	—	—	—
136	13d	—	0.34; 0.66	—	1.04; 0.82; 0.67–2.5	—
137	30y	—	0.52; 1.18	—	(0.662)	—
138	32m	—	3.4	—	1.43; 1.0; 0.46; 2.2; 0.13–3.3	—
139	9.5m	—	~4	—	+	—
140	66s	—	+	—	—	—
141	~1m	—	+	—	—	—
142	short	—	+	—	—	—
143	short	—	+	—	—	—
144	short	—	+	—	—	—

TABLE OF ISOTOPES—*Continued*

				NATURALLY OCCURRING ISOTOPES			RADIOACTIVE ISOTOPES						
Z	Name	Symbol	Atomic weight	A	σ Thermal	Abundance, %	A	Half life	Alpha α	Beta β	Positron β+	Gamma γ	Other
56	Barium σ 1.2	Ba	137.36	130	6	0.101	126	97m	—		(3.8)	0.22; 0.7; (0.38)	K
				132	3	0.097	127	~12m	—		(3.0)	0.27; (0.13–0.98)	Rad. ?
				134	<4	2.42	128	2.4d	—		1.6	+	K
				135	5	6.6	129	1.9h	—		—		e⁻ 0.13
				136	<1	7.8	131	11.6d	—		—	0.05; 0.122d; 0.214; 0.04–1.03	K
				137	4	11.3	133	39h	—		—	0.082d; 0.36; 0.03; 0.06; 0.07	I.T. 0.276; e⁻
				138	0.55	71.7	133	8y	—		—		K; e⁻
							135	29h	—		—		I.T. 0.268; e⁻
							137	2.6m	—		↑		I.T. 0.662; e⁻
							139	85m	—	2.22; 0.8; 2.38	—	0.165d; 1.43	e⁻
							140	12.8d	—	1.02; 0.48 (1.3–2.3)	—	0.54; 0.31; 0.16 (1.6; 0.1–2.5)	—
							141	18m	—	2.8	—	+	—
							142	6m	—	++	—		—
							143	<0.5m	—	++	—		—
							144	short	—		—		—
57	Lanthanum σ8.9	La	138.92	138*		0.089	131	58m	—	—	1.6	1.0	—
				139	8.9	99.911	132	4.5h	—	—	3.5	0.8	—
							133	4h	—	—	1.2	—	e⁻ 0.26; K
							134	6.5m	—	—	2.7	0.49; 0.66	K
							135	19h	—	—	—	—	K
							136	9m	—	—	2.1	—	K
							137	>10⁸y	—	—	—	—	Radiation ?
							138*	2 × 10¹¹y	—	1.0	—	1.4; 0.8; 0.5	K
							140	40.2h	—	1.34; 0.8–2.15	—	1.6; 0.11–2.9	—
							141	3.8h	—	2.43; 0.9	—	~1.5	—
							142	70m	—	>2.5	—	0.63; 0.87	—
							143	~19m	—	++	—		—
							144	short	—	++	—		—

Z	Element	Symbol	At. wt	Stable A	σ	Abundance %	Radioactive A	Half-life					Decay
58	Cerium σ 0.7	Ce	140.13	136	~2; ~20	0.19	133	6.3h	—	—	1.3	1.8	K
				138	1	0.26	134	72h	—	—	—	—	K
				140	0.6	88.47	135	22h	—	—	0.8	—	K
				142	1	11.08	137	35h	—	—	—	0.44	I.T. 0.26; e⁻
							137	9h	—	0.43; 0.57	—	1.65d	K; e⁻
							139	140d	—	1.09; 0.3–1.38	—	1.45d	—
							141	32d	—	0.3; (2.98)	—	0.29; 0.06–1.1	—
							143	33h	—	2.0	—	{0.03–1.4;	—
							144	285d	—	0.7	—	(0.7–2.18)	—
												+	
							145	3m	—	—	—	0.32; 0.05–0.22	—
							146	14m	—	—	—	—	—
59	Praseodymium σ11	Pr	140.92	141	11	100	135	22m	—	—	2.5	0.3; 0.22; 0.08	—
							136	70m	—	—	2.0	0.17; 0.8; 1.1	—
							138	2h	—	—	1.4	{1.0; 0.8	—
												0.3–1.7	
							139	4.5h	—	2.16; 0.6	1.0	1.3; 1.6; 0.17?	—
							140	3.4m	—	0.92	2.3	—	—
							142	19.1h	—	2.98; 0.8; 2.3	—	1.59	K
							143	13.8d	—	1.7	—	0.7; 2.18; 1.48	—
							144	17m	—	3.7; 2.3	—	0.07	—
							145	5.9h	—	—	—	0.46; 1.49; 0.74	—
							146	24m	—	—	—	—	—
60	Neodymium σ 48	Nd	144.27	142	17	27.1	138	22m	—	—	2.4	—	e⁻ (?)
				143	320	12.2	139	5.5h	—	—	3.1	1.3	K; e⁻ 0.28
				144*	5	23.9	140	3.3d	—	—	0.7	1.1	K
				145	44	8.3	141	2.4h	—	—	—	{0.092; 0.53	K
				146	2	17.2						0.12–0.69	
				148	4	5.7	144*	~2 × 10¹⁵y	1.8	—	—	—	—
							147	11.6d	—	0.81; 0.37	—	0.11; 0.03–0.65	—
				150	3	5.6	149	1.8h	—	1.5	—	0.08; 0.11; 0.42	—
							151	15m	—	1.9	—	0.7; 1.1	—

TABLE OF ISOTOPES—*Continued*

			NATURALL OCCURRING ISOTOPES				RADIOACTIVE ISOTOPES						
Z	Name	Symbol	Atomic weight	A	σ Thermal	Abundance, %	A	Half life	Alpha α	Beta β	Positron β+	Gamma γ	Other
61	Promethium	Pm					141	20m			~2.6		
							143	~300d				0.9	K
							144	~300d				0.7; 0.4; 0.2	K
							145	25y				0.068; 0.073	K; L
							146	~2y		0.7			
							147	2.6y		0.23			
							148	5.3d		2.5		0.8	
							148	42d		0.6; 2.4		1	
							149	50h		1.05		0.29; 1.3	
							150	2.7h		2.0; 3.0		{ 0.34; 0.92; 0.43; 1.0-3.0 }	
							151	27h		1.1		{ 0.34; 0.17; 0.06-1.5 }	
62	Samarium	SA	150.35	144	~0.03	3.1	143	8m			2.3		
				147*	2.18	15	145	1.0y				0.061	K
				148		11.2	146	~5 × 10⁷y	2.5				
				149	66,000	13.8	147*	1.3 × 10¹¹y	2.18				
				150	140	7.4	151	80y		0.076		0.02	
				152	5	26.8	153	47h		0.71; 0.64; 0.81		{ 0.102d; 0.069d; 0.08-0.54 }	
				154		22.7	155	23m		1.8		0.25; 0.105	
							156	~10h		0.9			
63	Europium σ 4300	Eu	152	151	1400; 7200	47.8	144	18m			2.4		
				153	400	52.2	145	5d				0.21; 0.12	K; e⁻ 0.2
							146	38h				0.57; 1.0	K; e⁻ 0.4
							147	24d	2.9			0.29; 0.57	K; e⁻ 0.2
							148	58d					K; e⁻
							149	120d					K; e⁻
							150	14h		1.1			
							152	9.3h		1.88		0.34d; 0.12d	K

Z	Element, σ	Symbol	At. wt.	Stable isotope	σ	Abundance %	Radioactive isotope	Half-life	β	β		γ	Decay
64	Gadolinium σ 38000	Gd	157.26	152	<160	0.20	152	13y	—	0.7	—	0.12d; 0.34; 1.1	—
				154		2.15	154	16y	—	1.5	—	0.123d; 1.42; 0.78; 1.12	—
				155	~70,000	14.70	155	1.7y	3.2	0.15; 0.25	—	0.019–0.137	K; e⁻ 0.3
				156	~180,000	20.50	156	15d	3.0	0.4; 2.4	—	2.0	K; e⁻
				157		15.70	157	15h	2.7	1.0; ~1.7	—	0.6; 0.2	K; e⁻
				158	4	24.90	158	60m	—	2.6	—	+	—
				160	0.8	21.90	159	20m	—	+	—	+	—
65	Terbium σ 45	Tb	158.93	159	45	100	148	>35y	—	—	—	—	K(?)
							149	9d	—	—	—	—	K(?)
							150	>10⁵y	—	—	—	0.26	K; e⁻ ~0.3
							151	~150d	—	—	—	0.102d; 0.069d; 0.097	K
							153	236d	—	—	—	0.36; 0.057; 0.23; 0.08	K; e⁻
							159	18h	3.95	0.95; 0.6	—	0.36; 0.1; 0.32	K
							161	3.7m	3.4	1.6	—	—	Rad.?
66	Dysprosium σ 1100	Dy	162.51	156	2700	0.052	149	4.1h	—	—	—	0.23; 1.2	—
				158		0.090	150	19h	—	—	—	—	—
				160		2.29	153	5.1d	—	—	2.75; 1.66	—	—
				161		18.9	154	7h	—	?	—	0.2–0.6	—
				162		25.5	154	17.2h	—	0.14	—	0.1–2.0	—
				163		25.0	156	5h	—	? 0.6; 0.2	—	0.96, 0.086–1.45	—
				164		28.2	160	5d	—	0.56; 0.85	—	0.049; 0.08	—
							161	72d	—	0.55	—		
							162	7d	4.2	—	—	0.32	K
								14m	4.1	~1	—	0.36; 0.16; 0.52	K; L
							153	7m	3.6	1.25	—	0.09–1.0	I.T. 0.108
							157	8.2h	—	0.3	—	<0.05	—
							159	134d					
							165	2.32h					
							166	82h					

TABLE OF ISOTOPES—*Continued*

			NATURALLY OCCURRING ISOTOPES				RADIOACTIVE ISOTOPES						
Z	Name	Symbol	Atomic weight	A	σ Thermal	Abundance, %	A	Half life	Alpah α	Beta β	Positron β⁺	Gamma γ	Other
67	Holmium σ 64	Ho	164.94	165	>0.007; 64	100	<157	~4m	4.2	—	—	—	—
							160	5.0h	—	—	—	0.19; 0.72; 0.96	K
							161	2.5h	—	—	—	0.09; 0.17	K
							162	22m	—	—	1.3	~1.2	K; e⁻ 0.17
							164	37m	—	0.99; 0.9	—	0.073; 0.09d; 0.037	I.T.(?) 0.046; K
							166	>30y	—	0.2	—	0.81d; 0.84	—
							166	27.2h	—	1.85	—	0.08d; 1.4-1.6	—
							167	3.0h	—	1.0; 0.28	—	0.35; 0.7	—
							169	1.6h	—	+	—	—	—
68	Erbium σ 170	Er	167.27	162		0.136	160	29h	—	—	—	0.82; 1.12	K
				164		1.56	161	3h	—	—	1.2	0.43; 1.1	K
				166		33.4	163	75m	—	—	—	—	K
				167	2	22.9	165	10h	—	—	—	—	K; e⁻ 0.1
				168		27.1	169	9.4d	—	0.33	—	—	—
				170	9	14.9	171	7.5h	—	1.06; 0.67; 1.48	—	0.113d; 0.31	—
							?	2.5s	—	—	—	0.12-0.81	I.T. 021; e⁻
69	Thulium σ 125	Tm	168.94	169	125	100	165	25h	—	—	—	0.20; 0.81; 1.16; 1.38	K
							166	7.7h	—	—	2.1	0.08d-1.32	K; e⁻
							167	9.6d	—	—	—	0.2; 0.72; 0.51; 0.11	K
							168	87d	—	0.5(?)	—	0.8; 0.2	—
							170	129d	—	0.97; 0.89	—	0.084d	—
							171	1.9y	—	0.1	—	—	—
							172	19m	—	+	—	—	—
							174	~2d	—	+	—	—	—

Z	Element	Sym	At. wt	Stable isotope	σ	Abundance	Radioactive isotope	Half-life		β		γ	Type
70	Ytterbium σ 37	Yb	173.04	168	11,000	0.14	165(?)	74m	—	—	—	—	K or r(?)
				170		3.03	166	54d	—	—	2.4	0.08–1.32	K
				171		14.3	167	18m	—	—	—	0.18(?); 0.33(?); 0.118	
				172		21.8	169	32d	—	0.47; 0.07; 0.36	—	0.064; 0.008d; 0.094–0.308d; 0.4; 0.28; 0.113; 0.14	K; e⁻
				173	~60	16.2	175	4.2d	—	1.3	—	0.146d; 0.119; 1.08; 1.23	—
				174		31.8	177	2h	—	—	—	0.46	—
				176		12.7	?	0.15s	—	—	—	0.10(?)	I.T.(?)
							?	6s	—	—	—	—	I.T. 0.21
							?	50s	—	—	—	—	I.T. 0.25
71	Lutetium σ 111	Lu	174.99	175	18; ?	97.40	170	1.7d	—	—	—	~2.5	K; e⁻ 0.1
				176*		2.60	171	8.5d	—	—	—	~1.2	K; e⁻ 0.17, 0.5
							171	1.6y	—	—	—	~1	K; e⁻ 0.1
							172	4h	—	—	1.2	1.2	K; e⁻ 0.13, ~0.6
							172	6.7d	—	—	—	—	
							173	1.4y	—	0.6	—	~2; 0.8	K; e⁻ 0.1, 0.2
							174	165d	—	1.2	—	~1	K
							176*	3.7h	—	—	0.42	0.089	e⁻
							176*	3 × 10^10 y	—	—	—	0.31; 0.2	K
							177	6.8d	—	0.5; 0.18; 0.39	—	0.113; 0.208; 0.07–0.32	—
72	Hafnium σ 105	Hf	178.50	174	~1000	0.18	178	22m	—	—	—	—	—
				176	<30	5.2	179	~5h	—	++	—	—	—
				177	370	18.5	170	1.8h	—	—	2.4	1.02; 0.63	K
				178	80	27.1	171	16h	—	—	—	0.8; 0.3	K; e⁻ 0.2
				179	65	13.8	172	~5y	—	—	—	0.12; 0.3	K
				180	10	35.2	173	24h	—	—	—	0.343; 0.089; 0.113–0.432	K
							175	70d	—	—	—	0.22	K
							179	19s	—	—	—	—	I.T. 0.16; e⁻
							180	5.5h	—	—	—	0.057–0.44	I.T.
							181	46d	—	0.41	—	0.13d–0.61d	e⁻

TABLE OF ISOTOPES—Continued

			NATURALLY OCCURRING ISOTOPES				RADIOACTIVE ISOTOPES						
Z	Name	Symbol	Atomic weight	A	σ Thermal	Abundance, %	A	Half life	Alpha α	Beta β	Positron β+	Gamma γ	Other
73	Tantalum σ22	Ta	180.95	180		0.12	176	8h	—	—	—	~2	K; e⁻ 0.1, 0.2
				181	0.07; 22		177	2.2d	—	—	—		~1
							178	9.3m	—	—	—	~1.4	K; e⁻ 0.1
							178	2.1h	—	—	1.1	~1.5	K; e⁻ 0.08
							179	~600d	—	—	~1	~1.4	K; e⁻ 0.1
							180	8.1h	—	0.7	—	0.7	K; e⁻ 0.1
							181	0.33s	—	—	—	0.093d; 0.102	K
							182	16m	—	?	—	—	I.T. 0.32;
							182	112d	—	0.51	—	1.1; 1.2	I.T. 0.18; e⁻
							183	5.2d	—	0.62	—	0.041-0.41	—
							184	8.7h	—	1.26; 0.15	—	0.4; 0.89; 0.24; 0.118; 0.11-0.78	—
							185	49m	—	1.7	—	0.13; 0.18; 0.24; 0.2; 0.73	e⁻
							186	10m	—	2.2	—	0.12-1.2	
74	Tungsten σ18 (Wolfram)	W	183.86	180*	<2.0	0.14	176	1.3h	—	—	—	~1.3	K; e⁻
				182	0.5; 2.0	26.2	177	2.2h	—	—	~2	~0.5; 1.2	K; e⁻ 0.13, 0.4
				183	11	14.3	178	21d	—	—	—	~0.3	K
				184	2.0	30.7	179	30m	—	—	—	—	K
				186	36	28.7	180	0.005s	—	—	—	0.35; 0.22	I.T.
							180*	~10¹⁴y	3(?)	—	—	—	
							181	140d	—	—	—	0.137; 0.153	K; L
							183	5.5s	—	—	—	0.11; 0.16	I.T.; e⁻
							185	1.7m	—	—	—	0.13; 0.16	I.T.; e⁻
							185	74d	—	0.43	—	0.056	—
							187	24h	—	0.62	—	0.072-0.87	—
							188	65d	—	+	—	—	—
75	Rhenium σ86	Re	186.22	185	105	37.1	180	2.4m	—	—	1.1	0.11; 0.88	K
				187*	75	62.9	182	13h	—	—	—	0.11; 0.35; ~1	
							182	64h	—	—	—	0.11-0.35; 1.5	K; e⁻
							183	150d	—	—	—	0.08; 0.25; 1	K; e⁻
							184	50d	—	—	—	0.11d; 0.79; 0.89	K; e⁻
							184	2.2d	—	—	—	0.04; 0.16	K; e⁻

At. No.	Element	A	σ (barns)	Abund. %	A	Half-life	α	β (MeV)	β⁺ (MeV)	γ (MeV)	Decay
76	Osmium Os 190.2 σ 15	184		0.018	186	91h	—	1.07; 0.93	—	0.137d; 0.123; 0.76; 0.63	K
		186	~20	1.59	187*	~5 × 10¹⁰ y	—	<0.008	—	—	I.T. 0.1; e⁻
		187		1.64	188	20m	—	2.12	—	0.06	—
		188		13.3	188	17h	—	—	—	0.155d; 0.44; 1.96	—
		189	8	16.1	189	~200d	—	0.2	—	1	—
		190	1.6	26.4	190	3m	—	1.7	—	0.19; 0.36; 0.56; 0.4–0.8	—
		192		41.0	191	10m	—	1.8	—	—	—
77	Iridium Ir 192.2 σ 460	191	250; 750	38.5	182	24h	—	—	—	0.14; 0.17; 1.1	K
		193	120	61.5	183	10h	—	—	—	0.11; 0.38	K
					183	15h	—	—	—	0.65; 0.88; 0.23; 0.16	K
					185	95d	—	—	—	—	K; L
					187	35h	—	—	—	?	I.T.
					190	9m	—	—	—	0.19–0.56	I.T. 0.62
					191	14h	—	—	—	(0.042; 0.129)	I.T. 0.074
					191	16d	—	0.14	—	0.073d; 0.14–	—
					193	31h	—	1.1	—	0.56	—
					194	~2y	+	—	—	—	—
					?	19m	—	—	—	0.12	K
					?	3h	—	—	2.2	0.3; 0.14; 0.44	K
					187	12h	—	—	2	0.155d; 0.63; 0.48	K; e⁻
					188	41h	—	—	—	0.24	K; e⁻
					189	11d	—	—	2.0	0.19; 0.36; 0.51; 0.62	K
					190	3h	—	—	—	0.19; 0.36–1.3	K
					190	11d	—	0.67	—	0.129	K
					191	5s	—	—	—	—	I.T. 0.042; e⁻
					192	1.4m	—	—	—	0.31; 0.47; 0.136–1.16	I.T. 0.057; e⁻
					192	74d	+	2.24; 1.91; 1.2; 2.1	—	0.33; 0.64	K
					194	19h	—	—	—	0.42; 0.66; 0.88; >1	—
					195	2.3h	—	—	—	0.58; 0.76; ~1	—
					196	9.7d	—	0.08	—		—
					197	7m	—	1.6	—	1.8	—
					198	50s	—	3.6	—	0.78	—

TABLE OF ISOTOPES—Continued

				NATURALLY OCCURRING ISOTOPES			RADIOACTIVE ISOTOPES						
Z	Name	Symbol	Atomic weight	A	σ Thermal	Abundance, %	A	Half life	Alpha α	Beta β	Positron β+	Gamma γ	Other
78	Platinum σ 10	Pt	195.09	190*	~90	0.012	187	3h	—	—	—		Rad.?
				192	8	0.78	188	10d				{0.192; 0.28; 0.043-0.4}	K
				194	1.2	32.8	189	11h	—	—	—	0.14	K
				195	27	33.7	190*	~10²y(?)	3.3(?)	—	—	—	—
				196	~0; 1.2	25.4	191	3d	—	—	—	{0.129; 0.042; 0.54; 0.047-0.63}	K; e⁻
				198	4	7.2	193	3.4d	—	—	—	—	I.T. 0.135
							193	Long	—	—	—	—	L
							195	~6d	—	—	—	0.99; 0.031	I.T. 0.13
							197	1.4h	—	—	—	—	I.T. 0.34; e⁻
							197	19h	—	0.67; 0.48; 0.47	—	{0.077d; 0.19; 0.28}	—
							199	30m	—	~1.2	—	0.07-0.96	—
79	Gold σ 98	Au	197.0	197	98	100	≤187	4.3m	5.1	—	+	—	K
							-187	~15m					Rad.?
							188	~10m					Rad.?
							-189	42m	—	—	—	0.29; 0.14	K
							191	3h	—	—	—	0.3; 0.048-0.6	K
							192	4.8d	—	—	1.9	{0.317; 0.296; 0.137-1.16}	K
							193	4s	—	—	—	0.258	I.T. 0.032, 0.29; e⁻
							193	17h	—	—	—	{0.11; 0.17; 0.19; 0.1-0.44}	K
							194	39h	—	—	1.55; 1.22	0.33; 1.48; 0.29-2.1	K; e⁻
							195	30s	—	—	—	0.261	I.T. 0.057, 0.318; e⁻

Mercury

Z	Element	Symbol	At. wt.	A (stable)	σ	Abundance %
80	Mercury σ 350	Hg	200.61	196	2500	0.15
				198	2000	10.0
				199	<50	16.9
				200	<50	23.1
				201	3	13.2
				202	0.4	29.8
				204		6.8

Radioactive isotopes:

A	Half-life	β⁺ / K	β⁻	γ and e⁻ energies (MeV)	Decay
<195	0.7m	5.6	—	—	—
<192	~3h	—	—	—	e⁻ 0.88
189	2.5m	+ or K	—	0.29	K or β⁺
190	90m	—	—	—	K; e⁻
191	57m	—	—	—	K; e⁻
192	6h	1.2	—	0.253	K
193	12h	—	—	0.031–0.275	I.T. 0.101; K
193	5h	—	—	0.039	K
194	0.4s	—	—	0.038; 0.032–1.63	I.T.(?)
194	~130d	—	—	0.048; 0.134	K
195	40h	—	—	0.26; 0.04–0.56	I.T. 0.123; e⁻; K
195	9.5h	—	—	0.061; 0.18; 0.6 / 0.37–1.15	K; e⁻
197	25h	—	—	0.134d; (0.28)	I.T. 0.165; e⁻; K
197	65h	—	—	(0.13)	K; e⁻
199	43m	—	—	0.077d; 0.191	I.T. 0.368; e⁻
203	48d	—	0.21	0.158d; 0.279d	e⁻
205	5.2m	—	1.6; 1.4	0.2	—
195	180d	—	—	0.099; 0.031; 0.14	K; e⁻
196	14h	—	—	0.354; 0.331	K or I.T.
196	5.6d	—	0.27	0.43	K
197	7.4s	—	—	0.279	I.T. 0.13, 0.409
198	2.70d	—	0.96; 0.28; 1.37	0.418d; 0.68; 1.09	—
199	3.15d	—	0.3; 0.25; 0.46	0.158d; 0.208d; 0.05d	—
200	48m	—	2.2	0.39; 1.13	—
201	2.6m	—	1.5	0.55	—
202	~25s	+	—	—	—
203	55s	—	1.9	0.69	—

TABLE OF ISOTOPES—*Continued*

			NATURALLY OCCURRING ISOTOPES				RADIOACTIVE ISOTOPES						
Z	Name	Symbol	Atomic weight	A	σ Thermal	Abundance, %	A	Half life	Alpha α	Beta β	Positron β+	Gamma γ	Other
81	Thallium σ 3.3	Tl	204.39	203	11	29.5	195	1.2h	—	—	—	0.43	Rad.?
				205	0.11	70.5	196	~4h	—	—	—	0.38	K
							197	0.54s	—	—	—		I.T.(?); e−
	(RaE″)	→		206*			197	2.8h	—	—	—	0.152; 0.43	K
	(AcC″)	→		207*			198	1.9h	—	—	—		I.T. 0.26
	(ThC″)	→		208*			198	5h	—	—	—	0.28; 0.049; 0.44–0.64	K
	(RaC″)	→		210*			199	7.4h	—	—	—	0.41d; 0.68 0.19–1.2 0.33; 0.155; 0.208;	K
							200	27h	—	—	+	0.247; 0.05–0.49 0.37; 1.2; 0.83	K
							201	3d	—	—	—	0.58; 0.116–1.52 0.167; 0.135; 0.032; 0.031	K; e−
							202	12d	—	—	—	0.44d	K; L; e−
							204	4.1y	—	0.76	—	—	K
							206*	4.2m	—	1.51	—	—	—
							207*	4.78m	—	1.45	—	—	—
							208*	3.1m	—	1.79; 1.28	—	2.615; 0.58d; 0.51; 1.28	—
							209	2.2m	—	1.8; 2.3	—	0.11–1.6; 0.12d	—
							210*	1.32m	—	1.9	—	+	—
82	Lead σ 0.17	Pb	207.21	204	0.9	1.3	197	42m		—		0.17; 0.22; 0.23 0.32; 0.39	I.T.(?); K
				206	0.03	26.0							
				207	0.73	21.0	198	2.3h		—		0.17; 0.29; 0.36 0.28–0.42	K
				208	0.00045	52.0	199	12m		—		—	
	(RaD)	→		210*			199	1.5h		—		0.37; 0.35; 0.72 0.148; 0.142;	I.T. 0.42; e−
	(AcB)	→		211*			200	21h		—		0.24	K
	(ThB)	→		212*									
	(RaB)	→		214*			201	1.0m		—		0.27; 0.033–0.45	I.T. 0.66; e−

(Lead, Z = 82 — continued from preceding page)

A	Half-life	α	β	γ	Other
201	9h	—	—	0.33; 0.36	K
202	35h	—	—	0.13–1.1	I.T. 0.79, 0.13;
				0.96; 0.42	K
202	~10^5y	—	—	0.39–0.66	L
203	6s	—	—	—	K
203	52h	—	—	0.28; 0.4; 0.68	I.T. 0.91; e⁻
205	>10^6y	—	—	0.37d; 0.89	L
207	0.8s	—	—	—	I.T. 1.06; e⁻
209	3.3h	—	0.62	0.57	—
210*	20y	—	0.02	0.047	e⁻
211*	36.1m	—	1.4; 0.5	0.83; 0.06–0.76	—
212*	10.64h	—	0.34; 0.58	0.2306; 0.3; 0.11–0.25	—
214*	26.8m	—	0.7	0.352; 0.2952; 0.053–0.259	—

83   Bismuth   σ 0.033

(RaE) (AcC) (ThC) (RaC)

Bi 209.00   100

209* → 210* → 211* → 212* → 214*   0.019; 0.14

A	Half-life	α	β	γ	Other
<198	1.7m	6.2	—	—	—
198	7m	5.83	—	—	K
199	~25m	5.47	—	—	K
200	35m	—	—	—	K
201	1.0h	5.15	—	—	K
201	~2h	—	—	—	K
202	1.6h	—	—	—	K
203	12h	4.85	—	0.03–1.6	K; e⁻
204	12h	—	—	0.22; 0.08–1.23; (0.91; 0.37; 0.89)	K
205	14d	—	—	0.7; 1.77; 1.04	K
206	6.4d	—	—	0.99; 0.11–1.91	K; e⁻
207	8y	—	—	0.84; 0.88d; 0.52d; 1.72	K; L
208*	?	3(?)	—	0.57; 1.77; (1.07; 0.57)	Rad.?
209*	3×10^{17}y(?)	4.94	—	—	—
210*	2.6×10^6y	6.62; 6.27; (9)	+	—	—
211*	2.15m	6.05; 6.09;	+	—	—
212*	60.5m	9.5–10.5	2.25	0.35	e⁻
213	47m	5.9	1.39; 0.96	0.04–2.2; 0.43	—
214*	19.7m	5.5; (8.3–10.5)	1.6; 3.17	0.61; 1.12; 1.76; 1.45–2.43	—
215	8m	—	+	—	—

TABLE OF ISOTOPES—Continued

NATURALLY OCCURRING ISOTOPES							RADIOACTIVE ISOTOPES						
Z	Name	Symbol	Atomic weight	A	σ Thermal	Abundance, %	A	Half life	Alpha α	Beta β	Positron β+	Gamma γ	Other
84	Polonium	Po	210	210*			197(?)	~4m	6.04	—	—	—	—
	(RaF)			211*			198(?)	~6m	5.94	—	—	—	—
	(AcC′)			212*			199	~11m	5.85	—	—	—	—
	(ThC′)			214*			200	~8m	5.77	—	—	—	K
	(RaC′)			215*			201	18m	5.67	—	—	—	K
	(AcA)			216*			202	56m	5.59	—	—	—	K
	(ThA)			218*			203	47m	—	—	—	—	K
	(RaA)						204	3.8h	5.37	—	—	—	K
							205	1.5h	5.2	—	—	—	K
							206	9d	5.22	—	—	0.06–1.03	K
							207	5.7h	5.10	—	—	0.41; 0.74; 0.99	K
							208	2.9y	5.11	—	—	0.28; 0.6	K
							209	~100y	4.88	—	—	0.9; 0.6; 0.29	K
							210*	138.4d	5.3	—	—	0.8	—
							211	25s	7.1; 8.7	—	—	1.06; 0.57	—
							211*	0.52s	7.43	—	—	0.89; 0.57	—
							212*	0.3μs	8.78	—	—	—	—
							213	4μs	8.34	—	—	—	—
							214*	160μs	7.68	—	—	—	—
							215*	0.0018s	7.36	+	—	—	—
							216*	0.16s	6.77	—	—	—	—
							217	<24m	6.5	—	—	—	—
							218*	3.05m	6.0	+	—	—	—
85	Astatine	At					<202	43s	6.5	—	—	—	—
							<203	6.7m	6.35	—	—	—	—
							203	7m	6.10	—	—	—	K
							204	~25m	—	—	—	—	K
							205	25m	5.90	—	—	—	K
							206	2.6h	—	—	—	—	K
							207	1.8h	5.75	—	—	—	K
							208	1.7h	5.65	—	—	0.18; 0.66	K

The table below covers elements 85 (top block, name not shown on this page), 86 (Emanation) and 87 (Francium). Columns: mass number, half-life, α-particle energy (Mev), β, γ-ray energy (Mev), orbital-electron capture.

Z	Element	Symbol	Genetic relation	Mass	Half-life	α (Mev)	β	γ (Mev)	Orbital e⁻ capture
				208	6h	5.64		—	K
				209	5.5h			0.195; 0.091; 0.55; 0.78; 1.18; 0.25; 0.047–2.6	K
				210	8.3h	5.35; 5.52			K
				211	7.5h	5.86; (7.43)		0.67; (0.89; 0.57)	K; L
				212	0.22s	+			
				213	<2s	9.2			
				214	<5s	8.78			
				215	$\sim 10^{-6}$s	8.0			
				216	$\sim 300\mu$s	7.79			
				217	0.018s	7.02			
				218	1.3s	6.63			
				219	0.9m	6.27	+		
86	Emanation (Actinon) (Thoron) (Radon)	Em (An) (Th) (Rn)	222 →219*, →220*, →222*	204(?)	3m	6.3			
				206	7m	6.22			
				207	11m	6.12			
				208	23m	6.14			
				209	30m	6.04			
				210	2.7h	6.04			
				211	16h	5.78; 5.85; 5.61		0.07; 0.15; 0.4; 0.60	K
				212	23m	6.26			K
				215	<1m	8.6			K
				216	<9m	8.01			K
				217	$\sim$0.001s	7.74			K
				218	0.019s	7.13; 6.53		0.61	
				219*	3.92s	6.82; 6.56		0.27; 0.40	
				220*	52s	6.28; 5.75	+		
				221	25m	+			
				222*	3.825d	5.48			
87	Francium (AcK)	Fr	→223*	212	19m	6.39; 6.41; 6.34			K
				217	<2s	8.3			
				218	<5s	7.85			
				219	0.02s	7.30			
				220	28s	6.69			
				221	4.8m	6.30; 6.07		0.22	
				222	15m	+	+		
				223*	22m	5.3	1.0; 1.3	0.05–0.31	

TABLE OF ISOTOPES—Continued

	NATURALLY OCCURRING ISOTOPES						RADIOACTIVE ISOTOPES						
Z	Name	Symbol	Atomic weight	A	σ Thermal	Abundance, %	A	Half life	Alpha α	Beta β	Positron β⁺	Gamma γ	Other
88	Radium (AcX) (ThX) (MsTh₁)	Ra	226.05 →	223* 224* 226* 228*	125 12 20 ~36		219	<1m	8.0	—	—	—	—
							220	<9m	7.43	—	—	—	—
							221	30s	6.71	—	—	—	—
							222	38s	6.55; 6.23	—	—	—	0.33	—
							223*	11.6d	5.7; 5.6; 5.42–5.86	—	—	0.026–0.44	—
							224*	3.64d	5.68; 5.44	0.32	—	0.24	—
							225	14.8d	—	—	—	0.04	—
							226*	1620y	4.78; 4.59	1.30	—	0.187	—
							227	41m	—	<0.02	—	0.29; 0.5	—
							228*	6.7y	—	+	—	—	—
							229	<5m	—	1.2	—	—	—
							230	1h	—	+	—	—	—
89	Actinium (MsTh₂)	Ac	227 →	227* 228*	~520		221	<2s	7.6	—	—	—	—
							222	5.5s	6.96	—	—	—	—
							223	2.2m	6.64	—	—	—	—
							224	2.9h	6.17	—	—	—	K
							225	10d	5.80	1.2	—	0.085	K
							226	29h	—	0.046	—	—	—
							227*	22y	4.94	1.11; 0.45–2.18	—	—	—
							228*	6.13h	—	—	—	0.058; 0.1; 0.91; 0.08–1.64	—
							229	66m	—	2.2 +	—	—	—
							230	<1m	—	—	—	—	—
90	Thorium σ 7.5 (RdAc) (RdTh) (Io) (UY)	Th	232.05 →	227* 228* 230* 231*	~1500b 120 35		223	<1m	7.5	—	—	—	—
							224	<9m	7.13	—	—	—	—
							225	8m	6.57	—	—	—	K
							226	31m	6.34; 6.23; 6.1	—	—	0.11; 0.24; 0.13; 0.19	—
							227*	18.2d	5.97; 5.65; 6.03	—	—	0.05; 0.87; 0.23; 0.03–0.64	—
							228*	1.90y	5.42; 5.34	—	—	0.09; 0.21; 0.13; 0.17	—

Element (σ)	At. wt	Genetic	σ	%	A	Half-life	α	β	(conv.)	γ	Decay
(UX₁)		→232*	7.5	100	229	7300y	4.85; 4.94; 5.02	—	—	0.068; 0.14–0.26	—
		→234*	1.8		230*	80,000y	4.68; 4.61	—	—	0.022d; 0.085d; 0.059–0.23	—
					231*	25.6h	—	0.09; 0.3; 0.22	—	0.06	—
					232*	1.39 × 10¹⁰y	3.99; 3.93	—	—	—	S.F.
					233	23.3m	—	1.23	—	0.098–0.66	—
					234*	24.1d	—	0.19; 0.1	—	0.093; 0.064; 0.029	—
					235	<5m	—	+	—	—	—
91 Protactinium σ 260	PA 231	231*	200		225	2.0s	6.81	—	—	—	K
(UX₂)		→234*			226	1.8m	6.46	—	—	—	K
(UZ)		→234*			227	38m	6.09; 5.85	—	—	0.58; 0.13	K
					228	22h	5.69	—	—	—	K
					229	1.5d	+	—	0.2; 0.4	—	—
					230	17d	5.0; 4.63–5.05	0.4	—	0.94; 0.3; 0.46 / 0.052–1.18	e⁻
					231*	34,000y	—	—	—	0.3; 0.027d–0.38	—
					232*	1.31d	—	0.28; 0.4–1.24	—	0.047–1.15	—
					233	27.4d	—	0.26; 0.14; 0.57	—	0.086; 0.31; 0.075; 0.016–0.42	—
					234*	1.18m	—	2.31	—	0.23–1.8	I.T.
					234*	6.66h	—	0.5	—	0.04–1.7	—
					235	24m	—	1.4	—	—	—
					237	10m	—	+	—	—	—
92 Uranium σ 3.5	U 238.07	→234*	80	0.0055	227	1.3m	6.8	—	—	—	K
(UII)		→235*	108	0.72	228	9.3m	6.67	—	—	—	K
(AcU)		→238*	2.8	99.27	229	58m	5.89; 5.82; 5.66	—	—	—	—
(UI)					230	21d	5.45	—	—	0.07; 0.16; 0.23	K
					231	4.3d	—	—	—	0.051; 0.064; 0.076	—
					232	74y	5.32; 5.26; 5.13	—	—	—	—
					233	1.62 × 10⁵y	4.82; 4.78; 4.73	—	—	0.058; 0.13; 0.27; 0.33	e⁻; S.F.
					234*	2.5 × 10⁵y	4.78	—	—	0.044; 0.05; 0.094	e⁻; S.F.
					235*	7.1 × 10⁸y	4.4; 4.56	—	—	0.05–0.12	S.F.
					236	2.39 × 10⁷y	4.5	—	—	0.19; 0.15	e⁻; S.F.
					237	6.75d	—	0.24	—	0.05	e⁻
					238*	4.51 × 10⁹y	4.18	—	—	0.21; 0.059 0.027–0.43	S.F.
					239	23.5m	—	1.21	—	0.05 0.074	—
					240	12h	—	0.36; 2.16	—	(0.56)	—

TABLE OF ISOTOPES—Continued

Z	Name	Symbol	Atomic weight	σ Thermal	Abundance %	A	Half life	Alpha α	Beta β	Positron β⁺	Gamma γ	Other
93	Neptunium σ 176	Np	237	170		231	50m	6.28	—	—	—	—
						232	~13m	—	—	—	—	K
						233	35m	5.53	—	—	+	K; e⁻ 0.3
						234	4.4d	—	—	0.8	0.8; 1.57	K; L
						235	1.1y	5.06	—	—	0.026; 0.085	K; L
						236	22h	—	0.52	—	0.043; 0.044	K
						236	>5000y	—	+	—	—	—
						237	2.2 × 10⁶y	4.79; 4.52; 4.87	—	—	0.087d; 0.02-0.2	—
						238	2.10d	—	1.26; 0.27	—	0.044; 0.99; 1.03	—
						239	2.33d	—	0.33-0.72	—	0.061d; 0.105d; 0.045-0.049	—
						240	7.3m	—	2.16	—	0.56; 0.91; 1.4	—
						240	60m	—	0.90	—	0.56; 0.43; 0.16-1.16	—
94	Plutonium σ 300	Pu	239.127	300		232	36m	6.58	—	—	—	K
						234	9h	6.19	—	—	—	K
						235	26m	5.85	—	—	—	K; L
						236	2.7y	5.75	—	—	0.047	e⁻; S.F.
						237	40d	5.49; 5.45	—	—	~0.064	K
						238	90y	5.15; 5.14; 5.10	—	—	0.044; 0.1; 0.15	S.F.
						239	24,300y	5.16; 5.12	—	—	0.052; 0.039	S.F.
						240	6600y	4.89; 4.85	—	—	0.045	S.F.
						241	13y	4.9; 4.85	0.02	—	0.1; 0.145	—
						242	3.8 × 10⁵y	—	—	—	—	S.F.
						243	5.0h	+	0.57; 0.48	—	0.085	e⁻
						244	8 × 10⁷y	—	—	—	—	S.F.
						245	11h	—	+	—	0.1; 0.22; 0.043	—
						246	11d	—	0.15	—	0.18	—
95	Americium	Am	237.124			237	~1h	6.01	—	—	—	K
			239.128			238	1.9h	—	—	—	0.98; 0.58; 0.102	K; e⁻
						239	12h	5.78	—	—	0.045-0.049	K
			241.132			240	47h	—	—	—	1.02; 1.4; 0.92	K
						241	470y	5.48; 5.38-5.54	—	—	0.06; 0.026-0.37	e⁻; S.F.

At. No.	Element	Symbol	At. mass	Mass No.	Half-life	α (Mev)	β (Mev)		γ (Mev)	Type	
				242	16h	—	0.62	—	0.04	K	—
			243.137	242	~100y	+	0.59	—	0.04	K	—
				243	~8000y	5.27; 5.22; 5.17–5.34	—	—	0.75	K	—
			244.141	244	26m	—	1.5	—	—	K	—
				245	2h	—	0.9	—	0.036; 0.12; 0.26; 0.06–0.23		—
				246	25m	—	1.22	—	1.07; 0.8; 0.1; 0.018		—
96	Curium	Cm	238.128	238	2.3h	6.50	—	—	—	K	—
				239	~3h	—	—	—	—	K	—
			240.131	240	27d	6.25	—	—	0.47; 0.59	S.F.	—
				241	35d	5.95	—	—	0.044; 0.102	K	—
			242.135	242	163d	611; 6.07	—	—	0.157	S.F.	—
			243.137	243	3.5y	5.78; 5.73; 5.99	—	—	0.23; 0.28; 0.21; 0.046–0.33		—
			244.139	244	18y	5.8; 5.76	—	—	0.043	S.F.	—
			245.142	245	11,000y	5.34	—	—	0.101; 0.17		—
			246.144	246	4,000y	5.36	—	—	—	S.F.	—
				247	≫1y	—	—	—	↑	Rad.?	—
				248	4×10⁵y	5.05	+	+		S.F.	—
				249	short	—	—	—	—		—
97	Berkelium	Bk	243.139	243	4.5h	6.55; 6.72; 6.20	—	—	0.74; 0.84; 0.96	K	—
				244	4.4h	6.66	—	—	0.90–1.72	K	—
				245	5d	6.17; 6.33; 5.90	—	—	0.25; 0.38; 0.16	K	—
				246	1.8d	—	—	—	0.8; 0.145; 0.98; 1.0; 1.1	K	—
			247.148	247	7000y	5.5; 5.67; 5.3	—	—	0.085; 0.26; 0.42		—
				248	~18h	—	0.67	—	—	K	—
				249	290d	5.4; 5.08	0.09	—	0.32		—
				250	3.1h	—	0.9; 1.9	—	1.0	S.F.	—

TABLE OF ISOTOPES—*Continued*

			NATURALLY OCCURRING ISOTOPES				RADIOACTIVE ISOTOPES						
Z	Name	Symbol	Atomic weight	A	σ Thermal	Abundance, %	A	Half life	Alpha α	Beta β	Positron β⁺	Gamma γ	Other
98	Californium	Cf	244.142				244	25m	7.17	—	—	—	K (?)
							245	44m	7.11	—	—	—	K
			246.146				246	36h	6.75; 6.71	—	—	0.044; 0.1; 0.15	e⁻; S.F.
							247	2.5h	—	—	—	0.28; 0.49	K
			248.150				248	225d	6.26	—	—	—	S.F.
							249	500y	5.81; 6.0	—	—	0.4; 0.34	S.F.
			250.155				250	10y	6.02; 5.98	—	—	0.043	S.F.
							251	~700y	+	—	—	—	—
							252	2.2y	6.11; 6.07	+	—	0.042; 0.10	S.F.
							253	18d	—	—	—	—	—
							254	70d	—	—	—	—	S.F.
99	Einsteinium	E	247.151				246	Short	—	—	—	—	K
							247	7.3m	7.35	—	—	—	K (?)
			249.154				249	2h	6.76	—	—	—	—
							251	15d	6.48	—	—	—	K
							252	~150d	6.64	—	—	—	—
							253	20d	6.64; 6.6; 6.55	—	—	0.042; 0.054; 0.39	S.F.
							254	37h	—	1.1	—	—	—
							254	~1y	6.44	+	—	0.68	K
							255	~30d	—	+	—	—	S.F.
							256	Short	—		—	—	—
100	Fermium	Fm	250.158				250	30m	7.43	—	—	—	—
			252.162				252	30h	7.1	—	—	—	—
							253	3d	—	—	—	—	K
			254.166				254	3.4h	7.22; 7.18	—	—	0.042; 0.094	S.F.
							255	20h	7.08	—	—	—	—
							256	3.1h	—	—	—	—	S.F.
101	Mendelevium	Mv					256	1h		—	—	—	K
102	Nobelium						251-253	10-12m	+				

Appendix II

Selected Symbols, Units and Definitions

A	Letter used to designate mass number or number of nuclear particles, both neutrons and protons
Å	Symbol for Angström unit, 10^{-8} cm.; used for wave length of higher energy electro-magnetic radiations, principally ultraviolet, x and gamma
Absolute temperature	Temperature in degrees centigrade beginning with absolute zero $(-273°)$
Alpha (α)	Greek letter used to designate "rays" consisting of helium nuclei. Mass of α particles $= 6.7 \times 10^{-24}$ gm.
AMU	Atomic Mass Unit. 1/16th the Mass of $_8O^{16}$; 931.162 Mev.
Anode	Positive electrode
Avogadro's number	6.02338×10^{23}. Number of atoms in a gram-atom or mole; also number of molecules in a gram-molecule
Barn (σ)	Unit of nuclear cross-section, 10^{-24} cm^2
Beta (β)	Greek letter used to designate "ray" consisting of electrons from radioactive elements
Boltzman constant	Universal gas constant used in some calculations, 1.371×10^{-16} ergs/degree
BTU (British thermal unit)	The amount of heat required to raise the temperature of one pound of water 1°F.; equivalent to 778 ft. pounds of energy, 252 calories or 1055 joules
c	Letter frequently used as symbol for speed of light, 2.99793×10^{10} cm./sec.
Calorie	Quantity of heat to raise 1 gm. water 1 degree C.
Cathode	Negative electrode

Coulomb	A unit of electrical charge equal to 3×10^9 esu and producible by a current of 1 ampere with 1 volt of potential flowing against a resistance of 1 ohm
Curie	3.7×10^{10} disintegrations/sec
Decay or disintegration constant	Decay factor derivable from equation:

$$\text{Log } A_0 - \log A = \frac{\lambda}{2.30} t$$

where A_0 = initial activity, A activity after interval of time t and λ the decay constant, when activity is measured in disintegrations per sec and t, or time, in seconds

Delta (Δ)	Greek letter freqently used to designate mass deficit
Dyne	Unit of force capable of producing an acceleration of 1 cm./sec. to 1 gm.
e, or e^-	Used as symbol for electron; electronic charge = 4.8029×10^{-10} esu
e^+	Used as symbol for positron
Eka	Prefix formerly used before names of certain elements to indicate a predicted new element next in the same group
Erg	Unit of work equal to that performed in moving an object 1 cm. against a force of 1 dyne
esu	Electrostatic unit of electrical charge; the amount of electric charge which in a vacuum will repeal a like charge at a distance of 1 cm. with a force of 1 dyne
ev (Electron Volt)	The amount of kinetic energy that is imparted to an electron by 1 volt. 1.6×10^{-12} ergs
F	The faraday = 9652.2 emu/mole (physical scale); 96,500 coulombs
Gamma (γ)	Greek letter designating electromagnetic radiation or photons of nuclear origin; similar in type to x-ray
gauss	Unit of flux density equal to one line of magnetic force per cm.
h	Symbol for Planck's constant: 6.624×10^{-27} erg/sec.
HVL	Half-value layer; thickness of a material required to reduce dosage rate to $\frac{1}{2}$ its initial value

Horsepower equivalent	746 watts
K	Symbol for "K" orbit and characteristic x-rays originating in the "K" orbital shell
L	Same for "L" orbit (See K)
Joule	Unit of work; 10^7 ergs (*see* BTU) and producible by electric current of 1 ampere in one second with resistance of 1 ohm
kev	Thousand electron volts
kv	Thousand volts
KWH	Kilowatt hour, practical electrical unit of work; the work available from 1000 watts an hr.: 1 kilowatt = 1.34 horsepower
Lambda (λ)	Greek letter in common use to designate wave length of light, x and gamma rays; also used to symbolize decay constant (q.v.)
m_e	mass of the electron, 9.1085×10^{-28} gm. or 0.000 54862 m.u.
m_p	mass of the proton, 1.6724×10^{-24} gm. or 1.00759 Amu
m_n	mass of the neutron, 1.6747×10^{-24} gm. or 1.00898 Amu
Mass energy equation (Einstein)	$E = MC^2$
M_H	Mass of hydrogen atom 1.67334×10^{-24} gm. = 1.008142 Amu
Mass energy equivalents	1 gram = 25.2×10^6 KWH or 8.5 billion BTU's or 21×10^{12} calories
	1 mass unit = 931 mev or
	1.49×10^{-3} ergs
	1 erg = 671 mass units
	1 lb uranium = 11.4×10^6 KWH

Mass frequency equation for particles (DeBroglie wave length): $\lambda = \dfrac{h}{m v}$

Mass frequency equation for photons: $M = \dfrac{h\nu}{c^2}$

Mass velocity equation: $m = \dfrac{mo}{\sqrt{1 - \left(\dfrac{v}{c}\right)^2}}$

where: ν = frequency
v = velocity

mo = resting mass
m = mass while in motion
c = velocity of light
h = Planck's constant

Mev	million electron volts
MPD	Maximum permissable dose of radiation
Mu (μ)	Greek letter designating term micro, or millionth part: 10^{-6}
Mv	Million Volts
n_o	Number of molecules in 1 cc. of gas under standard conditions = 2.688×10^{19}
n	Symbol for neutron
N	Avogadro's number 6.025×10^{23}
Nu (ν)	Greek letter in frequent use to designate frequency of radiation
Oersted	Unit of magnetizing force; 1 gilbert per cm., a gilbert being equal to 0.4 pi NI where N = no. of turns in coil and I = intensity electric current.
Photoelectric equation	$h\nu = \frac{1}{2} mv^2 + \phi$

where h = Planck's constant
m = mass
v = velocity of electron
ϕ (phi) = energy to expel electrons

Q	Often used to designate energy in nuclear equations
r	Symbol for "roentgen" unit of radiation
Rad	Unit of absorbed radiation; 100 ergs/gm.
RBE	Relative biological effectiveness
Rem	Roentgen equivalent man or the amount of radiation equal in biologic effect to 1 r of x or gamma rays
Rep	Roentgen equivalent physical, or amount of radiation equivalent in energy production to 1 r of x or gamma rays or 1.6×10^{12} ion pairs per gm./air; 87 ergs/gm air or 93 ergs/gm tissue (av)
rhm	Proposed unit: roentgen hour meter or number of r per hour at 1 meter from radioactive source
Roentgen or r	Unit of x or gamma rays; the amount which will produce 1 esu of charge in 1 cc. air under standard conditions
Rutherford	Proposed unit: Radioactivity from 1 million or 10^6 disintegrations/sec.

T (half life)	$\dfrac{0.693}{\lambda}$ where λ is the decay constant
Theta (θ)	Greek letter in common use to designate angles
Vo	Volume of 1 mole of gas under standard conditions $= 22{,}414.6$ cc.
Watt	Unit of electric power available from 1 ampere at 1 volt: 1 Watt hr is equivalent to 3.45 BTU/hr
Wien's displacement law:	$\lambda M T = $ constant

where $\lambda M = $ wave length of maximum intensity

$T = $ abolute temperature

constant $= 0.29$ cm./ degrees

Appendix III*

The Standard Man

1. Mass of Organs

Organs	Grams	Organs	Grams
Muscles	30,000	Brain	1,500
Skeleton:		Spinal cord	30
Bones	7,000	Bladder	150
Red marrow	1,500	Salivary glands	50
Yellow marrow	1,500	Eyes	30
Blood	5,000	Teeth	20
Gastrointestinal tract	2,000	Prostate	20
Lungs	1,000	Adrenals	20
Liver	1,700	Thymus	10
Kidney	300	Skin and subcutaneous tissues	8,500
Spleen	150	Other tissues and organs not sepa-	
Pancreas	70	rately defined	8,390
Thyroid	20		
Testes	40	Total body weight	70,000
Heart	300		
Lymphoid tissue	700		

2. Chemical Composition

Element	Proportion	Approximate mass in the body
	Per cent	g
Oxygen	65.0	45,500
Carbon	18.0	12,600
Hydrogen	10.0	7,000
Nitrogen	3.0	2,100
Calcium	1.5	1,050
Phosphorus	1.0	700
Potassium	0.35	245
Sulphur	.25	175
Sodium	.15	105
Chlorine	.15	105
Magnesium	.05	35
Iron	.004	3
Manganese	.0003	0.2
Copper	.0002	0.1
Iodine	.00004	0.03

The figures for a given organ may differ considerably from these averages for the whole body. For example, the nitrogen content of the dividing cells of the basal layer of skin is probably nearer 6 per cent than 3 per cent.

* From Bureau of Standards Handbook 47, 1950, Appendix I.

APPLIED PHYSIOLOGY

(3) *Water balance:*

Daily Water Intake

In food (including water of oxidation).......................... 1.0 liter
As fluids... 1.5 liters
                                                          _____
Total... 2.5 liters

Calculations of maximum permissible levels for radioactive isotopes in water have been based on the total intake figure of 2.5 liters a day.

Daily Water Output

Sweat.. 0.5 liter
From lungs... 0.4 liter
In feces... 0.1 liter
Urine.. 1.5 liters
                                                          _____
Total... 2.5 liters

(The total water content of the body is 50 liters)

(4) *Respiration:*

Area of Respiratory Tract

Respiratory interchange area...................................... 50m^2
Nonrespiratory area (upper tract and trachea to bronchioles)......... 20m^2
                                                          _____
Total... 70m^2

Respiratory Exchange

Physical activity	Hours per day	Tidal air (liters)	Respiration per minute	Volume per 8 hours, m³	Volume per day, m³
At work	8	1.0	20	10	20
Not at work	16	0.5	20	5	20

Carbon Dioxide Content (by Volume) of Air

Inhaled air (dry, at sea level).................................. 0.03%
Alveolar air... 5.5%
Exhaled air.. 4.0%

(5) *Retention of particulate matter in the lungs:*

In those cases where specific data are lacking, the convention has been adopted that 50 per cent of any aerosol reaches the alveoli of the lungs. If the particles are soluble, they have been considered to be completely absorbed; if insoluble, then the 50 per cent amount has been regarded as retained for 24 hours, after which only half of it, that is, 25 per cent of the inhaled amount, is retained *in situ* indefinitely.

INDEX